Planetary health approaches to understand and control vector-borne diseases

Ecology and control of vector-borne diseases

VOLUME 8

The titles published in this series are listed at *brill.com/ecvd*

Planetary health approaches to understand and control vector-borne diseases

Edited by

Kimberly M. Fornace
Jan E. Conn
Maria Anice M. Sallum
Leonardo Suveges Moreira Chaves
James Logan

BRILL | WAGENINGEN ACADEMIC

Cover illustration: Turbulence by Jan Conn, 2021.

Library of Congress Cataloging-in-Publication Data
Names: Fornace, Kimberly M., editor.
Title: Planetary health approaches to understand and control vector-borne diseases / edited by Kimberly M. Fornace, Jan E. Conn, Maria A.M. Sallum, Leonardo Suveges Moreira Chaves, James Logan.
Description: Leiden, The Netherlands ; [Boston] : Brill Wageningen Academic, [2024] | Series: Ecology and control of vector-borne diseases, 1875-0699 ; 8 | Includes bibliographical references and index.
Identifiers: LCCN 2023045426 (print) | LCCN 2023045427 (ebook) | ISBN 9789004687684 (hardback) | ISBN 9789004688650 (ebook)
Subjects: LCSH: Vector control. | World health. | Animals as carriers of disease. | Zoonoses. | Zoonoses—Prevention. | Zoonoses—Transmission.
Classification: LCC RA639.3 .P53 2024 (print) | LCC RA639.3 (ebook) | DDC 614.5/6—dc23/eng/20231031
LC record available at https://lccn.loc.gov/2023045426
LC ebook record available at https://lccn.loc.gov/2023045427

Typeface for the Latin, Greek, and Cyrillic scripts: "Brill". See and download: brill.com/brill-typeface.

ISSN 1875-0699
ISBN 978-90-04-68768-4 (hardback)
ISBN 978-90-04-68865-0 (e-book)
DOI 10.3920/9789004688650

This book is printed on acid-free paper and produced in a sustainable manner.

Contents

Ecology and control of vector borne diseases

1 The importance of vector control

Vector borne diseases account for 17% of all infectious diseases worldwide, causing 700,000 deaths annually. Although we have made significant progress towards understanding vector biology and ecology, vector control is facing many significant challenges. Current control almost entirely relies on insecticides and insecticide-treated bed nets, but many vector species have now developed resistance to insecticides and there is a significant dearth of alternative compounds. As a result of climate change, vectors are expanding their range and we face an ever-increasing and unpredictable threat of outbreaks with possible outcomes we don't fully understand. Malaria control is at a standstill. There are almost 100 million cases of dengue each year, with more than 3.9 billion people in more than 128 countries at risk. The Zika virus epidemic in 2015, was a wakeup call.

It is time for a revolution in vector control. We need to heighten our understanding of vector biology and ecology and we need a new generation of innovative and novel technologies for vector control that can be implemented quickly. This will include challenging the status quo, pushing boundaries and evaluating and implementing new tools more efficiently.

2 What we can do

We are living in an exciting point in history. Science has advanced such that we can not only think beyond conventional control methods, new and exciting technologies are on the horizon and have the capacity to transform the vector control landscape. Wiping out vector borne diseases could be a reality in our lifetime.

As scientists continue to innovate and develop better methods in molecular biology, we are beginning to unravel elements of vector biology and ecology that allow the development of potential game changing tools such as gene drive, including CRISPR and *Wolbachia*. As technology becomes smaller, smarter and more affordable, we are facing a future where the sort of technologies you might have only imagined could be possible in sci-fi movies, is now becoming a reality. Drones are being developed that seek out breeding sites, solar powered traps are being developed with automated vector identification technologies using machine learning. Although there are significant hurdles to overcome, we have the capacity to collect data on a scale never seen before and model it for evidence-based predictions to respond to disease outbreaks. It is probably one of the most exciting times for vector researchers with opportunities to be profoundly impactful.

3 How the book series helps

This series of books aims not only to educate and showcase the latest advances in understanding vector ecology and vector control, but to inspire, promote and stimulate new and innovate ideas.

Our past topics have already explored complex and important issues like ticks and Lyme disease, olfaction and emerging vector borne diseases in Europe. Going forward, the series will explore state-of-the-art thinking and science, including game changing technologies and interventions, based on molecular biology and genetics, digital technology and artificial intelligence, study design for efficient and robust evaluation of control tools, social science and the need for multisectoral collaboration. The series will also be tackling some of the biggest issues, including the environment and minimising the use of toxic insecticides, and exploring how climate change and the concept of planetary health, will impact on vector ecology and control.

Dedication

We would like to dedicate this book to our friend and co-editor, Leonardo Suveges Moreira Chaves, who died unexpectedly on January 20, 2023. Leonardo was the first and corresponding author of the chapter 'Malaria in the Amazon Basin: how climate change and natural disasters create new challenges for an old disease', included in this volume. He was a vibrant young mosquito ecologist at the beginning of his career.

Leonardo's research spanned epidemiology, environmental science and economics and his vision for planetary health shaped the focus of this book.

Notes on Editors

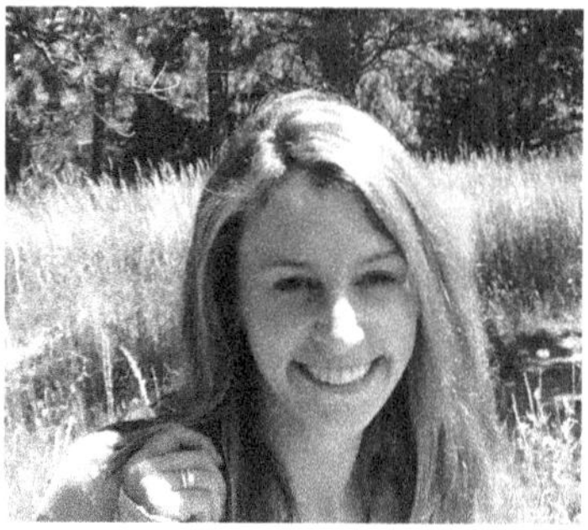

Kimberly M. Fornace
is a Wellcome Trust/ Royal Society Sir Henry Dale Fellow at the University of Glasgow and a Visiting Senior Research Fellow at the Saw Swee Hock School of Public Health at the National University of Singapore. From 2006–2010, she worked for the Harvard School of Public Health and was based at the Medical Research Council in The Gambia coordinating a project on environmental risk factors for childhood respiratory diseases. Subsequently, she completed a PhD at the London School of Hygiene and Tropical Medicine in 2018 on the spatial epidemiology of the zoonotic malaria *Plasmodium knowlesi*. Throughout her PhD, she was the coordinator for a multidisciplinary project in Malaysia and the Philippines on the emergence of this malaria species and described the first links between *P. knowlesi* risks and deforestation. She currently leads a large project in Malaysia conducting integrated field and mathematical modelling studies to identify new strategies for environmentally targeted disease surveillance and contributes to projects on zoonotic and vector-borne diseases in South America, Africa and Southeast Asia. A key focus of her work is applying novel technologies to monitor socio-ecological systems, using new sources of Earth Observation data, emerging technologies (e.g. acoustic monitoring, mobile applications) and geostatistical approaches to identify the mechanisms underlying disease transmission.

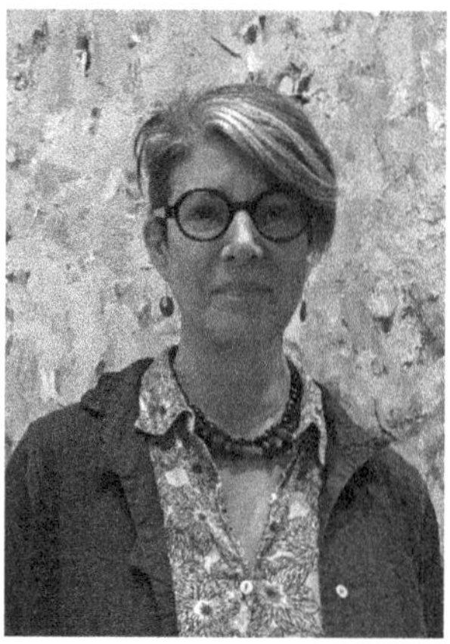

Jan E. Conn
is Research Scientist at the Wadsworth Center, Division of Infectious Diseases at the New York State Department of Health in Albany, New York and Professor in the Department of Biomedical Sciences at the School of Public Health, State University of New York-Albany. Her field is vector biology and population genetics. She earned a MS in entomology from Simon Fraser University in Burnaby, B.C., Canada working on the chemical ecology of mountain pine beetles, and a PhD in population genetics and systematics from the University of Toronto, Canada in 1987. Her doctoral studies took her to Guatemala and Mexico where she conducted field work on the Simuliidae (black flies) that transmit the nematode parasite *Onchocerca volvulus*, responsible for onchocerciasis in Latin America and

Africa. After a Postdoctoral Fellowship at the Universidad Central de Venezuela, Caracas, Venezuela in mosquito population genetics and malaria, and a Postdoctoral Associateship at the University of Florida-Gainesville, she was hired as an Assistant Professor at the Biology Department at the University of Vermont where she was promoted to Associate Professor. Since her move to the Wadsworth Center in 2002, her research has focused on population genomics, entomology and ecology. Her goals have been to broaden and deepen the field of vector biology by combining and integrating these disciplines to be of practical value in moving the field of malaria eradication forward. She has conducted field studies with collaborators in Brazil, Colombia, Panama, Peru and Venezuela, demonstrating the need for an increased focus on the quantification of entomological and ecological parameters locally, and on the underlying broad-scale ecological processes, together with local adaptation, that influence malaria transmission. She has published nine books of poetry, with a tenth, *Peony Vertigo*, forthcoming from Brick Books (Canada), in the fall of 2023. She is a visual artist, whose work has been shown in Toronto, Albany, NY, and in several cities in Massachusetts. One of her paintings, *Turbulence*, is on the cover of this book. Please visit www.janconn.com. Her Instagram handle is artistatplay001.

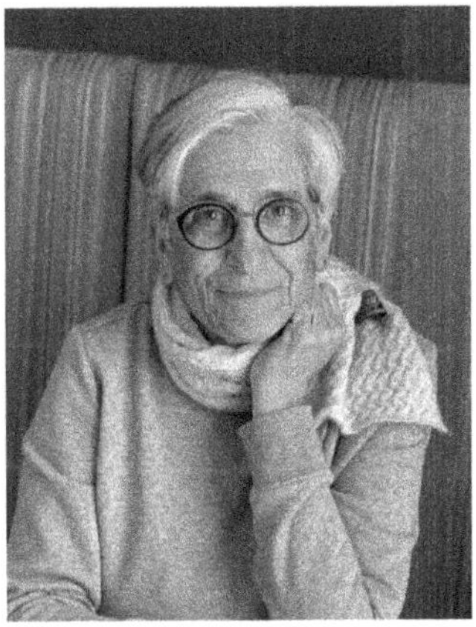

Maria Anice M. Sallum
is a professor in Epidemiology, Ecology in Public Health, and Biology, Ecology and Taxonomy of Culicidae in the School of Public Health at the University of São Paulo, Brazil. She studied at the University of Sao Paulo and obtained her PhD degree in 1994 based on research on the systematics of the Spissipes Section of *Culex* (*Melanoconion*) (Culicidae). She continued her education in the United States, with post-doctoral studies in molecular phylogeny of Anophelinae mosquitoes at the Natural Museum of Natural History at the Smithsonian Institution in Washington, DC, and a one-year position as a Senior Visiting Researcher at The Walter Reed Biosystematics Unit, Suitland, MD. Her work there involved the revision of species of the Leucosphyrus Group of *Anopheles*, subgenus *Cellia*, with a description of six new species in collaboration with EL Peyton and Rick Wilkerson. Upon her return, she coordinated several projects in biology and systematics of Culicidae with an emphasis on Anophelinae. Later, she expanded her focus on field research to include malaria across the Amazon River basin, with a special focus on ecology, the impact of environmental change on mosquito assemblages and increased risk of acquiring *Plasmodium* infection. She has a broad background in biology, ecology, and public health, with specific training and expertise in key research areas for vector-borne diseases. During her university career, she has

built strong collaborations with other institutions and has an extensive network of national and international collaborators. In 2008, she was awarded with John Belkin Award by the American Mosquito Control Association for her meritorious contribution to biology and/or systematics of Culicidae.

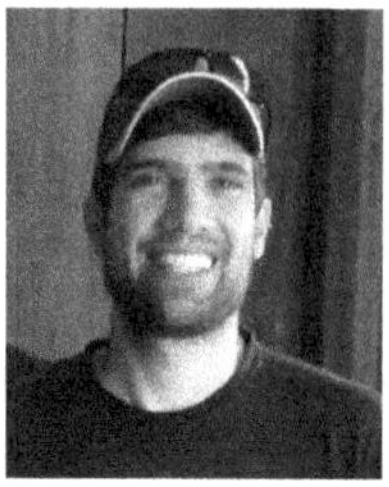

Leonardo Suveges Moreira Chaves
studied biology at the University of Taubaté, Brazil, in 2007, and received a degree in Business Administration from the International Association of Continuing Education (2010). He earned a specialist degree in Environmental Engineering from the School of Engineering of Lorena (EEL-USP) 2010. After this, he obtained both a Masters (2012) and a Doctoral (2018) degree in Sciences from the Department of Epidemiology of the Faculty of Public Health of the University of São Paulo. For his Ph.D. thesis, he carried out field work on the impact of environmental change on the risk of malaria in the Amazon River basin. During his Ph.D. he took a short training in mathematical modeling at the University of Sydney, Australia, with Professor Manfred Lenzen. He was a researcher in the field of medical entomology with a focus in the landscape epidemiology and the ecology of human malaria. He also worked as a consultant in environmental impact associated with anthropogenetic changes in natural ecosystems. He died unexpectedly on January 20, 2023, at the beginning of a productive scientific career, leaving a legacy of important contributions to the field of malaria epidemiology in the Amazon.

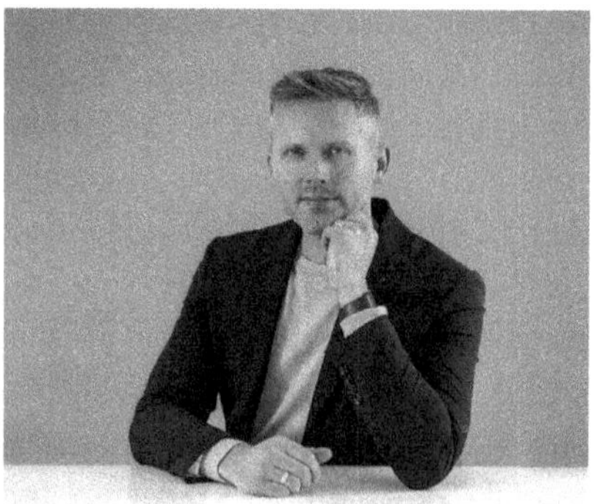

James Logan
is a Professor at the London School of Hygiene & Tropical Medicine (LSHTM), United Kingdom and was Head of the Department of Disease Control for 4 years. He is also Co-Founder and CEO of Arctech Innovation, a world-leading innovation centre for breakthrough research, evaluation and commercialisation of new, game-changing products for the surveillance and control of diseases. He is the Principal Investigator of a large research portfolio, investigating novel surveillance and control technologies for diseases including malaria, Zika, dengue, trachoma and Lyme disease. Professor Logan's research group explores the complex interaction between arthropod vectors, and his ground-breaking research has led to the discovery of novel methods for the control of vectors that transmit pathogens that cause diseases such as malaria, Zika, dengue, trachoma and Lyme disease. His work extends into field evaluation

of vector control tools in developing countries. His work also aims to identify and understand chemical signals given off by the human body during infection and use these as biomarkers of diseases for the development of non-invasive diagnostics, and his recent research discovered that malaria infection causes changes in our body odour, making us more attractive to mosquitoes. He's now working on translating that to develop a novel, non-invasive diagnostic for malaria and other infections. James has more than 150 publications, and is the UK's leading expert on insect repellents and methods of personal protection against arthropod vectors.

Contributors

Tilly Alcayna
Centre for Mathematical Modelling of Infectious Diseases, London School of Hygiene & Tropical Medicine, London, United Kingdom; Centre on Climate Change and Planetary Health, London School of Hygiene & Tropical Medicine, London, UK; and Red Cross Red Crescent Climate Centre, The Hague, the Netherlands
Email: tilly.alcayna@lshtm.ac.uk

Martin Lotto Batista
Epidemiology Department, Helmholtz Centre for Infection Research (HZI), Braunschweig, Germany and Barcelona Supercomputing Center (BSC), Barcelona, Spain
Email: martin.lotto@bsc.es

Jacob Brockmann
Department of Anthropology, University College London, 14 Taviton St, London WC1H 0BW, United Kingdom
Email: jacob.brockmann.20@ucl.ac.uk

Isabel Byrne
Faculty of Infectious and Tropical Diseases, London School of Hygiene and Tropical Medicine, Keppel Street, London WC1E 7HT, United Kingdom
Email: isabel.byrne@lshtm.ac.uk

Jaimie M. Caldwell
High Meadows Environmental Institute, Princeton University, Guyot Hall, Princeton, NJ 08540, USA
Email: jc6991@princeton.edu

Gabriel Carrasco-Escobar
Health Innovation Laboratory, Institute of Tropical Medicine 'Alexander von Humboldt, Universidad Peruana Cayetano Heredia, Lima, Peru and School of Public Health, University of California San Diego, La Jolla, CA, USA
Email: gabriel.carrasco@upch.pe

Kallista Chan
Faculty of Infectious and Tropical Diseases, London School of Hygiene and Tropical Medicine, Keppel Street, London WC1E 7HT, United Kingdom
Email: kallista.chan@lshtm.ac.uk

Leonardo Suveges Moreira Chaves (deceased)
Departamento de Epidemiologia, Facultade de Saúde Publica, Universidade de São Paulo, Sao Paulo, SP, Brazil

Luis F. Chaves
Department of Environmental and Occupational Health, School of Public Health, Indiana State University, Bloomingdale, IN 47405, USA
Email: lfchaves@iu.edu

Gillian Eastwood
Department of Entomology, Center of Emerging Zoonotic & Arthropod-borne Pathogens (CeZAP), Virginia Polytechnic Institute & State University, Blacksburg, VA 24060, USA, Global Change Center, Virginia Tech, Blacksburg, VA, USA
Email: geastwood@vt.edu

Emilie Finch
Centre for Mathematical Modelling of Infectious Diseases, London School of Hygiene & Tropical Medicine, London, United Kingdom and Centre on Climate Change and Planetary Health, London School of Hygiene & Tropical Medicine, London, UK
Email: emilie.finch1@lshtm.ac.uk

Isabel K. Fletcher
Data for Science & Health, Wellcome Trust, London, United Kingdom
Email: i.fletcher@wellcome.org

Kimberly M. Fornace
School of Biodiversity, One Health and Veterinary Medicine, Graham Kerr Building, College of Medical, Veterinary & Life Sciences, University of Glasgow, Glasgow G12 8QQ United Kingdom and Saw Swee Hock School of Public Health, National University of Singapore and National University Health System, Singapore
Email: kimberly.fornace@glasgow.ac.uk

Natasha Glendening
Program in Public Health, College of Health Sciences, University of California at Irvine, Irvine, CA 92697, USA
Email: nglenden@uci.edu

Maria-Eugenia Grillet
Instituto de Ecologia y Zoologia Tropical, Facultad de Ciencias, Universidad Central de Venezuela, Caracas 1053, Venezuela
Email: mariaeugenia.grillet@gmail.com

Sandra de Souza Hacon
Departamento de Endemias Samuel Pessoa (DENSP), Sergio Arouca National School of Public Health (ENSP), Fundação Oswaldo Cruz – FIOCRUZ, Rio de Janeiro, RJ, Brazil
Email: sandrahacon@gmail.com

Werissaw Haileselassie
School of Public Health, Addis Ababa University, Ethiopia
Email: werissawhaileselassie@yahoo.com

Andy Hardy
Department of Geography and Earth Sciences, Aberystwyth University, Aberystwth, United Kingdom
Email: ajh13@aber.ac.uk

Paul J. Huxley
Department of Statistics, Virginia Polytechnic and State University, 250 Drillfield Drive, Blacksburg, VA 24061, USA
Email: phuxley@vt.edu

Dalia Iskander
Department of Anthropology, University College London, 14 Taviton St, London WC1H 0BW, United Kingdom
Email: dalia.iskander@ucl.ac.uk

Emilia Johnson
School of Biodiversity, One Health and Veterinary Medicine, Graham Kerr Building, College of Medical, Veterinary & Life Sciences, University of Glasgow, Glasgow G12 8QQ United Kingdom and Centre for Climate Change and Planetary Health, London School of Hygiene and Tropical Medicine, London, United Kingdom
Email: emilia.johnson@glasgow.ac.uk

Alexander C. Keyel
Division of Infectious Diseases, Wadsworth Center, New York State Department of Health, 120 New Scotland Rd, Albany NY 12208, USA and Department of Atmospheric and Environmental Sciences, University at Albany, 1400 Washington Avenue, Albany, NY 12222, USA
Email: akeyel@albany.edu

Nikolas Kuschnig
Vienna University of Economics and Business, Welthandelsplatz 1, 1020 Vienna, Austria
Email: nikolas.kuschnig@wu.ac.at

Gabriel Z. Laporta
Centro Universitário FMABC, Santo Andre, São Paulo, SP, Brazil
Email: gabriel.laporta@fmabc.br

Sophie A. Lee
Centre for Mathematical Modelling of Infectious Diseases, London School of Hygiene & Tropical Medicine, London, United Kingdom and Centre on Climate Change and Planetary Health, London School of Hygiene & Tropical Medicine, London, UK
Email: sophie.lee@lshtm.ac.uk

Catherine A. Lippi
Emerging Pathogens Institute, University of Florida, P.O. Box 100009, 2055 Mowry Road, Gainesville, FL 32610, USA
Email: clippi@ufl.edu

Jose R. Loaiza
Instituto de Investigaciones Cientificas y Servicios de Alta Tecnologia (INDICASAT AIP), P.O. Box 0843–01103, Panama, Republica de Panama
Email: jloaiza@indicasat.org.pa

Rachel Lowe
Centre for Mathematical Modelling of Infectious Diseases, London School of Hygiene & Tropical Medicine, London, United Kingdom; Centre on Climate Change and Planetary Health, London School of Hygiene & Tropical Medicine, London, UK; Barcelona Supercomputing Center (BSC), Barcelona, Spain; and Catalan Institution for Research and Advanced Studies (ICREA), Barcelona Spain
Email: rachel.lowe@bsc.es

Jorge E. Moreno
Centro de Investigaciones de Campo 'Dr. Francesco Vitanza,' Servicio Autónomo Instituto de Altos Estudios 'Dr. Arnoldo Gabaldón,' MPPS. Tumereno, Bolívar, Venezuela
Email: jorermo@gmail.com

Marta Moreno
Department of Biology, London School of Hygiene and Tropical Medicine, Keppel Street, London WC1E 7HT, United Kingdom
Email: marta.moreno@lshtm.ac.uk

Juan Carlos Navarro
Research Group of Emerging Diseases, Ecoepidemiolgy and Biodiversity, Health Sciences Faculty, Universidad Internacional SEK, Quito 170134, Ecuador and Instituto de Ecologia y Zoologia Tropical, Facultad de Ciencias, Universidad Central de Venezuela, Caracas 1053, Venezuela
Email: juancarlos.navarro@uisek.edu.ec

Alberto Paníz-Mondolfi
Department of Pathology, Molecular and Cell-Based Medicine, Icahn School of Medicine at Mount Sinai, 1425 Madison Ave Room L9–52B, New York, NY 10029, USA
Email: alberto.paniz-mondolfi@mountsinai.org

Daniel M. Parker
Program in Public Health, College of Health Sciences, University of California at Irvine, Irvine, CA 92697, USA
Email: dparker1@hs.uci.edu

Luiz Carlos Ferreira Penha
Programa VigiFronteiras Brasil, Fundação Oswaldo Cruz – FIOCRUZ, Rio de Janeiro, RJ, Brazil
Email: luizsgc@gmail.com

Rafael Piovezan
Facultade de Saúde Publica, Universidade de São Paulo, São Paulo, SP, Brazil and Secretary of the Environment, Santa Barbara d'Oeste, SP, Brazil
Email: piovezan.rafael@gmail.com

Paula Ribeiro Prist
EcoHealth Alliance, 520 Eight Avenue, Ste. 1200, New York, NY 10018, USA
Email: pprist@hotmail.com

Thiago Salomão-Azevedo
Facultade de Saúde Publica, Universidade de São Paulo, São Paulo, SP, Brazil and Secretary of Health, Municipality of Santa Barbara d'Oeste, São Paulo, Brazil
Email: azevedots@gmail.com

Marta S. Shocket
Department of Geography, University of Florida, 3141 Turlington Hall, 330 Newell Dr, Gainesville, FL 32611, USA
Email: marta.shocket@gmail.com

Tatiane Moraes de Sousa
Departamento de Endemias Samuel Pessoa (DENSP), Sergio Arouca National School of Public Health (ENSP), Fundação Oswaldo Cruz – FIOCRUZ, Rio de Janeiro, RJ, Brazil
Email: taticmsousa@gmail.com

Lukas Vashold
Vienna University of Economics and Business, Welthandelsplatz 1, 1020 Vienna, Austria
Email: lukas.vashold@wu.ac.at

Francis A. Windram
Department of Life Sciences, Imperial College London, Silwood Park, Ascot, Berkshire, United Kingdom
Email: francis.windram17@imperial.ac.uk

Introduction

Jan E. Conn[1,2*], *Maria Anice M. Sallum*[3] *and Kimberly M. Fornace*[4,5,6]

[1]The Wadsworth Center, New York State Department of Health, Griffin Laboratory, 2659 State Farm Rd, Slingerlands NY 12159, USA, [2]Department of Biomedical Sciences, School of Public Health, State Universitty of New York at Albany, Albany, NY, USA; [3]Departamento de Epidemiologia, Faculdade de Saúde Pública, Universidade de São Paulo, São Paulo, SP 01246-904, Brazil; [4]School of Biodiversity, One Health and Veterinary Medicine, University of Glasgow, Glasgow, United Kingdom, [5]Saw Swee Hock School of Public Health, National University of Singapore, Singapore, [6]Faculty of Infectious and Tropical Diseases, London School of Hygiene and Tropical Medicine, London, United Kingdom; *jan.conn@health.ny.gov

Current levels of global environmental change are unprecedented, causing widespread and rapid changes to the natural and human systems. As global greenhouse gas emissions continue to increase, disruptions of environmental systems will have profound impacts on human health and well-being (IPCC 2023). The concept of planetary health developed in response to these challenges, recognising that human health is dependent on natural systems and safeguarding natural systems is a core public health need. Planetary health extends outside traditional health sectors to consider the health of both human populations and the natural systems on which they depend (Whitmee *et al.* 2015). This requires an integrated approach to address social, economic and environmental determinants of health, understanding the complex interactions between these factors to identify sustainable solutions that support health. As some of the most environmentally sensitive infectious diseases, vector-borne diseases (VBD) are a key focus of planetary health. Within this book, we explore the impacts of environmental change on VBD ecology, the impacts of these changes on both social and natural systems and opportunities for integrated surveillance and control.

1 Part 1: Impacts of environmental change on VBD ecology

The major impetus for this book was our concern about the far-reaching effects of current and future climate change on the trifecta of humans, vectors, and pathogens. Landscapes *per se*, whether local, regional, or continental, are major players in pathogen transmission, and are remarkably sensitive to small changes in

 | DOI:10.3920/9789004688650_002

temperature, humidity and rainfall. All landscapes are anthropogenic to greater or lesser degrees, and constitute the building blocks of ecology and epidemiology, extended to the sister-disciplines of landscape ecology and ecoepidemiology (Begon and Townsend 2021). The negative effects of climate and land-use and land-cover (LULC), mainly deforestation, on many landscape types, are documented in several chapters (1–4, 5, 9).

Because mosquitoes have been recognised as one of the most dangerous animals on Earth, (Gates 2016) mosquito vector species are the main feature in several chapters (1–4). Various aspects of malaria are a focus (Chapters 1–3, 5–7, 10–11, 13) as it remains, despite enormous progress, the most devastating of the parasitic vector-borne diseases globally (WHO 2022) and the third largest globally (after HIV/AIDS and tuberculosis) in direct cost (Chapter 6). Furthermore, nearly half of the world's population is considered to be at risk of acquiring malaria, according to the World Malaria Report (2021). The recent invasion and spread of the competent Asian malaria vector *An. stephensi* into several eastern African countries has been causing considerable alarm (WHO 2019; Whittaker *et al.* 2023), and is briefly discussed in Chapters 10–11, 13. Collectively, mosquito species transmit a wide range of viruses (especially dengue, Zika, chikungunya and West Nile) to an estimated 350 million people annually, with *Aedes aegypti* and *Aedes albopictus* responsible for most dengue virus transmission in urban/periurban areas (Chapters 4, 8, 10, 12) (Baker *et al.* 2022). An observation that deserves attention has been the increase in Yellow Fever virus (YFV) transmission in several countries, notably Brazil's Atlantic Forest, Peru, and Venezuela (Chapters 1, 2). As YFV is globally restricted to Africa and South America, any increase or potential spread within these regions is important to underscore, given historically lower adherence to vaccines generally (Nuwarda *et al.* 2022) among other pressing public health issues.

Prist and Laporta (Chapter 1) analysed temporal epidemiological data from three vector-borne diseases in Brazilian Amazonian municipalities transmitted by three different insect vectors: malaria – anopheline mosquitoes; Chagas disease – triatomines bugs; and cutaneous leishmaniasis – sandflies. The aims were to identify disease case incidence clusters and temporal trends relative to changes in landscape structure, and to evaluate trade-offs relative to differences in these three diseases. The clusters differed spatially by disease with very little geographic overlap. The main finding is that for malaria and cutaneous leishmaniasis, municipalities at highest risk are those with greater than 50% forest cover that are experiencing deforestation. In contrast, the landscape of greatest risk for Chagas disease consists of continuous forest in a matrix of deforested non-pasture. Nevertheless, in general, loss of biodiversity of the most preserved Amazonian landscapes (those with up to 50% remaining forest cover) increases the risk of VBD. Managing landscape structure to become less deforested and fragmented (a multifunctional landscape approach) is recommended to prevent known diseases and new pandemics.

Even though there has been increased awareness of Venezuela's health crisis, the situation on the ground remains dire (Chapter 2). Grillet and colleagues highlight the egregious malaria circumstances, with the nexus of economic crisis-driven migration identified as unregulated gold extraction in the south, deforestation, and malaria endemicity, resulting in the highest levels of reported malaria cases (467,421 in 2019) in the Americas in decades (WHO 2021). Further complications include migrant miners from the south who may return to states in the north and west (where competent malaria vectors exist) and thus inadvertently precipitate new or renewed malaria transmission foci. A disturbing international epidemiological threat is a novel migrant corridor among countries that make up the Guyana Shield that may spread artemisinin-resistant mutations. Increased arbovirus transmission in Venezuela is less-well understood and documented, but also of great concern. The authors provide practical, reasonable local and regional actions that could be undertaken to help mitigate this crisis, although the appropriate political will would be needed for implementation.

In Chapter 3 by Chaves and colleagues, the diverse and vital Amazon Basin is the primary exemplar; however, changes there and in the Congo-Gabonese region of Africa and the Greater Mekong in Southern Asia will affect every corner of the globe. In the Amazon, predicted 60% reduction in rainfall and 2^{0}C increase in air temperature would trigger weather pattern shifts, reduce biodiversity, and carbon storage, and increase human migration, complex socioeconomic damage, and VBD prevalence. The primary driver of loss of forested areas is directly attributable to agropastoral activity (Garret *et al.* 2021). Direct and lateral damage includes the amplification of several types of disasters, i.e., in the Amazon, wildfires and dam collapses; globally, tropical cyclones and a range of hydrometeorological events (in South East Asia, see Chapter 9, and across the African continent, see Chapter 13). Extreme weather events and their multiple effects on VBD are discussed in Chapter 12, relative to the design of early warning systems (EWS). A crucial final section of Chapter 3 documents the history and causes of the extreme vulnerabilities of Amazonian indigenous peoples to malaria. This chapter's sobering assessment can be mitigated somewhat by solutions proposed in other chapters: e.g. creating healthy landscapes (Chapter 1); local and regional actions to provide pragmatic and rational solutions to the VBD crisis in Venezuela (Chapter 2); proactive use of spatial association analysis to locate, monitor and eliminate urban breeding sites for *Aedes* and *Culex* arbovirus vectors (Chapter 4); inclusion of transient and under-the-radar extraction-based settlements in local, regional and/or national healthcare systems (Chapter 5); incorporation of economic research findings into a more interdisciplinary approach to malaria eradication and intervention (Chapter 6); better recognition of the patchiness of heterogeneous malaria-endemic environments and novel uses of drone technologies (Chapter 7); approaches and recommendations to maintain vector-borne surveillance and interventions during pandemics (Chapter 8); expansion of the concept of 'co-benefits' (Crumpler and Meybeck 2020), designed initially to foster climate-resilient agriculture, to include health outcomes, especially those linked to VBD (Chapter 9); improvements in mathematical and statistical modelling to better understand VBD in the context of climate and environmental change (especially temperature and rainfall) at various temporal and spatial scales (Chapter 10); application of Earth Observation data to improve VBD surveillance and control, particularly for detection of water bodies and development of predictive models applicable to deployment of targeted control interventions (Chapter 11); creation of climate-informed early warning systems (EWS) for vector borne disease globally, at a range of scales (Chapter 12); and reassessment of the effectiveness and impact of mainstay interventions to prevent malaria transmission in Africa (insecticide treated nets, insecticide residual spray, larval source management) in the face of the complex effects of climate change (Chapter 13).

In some ways in parallel with the focus in Chapter 3, environmental degradation that accompanies the unchecked growth of sprawling global urban centres or megacities frequently leads to the proliferation of breeding sites suitable for immature *Aedes* and *Culex* arbovirus vector mosquitoes. The most obvious examples of arboviruses that have increased in part from urban sprawl are dengue, Zika, chikungunya and yellow fever (Chapter 4). This chapter by Salomao de Azevedo and Piovezan emphasises the critical role of mosquito surveillance and control in public health policy (see also Chapter 12 for case studies of dengue early warning systems (EWS) in Brazil, Singapore, and Vietnam), provides brief overviews of the importance and roles in virus transmission of *Aedes aegypti* and *Aedes albopictus* as well as a thumbnail sketch of the *Culex pipiens* group and its transformation into a significant vector of the West Nile virus in many countries. The final section of Chapter 4 includes a detailed example in a municipality in São Paulo state of the use of the normalised difference vegetation index (NDVI) combined with spatial association analysis and local temperature fluctuation to track probable breeding sites of *Ae. aegypti*, *Ae. albopictus* and *Cx. quinquefasciatus*, to predict and intervene to prevent viral transmission.

2 Part 2: Coupled human and natural systems

In their noteworthy blueprint for re-envisioning how various types of extractive settlements (i.e. agriculture, mining, timber) could provide or substantially improve healthcare services for human community members, Glendening and colleagues (Chapter 5) conducted a pilot case-study within an artisanal and small-scale gold-mining settler community in western Ethiopia near the beginning of its establishment by pioneer migrants (2017–2018). The authors used a three-pronged approach to determine settler origin, current occupation, and general healthcare plus an evaluation of the malaria situation. Focused on household questionnaires and Landsat image data to track forest loss, authors provide a succinct report of local environmental degradation (mainly forest loss and landscape fragmentation linked to road construction and mining) and health of the mostly young adult population in their representative sampling. Their data support the concern that the informal nature of such in-country migration, an increasingly global problem, usually results in limited access to healthcare and subsequent worse health outcomes for the settlers. As such settlements are often overlooked or discounted by government healthcare providers, in addition to being remote and/or in conflict zones in this malaria endemic region, most study participants did not own a mosquito net to protect against malaria transmission. In line with documentation in Chapters 1–4, 9, 13, the ensuing environmental damage and changes frequently result in increased VBD within settlements and sometimes beyond. The solutions offered by Glendening *et al.* (Chapter 5) require some measure of government awareness and action: traveling community workers should be recruited as soon as a group of humans settles; then as (if) the settlement grows and stabilises the authors advocate strongly for establishment of a community healthcare system with at least one resident healthcare worker. The third imperative is to ensure safe drinking water and healthy housing, and to work toward creation of healthy communities, as recommended in Chapter 1.

One of the most commonly held assumptions about malaria globally is that it is intimately associated with poverty and development; yet there exist some major studies that contradict this perception and underscore a lack of causality (Chapter 6). While there is no doubt about the direct health burden of malaria and the economic impact at the individual and community levels, Kuschnig and Vashold argue that an interdisciplinary approach to eradication and intervention strategies that takes economic research findings into account is likely to improve outcomes by providing a deeper understanding of the many indirect economic impacts of malaria (Chapters 2, 5). A key aspect to disentangling the myriad interaction factors that affect the cost of the malaria burden is to focus on either microeconomic or macroeconomic studies, the former invoking identification strategies with narrow causal pathways (one example, apart from contemporaneous morbidity and mortality, is the extensive lifelong effects of reduced educational capacity for children). In contrast, macroeconomic impact studies function at country, region, or global scales, and as such, utilise a range of theories to provide broader snapshots; these are often more appropriate for national policymakers' decisions. Another important facet under brief consideration is the enormous cost of eradication programmes, that to date have been successful mainly in more temperate regions. Gaps and near-term challenges are clearly identified, particularly the need for better data on malaria resurgence in the face of increasing temperatures, spillover effects relative to location and socioeconomic status, and interactions between VBD and the environment.

Anthropologists Brockmann and Iskander (Chapter 7) interviewed malaria researchers who teamed up in a global network called MACONDO to apply drone technologies in heterogeneous landscapes to gain insights into their potential to augment surveillance, risk-mapping, and interventions to reduce malaria transmission. One of the clearest motivations for the use of drones for malaria research has been the recognition that extensive transmission by exophagic (outdoor biting) mosquito species occurs in diverse landscapes, work and social situations, and the concomitant need for additional, complementary environmentally-based approaches. Various ways of collecting data were revealed, such as the use of a thermal camera to locate primates that cut through the visual noise of a drone image to spotlight a very particular aspect of importance to malaria transmission. Analogous to the focus on NDVI, spatial association analysis and fluctuating temperature to predict, locate and treat potential Culicine and Aedine arbovirus vector breeding sites (Chapter 4), another MACONDO researcher focused on Larval Source Management (LSM) as an approach to locate potential malaria mosquito breeding sites with a drone and then conduct precision larviciding on the ground in the back streets of the capital of Tanzania. Such an approach was tailored for this uban/periurban landscape but would have been overwhelming in the Amazon, a landscape that includes thousands of water bodies. In the latter case, Carrasco-Escobar *et al.* (2019) characterised and quantified water bodies that were suitable for the vector species, enabling them to recommend treatment of a portion of the total. An overall observation was that all malaria-transmission landscapes are patchy, that the limits of drone flight time imposed a need to make rapid, informed decisions about where to conduct surveys, and that multidisciplinary teams were optimal for providing a more nuanced series of views and foci to help guide intervention measures.

Narrowing the VBD view to aspects of vector intervention and surveillance that should be maintained during pandemics such as COVID-19, Loaiza and colleagues (Chapter 8) note that the extensive containment tactics at the beginning of this pandemic in the Americas in 2020 often resulted in increased VBD outbreaks that went unrecorded (e.g. a coronavirus-VBD syndemic). In the US, increased outdoor activity combined with reduced avoidance of visits to medical facilities led in some regions to artificially low reporting of Lyme disease, and many mosquito and tick surveillance operations across the country were reduced or even ended due to redeployment of staff or funding to cope with COVID-19 prevention, testing and treatment. This chapter includes recommendations for different categories of transmission of a range of VBD systems in the form of tables suggested for: (1) vector personnel to enable them to protect themselves from contracting an infectious pathogen while maintaining modified surveillance and interventions; and (2) for people to protect themselves from transmission. There are brief descriptions of ways that citizen science programs can be implemented including crowdsourced data and online platforms, community involvement, and the use of drones to help locate mosquito breeding sites and trash accumulation including tire dumps, similar if less detailed than drone use described in Chapter 7. There is an excellent emphasis on the importance of community involvement and engagement to achieve sustainable VBD mitigation, and a section describing state-of-the-art methods for rapid identification of vector pathogens and bloodmeal hosts at scale.

Two major environmental drivers of agriculture, deforestation, and irrigation, are tackled by Bryne and Chan (Chapter 9). These two (among many) add another level of concern to the severe consequences of extensive deforestation and the resultant ecological change viz-a-viz temperature increase, inadvertent creation of mosquito breeding sites, loss of/changes in plant and animal diversity, modified microclimate conditions, soil composition and erosion, and increased vector-human interaction as discussed in several chapters (1–4, 5, 13). A significant, often overlooked health and VBD issue has arisen in agricultural practices that promote a more diverse range of crops and foodstuffs, namely there is less regard for the increasing risk of VBD transmission to agricultural workers. On the plus side, food production is increasingly conducted with sustainable environmental mandates at the forefront. Water redistribution that benefits agricultural development via reservoirs, dams and irrigation canals/networks is also strongly linked – particularly irrigation for rice production – to increased abundance of malaria vectors and *Plasmodium* transmission globally, along with greater incidences of schistosomiasis and leishmaniasis in some regions. In addition to increased dengue, chikungunya and malaria, the creation of thousands of monoculture-based plantation farms across South East Asia for palm oil, rubber, sugarcane and cassava are increasing the incidence of lymphatic filariasis, scrub typhus, and simian malaria (*Plasmodium knowlesi*). Several examples and case studies exemplifying co-benefits or 'win-win' strategies focused on rice irrigation are provided such as alternate wetting and drying, intermittent, and drip irrigation, along with system of rice intensification (SRI). Considering the need for rice fertilisation, especially interesting strategies are the use of fertiliser + biolarvicides (*Bti*) and organic materials such as *Azolla* (mosquito fern) and *Azadirachta indica* (neem), rice-fish and rice-duck co-culture systems. The final section is a powerful summary of mechanisms that could overcome the barriers between agriculture and health sectors.

3 Part 3: VBD surveillance and control in changing environments

Pathogen transmission, temperature (fluctuating vs constant, heterogeneity at fine spatial scales), rainfall, humidity/wind/tides, and non-climatic factors (such as LULC, reservoir hosts, population densities, predators, competitors, food resources) are featured as the primary biological mechanisms that affect transmission patterns of mosquito-borne disease (MBD) via climate in Chapter 10 by Shocket and co-authors. Rainfall and temperature are especially important for modeling as both have nonlinear impacts on vector abundance and transmission (see also Chapters 11–13). Major differences in lifecycle and physiology of tick vs mosquitoes hosts that strongly differentiate climatic effects on their transmission of pathogens and population dynamics, are discussed here and in Chapter 8. A concise review of the differences, strengths, uses, and limitations of each of the two main MBD climate change transmission model types – mechanistic (process or trait-based, better for comprehending biological processes) and statistical (phenomenological/correlative, better as predictors) – is that they provide complementary forms of illumination such that the use of both seems to be optimal. Use of Table 1 to characterise multiple kinds of statistical approaches is excellent, and pains were taken to highlight the importance of acquiring appropriate climate data, depending on the scale of the inquiry. The need for output from a general circulation model (GMC) that predicts future climatic conditions based on Earth's atmospheric processes is stressed, along with choice of which of several phases of Coupled Model Intercomparison Project (CMIP) to use as a best-match scenario. Model selection and validation are also fortified by descriptions in Table 2. Three case studies at different scales: dengue fever in the city of San Juan, Puerto Rico (see also dengue in southern Sao Paulo state in Chapter 4); regional models of West Nile virus in the US (especially the excellent summary in Table 3); and large-scale models for the impact of climate change on malaria (see also Chapter 13 for malaria and Africa) and dengue, are each lucidly articulated and summarised, and provide many useful references. The last section acknowledges three categories of challenges: data generation and availability; model construction; and ways to put model output into action to reduce MBDs.

Significant advances in the use of Earth Observation (EO) data, i.e. the collection of physical and biological data from Earth's surface, in addition to remote sensing, computing advances and imagery analysis methods to integrate these data successfully into vector-borne disease surveillance and intervention programmes, are detailed in Chapter 11 by Fornace and colleagues. The importance of assessing environmental change at a local scale (see also Chapters 4–5) is underscored relative to human settlements, vegetation type and density, land cover, and distribution of water bodies. This chapter also stresses the usefulness of seasonal, local vector ecology data for informed VBD data selection and applications. Characteristics of EO are determined by specific sensor type (e.g. from visible to near infrared and shortwave), the latter being especially suitable for complex habitat types. Both spatial (pixel size of collected data) and temporal (seasonal, monthly) resolution are key factors to consider. A useful comparison of the strengths and limitations of optical satellite-based systems vs. drones is provided (see also Chapter 7 for the latter). An important aspect of EO data is the ability to identify high-risk areas or populations of animal hosts or reservoirs, such as wild ungulates infected with Rift Valley virus in Kenya, or non-human primates in Malaysia that may harbour *Plasmodium knowlesi*, that could benefit from surveillance and potential interventions. Other relevant applications include spatial distribution of vectors and pathogens under models of climate change and predictions of habitat-specific locations where invasive species such as *An. stephensi* (from Asia into the Horn of Africa) would most likely become established. Neatly summarised case studies in the malaria endemic countries of Zanzibar, Cote d'Ivoire, and Peru provide examples of methods and approaches that enhanced detection, surveillance, and treatment of water bodies for effective mosquito larvae control. A different but analogous approach is used to track and predict larval breeding sites of arbovirus vectors *Ae. aegypti*, *Ae. albopictus* and *Cx. quinquefasciatus* in southern São Paulo state, Brazil in Chapter 4.

Finch and co-authors describe and recommend a pathway to create climate-informed early warning systems (EWS) for VBDs at a range of scales in Chapter 12. It is evident that EWS are increasingly essential for public health systems to function to prevent or mitigate disease outbreaks with adequate lead-time as climate extremes increase in frequency (WHO 2021). There is a significant gap in the existence of operationalised tools for EWS within the health sector, and major barriers include: (1) a lack of formal partnerships between climate and health sectors in most countries (see also Chapter 13 for a fruitful discussion); and (2) sharing of local and global datasets (notably epidemiological and health data). A series of steps is articulated that, while not prescriptive, offers useful starting points for a complex transdisciplinary process, comprising engagement, feasibility study, tool development, implementation, monitoring, and finally, evaluation. As there are alternative EWS models, rigorous statistical evaluation of each in terms of predictive accuracy forecasts is essential. Starting with data that are available and regularly assessed in a country (e.g. routine epidemiology data; local or regional meteorological stations) increases the likelihood of creating a viable EWS, especially if stakeholders advocate for appropriate technology, financial resources, training, and capacity building at the outset. Also important is understanding the varied regional influences of interannual climatic phenomena: in the Pacific Ocean, *El Niño Southern Oscillation Event* (ENSO – increases temperature and rainfall) and La Niña (decreases temperature, increases flooding and/or tropical storms) on VBD transmission; and for parts of Asia, the Indian Ocean Dipole (oscillations in sea surface temperature). For model development, there are several non-climatic aspects that can also drive outbreaks, such as lack of immunity of human populations to introduced pathogen(s), multiple serotypes (dengue, for example), LULC, connectivity among populations, among other socioeconomic and environmental factors. Model approaches (statistical, mechanistic, semi-mechanistic and ensemble) for VBD outbreak risk prediction described in text and Table 2, nicely complement approaches and models described in Table 1 and 2 of Chapter 10.

Ferguson and Govella in Chapter 13 think outside the box and consider the consequences of alternatives interventions as the mainstays for malaria in Africa (indoor residual spray; IRS, insecticide treated nets; ITN and larval source management; LSM) become increasingly ineffective. In general, across Africa, direct climate change impacts will consist mainly of increasing temperature, rainfall shifts and increased extreme weather events with little expansion of transmission area; recent models consider that increased exposure within stable transmission areas may be the most likely scenario (Mordecai *et al.* 2020). Climate change will modify vector species composition, abundance, and distribution; rising temperatures will impact vector susceptibility and competence for *Plasmodium*, along with *Plasmodium* sporogonic success, which is temperature dependent. Each of the major malaria vectors in Africa (*An. gambiae*, *An. coluzzii*, *An. arabiensis*, *An. funestus*, and the invasive *An. stephensi*) differs in breeding site characteristics, feeding behaviour and/or host preference, and other ecological traits. Some of the current interventions already display limited effectivity – the more zoophagic *An. arabiensis* encounters ITN and IRS less frequently and is consequently more difficult to suppress; should the mainly invasive, urban, exophilic and exophagic *An. stephensi* continue expanding in Africa, malaria interventions, historically more rural, will need to shift in focus, infrastructure, and type to include urban centres (see also Chapter 10). Insecticides used for IRS and ITN to control adult anophelines are known to be heterogeneous in their effectiveness across Africa, even for the same species, suggesting possible insecticide resistance, temperature effects and/or differences in local mosquito ecology. Although LSM has been highly successful, studies of potential effects of extreme flooding or drought on its continued feasibility have not been a priority. There are also 'indirect climate change impacts' that could be overlooked easily. Newer strategies such as house eaves (used with insecticidal netting to kill anophelines as they enter houses) and ivermectin (an endectocide used to treat [mainly] cattle), that kills mosquitoes feeding on cattle and humans (the latter in the case of mass administration), also need to be reconsidered in the light of the effects of increased temperature on both acceptability and impact. Severe effects on agricultural and food security (a focus of Chapter 9) are expected to lead to additional needs for irrigation, dam construction, crop diversification, increased pesticide use, and human migration to relatively unstable informal settlements surrounding urban centres (that, like extraction-based settlements (Chapter 5), often become hotspots of VBD transmission due to inadequate housing, electricity, water and infrastructure). Humanitarian and socio-economic crises are in danger of accompanying severe climate change, and without political will and economic security, major resurgences of VBDs as in Venezuela (Chapter 2) could overwhelm other countries in Africa and beyond.

Acknowledgements

Thanks to the following for support for the introduction: JEC and MAMS were partially funded by US National Institutes of Health grant 2R01AI110112. KMF was supported by a Sir Henry Dale fellowship jointly funded by the Wellcome Trust and the Royal Society (Grant no. 221963/Z/20/Z).

References

Baker RE, Mahmud AS, Miller IF, Rajeev M, Rasambainarivo F, Rice BL, Takahashi S, Tatem AJ, Wagner CE, Wang LF, Wesolowski A and Metcalf CJE (2022) Infectious disease in an era of global change. Nature reviews. Microbiology, 20(4), 193–205. https://doi.org/10.1038/s41579-021-00639-z.

Begon M and Townsend CR (2021) Ecology: from individuals to ecosystems, 5th edition, Wiley-Blackwell Pub, Hoboken NJ.

Carrasco-Escobar G, Manrique E, Ruiz-Cabrejos J, Saavedra M, Alava F, Bickersmith S, Prussing C, Vinetz JM, Conn JE, Moreno M and Gamboa D (2019) High-accuracy detection of malaria vector larval habitats using drone-based multispectral imagery. PLoS neglected tropical diseases, 13(1), e0007105. https://doi.org/10.1371/journal.pntd.0007105.

Crumpler K and Meybeck A (2020) Adaptation in the agriculture sectors: leveraging co-benefits for mitigation and sustainable development. Tech. Report. Food and Agriculture Organization of the United Nations, Rome. 18 pp. https://doi.org/10.13140/RG.2.2.35243.87842.

Garret RD, Cammelli F, Ferreira J, Levy SA, Valentim J and Veira I (2021) Forests and sustainable developments in the Brazilian Amazon: history, trends and future prospects. Annual Rev Environment and Resources. 46: 625–652. https://doi.org/10.1146/annurev-environ-012220-010228.

Gates B (2016) The deadliest animal in the world. Artroópodos y Salud Vol. 6, No. 2. Pp. 4–5. Available at: https://www.gatesnotes.com/Health/Most-Lethal-Animal-Mosquito-Week.

Intergovernmental Panel on Climate Change (IPCC) (2023). Available at: https://www.ipcc.ch/report/ar6/syr/.

Mordecai EA, Ryan SJ, Caldwell JM, Shah MM and LaBeaud AD (2020) Climate change could shift disease burden from malaria to arboviruses in Africa. The Lancet. Planetary health, 4(9), e416–e423. https://doi.org/10.1016/S2542-5196(20)30178-9.

Nuwarda RF, Ramzan I, Weekes L and Kayser V (2022) Vaccine hesitancy: contemporary issues and historical background. Vaccines, 10(10), 1595. https://doi.org/10.3390/vaccines10101595.

Whitmee S, Haines A, Beyrer C, Boltz F, Capon AG, Ferreira de Souza Dias B, Ezeh A, Frumkin H, Gong P, Head P, Horton R, Mace GM, Marten R, Myers SS, Nishtar S, Osofsky SA, Pattanayak SK, Pongsiri MJ, Romanelli C, Soucat A, Vega J and Yach D (2015) Safeguarding human health in the Anthropocene epoch: report of The Rockefeller Foundation-*Lancet* Commission on planetary health. Lancet, 386, 1973. http://dx.doi.org/10.1016/S0140-6736(15)60901-1.

Whittaker C, Hamlet A, Sherrard-Smith E, Winskill P, Cuomo-Dannenburg G, Walker PGT, Sinka M, Pironon S, Kumar A, Ghani A, Bhatt S and Churcher TS (2023) Seasonal dynamics of *Anopheles stephensi* and its implications for mosquito detection and emergent malaria control in the Horn of Africa. Proceedings of the National Academy of Sciences of the United States of America, 120(8), e2216142120. https://doi.org/10.1073/pnas.2216142120.

World Health Organization. (2019) World malaria report 2019. Geneva: World Health Organization. Available at: https://apps.who.int/iris/handle/10665/330011.

World Health Organization. (2021) World malaria report 2021. Geneva: World Health Organization. Available at: https://apps.who.int/iris/handle/10665/350147.

World Health Organization. (2022) World malaria report 2022. Geneva: World Health Organization. 2022. Available at: https://www.who.int/publications/i/item/9789240064898.

PART 1

Impacts of environmental change on VBD ecology

CHAPTER 1

Landscape ecology and vector-borne diseases in the Amazon

Paula R. Prist[1]* *and Gabriel Zorello Laporta*[2]

[1]EcoHealth Alliance, 520 8th Avenue, Suite 1200, New York, NY 10018, USA;
[2]Setor de Pós-graduação, Pesquisa e Inovação, Centro Universitário FMABC, Fundação ABC, Av. Lauro Gomes, 2000 – Vila Sacadura Cabral, Santo André, SP 09060–870, Brazil; *prist@ecohealthalliance.org

Abstract

Malaria, Chagas disease, and cutaneous leishmaniasis are endemic in the Amazon. Changes in landscape caused by deforestation and fragmentation can support transmission of malarial parasites through the increased dominance of anopheline vectors that augments human exposure to infectious bites. As for Chagas disease and cutaneous leishmaniasis, accumulated knowledge on this respect is still scant. Here the relationships between each of these diseases and changes in the landscape structure of 773 municipalities in the Brazilian Amazon were assessed from 2007 to 2019. Disease specific responses to forest cover loss and fragmentation were observed. As expected, deforestation and fragmentation of preserved municipal landscapes were drivers of the highest number of malaria cases. Deforestation, but not fragmentation, was determinant of increased numbers of cases of cutaneous leishmaniasis in preserved (≥ 50% forest cover) municipal landscapes. Municipalities with remaining forests contiguous to deforested areas modified into crops of Açai trees represent the microcosm of Chagas disease in the Amazon. Interpretations from these results allowed us to distil a general pattern. The loss of biodiversity in preserved landscapes can increase the risk of vector-borne disease in the Amazon up to a given threshold (50% of forest cover). Below this level, the risks might be lower, but there will be no biodiversity left to be preserved in the degraded landscape (< 50% forest cover). One further idea can be logically deducted from this general pattern. The concept of 'healthy landscapes' depends on the disease under study. In this respect, malaria and cutaneous leishmaniasis can both be prevented if deforestation and fragmentation of preserved landscapes are controlled. This leads to the concept of multifunctional landscapes, where landscape-based interventions have multiple functions, including precluding cases of two or more diseases. A multifunctional landscape approach will help in the landscape management and restoration to prevent endemic diseases and future pandemics.

 | DOI:10.3920/9789004688650_003

Keywords

diseases – fragmentation – human health – healthy landscapes – landscape management – multifunctional landscapes – pandemics

1 Introduction

Landscape is a physical environment in which the relationship between nature and humans evolves (Simpson *et al.* 1989). Natural landscape is defined as an ecosystem free of the interference from human activities (Carson 2002). Although truly pristine or natural landscape spots are becoming scarcer in the 21st century, Amazon has the largest area of intact forest landscapes (4 million km^2) among all continents, followed by Congo basin and Southeast Asia (Potapov *et al.* 2017). However, these areas remain under strong threat. In 2020 alone, the planet lost an area of tree cover larger than the United Kingdom, including more than 4.2 million hectares of primary tropical forests, led by the increasing deforestation and incidence of fires in the Amazon (IPBES 2020; Weisse and Goldman 2021). When any disturbance from human activities occurs in a natural landscape, temporally subsequent landscapes from this natural landscape becomes anthropic or humanized. This concept of a human-modified natural landscape is central in disciplines of ecology and epidemiology, including landscape ecology and ecoepidemiology (Forman and Godron 1986; Begon *et al.* 2006).

The Amazon biome has the largest amount of intact forest landscapes in the world (Potapov *et al.* 2017). These last frontiers of wilderness are mainly clustered in partially continuous areas of forests in eastern Peru, southeastern Colombia, southern Venezuela, Suriname, Guyana, French Guiana, and in the Brazilian states of Acre, Amapá, Amazonas, Pará, Rondônia, and Roraima. Notwithstanding, these authors (Potapov *et al.* 2017) also have measured forest cover loss in these Amazonian natural landscapes, whose magnitude of loss was 320,000 km^2 between 2000–2013 (4.43 to 4.11 million km^2) which approaches to the area of Germany in Europe. Several consequences from this loss can be listed, including Amazonian biodiversity depletion, shortcomings in ecosystem services, slowed progress of new therapeutics discovery, decreased locals' quality of life, and heightened vector-borne disease risk (Vittor *et al.* 2021). In the present work, we are dealing with landscape ecology of vector-borne diseases in the Amazon, trying to understand how these landscape changes modulate the transmission risk of these diseases, and what could be considered a healthy landscape under the perspective of vector-borne diseases.

1.1 *Landscape ecology and vector-borne diseases*

Landscapes, in the landscape ecology perspective, are spatially heterogeneous areas formed by interacting mosaics of elements relevant to some phenomenon under consideration (Turner *et al.* 2001). Thus, a landscape is simply an area of land containing an interesting pattern that affects and is affected by an ecological process of interest (Turner *et al.* 2001). The discipline of landscape ecology is the science and art of studying and improving the relationship between spatial pattern and ecological processes on a multitude of scales and organizational levels (Wu 2008). In summary, it is the study of scale and structure, defined by composition and configuration, of human-modified natural landscapes (Forman and Godron 1986). Scale refers to the spatial scale whose event of interest occurs. Composition is the set of elements that compose a landscape and thus forest cover means the respective area (%) this element covers within each spatial scale. Configuration is how elements composing a landscape are spatially distributed over the spatial scale. Forest cover loss or deforestation is the proportion of cleared land previously covered by forest. Forest fragmentation is defined as a process during which a large expanse of habitat is transformed into a series of smaller patches of smaller area, isolated from each other by a habitat matrix different from the original (Wilcove *et al.* 1986; van den Berg *et al.* 2001; Ewers and Didham 2005), being different from forest loss in that it reflects aspects of configuration (e.g. number of habitat patches, edge density, patch shape), not just the total amount of habitat in a landscape (Swift and Hannon 2010).

Both deforestation and fragmentation have the potential to impact the dynamics of vector-borne diseases, with land use change being the leading driver of emerging zoonoses (Loh *et al.* 2015) and being linked to more than 30% of the new diseases since 1960 (IPBES 2020). It alters the niche of vectors, hosts and pathogens, cause changes in the community composition of both hosts and vectors, in the behavior or movement of vectors and hosts and affect their spatial distribution (Gottdenker *et al.* 2014). However, these effects can be scale dependent. A study in Southeast Asia found distinct effects from each spatial scale on zoonotic malaria occurrence (Brock *et al.* 2019). In this study, the most parsimonious scale of deforestation in the transmission dynamics of zoonotic malaria was assessed by testing effects from eleven spatial scales in Southeast Asia (Brock *et al.* 2019). Transmission dynamics of zoonotic malaria occurs among humans who live in settlements in deforested sites where the malarial parasite, *Plasmodium knowlesi*, is harboured by macaques (*Macaca*) and transmitted by anopheline vectors. The influence of composition and configuration within 0.1 to 20 km of households on *P. knowlesi* occurrence was tested (Brock *et al.* 2019). Forest cover loss in the previous year influenced *P. knowlesi* occurrence most strongly at smaller scales (within 0.5 km of households, or 0.78-km^2), while fragmentation of deforested areas in the previous year had higher levels of influence at larger scales (5 km, or 78-km^2).

It is reasonable to suppose that each vector-borne disease has its own signature of scale, composition, and configuration in the human-modified natural landscape. The dispersion of yellow fever virus (YFV) is an astonishing example of connectivity in-between forested patches in highly fragmented landscapes in the Brazilian Atlantic Forest biome (Prist *et al.* 2021). The authors evaluated the dispersion of YFV by considering 243 georeferenced sites of PCR-positive dead monkeys (*Alouatta*) in São Paulo state. These nonhuman primates' cases were analysed using a network approach to model the movement of the epizootic events in time and space. In this network analysis, epizootic events portraited nodes and the goal was to establish potential links (dispersion) between each pair of nodes. Parameters that conditioned to the establishment of those links were the date of each epizootic event, the distance among the nodes, and the permeability of the landscapes' composition. Results obtained showed incredible dispersion rate per day of YFV across landscapes. On average YFV could disperse 1.42 km per day, but it could be seen with larger movements, being up to 6.9 km/day. As expected, dispersions were five times longer in summer than in winter (1.2 vs 0.22 km/day). Additionally, most dispersions (73%) occurred within a week after the arrival of YFV in the node, but in winter they occurred within two or three weeks. Lastly, YFV disperses via roads nearby forest or along forest edges in interface with agriculture, water, and forestry. Important barriers for virus movement were the core of urban, agricultural, and forest regions (Prist *et al.* 2021). In the following paragraphs, we will highlight landscape ecology of key vector-borne diseases, including malaria, Chagas disease, and cutaneous leishmaniasis in the Amazon.

1.2 *Malaria in the Amazon*

The malaria microcosm is highly clustered in the human-modified natural landscape in the Amazon. Malaria is an endemic transmissible disease in the Amazon, where *Plasmodium vivax* and *Plasmodium falciparum* are the most prevalent malarial parasites, and *Anopheles darlingi* is the main vector. The disease is an interesting study system to apply the concepts of landscape ecology. This is because of the association between malaria risk to population and deforestation in recently colonized settlements (Laporta *et al.* 2021). Pioneers inhabit in poor housing on the forest edges in these recently deforested settlements. Settlers usually store ground waters that are employed to prepare meals, wash clothes, and take baths. In these waters the principal vector, *An. darlingi*, breeds as immatures until the completion of their development to the adult stages. These anophelines seek blood in the houses nearby and, if any settler is already *Plasmodium*-infected, transmission cycle of malaria successfully starts (Oliveira *et al.* 2021).

Composition and configuration of the human-modified natural landscapes that favour malaria risk have been recently estimated by using 79 landscape-sites in the Amazon (Chaves *et al.* 2021). A conspicuous pattern was identified from this dataset (Figure 1). Landscapes having intermediate forest cover (~70–30%) and higher levels of forest fragmentation have the highest risk of malaria transmission risk to humans. This high landscape-score in Figure 1 means intensification of the contact between humans and *An. darlingi*. This occurs because forest cover loss from pristine to intermediate disturbance, and augmented levels of forest edge density in the

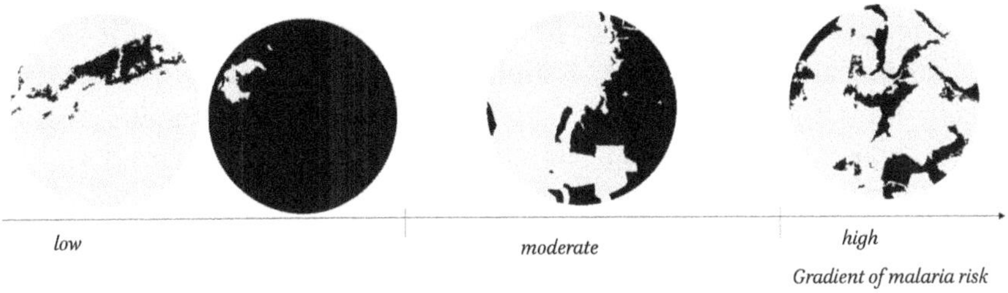

FIGURE 1 Gradient of malaria risk per composition and configuration of human-modified natural landscapes in the Amazon. Low risk occurs in highly deforested (light grey colour) or forested preserved sites (black colour). Moderate and high risks are supported by a combination of composition (30–70% forest cover) and configuration (higher levels of forest edge densities). The spatial scale of the landscape is within 1-km of households. Adapted from (Chaves *et al.* 2021)

landscape (Figure 1, moderate and high), can decrease the Shannon diversity index in mosquito assemblage. Lowered diversity in mosquito assemblage reduces diffuse competition to *An. darlingi*, which in turn can increase abundance of this malaria vector (Chaves *et al.* 2021). This can ultimately result in rise of malaria transmission.

1.3 *Chagas disease in Brazil*

Chagas disease or American trypanosomiasis is a chronic and potentially fatal infection caused by *Trypanosoma cruzi* transmitted by triatomines (Chagas 1909). Symptoms are characterized by heart failure and gastrointestinal complications. Although it is a vector-transmitted disease, transmission can also occur congenitally, or via blood transfusion, organ transplantation, and ingestion of foods contaminated with *T. cruzi* (Coura and Viñas 2010). When infected by *T. cruzi*, the chronic disease persists throughout the host's life. No vaccines or efficient treatments are available. Control of triatomine vectors is the main strategy to prevent infections in humans. In 2006 the World Health Organization (WHO) certified Brazil as a country free from vector transmission by the dominant Chagas vector *Triatoma infestans* (Schofield *et al.* 2006). The estimated number of *T. cruzi*-infected people today is six times lower (~1 million) than that in the 1980s (~6 millions) (Brazilian Ministry of Health 2021). However, outbreaks of Chagas disease still occur in Brazil, mainly in the Amazon, where it is a zoonotic endemic disease, whose transmission dynamics of *T. cruzi* involves sylvatic triatomines and wild reservoirs. These outbreaks are mainly related to contaminated food by triatomines infected with *T. cruzi*. Açai juice, which is a major Amazonian nourishment, can become easily contaminated. The consumption of *T. cruzi*-contaminated Açai juice can lead to orally-transmitted acute Chagas disease (Nolan *et al.* 2020).

The landscape ecology of Chagas disease has gone largely neglected in the specialized literature; yet one should expect critical landscape interactions of *T. cruzi* with triatomines conditioned to the presence and relative abundance of mammal hosts. Perhaps the most comprehensive study in this respect was carried out in the village of Zoh Laguna, nearby the Calakmul Biosphere Reserve in the southern Yucatan Peninsula (López-Cancino *et al.* 2015). This study analysed a human-modified natural landscape composed of a biosphere reserve, adjacent to crop and farming areas with reported Chagas disease cases. Bats, rodents, marsupials, livestock, pets, triatomines, and humans were tested for *T. cruzi* infections in sylvatic, ecotone, and domestic habitats. Two genotypes (I and II) of *T. cruzi* were obtained, with both genotypes occurring in all animals and habitats, except in humans who were found to be exclusively infected by genotype II. Intriguingly, bats showed a key role in the dispersal of genotype II of *T. cruzi* from the sylvatic habitat, while dogs, sheep, and humans appeared to be drivers of this genotype between domestic and ecotone habitats. Overall, disease risk of *T. cruzi* transmission thrives in highly permeable landscapes and is dependent upon host assemblage properties of the landscape (López-Cancino *et al.* 2015). It should be therefore expected a high landscape-score for Chagas disease transmission in landscapes having a massive forest land cover tied with cattle ranching at a large spatial scale. Notwithstanding, there should be other landscape interactions with Chagas disease that are still unknown.

1.4 *Cutaneous leishmaniasis in Brazil*

The leishmaniases are devastating and poorly recognized diseases vectorized by sand flies to humans and several other mammal species (Antinori *et al.* 2012). The causative agent *Leishmania* is a protozoan parasite that can induce the human host to manifest various symptoms, from cutaneous and mucocutaneous processes (cutaneous leishmaniasis) to internal organ abnormalities, including splenomegaly (visceral leishmaniasis), which can become a fatal outcome if not treated timely (Alvar *et al.* 2012). In 2020, 208,357 new cutaneous leishmaniasis cases and 12,838 new visceral leishmaniasis cases were reported (World Health Organization 2021). Cutaneous leishmaniasis cases from Afghanistan, Algeria, Brazil, Colombia, Iraq, Pakistan, and the Syrian Arab Republic, represented more than 80% of all cases in 2020 (World Health Organization 2021).

The epidemiology of cutaneous leishmaniasis in the Americas is exceptionally complex, exposing a multitude of transmission cycles, reservoir hosts, sandfly vectors, clinical manifestations, and circulating *Leishmania* species in the same geographical area. The greatest diversity of species of *Leishmania* in Brazil is found in the Amazon, with *Leishmania braziliensis* as the most prevalent, followed by *Leishmania amazonensis* and *Leishmania guyanensis*. Transmission of cutaneous leishmaniasis in the Amazon has an aggregated spatial distribution around the natural focus of *Leishmania*, which is clustered in the forest. Transmission of *L. braziliensis* in Brazil is perpetrated by sandflies *Nyssomyia intermedia* and *Nyssomyia whitmani* from wild or domestic animals to humans (Rangel and Lainson 2009). Reservoirs of *L. amazonensis* and *L. guyanensis* are exclusively wild animals. Interestingly, the transmission of *L. guyanensis* is distinctly dependent on the forest cover in the landscape because its reservoirs are sloths (*Choloepus didactilus*), which live in the forest canopy, and its leading vector is a forest-specialized sandfly (*Nyssomyia umbratilis*) (Rangel and Lainson 2009). Studies on transmission of cutaneous leishmaniasis and landscape associations are somewhat scant, but an emblematic study case was demonstrated in the Chico Mendes Reserve, Xapuri municipality, Acre state, Brazil (Brilhante *et al.* 2021). Both *L. braziliensis* and *L. amazonensis* were identified from diverse species of sand flies in the well-preserved areas of Xapuri, in where latex extraction from rubber trees and tourism in the forest are the main economic activities (Brilhante *et al.* 2021).

1.5 *Study goals and significance*

Considering the lack of vaccines or efficient treatments against the major parasites in malaria, Chagas disease, and cutaneous leishmaniasis in Brazil, and the links between land use change and the incidence of vector-borne diseases, we sought to tackle this problem by undertaking an ecological study in epidemiology to depict the big picture in disease incidence case per landscape metrics in 773 Amazonian municipalities in Brazil 2007–2019. The study goals are: (1) to identify clusters of disease case incidence; (2) to analyse temporal trends in disease case incidence; (3) to assess how changes in landscape structure (such as deforestation and fragmentation) affect the case incidence of these diseases; (4) to evaluate trade-offs for the different diseases analysed. We believe that the knowledge obtained here can help in the control and surveillance of these diseases in Brazil and beyond and contribute to the management of multifunctional landscapes that allow the maintenance of different ecosystem services, especially the regulation of diseases.

2 Methods

2.1 *Epidemiological data and landscape variables*

Case incidence of malaria, Chagas disease, and cutaneous leishmaniasis from 2007 to 2019 per 773 Amazonian municipalities were obtained from the Brazilian Malaria Control Programme (SIVEP-malaria) and from the Brazilian Unified Health System Database (DATASUS). They are reportable diseases in Brazil, which means every country's health unit that can undertake clinical and/or laboratory-based diagnostics, from hospitals to outposts, either public or private, must report patient cases to the Brazilian Ministry of Health. The gold standard for malaria diagnostics is the observation of malaria parasites on blood smear slides under light microscopy. Case incidence of malaria here represents the sum of all malaria parasites identified, mainly *P. vivax* and *P. falciparum*. As for Chagas disease, only acute, oral events were considered because these events have become systematically frequent in the last 15 years, especially in the Amazon region, due to ingestion of *T. cruzi*-contaminated food accidentally exposed to sylvatic triatomines. In the acute phase of Chagas disease, laboratory diagnosis is based on observing *T. cruzi* present in a patient's blood. Lastly, diagnostics of cutaneous leishmaniasis relies on parasitological tests to identify *Leishmania* in skin wound scrapings associated with a featured skin active ulcer.

Landscape variables Percentage of Landscape, Patch Density, Edge Density, Aggregation Index, Land Use Land Cover, and Largest Patch Index from 2007 to 2019 per 773 Amazonian municipalities were obtained from MAPBIOMAS v.6.0. The Mapbiomas Collection is based on Landsat images, with 30-meters spatial resolution, and generates annual maps of land use and land cover for 35 years (1985 to 2020). All Landsat images available for this period (Landsat 5; L5, Landsat 7; L7, and Landsat 8; L8) were used with Cloud Cover (CC) less or equal 50%. The final maps have 41 land cover classification of the main uses: forest, savanna, grassland, pasture agriculture, other non-vegetated areas and river, lakes, and oceans. A detailed methodology about the mapping can be found in https://mapbiomas.org/download-dos-atbds.

Percentage of Landscape is the quantification of the proportion of each element in the municipal landscape. Patch Density is the number of patches of an element on municipal area. Edge Density is the sum of the lengths of all edge segments of an element, divided by the municipal landscape area. Aggregation Index is the number of like adjacencies of an element, divided by its maximum possible number of like adjacencies. Land Use Land Cover is the composition of elements in the municipal landscape. Largest Patch Index is the area of the largest patch divided by municipal landscape area.

2.2 *Spatial analysis*

To identify clustering patterns of disease case incidence we performed a hotspot analysis using the Getis-Ord Gi* statistics with contiguity edges distance matrix. This is a spatial autocorrelation method widely used in health research (Wubuli *et al.* 2015) that measure the degree of correlation of weighted features within the specified distance threshold (Anselin and Getis 1992; Songchitruksa and Zeng 2010). The local sum for a feature and its neighbours is compared accordingly to the sums of all features (Haque *et al.* 2012), following the above equation:

$$G_i^* = \frac{\sum_{j=1}^{n} w_{ij} x_j}{\sum_{j=1}^{n} x_j}$$

Where, G_i^* is the spatial autocorrelation (spatial dependency) statistics of an event i over n events. The term x_j defines the magnitude of variable x at events j over all n, and the term w_{ij} defines the weight value between the event *i* and *j* that represent their spatial interrelationship. A cluster was considered permanent, if it occurred in at least 75% of the time of analysis (10 of the 13 analysed years); otherwise, it was considered sporadic. Hotspots and both permanent and sporadic clusters were mapped.

2.3 *Temporal trends*

Temporal trends were accessed through graphs summarizing the total number of cases reported for each year, and the autocorrelation function (acf). This function was employed to assess how the total number of cases reported in a given year were related, on average, to the total number of cases in the preceding years (Box *et al.* 2008).

2.4 *Disease and landscape relationships*

A model selection approach was undertaken to assess the relationships between cases of malaria, Chagas disease and cutaneous leishmaniasis and changes in the structure of municipal landscapes. Model fitting was done using generalized linear models (GLM) with a negative binomial distribution for malaria and cutaneous leishmaniasis and binomial for Chagas disease. The predictor variables used were percentage of forest cover, amount of deforestation, amount of forest restoration, the size of the largest fragment, forest edge density and the percentage of pasture. A null model was built in which disease cases vary at random and has no influence of landscape parameters. Correlation between landscape metrics was low (Pearson's $r < 0.50$). For model selection, we conducted a maximum likelihood model selection procedure, considering the second order Akaike's information criterion (AIC) (Burnham and Anderson 2010), choosing the model with the lower AIC.

The residuals of the best supported model per each disease were tested for spatial autocorrelation and temporal autocorrelation. The results showed that residuals had spatial autocorrelation (Moran's *I*, $P = 0.0001$), but not temporal autocorrelation. These models were then re-analysed as spatial models using a Bayesian modelling approach with non-informative priors, four chains of Markov Chain Monte Carlo (MCMC), 5,000 burn in values and 2,000 iterations. Model convergence was checked through R-hat values, and a reliable convergence occurred when R-hat values ranged from 0.9 to 1.05. In each model the average values of disease landscape relationships were estimated.

2.5 *Software and resources*

All analyses were carried out in the *R* programming environment *v.* 4.1.2 and the spatial model using a Bayesian approach was run using the package *glmmfields v.* 0.1.4 (Anderson and Ward 2019).

3 Results and discussion

3.1 *Clusters of disease case incidence*

The cluster analysis for malaria showed that there are no coldspots in the Amazon region for any of the years analysed. In addition, hotspots areas, i.e. municipalities that require more attention from public health services, are more intense in the west and central part for most of the analysed years. The other municipalities, i.e. white colour, showed that malaria cases are randomly spread across the region. Moreover, over the years there has not been a sharp change in the paradigm of locating malaria hotspots, showing that 23% of the municipalities (n = 30) are permanent hotpots, being at high risk in at least 75% of the years analysed (Figure 2), and being concentrated in the west part of the Amazon.

The cluster analysis for Chagas disease also showed that there are no coldspots in the Amazon region for any of the years analysed. Unlike malaria, the municipalities indicated as hotspots for Chagas disease, in most years, comprise only a few municipalities in the Amazon region, which shows that this zoonosis does not have such high number of cases in the region when compared to malaria. In 2010, the largest number of hotspots were seen, followed by 2007 and 2014. In all the years analysed, some municipalities in north-eastern Pará were indicated as clusters, indicating that these locations require more attention from public health services (Figure 3). In fact, this region is the one with permanent hotspots, indicating that preventive measures should be taken in place in these municipalities.

The cluster analysis for cutaneous leishmaniasis presented only one coldspot when analysing all years together, in the municipality of Peixe, in Tocantins state. Cutaneous leishmaniasis hotspots showed a spatial pattern more similar to malaria, with a high number of municipalities being considered of concern, and with little variation over the years. The central part of the Amazon, i.e. much of the state of Pará, were classified in this category in all 14 years. In addition, parts of the states of Amapá and Maranhão also fell into this category in most years (Figure 4), with a total of 68 municipalities (~30% of the total) being considered permanent hotspots.

When looking at the three zoonoses together, the aggregation patterns are different for each one, and few municipalities were considered critical for one or more zoonoses. Most of the Chagas disease clusters are in the northeast part of the Amazon, while the malaria ones are in the northwest and in the central part of the Amazon. The exception is the year of 2007, that presented clusters for both malaria and Chagas disease in the municipalities of Coari, Tapauá and Tefé, in Amazonas state. Cutaneous leishmaniasis is more present in Pará state and only few states, i.e. Presidente Figueiredo and Novo Airão, presented clusters for both malaria and cutaneous leishmaniasis.

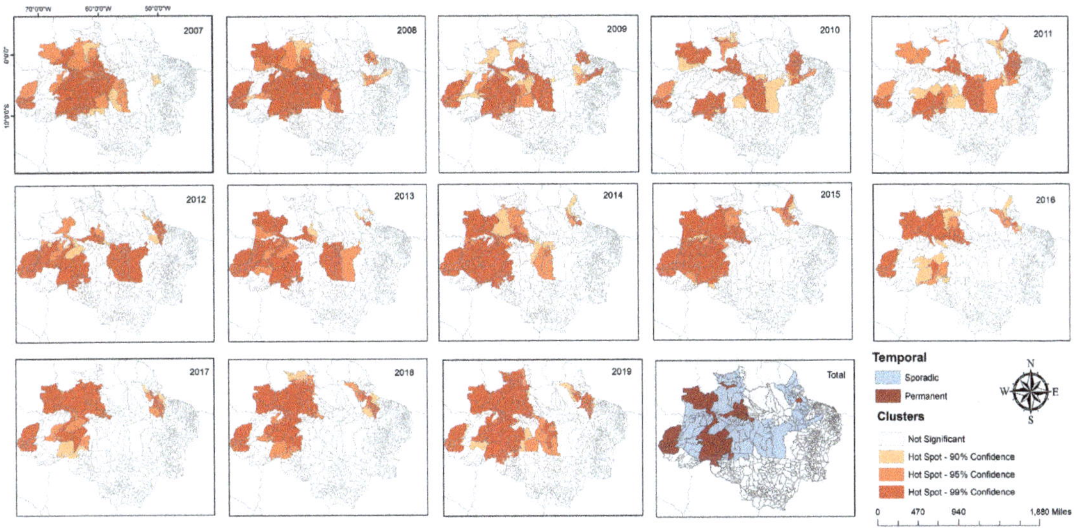

FIGURE 2 Clusters of malaria disease cases from 2007 to 2019 and a last map showing permanent and sporadic cluster for the total time-series

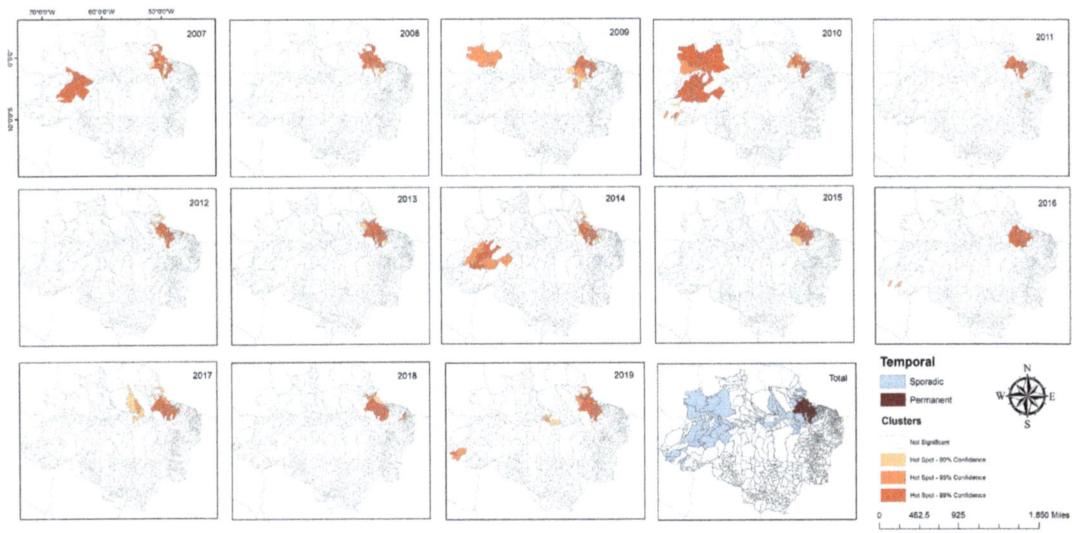

FIGURE 3 Clusters of Chagas disease cases from 2007 to 2019 and a last map showing permanent and sporadic cluster for the total time-series

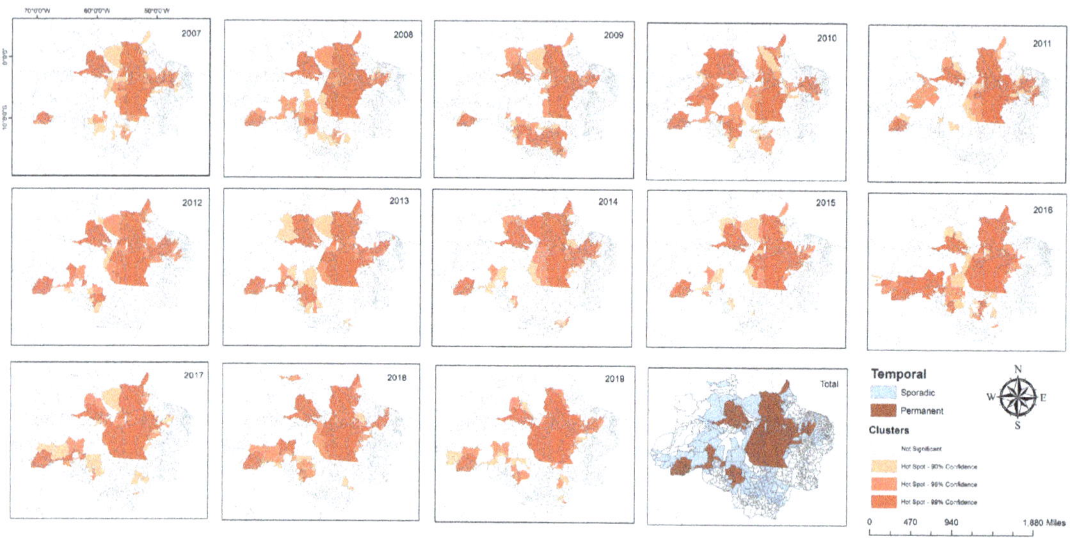

FIGURE 4 Clusters of cutaneous leishmaniasis cases from 2007 to 2019 and a last map showing permanent and sporadic cluster for the total time-series

3.2 *Temporal trends of disease case incidence*

The temporal variation in the number of cases was greater for malaria and Chagas disease than for cutaneous leishmaniasis, with the former showing a downward behaviour and the latter increasing over the years. The total annual number of malaria cases during the study period ranged from a high of 448,435 in 2007 to a low of 119,510 in 2016, showing overall decreasing behaviour over the years, but with some slight increases in occasional years. Chagas disease presented a general behaviour of increase over the years, reaching a peak in 2018 with 333 cases. Cutaneous leishmaniasis showed the least variation among the three zoonoses, but again trended downward over the years, ranging from a high of 14,123 in 2007 to a low of 7,049 in 2016 (Figure 5). The temporal autocorrelation analysis (acf) showed

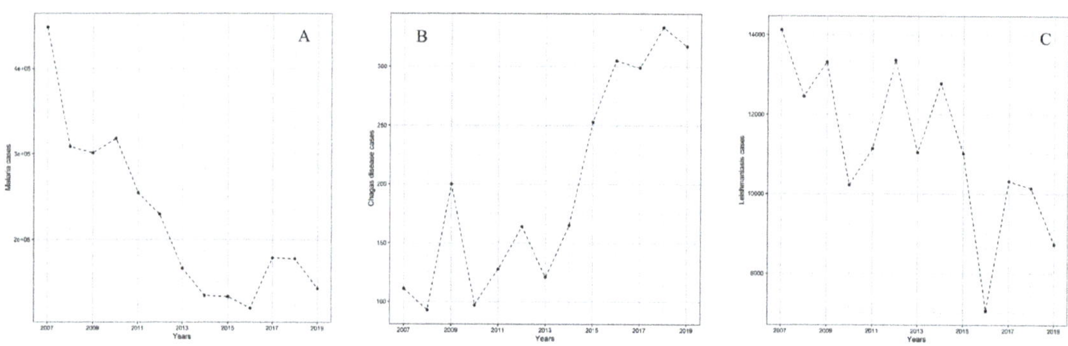

FIGURE 5 Temporal trends of malaria (A), Chagas disease (B) and cutaneous leishmaniasis (C) in the Brazilian Amazon, from 2007 to 2019

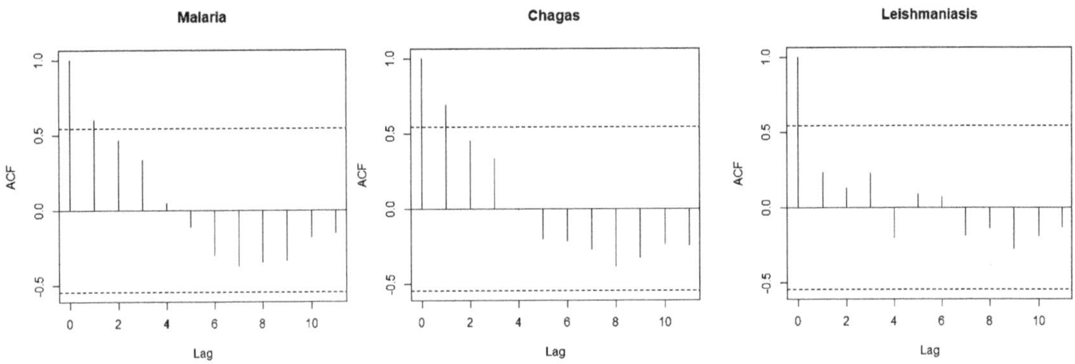

FIGURE 6 Temporal autocorrelation analysis (acf) for malaria, Chagas disease and cutaneous leishmaniasis in the Brazilian Amazon, from 2007 to 2019

that malaria and Chagas disease cases have significant correlations only in the first and second years (2007 and 2008), being non-significant in the following years. For cutaneous leishmaniasis, the pattern found was of correlation only for the first year (2007), which shows that there is no temporal autocorrelation of the number of reported cases (Figure 6).

3.3 *How do changes in the municipal landscape structure affect the cases of each disease?*

Three models were equally plausible to explain the variation in the number of malaria cases, all of which included the percentage of forest cover (Table 1). The first-ranked model contained only this variable, while the second-ranked model had this plus the amount of cleared forest. The third one, again, had the percentage of forest cover together with the fragmentation index (patch density). For this disease, the higher a forest percentage in a given municipality, the higher the number of expected cases. Deforestation also seems to affect the number of cases, especially when the municipalities have a high amount of forest cover. In addition, the fragmentation index was also selected, showing that forest areas in a fragmented state can also increase malaria risk. For this disease, municipalities considered as 'high risk' are the ones with more than 50% of forest cover, and that present deforestation and fragmentation. In other words, deforestation and fragmentation have a high-risk effect for malaria when they occur in municipalities with more than 50% preserved forest. The same effect was seen in previous studies, including (Chaves *et al.* 2021; Laporta *et al.* 2021; Oliveira *et al.* 2021). Deforestation and fragmentation favour the dominance of the main malaria vector in anthropogenic landscapes (Chaves *et al.* 2021), thus increasing the malaria transmission risk.

Analogously to malaria, two models were equally plausible to explain the variation in the number of cutaneous leishmaniasis cases, all of which included the percentage of forest cover. The first-ranked model contained this variable plus the

TABLE 1 Parameter estimates for spatial model. Gp_sigma and gp_theta are the spatial parameters[a]

Disease	Parameter	Mean	SE mean	SD	R-hat
Malaria	gp_sigma	4.16	0.50	1.14	1.26
	gp_theta	3.82	1.57	2.23	12.13
	Intercept	5.53	0.03	0.06	2.28
	% of forest cover	0.98	0.03	0.06	1.28
	Deforestation	0.00	0.00	0.03	1.0
	Patch density	0.02	0.07	0.24	1.01
Chagas disease	gp_sigma	2.69	0.02	0.74	1
	gp_theta	3.32	0.01	0.37	1
	Pasture	−0.87	0.00	0.13	1.00
	Patch density	−3.07	0.13	3.22	1
	Edge density	−3.75	0.33	5.08	1.02
Cutaneous leishmaniasis	gp_sigma	2.03	0.01	0.47	1
	gp_theta	0.76	0.00	0.02	1
	% of forest cover	3.21	0.00	0.03	1
	Deforestation	0.39	0.00	0.02	1

a SD = standard deviation; SE = standard error; R-hat = model convergence when values range 0.9–1.05.

amount of forest deforested (Table 1), while the second-ranked model had only the amount of forest cover. For this disease, the higher the forest percentage in a municipality, the higher the number of expected cases. In addition, deforestation also seems to affect the incidence of cases, especially when the municipalities have a high amount of forest cover. Municipalities facing deforestation, in situations of high forest cover, represent a high risk for cutaneous leishmaniasis. This result is supported by the studies undertaken in Xapuri municipality, Acre state (Brilhante *et al.* 2021). Most of the area of this municipality is covered by forests that has been deforested in a piecemeal fashion annually. In consequence, vectors and agents of cutaneous leishmaniasis are being frequently found in this municipality.

For Chagas disease three models were also equally plausible to explain the variation in the number of cases, all of which included the percentage of pasture present in a municipality. For this disease the higher the amount of pasture, the lower the chance of the disease to occur. Patch density and the amount of edge density were also selected, showing that higher the amount of edge density and the fragmentation index of a municipality, lower the chances of Chagas disease to occur. For this zoonosis, apparently, municipalities formed by forest areas with a low fragmentation and with a small quantity of edges, immersed in a matrix of non-pasture, are the ones most at risk.

The Chagas disease microcosm in Amazon occurs in landscapes having a matrix of crops of Açai trees. Chagas agents, reservoirs, and vectors interact to each other in the canopies of these trees. These crops usually occur in regions that do not contain pastures, because pastures make the soil inviable to the production of trees. In fact, crops of Açai trees occur mixed with continuous preserved forests. The closer geographic relationship between forests and Açai trees is related to the ease of pollination. Majority of flowers of Açai trees are pollinated by native bees that are found in forest.

The crops of Açai trees represent a change in the landscape structure. Continuous forests are deforested and modified into these crops that in the long-term support a homogenization of the local biodiversity. Such changes in the landscape structure are underlying the increased risks of Chagas disease in the Amazon. This relationship has been supported by (Santos *et al.* 2018).

3.4 *What are the trade-offs for the different diseases analysed?*

Two of the three zoonoses analysed showed similar response patterns, with risk landscapes that can be considered alike. Both malaria and cutaneous leishmaniasis presented as high-risk municipalities that have a high amount of forest cover and that are experiencing forest loss (deforestation), with the latter effect being much stronger for cutaneous leishmaniasis. Even though deforestation showed up for malaria, the most important variable was forest cover. For malaria, fragmentation was also important, with higher fragmentation equating to a higher number of reported cases. Therefore, for both zoonoses, municipalities at risk should be considered those with more than 50% of forest cover and that are experiencing deforestation.

Chagas disease showed a similar result to these zoonoses, but in a different way. Landscapes consisting of continuous forests and immersed in a matrix of non-pasture (i.e. crops of Açai trees) are the ones that bring the highest risk of transmission.

4 Conclusions

Considering the study goals, it was possible here to identify clusters of cases per each disease. Each disease has specific clusters in the Amazon. Malaria is clustered in the north-western Amazon in the states of Amazonas, Acre, and Roraima; Chagas disease clusters mostly occur in Pará state, and cutaneous leishmaniasis clusters are widespread in the Amazon. While spatial clustering was noted, there was no critical temporal trend observed for any of the diseases.

Specific changes in landscape structure affected the number of cases per disease. Malaria cases occur in municipalities having 50% or more forest cover preserved under the effects of deforestation and fragmentation. Cutaneous leishmaniasis cases occur in the same landscape settings as malaria, but the deforestation effect is greater, and fragmentation is not needed. Chagas disease occur in municipalities with continuous forests adjacent to deforested sites modified into crops of Açai trees.

Overall, despite a disease specific response with the landscape structure, the general pattern is clear. The loss of biodiversity of the most preserved landscapes in general increases the risk of vector-borne diseases in the Amazon, up to a certain level of forest cover remained (~50%). Below this threshold (50% of forest cover), in a more degraded landscape, that risk may be lower, but there will be no biodiversity or remaining forest left to preserve.

5 Closing remarks for bright opportunities

This chapter shows that 'healthy landscapes' depend on the disease under study. For instance, a 'healthy' landscape for Chagas disease with fragmented and deforested forests may be a 'risky' landscape for malaria or cutaneous leishmaniases. Managing the landscape structure to become less deforested and fragmented play a multifunctional role that prevents the latter diseases. The multifunctional landscape concept is therefore herein proposed for landscape management and restoration that will be needed for preventing old diseases and new pandemics.

Acknowledgements

GZL was supported by São Paulo Research Foundation (FAPESP grant n. 21/06669–6); PRP was funded by the US National Science Foundation grant 2225023 and USAID – Conservation Works Liberia.

References

Alvar J, Vélez ID, Bern C, Herrero M, Desjeux P, Cano J, Jannin J, Boer M den, and the WHO Leishmaniasis Control Team (2012) Leishmaniasis Worldwide and Global Estimates of Its Incidence. PLoS ONE 7: e35671.

Anderson SC, and Ward EJ (2019) Black swans in space: modeling spatiotemporal processes with extremes. Ecology 100.

Anselin L, and Getis A (1992) Spatial statistical analysis and geographic information systems. Ann Reg Sci 26: 19–33.

Antinori S, Schifanella L, and Corbellino M (2012) Leishmaniasis: new insights from an old and neglected disease. Eur J Clin Microbiol Infect Dis 31: 109–118.

Begon M, Townsend CR, and Harper JL (2006) Ecology: from individuals to ecosystems, 4th ed, Blackwell Pub, Malden, MA.

Box GEP, Jenkins GM, and Reinsel GC (2008) Time series analysis: forecasting and control, 4th ed, John Wiley, Hoboken, N.J.

Brazilian Ministry of Health (2021) Boletim Epidemiológico – Doença de Chagas, Ministério da Saúde, Secretaria de Vigilância em Saúde.

Brilhante AF, Lima L, de Ávila MM, Medeiros-Sousa AR, de Souza JF, dos Santos NP, de Paula MB, Godoy RE, Sábio PB, Cardoso C de O, Nunes VLB, Teixeira MMG, and Galati EAB (2021) Remarkable diversity, new records and Leishmania detection in the sand fly fauna of an area of high endemicity for cutaneous leishmaniasis in Acre state, Brazilian Amazonian Forest. Acta Tropica 223: 106103.

Brock PM, Fornace KM, Grigg MJ, Anstey NM, William T, Cox J, Drakeley CJ, Ferguson HM, and Kao RR (2019) Predictive analysis across spatial scales links zoonotic malaria to deforestation. Proc R Soc B 286: 20182351.

Burnham KP, and Anderson DR (2010) Model selection and multimodel inference: a practical information-theoretic approach, 2. ed, Springer, New York, NY.

Carson R (2002) Silent spring, 40th anniversary ed., 1st Mariner Books ed, Houghton Mifflin, Boston.

Chagas C (1909) Nova tripanozomiaze humana: estudos sobre a morfolojia e o ciclo evolutivo do Schizotrypanum cruzi n. gen., n. sp., ajente etiolojico de nova entidade morbida do homem. Mem Inst Oswaldo Cruz 1: 159–218.

Chaves LSM, Bergo ES, Conn JE, Laporta GZ, Prist PR, and Sallum MAM (2021) Anthropogenic landscape decreases mosquito biodiversity and drives malaria vector proliferation in the Amazon rainforest. PLoS One 16: e0245087.

Coura JR, and Viñas PA (2010) Chagas disease: a new worldwide challenge. Nature 465: S6–7.

Ewers RM, and Didham RK (2005) Confounding factors in the detection of species responses to habitat fragmentation. Biol Rev 81: 117.

Forman RTT, and Godron M (1986) Landscape ecology, Wiley, New York.

Gottdenker NL, Streicker DG, Faust CL, and Carroll CR (2014) Anthropogenic Land Use Change and Infectious Diseases: A Review of the Evidence. EcoHealth 11: 619–632.

Haque U, Scott LM, Hashizume M, Fisher E, Haque R, Yamamoto T, and Glass GE (2012) Modelling malaria treatment practices in Bangladesh using spatial statistics. Malar J 11: 63.

IPBES (2020) Intergovernmental Science-Policy Platform On Biodiversity And Ecosystem Services (IPBES), Zenodo.

Laporta GZ, Ilacqua RC, Bergo ES, Chaves LSM, Rodovalho SR, Moresco GG, Figueira EAG, Massad E, de Oliveira TMP, Bickersmith SA, Conn JE, and Sallum MAM (2021) Malaria transmission in landscapes with varying deforestation levels and timelines in the Amazon: a longitudinal spatiotemporal study. Sci Rep 11: 6477.

Loh EH, Zambrana-Torrelio C, Olival KJ, Bogich TL, Johnson CK, Mazet JAK, Karesh W, and Daszak P (2015) Targeting Transmission Pathways for Emerging Zoonotic Disease Surveillance and Control. Vector-Borne and Zoonotic Diseases 15: 432–437.

López-Cancino SA, Tun-Ku E, De la Cruz-Felix HK, Ibarra-Cerdeña CN, Izeta-Alberdi A, Pech-May A, Mazariegos-Hidalgo CJ, Valdez-Tah A, and Ramsey JM (2015) Landscape ecology of *Trypanosoma cruzi* in the southern Yucatan Peninsula. Acta Trop 151: 58–72.

Nolan MS, Tonussi Mendes JE, Perez Riera AR, and Laporta GZ (2020) Oral *Trypanosoma cruzi* Transmission Resulting in Advanced Chagasic Cardiomyopathy in an 11-Month-Old Male. Case Rep Infect Dis 2020: 8828950.

Oliveira TMP, Laporta GZ, Bergo ES, Chaves LSM, Antunes JLF, Bickersmith SA, Conn JE, Massad E, and Sallum MAM (2021) Vector role and human biting activity of Anophelinae mosquitoes in different landscapes in the Brazilian Amazon. Parasit Vectors 14: 236.

Potapov P, Hansen MC, Laestadius L, Turubanova S, Yaroshenko A, Thies C, Smith W, Zhuravleva I, Komarova A, Minnemeyer S, and Esipova E (2017) The last frontiers of wilderness: Tracking loss of intact forest landscapes from 2000 to 2013. Sci Adv 3: e1600821.

Prist PR, Tambosi LR, Filipe Mucci L, Pinter A, Pereira de Souza R, Muylaert RL, Rhodes JR, Henrique Comin C, da F. Costa L, Lang D'Agostini T, Telles de Deus J, Pavão M, Port-Carvalho M, Del Castillo Saad L, Mureb Sallum MA, Fernandes Spinola RM, and Metzger JP (2021) Roads and forest edges facilitate yellow fever virus dispersion. Journal of Applied Ecology 1365-2664.14031.

Rangel EF, and Lainson R (2009) Proven and putative vectors of American cutaneous leishmaniasis in Brazil: aspects of their biology and vectorial competence. Mem Inst Oswaldo Cruz 104: 937–954.

Santos VRCD, Meis J de, Savino W, Andrade JAA, Vieira JRDS, Coura JR, and Junqueira ACV (2018) Acute Chagas disease in the state of Pará, Amazon Region: is it increasing? Mem Inst Oswaldo Cruz 113: e170298.

Schofield CJ, Jannin J, and Salvatella R (2006) The future of Chagas disease control. Trends Parasitol 22: 583–588.

Simpson JA, Weiner ESC, and Oxford University Press (eds) (1989) The Oxford English dictionary, 2nd ed, Clarendon Press; Oxford University Press, Oxford: Oxford; New York.

Songchitruksa P, and Zeng X (2010) Getis – Ord Spatial Statistics to Identify Hot Spots by Using Incident Management Data. Transportation Research Record 2165: 42–51.

Swift TL, and Hannon SJ (2010) Critical thresholds associated with habitat loss: a review of the concepts, evidence, and applications. Biological Reviews 85: 35–53.

Turner MG, Gardner RH, and O'Neill RV (2001) Landscape ecology in theory and practice: pattern and process, Springer, New York.

van den Berg LJL, Bullock James M, Clarke RT, Langston RHW, and Rose RJ (2001) Territory selection by the Dartford warbler (Sylvia undata) in Dorset, England: the role of vegetation type, habitat fragmentation and population size. Biological Conservation 101: 217–228.

Vittor AY, Laporta GZ, Sallum MAM, and Walker RT (2021) The COVID-19 crisis and Amazonia's indigenous people: Implications for conservation and global health. World Development 145: 105533.

Weisse M, and Goldman E (2021) Primary rainforest destruction increases 12% from 2019 to 2020, World Resource Institute.

Wilcove D, McLellan C, and Dobson A (1986) Habitat fragmentation in the temperate zone, in *Conservation Biology* pp. 237–56, Sinauer, Sunderland, MA.

World Health Organization (2021) Global leishmaniasis surveillance: 2019–2020, a baseline for the 2030 roadmap, World Health Organization.

Wu J (2008) Landscape Ecology, in *Encyclopedia of Ecology* pp. 2103–2108, Elsevier.

Wubuli A, Xue F, Jiang D, Yao X, Upur H, and Wushouer Q (2015) Socio-demographic predictors and distribution of pulmonary tuberculosis (TB) in Xinjiang, China: a spatial analysis. PLoS ONE 10: e0144010.

CHAPTER 2

The emerging epidemiology and changing landscape of mosquito-borne infectious diseases in Venezuela

Maria E. Grillet[1*], *Jorge E. Moreno*[2], *Alberto Paníz-Mondolfi*[3,4] *and Juan C. Navarro*[5,1]

[1]Laboratorio de Biología de Vectores y Parásitos, Instituto de Zoología y Ecología Tropical, Facultad de Ciencias, Universidad Central de Venezuela, Avenida Los Ilustres, Los Chaguaramos, Caracas 1041-A, Venezuela; [2]Centro de Investigaciones de Campo Dr Francesco Vitanza, Servicio Autónomo Instituto de Altos Estudios Dr Arnoldo Gabaldón, MPPS, Tumeremo 8057, Venezuela; [3]Infectious Diseases Research Branch, Venezuelan Science Incubator and the Zoonosis and Emerging Pathogens Regional Collaborative Network, Cabudare 3023, Lara, Venezuela; [4]Direction of Microbiology, Department of Pathology, Molecular and Cellbased Medicine, The Mount Sinai Hospital-Icahn School of Medicine at Mount Sinai, 1425 Madison Ave Room L9–52B, New York, NY 10029 USA; [5]Research Group of Emerging Diseases, Ecoepidemiology and Biodiversity, Health Sciences Faculty, Universidad Internacional SEK, Calle Alberto Einstein 5ta Transversal, Quito, Ecuador; *mariaeugenia.grillet@gmail.com

Abstract

In recent decades, Venezuela has faced a severe economic and social crisis, precipitated by political instability, which in turn has particularly affected public health provision. Here, we assess how Venezuela's health crisis has impacted mosquito-borne infectious diseases (MBIDs), placing Venezuela as the hotspot of malaria in the region and one of the countries currently reporting yellow fever outbreaks in the Americas. We describe the reshaping of the MBID epidemiological landscape in the midst of a changing environmental setting, highlighting the main knowledge gaps. The rise of MBID in Venezuela has the potential to severely undermine regional disease elimination efforts. Therefore, national, and regional measures must be taken to address these worsening epidemics and prevent their spread beyond country borders.

Keywords

malaria – arboviruses – hotspots – outbreaks – mining – deforestation – Venezuela

 | DOI:10.3920/9789004688650_004

1 Introduction

During the last 20 years, Venezuela has witnessed a significant increase in the incidence of infectious diseases mediated by mosquito vectors (Grillet *et al.* 2019). Among these, and at center stage, is malaria, a parasitic disease that has re-emerged in Venezuela after being successfully eliminated countrywide in the early 1960s (Gabaldon 1983). Currently, the disease has propagated to new geographic areas or intensified in previously endemic regions (Grillet *et al.* 2021), creating a new epidemiological landscape in terms of diversity of vector species and transmission contexts. Intermittent signs of the potential reemergence of yellow fever include six specific outbreaks recorded in endemic areas after a period of epidemiological silence that followed its effective control at the end of the 70s (Chavero *et al.* 2021, Rodríguez-Morales *et al.* 2021). During this same period, new and emerging arboviruses such as chikungunya and Zika have been established in Venezuela (Grillet *et al.* 2019; Lizarazo *et al.* 2019), following expansive initial epidemics. Others, such as Mayaro (Muñoz & Navarro 2012) and Oropouche (Navarro *et al.* 2016), have been detected, but their current status of occurrence remains unknown, constituting a potential threat for disease emergence events in the coming years. Furthermore, over a decade ago, *Aedes albopictus* was first detected in Venezuela (Navarro *et al.* 2009), but since then its status regarding geographical spread, population level, and role as a vector remains unknown.

Here, we will review and describe how specific social and environmental determinants have promoted the increase and spread of malaria and arboviruses in Venezuela, with special emphasis on how their current occurrence may have changed or is changing in a local and regional context of unprecedented re-emergence and emergence of pathogens and anthropogenic transformations. Specifically, we will describe how the impact of the social crisis and changes in land use (deforestation) may have contributed to local changes in the distribution, abundance, disease transmission dynamics and mosquito vector competence in Venezuela in the past 20 years, generating a new epidemiological landscape that could impact the effectiveness of current and developing vector control strategies. We conclude by suggesting recommendations that could mitigate but also serve to evaluate and understand the current status of these mosquito-borne infectious diseases in Venezuela.

2 Resurgence of malaria in Venezuela: a *Plasmodium* hotspot in the Americas

2.1 *The local epidemiological landscape and regional menace*

In 2020, 241 million annual cases and 627,000 deaths due to malaria were estimated globally (WHO 2021). The elimination agenda of this parasitic disease has been outlined by the World Health Organization (WHO) in the Global Technical Strategy

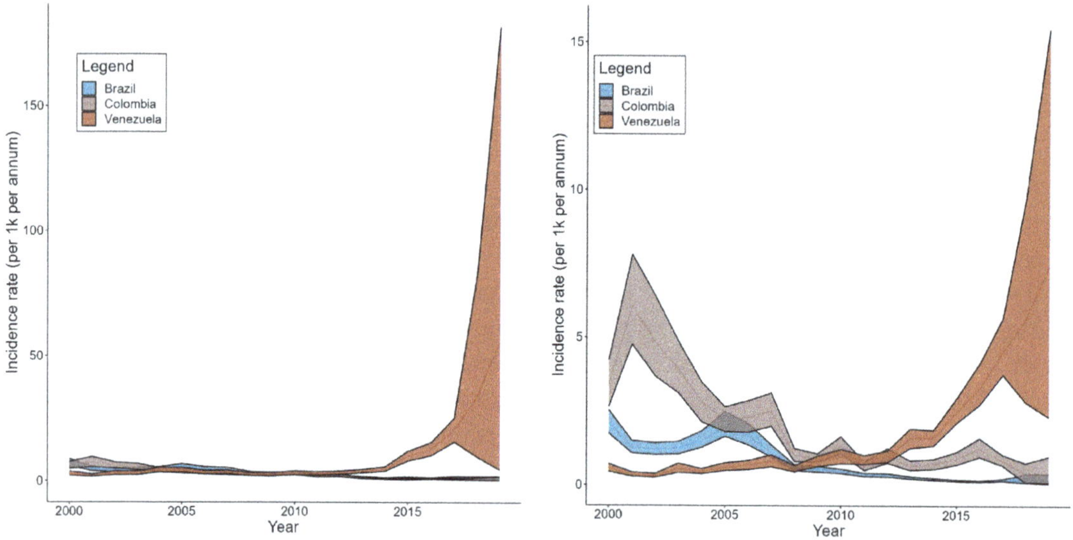

FIGURE 1 Annual malaria incidence in Brazil, Colombia and Venezuela during the last 20 years. (A) *Plasmodium vivax*. (B) *Plasmodium falciparum*
DATA SOURCE: HTTPS://WWW3.PAHO.ORG/DATA/INDEX.PHP/EN/MNU-TOPICS/INDICADORES-MALARIA-EN.HTML

(GTS) for malaria 2016–2030. In line with this goal, the region of the Americas has made significant advances, reducing disease cases and incidence by 58% and 67%, through 2000 and 2020, respectively (WHO 2021). During the same period, malaria deaths and mortality rates decreased by 56% and 66%, correspondingly. However, progress stalled due to the behavior of malaria in Venezuela, a country that reported 467,421 cases in 2019, representing an increase of 1,200% compared to the year 2000. Mortality figures are similarly conspicuous, with 351 deaths in 2019, accounting for 73% of the total deaths from malaria estimated in South America. Venezuela has contributed the most to the regional malaria trends since 2016 (Figure 1).

Plasmodium vivax leads the majority of reported cases (77%) in Venezuela, followed by *Plasmodium falciparum* (17%), mixed *P. vivax* /*P. falciparum* infections (6%) and *Plasmodium malariae* < 1% (WHO 2021). During the early 1960s, Venezuela successfully achieved malaria elimination in approximately 68% of its territory (Gabaldon 1983). However, low to moderate malaria transmission by *P. vivax* and *P. falciparum* persisted mainly in the lowland Amazon rainforests and savannas of the remote Guayana region, south of the Orinoco River. During the 1980s, *P. vivax* malaria reemerged along the coastal wetlands of the country's northeastern region, but its transmission was interrupted twenty years later (Grillet *et al.* 2014). Consequently, malaria transmission in the south persisted as the most important endemic area remaining in the country until 2013, with the southeastern region bordering Brazil and Guyana contributing > 60% (1992–1995) to 88% (2000–2014) of Venezuela's total malaria cases (Grillet *et al.* 2021). Since then, a growing epidemic

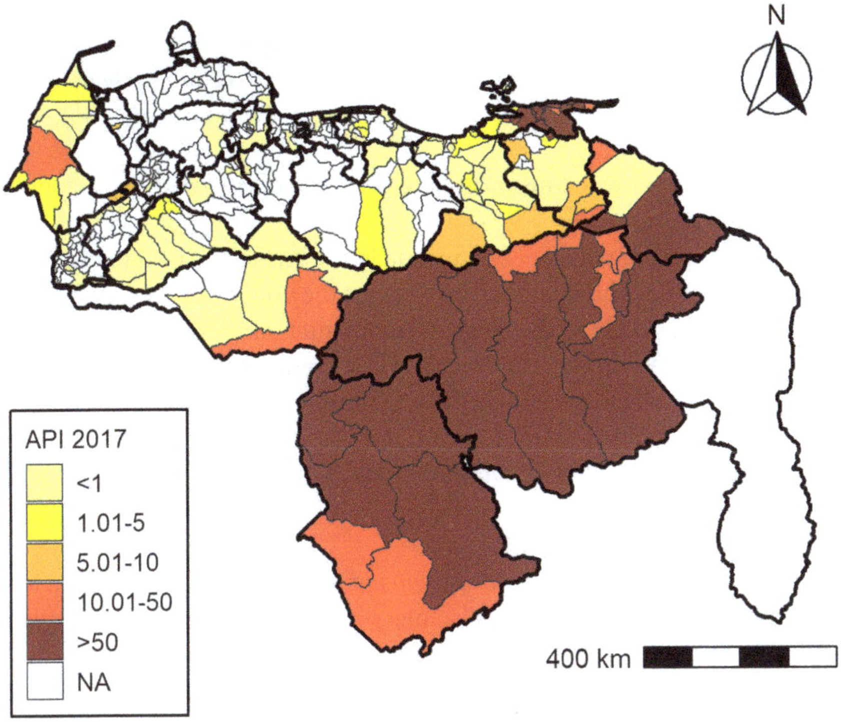

FIGURE 2 Map of malaria incidence in Venezuela during 2017 (API: Number of confirmed malaria cases by Municipality/at-risk population × 1000 inhabitants)
DATA SOURCE: HTTPS://WWW3.PAHO.ORG/DATA/INDEX.PHP/EN/MNU-TOPICS/INDICADORES-MALARIA-EN.HTML

has been unleashed, spreading later in 2014 further to the north-central-western areas (Figure 2), establishing new transmission foci in urban or peri-urban areas not previously known to be endemic, and with an increased population at-risk of around 50% compared to the 34.4% in 2010. Similarly, sporadic autochthonous cases of *P. falciparum* began to emerge along the northeastern coast, revealing a new pattern of transmission of a parasite species that had been eliminated north of the Orinoco River over half a century ago.

Currently, the uncontrolled increase of malaria in Venezuela, coupled with the massive migration of Venezuelans to neighboring countries due to the humanitarian crisis, poses a serious epidemiological threat to the region (Grillet *et al.* 2019), particularly endangering disease control efforts in border endemic countries (Brazil and Colombia) and jeopardizing the hard-won gains in the malaria elimination agenda of the Americas (Laporta *et al.* 2022). Furthermore, frequent movements of the human population between the Amazonian countries included in the Guiana Shield (Guyana, French Guiana, Suriname, and parts of Colombia, Venezuela, and Brazil) could be amplifying the regional impact of increased malaria in southern Venezuela (cross-border malaria), with a latent risk of establishing a regional malaria corridor. A growing concern is the presence and possible regional spread of novel mutations linked to artemisinin resistance in Guyana with Venezuela acting as a hub. Specifically, these mutations have been linked to delayed clearance of drug-resistant parasites and artemisinin in *P. falciparum* (Pacheco *et al.* 2020).

2.2 *Known and unknown transmission scenarios in the midst of changing ecology*

To explore whether the reemergence of malaria in Venezuela has meant new transmission scenarios, it is worth updating the status of the vector species. New scenarios could have arisen in light of the deep environmental transformations that have occurred in some regions of the country in the last twenty years. Of 46 anopheline species identified to date in Venezuela, four of the genus *Anopheles* are the main vectors of malaria (Rubio-Palis 2005, 2022): *Anopheles* (*Nyssorhynchus*) *darlingi*, *An.* (*Nys.*) *albitarsis* s.l., *An.* (*Nys.*) *nuneztovari* s.l. and *An.* (*Nys.*) *aquasalis*.

2.3 *Anopheles darlingi*

This species is the main vector of *P. falciparum* and *P. vivax* in the lowland rain forest and savannahs of southern Venezuela. Infection Rates (IR) of *Plasmodium* spp. ranging from 0.76 to 4.0% have been reported, whereas the entomological inoculation rates (EIR) vary between 2.21 and 70.1 infective bites per person/year (Abou *et al.* 2017, Magris *et al.* 2007, Moreno *et al.* 2009, Rubio-Palis *et al.* 2013). *Anopheles darlingi* is a colonizing species associated with wooded riverine habitats and modified (often deforested) habitat patches whose hematophagous behaviour is usually variable and opportunistic; however, its behaviour can be classified as mainly exophilic and exophagic (Conn *et al.* 2018). In southern Venezuela, it has been collected generally in shaded aquatic habitats, such as natural lagoons or those associated with gold mining, and/or in clusters of floating vegetation in the rivers of Bolívar state (Moreno *et al.* 2015, 2018). *Anopheles darlingi* is common at altitudes below 500 m in southern Venezuela, but has also been collected in highlands on the southeastern border with Brazil (Berti *et al.* 2015), a region where an increase in malaria has been recorded recently. Its role as a vector in this cross-border region remains to be elucidated along with other potential vectors such as *Anopheles* (*Nyssorhynchus*) *braziliensis* and *Anopheles* (*Anopheles*) *peryassui* (Berti *et al.* 2015). Since the mid-20th century, *An. darlingi* has contracted its distribution to the south of the Orinoco River, with sporadic records in the western piedmont ecoregion of Venezuela (Osborn *et al.* 2004). Studies are urgently needed to update its distribution north of the Orinoco River, and to evaluate how its current geographic pattern is related to recent environmental transformation in Venezuela.

2.4 *The Albitarsis complex*

The *Albitarsis* Complex comprises ten species described so far distributed across Central and South America (Motoki *et al.* 2021; Zuñiga *et al.* 2021). Zuñiga *et al.*

(2021) suggested that all previous and more recent reports of *An. albitarsis* s.l. in Venezuela, including those that have found the species infected with *Plasmodium*, correspond to *An. albitarsis* F on the basis of geographic distribution, bionomics, and molecular analysis. In agreement with these findings, *An. albitarsis* F has been incriminated as the main malaria vector (Abou *et al.* 2017, Moreno *et al.* 2005) in the southern gold mining malaria hotspots, with its role in transmission rivaling that of *An. darlingi*. Here, in this region of lowland rain forests and savannas, *An. albitarsis* F has been found positive for *P. falciparum* and *P. vivax*, with an overall sporozoite rate of 1.27 and an EIR of 1.25 infective bites per person/year (Moreno *et al.* 2005, 2007, 2009). Recently, IR values of 5.4% have been detected for this species compared with 4% for *An. darlingi* (Abou *et al.* 2017). *Anopheles albitarsis* F is anthropophilic in this region and bites throughout the night, mainly outdoors (Abou *et al.* 2017; Moreno *et al.* 2009). It has a wide geographic distribution at altitudes below 1,000 m (Osborn *et al.* 2004), and immature stages are associated with grasses and aquatic vegetation in rice fields, streams, swamps, flooded savannahs, river margins, and pools in the riverbeds. Similar to *An. darlingi*, *An. albitarsis F* colonizes disturbed habitats such as wells left by the gold miners in the forest (Moreno *et al.* 2007, 2015). Land use changes, especially deforestation, are likely responsible for the increased abundance and distribution of this species since 1992, which has also increased its *Plasmodium* spp. vectorial capacity more than three times in the last ten years (Abou *et al.* 2017).

2.5 *The Nuneztovari complex*

The *Nuneztovari* Complex includes *An. nuneztovari s.s.*, *An. nuneztovari* A, *An. dunhami*, and *An. goeldii* (Conn *et al.* 2018, Martin dos Santos *et al.* 2019). *Anopheles nuneztovari s.s.* is mostly restricted to western Venezuela (Rubio-Palis 2005, Rubio-Palis *et al.* 1992), but in 2004, it was first reported south of the Orinoco River (Moreno *et al.* 2004). Here, it was found to harbor *P. vivax* (IR = 0.52%), however, its role as main malaria vector in the mining areas along with *An. darlingi* and *An. albitarsis* F remains unexplored (Abou *et al.* 2017). *Anopheles nuneztovari s.s.* has also been found in other areas with a high malaria incidence (e.g. the lower Caura River Basin, Venezuela), but not infected with *Plasmodium* (Rubio-Palis *et al.* 2013). In Venezuela, research has focused mainly on this species' adult habits. Most commonly, wetlands serve as larval habitat, although the immatures can also be collected in a variety of diverse water bodies (Moreno *et al.* 2015, 2018).

2.6 *Anopheles aquasalis*

Endemic *P. vivax* malaria transmission in northeastern Venezuela has been maintained historically by *Anopheles aquasalis* (Berti *et al.* 1993; Grillet 2000; Grillet *et al.* 2014). This species is restricted to the coastal eco-region of the country, along the Caribbean, and is associated with brackish and freshwater wetlands such as mangroves, lagoons, herbaceous and woody swamps where it generally coexists with *Anopheles* (*Nyssorhynchus*) *albimanus* or *Anopheles* (*Nyssorhynchus*) *oswaldoi* (Grillet 2000). However, it is still unclear what influence this species played in recent *P. vivax* malaria outbreaks in Zulia state (western Venezuela), urban *P. vivax* malaria in Miranda state (north-central Venezuela), and sporadic *P. falciparum* malaria outbreaks in coastal Sucre state. Other anopheline species, such as *Anopheles pseudopunctipennis* or *Anopheles albimanus*, may play a role in the current outbreaks of malaria transmission, but this is questionable.

3 Arboviruses: a silent threat

Arboviruses can arise or reappear through a complicated epidemiological process that involves the adaptation of zoonotic viruses to amplified animal hosts, mosquito vectors, and people, all of whom are intertwined in a web of intricate reciprocal connections (Weaver *et al.* 2004). Shifts in human pressures, environmental, climatic or socioeconomic conditions can bring about sudden onsets of epidemic outbreaks of limited duration and indeterminate periodicity, making these events difficult to predict and manage (Navarro *et al.* 2017). In this sense, arboviral infections evolve insidiously as silent threats. Beyond dengue, the archetypical arboviral representative, other emerging and re-emerging viruses such as Venezuela equine encephalitis (VEEV), Eastern equine encephalitis (EEEV), Yellow Fever (YFV), Mayaro Fever (MAYV) and Oropouche Fever (OROV) viruses, are currently hard to trace and predict in time and space in Venezuela (Auguste *et al.* 2015a, Navarro *et al.* 2005b, 2016).

From a taxonomic perspective, three main groups stand out: the Alphaviruses (VEEV, EEEV, MAYV), Flaviviruses (YFV, DENV and ZIKV) and Orthobunyaviruses (OROV – Madre de Dios virus). However, an alternative classification has been suggested that captures the diversity and complexity of the transmission cycles involved and could facilitate a better understanding ecologically (Arrigo *et al.* 2010; Navarro *et al.* 2017). This would include first, mostly urban and/or rural simpler cycles-virus circulation by *Aedes* (mosquito-human-mosquito), such as those of dengue, chikungunya (CHIKV) and Zika (ZIKV) viruses; second, the occasional re-emergence of jungle-rural viruses displaying more complex cycles (several hosts and vectors) including VEEV, EEEV or the Madariaga virus (MADV); and finally, sylvatic cycles which include non-human primates such as YFV, MAYV and OROV. Yellow Fever Virus exhibits a persistence enzootic circulation and has been the focus of recent re-emergence events (Auguste *et al.* 2015a, Rodríguez-Morales *et al.* 2021), whereas MAYV and OROV are newly emerging in Venezuela (Auguste *et al.* 2015b, Navarro *et al.* 2016a) for which many of their ecologic features and transmission dynamics drivers remain poorly understood.

3.1 *Alphavirus and its complex transmission cycle: Venezuela equine encephalitis ecoepidemiology*

Alphaviruses have complex transmission cycles, with VEEV being the most intricate. Venezuela equine encephalitis is an RNA single-stranded mosquito-borne zoonotic pathogen transmitted throughout the Americas (Weaver *et al.* 2004). *Culex* mosquito species of the subgenus *Melanoconion* have been involved in enzootic transmission, as well as *Aedes, Mansonia* and *Psorophora* species, which have been linked to epizootic cycles (Weaver *et al.* 2004). Venezuela equine encephalitis has caused periodic outbreaks in western and central regions of Venezuela involving tens to hundreds of thousands of equine and human cases. This virus was first detected in horses in 1938 (enzootic circulation). From 1960–1973, there were active epizoodemics, followed by a 19-year epidemic silence. In 1993, an epizootic/epidemic outbreak that began in 1992 in western Venezuela (Trujillo state, Rico-Hesse *et al.* 1995) continued to spread discontinuously westward. Then, the largest VEE epizootic and epidemic on record emerged in 1995, affecting an estimated 75,000 to 100,000 people (Weaver *et al.* 2004), spreading as far west as the Colombian border.

Over the last two decades, in the enzootic transmission cycle in the flooded forest of Catatumbo river, vectors involved in virus circulation have been identified as *Culex (Melanoconion) pedroi, Cx. (Mel) vomerifer* and *Cx. (Mel) spissipes*, and rodent hosts as well as other possible vertebrate reservoirs identified, such as *Proechymys guairae* and *Sigmodon hispidus* (Alfonzo *et al.* 2005, Barrera *et al.* 2002, Mendez *et al.* 2001). In this area, the flooded environment maintains the main vector breeding sites, while palm fruits sustain the rodent population. These players along with *Mansonia* spp. and *Psorophora* spp. maintain the forest cycle, exporting it to open areas and transmitting it to horses (Alfonzo *et al.* 2005, Barrera *et al.* 2002, Mendez *et al.* 2001). Molecular phylogenetic studies have identified the Section Spissipes of *Melanoconion*, composed of 23 species, as the evolutionary group involved in the enzootic transmission of VEEV, within the highly diverse subgenus *Melanoconion* (Navarro and Weaver 2004). Later studies were carried out during the 2000's after the identification of isolated cases of horses in Carabobo and Barinas north-western states. These outbreaks seem to be associated with edge effects of the highly deforested relict forests in Barinas state and possibly with distinct silent cycles that involved birds and/or bats as vertebrate hosts and species of *Psorophora* spp. as epizootic vectors (Navarro *et al.* 2005a).

3.2 *Eastern equine encephalitis and Madariaga virus: unknown and pending detection*

The EEEV is an RNA single strand virus circulating in North American, Caribbean (EEEV/NA) and South American (EEEV/SA) regions. New evidence found that EEEV/NA and EEEV/SA variants can be separated leading to a new classification of the EEEV/SA complex as a new species group called Madariaga Virus (MADV). This group is composed of three distinct genetic lineages, one of which circulates in Venezuela (Arrigo *et al.* 2010). *Culex* (*Mel.*) *taeniopus* and *Cx.* (*Mel.*) *pedroi* are the main enzootic vectors of MADV in Central and South America, respectively (Sunthorn *et al.* 1967, Turell *et al.* 2005). However, in Venezuela, EEEV has been isolated from *Cx.* (*Mel.*) *dunni* and *Cx.* (*Mel*) *panocossa* (Walder *et al.* 1984). With few reports so far, many of the epidemiological details of EEEV in Venezuela remain largely unknown.

3.3 *Dengue, Zika, chikungunya, and Aedes species as protagonists*

Three viruses of African origin belonging to two families, along with *Aedes* vectors that share the same urban transmission cycle, define dengue (DENV), Zika (ZIKV) and chikungunya (CHIKV) viruses. Thus, the eco-epidemiological patterns of DENV transmission, in principle, could be extrapolated to ZIKV and CHIKV in the absence of specific data analysis for the latter. Four dengue virus serotypes (DENV-1-4) co-circulate in Venezuela. In the last decade, the incidence, frequency and magnitude of dengue epidemics have increased over five-fold, and are now more widespread across urban and rural settings. The average incidence between 2010–2016 was 211 cases/ 100,000 and a total of six increasingly large epidemics were recorded from 2007–2016, compared with four in the previous 16 years (Grillet *et al.* 2019). The largest reported epidemic occurred in 2010, with approximately 125,000 cases, including 10,300 (8.24%) classified as severe. During that year, Venezuela ranked third in case reporting and second in case severity in the Americas. CHIKV was introduced in 2014 (Lizarazo *et al.* 2019) and ZIKV in 2016 (Grillet *et al.* 2019), resulting in co-circulation of all 3 viruses transmitted by *Aedes aegypti* for the first time in Venezuela.

The vectorial role of *Ae. albopictus* remains largely under-investigated since its introduction into South America in the 1980's (Garcia-Rejon *et al.* 2021) and in 2009 in Venezuela (Navarro *et al.* 2009). *Aedes aegypti* is widely distributed in Venezuela (Del Ventura *et al.* 2013, Navarro *et al.* 2010), and *Ae. albopictus* has spread extensively across the country. A recent review suggests that beyond its high potential vector competence, *Ae. albopictus* could act as a viral reservoir during dengue interepidemic periods, due to vertical transmission (Garcia-Rejon *et al.* 2021). Adding to the complexity of the epidemiological picture, *Aedes vitattus* has emerged recently in the Caribbean region (Pagac *et al.* 2021), although it is not known to be present to date in Venezuela. Active surveillance and ecological information of these three vectors are needed in order to be incorporated into integrated *Aedes* management in Venezuela.

The interaction of socioeconomic factors, such as increasingly crowded living conditions, growing population density, precarious homes, and long-term deficits in public services including frequent and prolonged interruptions in water supply, have been linked with a greater risk of acquiring dengue virus infection in Venezuela (Barrera *et al.* 1995, Vincenti *et al.* 2017). Since 2015, the true burden of DENV, CHIKV and ZIKV remains unknown due to significant underreporting. Although no evidence is available to suggest that dengue incidence is higher in Venezuela than in other countries, the current situation has increased local risk factors, hence, a high abundance and spread of cases is presumed, especially considering the asymptomatic nature of this disease.

3.4 *Mayaro, a threat at the door*

The MAYV has been isolated in different regions of Latin America, including Venezuela (Navarro *et al.* 2017). An outbreak of 77 suspected cases was detected in western Venezuela during 2010 (Auguste *et al.* 2015b). Two further isolations have been reported, an enzootic strain in a rodent from southern Zulia state (Medina *et al.* 2015), and a human case from central-western Venezuela (Lara state, Blohm *et al.* 2019). Although typically primary forest is the habitat of enzootic transmission of MAYV, perhaps in Venezuela other perturbed forest such as secondary gallery forest, could serve as alternative sites of virus-human-mosquito (*Haemagogus-Sabethes*) interaction (Muñoz and Navarro 2012). However, little is known about the nature and persistence of enzootic transmission cycles of MAYV. Its isolations in other mosquito genera and/or species such as *Psorophora, Mansonia,* and *Culex* (*Mel*) *vomerifer* (Caicedo *et al.* 2021) suggest there is a diversity of secondary vectors, and more complex epidemiological cycles remain to be elucidated. Given the recent isolation of MAYV in *Ae. aegypti* in Brazil (Caicedo *et al.* 2021), *Ae. aegypti* and *Ae. albopictus* could be also involved in transmission in Venezuela.

3.5 *Oropouche-Madre de Dios virus: at the outer limit of its known distribution*

In Venezuela, a new OROV reassortment Orthobunyavirus strain related to Madre de Dios virus (MDDV) was isolated from the non-Human primate *Cebus olivaceus* Schomburgk in Atapirire, Central Llanos (Anzoátegui state), during an epizootic of monkey deaths in 2010. This virus has been associated previously with human illness in Peru. Atapirire is a small rural village with a population of ~800, surrounded by gallery and secondary forests near the Orinoco River. The mosquito vector(s) are not known, however, species such as *Aedes serratus* (in ephemeral ground water bodies) and *Coquillettidia venezuelensis* (in small lagoons with floating aquatic plants) are common regionally, suggesting a possible role (Del Ventura *et al.* 2013).

3.6 *Recurring Yellow Fever*

YFV is one of the most important global human arboviral pathogens and the oldest arbovirus on record in Venezuela, with the first case reported officially in 1941. YFV emergences have been periodic, causing sporadic outbreaks during the 1940's,

1950's, 1960's, 1970's, then from 1997–1999, followed by a 20-year silent period and a new upsurge in 2003–2005 (highest rate of cases), and two very recent outbreaks, in 2019 and 2021 (Chavero *et al.* 2021, Rodríguez-Morales *et al.* 2021). The success of the Yellow Fever vaccination program in Venezuela may have been the reason for the long period between epidemics (1970–1990). The YFV deaths coincide with the outbreak years, with a case fatality rate of approximately 40%, except in the last decade and the recent 2021 outbreak in the east of the country that have shown zero case fatality. Mosquito genera and/or species confirmed as vectors of YFV (Barrett and Higgs 2007) are *Ae. aegypti* (urban cycle), *Haemagogus* and *Sabethes* (forest cycle). There is no clear evidence of the role of these mosquito species in the Venezuelan epidemics to date but it is hypothesized that *Ae. aegypti* was involved in the 2005 YFV outbreak (Muñoz-Rodríguez *et al.* 2010). Three foci have been identified and associated with three routes of virus dispersal or epidemiological waves with cyclical occurrences: two in the west, south of Maracaibo Lake, and San Camilo Forest (Apure state). The third is restricted to the east in the states of Bolívar, Monagas and Anzoátegui. Currently, Venezuela is the third country along with Brazil and Peru reporting recent outbreaks of YFV in the Americas region.

4 Main drivers of the surge of mosquito-borne infectious diseases in Venezuela

4.1 *A complex health emergency*

Venezuela has experienced an economic crisis of historic proportions during the past ten years, with pronounced negative economic growth and high rates of inflation (Grillet *et al.* 2019). An ongoing humanitarian crisis with serious societal repercussions for the nation and the region has been caused by this circumstance, which has led the general breakdown of Venezuela's healthcare system and the mass exodus of medically educated personnel. Prior to the steep decline of Venezuela's economy (beginning in 2013), lack of investment in healthcare infrastructure and public health prevention efforts began to generate an inefficient and neglected public health system that has engendered the re-emergence, spread and expansion of MBIDs such as malaria, dengue, or Yellow Fever. Immediate causes of this crisis include: (1) shortages of insecticides, essential medicines, medical equipment, supplies for diagnostics and fuel which hinder vector-control and disease-treatment efforts; (2) lapses in support for government health workers and vector-control efforts; and (3) partial interruption or weakening of immunization programs. Additionally, the depletion of the health system has reduced epidemiological surveillance and reporting activities causing a significant level of infectious disease underreporting since 2015. The malaria epidemic has been fueled particularly by a lack of malaria commodities such as insecticides, drugs, diagnostic supplies, mosquito nets, and lack of efficient surveillance and vector control activities (Grillet *et al.* 2018). Additionally, the absence of regular access to water supplies has led to an increase in stored water hoarding, which has caused a significant rise in the percentage of homes with *Ae. aegypti* infestations, above the WHO transmission threshold (Grillet *et al.* 2019). Such conditions preceded the arboviral epidemics in Venezuela in 2014 (CHIKV) and 2016 (ZIKV). The recent reemergence of YF cases in Venezuela is mainly the consequence of a low vaccination rate among adults, estimated to be 12.02% by 2019 (Rodríguez-Morales *et al.* 2021). VEEV control through equine vaccination has been conducted through private initiatives rather than a national vaccination program. Yellow Fever surveillance in populations at risk, vectors and reservoirs, has been impacted additionally by the absence of a robust epidemiological arbovirus surveillance program which Venezuela had in past decades. YF and dengue surveillance, on the other hand, has faced limited availability of laboratories to carry out molecular and/or immuno-serological assays for diagnosis.

4.2 *Land use change: gold fever, mining malaria and deforestation*

In Venezuela, illegal gold mining is the primary local socioeconomic cause of malaria and a significant contributor to the country's overall rise in the past 20 years (Fletcher *et al.* 2022). The humanitarian crisis has ignited illegal gold mining in the south as one of the country's fastest-growing shadow economies. Recent evidence has demonstrated clearly that specific areas deforested for gold extraction have more cases of malaria compared to nearby non-mining areas. The former contribute to 80% of malaria cases in Venezuela (Grillet *et al.* 2021; Fletcher *et al.* 2022). The economic crisis has promoted migration of human populations from different regions of Venezuela in search of economic opportunities to regions where gold mining activities and malaria are clustered. Some of these internal migrants return to their original community facilitating parasite diffusion and local transmission where susceptible *Anopheles* vector populations exist. Consequently, malaria has reemerged and been reintroduced to areas where autochthonous transmission had been eliminated previously, resulting in a shift in malaria epidemiology (Figure 2). Illegal gold mining and its associated deforestation have increased and expanded in southern Venezuela since 1997 (Fletcher *et al.* 2022), with a marked annual increment since 2004.

Of all regions in the south, Sifontes Municipality, the main malaria hotspot in Venezuela (Grillet *et al.* 2021), has exhibited a statistically significant trend in annual forest loss, with an estimated annual increase in loss of 120 Hectare/year and an accumulated loss rate of 30,265 Ha/year from 2000–2020. During the same period, the area occupied by gold mining activities increased from 14,797 Ha (2000) to 34,465 Ha in 2020 and both *P. vivax* and *P. falciparum* have increased in incidence (4-8-fold) with a concomitant decrease (3-6-fold) of vegetation cover (Grillet *et al.* 2021; Fletcher *et al.* 2022). Overall, environmental degradation caused by mining activity can facilitate the spread of vector-borne diseases, such as malaria, by altering the ecological landscape and increasing exposure to mosquito vectors, especially in human settlements located near the fragmented forest fringe (Grillet *et al.* 2021; Fletcher *et al.* 2022).

Earlier studies in southern Venezuela indicated that the most productive breeding site types for *An. albitarsis* F and to a lesser degree for *An. darlingi*, are abandoned open mining dug-outs left after clearing vegetation (Moreno *et al.* 2007, Moreno *et al.* 2015). How the fragmentation of forests generated by mining influences mosquito ecology and vectorial capacity are essential knowledge gaps in this region. In the past two decades, there have also been considerable changes in the forest cover north of the Orinoco River, particularly in the central and western areas where the majority of arboviruses are found. Changes in land use could alter the intricate reciprocal relationships among pathogens, human, non-human vertebrate hosts, and mosquito vectors, which in turn could alter the risk of sylvatic and jungle-rural arboviruses (Franklinos *et al.* 2019; Ilacqua *et al.* 2021; Wilk-da-Silva *et al.* 2020). However, there is little information on how the current land-use changes are causing arboviruses to develop or reappear in Venezuela.

5 Final remarks

Poverty is a major social determinant of neglected tropical diseases (NTDs), (see Chapter 5, The economic impacts of malaria: past, present and future, by Kuschnig and Vashold for a more nuanced micro-and macroeconomics perspective) but during recent decades, we have also seen how socio-political conflict can accelerate economic decline and promote a substantial increase in the incidence and prevalence of NTDs. Some examples include the emergence of visceral leishmaniasis in East Africa, cutaneous leishmaniasis in the Middle East and North Africa, and more recently, the resurgence of MBIDs in Venezuela (Hotez *et al.* 2017). Deforestation, on the other hand, is among the most pressing anthropogenic environmental impacts in the Amazon Forest. Between 2000 and 2012, tropical rainforest ecozones totaled 32% of global forest cover loss, nearly half of which occurred in South America (Hansen *et al.* 2013). Most malaria cases in South America occur in the Amazon rainforest (WHO 2021) and deforestation by mining has caused the surge of malaria in recent decades in countries such as Peru, Brazil and Venezuela (Conn *et al.* 2018). Transmission in such settings is currently considered a Gordian knot for achieving malaria elimination (Fornace *et al.* 2021, Grillet *et al.* 2021). Therefore, the GTS target for the elimination of malaria in the Americas will not be achieved by 2030 if the malaria epidemic in Venezuela continues (Laporta *et al.* 2022; WHO 2021).

Dengue outbreaks are increasing in frequency and magnitude throughout Latin America. Considering the few possibilities for detection and cure of arboviral diseases in Venezuela combined with the high level of population displacement, emigrating infected individuals could be unwittingly causing a spillover of these diseases to neighboring countries, a process that requires careful quantification. The current panorama leaves the at-risk population unprotected and makes it less probable that Venezuela has the capacity to evaluate the current burden and to detect early indicators of the potential emergence or reemergence of a range of arboviruses (such as MAYV, OROV, dengue, or YFV), new pathogens or invasive vectors. Indeed, the occurrence of epizootic strains of VEEV and MAYV along with cryptic transmission cycles of these viruses, combined with a lack of immunization programs, pose further threats in Venezuela. Finally, the rise of MBIDs in Venezuela is occurring in the context of a complex situation, which includes the COVID-19 pandemic and its disruption of access to health care (Lampo *et al.* 2021). To effectively control epidemics and prevent future outbreaks, it is necessary to recover and strengthen the surveillance and control program in Venezuela. The following recommendations may be part of the vital actions needed to mitigate and assess the real impact, as well as address some key questions about the transmission of mosquito-borne infectious diseases in Venezuela.

Local actions:

- Actions focused on rapid diagnosis and timely treatment, vector control, and monitoring for drug/insecticide resistance in the main malaria hotspots are urgent and essential. Increased enforcement of the control program in the rest of the country is pivotal to lower the risks of reintroduction to vulnerable areas.
- Epidemiologic surveillance programs, early outbreak reporting, and rapid response systems should be implemented immediately to ensure timely outbreak response and / or prevent the risk of forthcoming arboviral emergence events.
- In at-risk areas comprising modified environments (such as gold mining regions) or areas with ever-increasing trends towards urbanization, improving surveillance strategies for early case detection should be mandatory.
- Strengthening genomic surveillance systems countrywide is another crucial factor for tracking pathogen transmission and outbreak dynamics providing a near real-time response in emergence events.

Regional actions:

- Given the current context, successful control of the ongoing malaria epidemic in Venezuela requires not only national but regional coordination.
- Intercountry surveillance initiatives should be put into effect across borders along with healthcare authorities in Brazil and Colombia to mitigate the effects of massive migration and spillover and / or spread of arboviruses or malaria.
- As Venezuela becomes an increasingly high-risk area for malaria and arboviral emergence, decisive actions must be adopted alongside regional and national partners to tackle a potential regional crisis and prevent future establishment of transmission routes and expansion among countries bordering Venezuela.

Acknowledgements

We acknowledge funds provided by the National Institute of Health (USA), grant 2R01AI110112 to MEG, and the NIH Fogarty International Center Grant R03TW415640, FONACIT-S1-2001000921 and DII-UISEK-P011617-2 grants to JCN. This work was supported in part by the Scottish Funding Council Global Challenges Research Fund (Small Grants Fund SFC/AN/12/2017) as well as the GCRF Vector-borne disease control in Venezuela Network – www.vbdvenezuelanetwork.com (EP/T003782/1) to MEG and APM. We acknowledge the data visualization provided by Napoleon Malpica and Juan Vicente Hernandez-Villena.

References

Abou Orm S, Moreno JE, Carrozza M, Acevedo P, Herrera F (2017) Tasas de infección de *Plasmodium* spp. para algunos *Anopheles* spp. del municipio Sifontes, Estado Bolívar, Venezuela. Bol Mal Salud Amb 57: 17–25.

Alfonzo D, Grillet ME, Liria J, *et al.* (2005) Ecological characterization of the aquatic habitats of mosquitoes (Diptera: Culicidae) in enzootic foci of Venezuelan equine encephalitis virus in western Venezuela. J Med Entomol. 42(3): 278–284. https://doi.org/10.1093/jmedent/42.3.278.

Arrigo NC, Adams AP, Weaver SC (2010) Evolutionary patterns of eastern equine encephalitis virus in North versus South America suggest ecological differences and taxonomic revision. J Virol 84: 1014–25. https://doi.org/10.1128/JVI.01586-09.

Auguste AJ, Lemey P, Bergren NA, *et al.* (2015a) Enzootic Transmission of Yellow Fever Virus, Venezuela. Emerg Infect Dis 21: 99–102. https://doi.org/10.3201/eid2101.140814.

Auguste AJAJ, Liria J, Forrester NL, *et al.* (2015b) Evolutionary and Ecological Characterization of Mayaro Virus Strains Isolated during an Outbreak, Venezuela, 2010. Emerg Infect Dis 21: 1742–1750. https://doi.org/10.3201/eid2110.141660.

Barrera R, Ferro C, Navarro J-C, *et al.* (2002) Contrasting sylvatic foci of Venezuelan equine encephalitis virus in northern South America. Am J Trop Med Hyg. 2002 Sep;67(3): 324–334. https://doi.org/10.4269/ajtmh.2002.67.324.

Barrera R, Navarro JC, Mora JDD, *et al.* (1995) Public service deficiencies and *Aedes aegypti* breeding sites in Venezuela. Bull Pan Am Health Organ 29: 193–205. PMID: 8520605.

Barrett ADT, Higgs S (2007) Yellow fever: A disease that has yet to be conquered. Annu Rev Entomol 52: 209–229. https://doi.org/10.1146/annurev.ento.52.110405.091454.

Berti J, Zimmerman R, Amarista J (1993) Adult abundance, biting behavior and parity of *Anopheles aquasalis*, Curry 1932 in two malarious areas of Sucre State, Venezuela. Mem Inst Oswaldo Cruz 88(3): 363–369. https://doi.org/10.1590/s0074-02761993000300004.

Berti J, Guzmán H, Estrada Y, Ramírez R (2015) New records of mosquitoes (Diptera: Culicidae) from Bolívar state in South eastern Venezuela, with 27 new species for the state and 5 of them new in the country. Front Public Health 2: 268. https://doi.org/10.3389/fpubh.2014.00268.

Blohm GM, Márquez-Colmenarez MC, Lednicky JA, *et al.* (2019) Isolation of Mayaro Virus from a Venezuelan Patient with Febrile Illness, Arthralgias, and Rash: Further Evidence of Regional Strain Circulation and Possible Long-Term Endemicity. Am J Trop Med Hyg 101: 1219–1225. https://doi.org/10.4269/ajtmh.19-0357.

Caicedo EY, Charniga K, Rueda A, *et al.* (2021) The epidemiology of mayaro virus in the Americas: A systematic review and key parameter estimates for outbreak modelling. PLoS Negl Trop Dis 15: 1–19. https://doi.org/10.1371/journal.pntd.0009418.

Chavero M, Guevara O, Figuera L *et al.* (2021) Re-emergence of yellow fever in Venezuela: Report of the first case after 14 years. Travel Med Infect Dis 41: 102025. https://doi.org/10.1016/j.tmaid.2021.102025.

Conn JE, Grillet ME, Correa M, Sallum MAM (2018) Malaria Transmission in South America – Present Status and Prospects for Elimination. In: Manguin S, Dev V, editors. Towards Malaria Elimination – A Leap Forward. IntechOpen, London. pp. 281–313. https://doi.org/10.5772/intechopen.76964.

Del Ventura F, Liria J, Navarro JC (2013) Determinación de áreas de endemismo en mosquitos (Diptera: Culicidae) en Venezuela, mediante criterios explícitos de optimización. Bol Malariol Salud Amb LIII: 165–182.

Dos Santos MMM, Sucupira IMC, Dos Santos TV, Dos Santos ACF, Lacerda RNDL, Póvoa MM (2019) Morphological identification of species of the Nuneztovari Complex of *Anopheles* (Diptera: Culicidae) from an area affected by a Brazilian hydroelectric plant. Zootaxa 4565(2): 4565.2.7. https://doi.org/10.11646/zootaxa.

Fletcher IK, Grillet ME, Moreno JE, Drakeley C, Hernández-Villena J, Jones KE, Lowe R (2022) Synergies between environmental degradation and climate variation on malaria re-emergence in southern Venezuela: a spatiotemporal modelling study. Lancet Planet. Health. 6(9): e739–e748. https://doi.org/10.1016/S2542-5196(22)00192-9.

Fornace KM, Diaz AV, Lines J, Drakeley CJ (2021) Achieving global malaria eradication in changing landscapes. Malar J. 20(1): 69. https://doi.org/10.1186/s12936-021-03599-0.

Franklinos LHV, Jones KE, Redding DW, Abubakar I (2019) The effect of global change on mosquito-borne disease. Lancet Infect Dis. 19(9): e302–e312. https://doi.org/10.1016/S1473-3099(19)30161-6.

Gabaldon A (1983) Malaria eradication in Venezuela: doctrine, practice, achievements after twenty years. Am J Trop Med Hyg. 1983; 32: 203–211. https://doi.org/10.4269/ajtmh.1983.32.203.

Garcia-Rejon JE, Navarro JC, Cigarroa-Toledo N, Baak-Baak CM (2021) An updated review of the invasive *Aedes albopictus* in the Americas; geographical distribution, host feeding patterns, arbovirus infection, and the potential for vertical transmission of dengue virus. Insects 26;12(11): 967. https://doi.org/10.3390/insects12110967.

Grillet ME (2000) Factors associated with distribution of *Anopheles aquasalis* and *Anopheles oswaldoi* (Diptera: Culicidae) in a malarious area, northeastern Venezuela. J Med Entomol 37(2): 231–238. https://doi.org/10.1603/0022-2585-37.2.231.

Grillet ME, El Souki M, Laguna F, León JR (2014) The periodicity of *Plasmodium vivax* and *Plasmodium falciparum* in Venezuela. Acta Trop 129: 52–60. https://doi.org/10.1016/j.actatropica.2013.10.007.

Grillet ME, Villegas L, Oletta JF, Tami A, Conn JE (2018) Malaria in Venezuela requires response. Science. 359: 528. https://doi.org/https://doi.org/10.1126/science.aar5440.

Grillet ME, Hernández-Villena JV, Llewellyn MS *et al.* (2019) Venezuela's humanitarian crisis, resurgence of vector-borne diseases, and implications for spillover in the region. Lancet Infect Dis. 19(5): 149–161. https://doi.org/10.1016/S1473-3099(18)30757-6.

Grillet ME, Moreno JE, Hernández-Villena JV *et al.* (2021) Malaria in Southern Venezuela: The hottest hotspot in Latin America. PLoS Negl Trop Dis 15(1): e0008211. https://doi.org/10.1371/journal.pntd.0008211.

Hansen MC, Potapov PV, Moore R *et al.* (2013) High-resolution global maps of 21st-century forest cover change. Science 15;342(6160): 850–853. https://doi.org/10.1126/science.1244693.

Hotez PJ, Basáñez MG, Acosta-Serrano A, Grillet ME (2017). Venezuela and its rising vector-borne neglected diseases. PLoS Negl Trop Dis 11(6): e0005423. https://doi.org/https://doi.org/10.1371/journal.pntd.0005423.

Ilacqua RC, Medeiros-Sousa AR, Ramos DG, Obara MT, Ceretti-Junior W, Mucci LF, Marrelli MT, Laporta GZ (2021) Reemergence of yellow fever in Brazil: The Role of Distinct Landscape fragmentation thresholds. J Environ Public Health. 2021: 8230789. https://doi.org/10.1155/2021/8230789.

Lampo M, Hernández-Villena JV, Cascante J *et al.* (2021) Signatures of the Venezuelan Humanitarian Crisis in the First Wave of COVID-19: Fuel Shortages and Border Migration. Vaccines (Basel) 9(7): 719. https://doi.org/10.3390/vaccines9070719.

Laporta GZ, Grillet ME, Rodovalho SR *et al.* (2022) Reaching the malaria elimination goal in Brazil: a spatial analysis and time-series study. Infect Dis Poverty 11: 39. https://doi.org/10.1186/s40249-022-00945-5.

Lizarazo E, Vincenti-Gonzalez MF, Grillet ME, Tami A (2019) Spatial dynamics of chikungunya transmission in northern Venezuela: The first six months of the epidemic outbreak. Emerg Infect Dis 25(4): 672–680. https://doi.org/10.3201/eid2504.172121.

Magris M, Rubio-Palis Y, Menares C, Villegas L (2007) Vector bionomics and malaria transmission in the Upper Orinoco River, Southern Venezuela. Mem Inst Oswaldo Cruz 102(3): 303–311. https://doi.org/10.1590/s0074-02762007005000049.

Motoki MT, Linton YM, Conn JE, Ruiz-Lopez F, Wilkerson RC (2021) Phylogenetic Network of Mitochondrial COI Gene Sequences Distinguishes 10 Taxa Within the Neotropical Albitarsis Group (Diptera: Culicidae), Confirming the Separate Species Status of *Anopheles albitarsis* H (Diptera: Culicidae) and Revealing a Novel Lineage, *Anopheles albitarsis* J. J Med Entomol 58(2): 599–607. https://doi.org/10.1093/jme/tjaa211.

Medina G, Garzaro DJ, Barrios M, *et al.* (2015) Genetic diversity of Venezuelan alphaviruses and circulation of a Venezuelan equine encephalitis virus subtype IAB strain during an interepizootic period. Am J Trop Med Hyg 93: 7–10. https://doi.org/10.4269/ajtmh.14-0543.

Mendez W, Liria J, Navarro J-CC, *et al.* (2001) Spatial dispersion of adult mosquitoes (Diptera: Culicidae) in a sylvatic focus of Venezuelan equine encephalitis virus. J Med Entomol 38: 813–821.

Moreno J, Rubio-Palis Y, Sánchez V, Mariany D (2004) Primer registro de *Anopheles* (*Nyssorhynchus*) *nuneztovari* Gabaldon, 1940 (Diptera: Culicidae) en el estado Bolívar y sus implicaciones eco-epidemiológicas. Entomotrópica. 19: 55–58.

Moreno JE, Rubio-Palis Y, Páez E, Pérez E, Sánchez V, Vaccari E (2005) *Anopheles* (*Anopheles*) *neomaculipalpus*: a new malaria vector in the Amazon basin? Med Vet Entomol 19(3): 329–332. https://doi.org/10.1111/j.1365-2915.2005.00572.x.

Moreno JE, Rubio-Palis Y, Paez E, Perez E, Sanchez V (2007) Abundance, biting behavior and parous rate of anopheline mosquito species in relation to malaria incidence in gold-mining areas of southern Venezuela. Med Vet Entomol 21(4): 339–349. https://doi.org/10.1111/j.1365-2915.2007.00704.x.

Moreno JE, Rubio-Palis Y, Paez E, Perez E, Sanchez V, Vaccari E (2009) Malaria entomological inoculation rates in gold mining areas of Southern Venezuela. Mem Inst Oswaldo Cruz 104(5): 764–768. https://doi.org/https://doi.org/10.1590/S0074-02762009000500017.

Moreno JE, Rubio-Palis Y, Sánchez V, Martínez Á (2015) Caracterización de hábitats larvales de anofelinos en el municipio Sifontes del estado Bolívar, Venezuela. Bol Mal Salud Amb 55: 117–131.

Moreno JE, Rubio-Palis Y, Bevilacqua M, Sanchez V, Guzman H (2018) Caracterización de hábitats larvales de Anofelinos en el bajo Rio Caura, región malárica del Estado Bolívar, Venezuela. Bol Mal Salud Amb 58: 17–30.

Muñoz-Rodríguez M, Arrivillaga J, Navarro J (2010) Casos de Fiebre Amarilla en Portuguesa, Venezuela: ¿un brote selvático espurio? 21: 163–177.

Muñoz M, Navarro JC (2012) Mayaro: A re-emerging arbovirus in Venezuela and Latin America, Virus Mayaro: Un arbovirus reemergente en Venezuela y Latinoamérica. Biomedica 32(2): 286–302. https://doi.org/10.1590/S0120-41572012000300017.

Navarro J-C, Carrera J-P, Liria J, *et al.* (2017) Alphaviruses in Latin America and the Introduction of Chikungunya Virus. In: Human Virology in Latin America. Springer International Publishing, Cham, pp. 169–192.

Navarro J-C, Giambalvo D, Hernandez R, *et al.* (2016a) Isolation of Madre de Dios virus (Orthobunyavirus; Bunyaviridae), an oropouche virus Species Reassortant, from a Monkey in Venezuela. Am J Trop Med Hyg. 95(2): 328–338. https://doi.org/10.4269/ajtmh.15-0679.

Navarro J-C, Weaver SC (2004) Molecular phylogeny of the Vomerifer and Pedroi Groups in the spissipes section of the subgenus *Culex* (*Melanoconion*). J Med Entomol. 41(4): 575–581. https://doi.org/10.1603/0022-2585-41.4.575.

Navarro J-C, Medina G, Vasquez C, *et al.* (2005a) Postepizootic Persistence of Venezuelan Equine Encephalitis Virus, Venezuela. Emerg Infect Dis 11: 1907–1915. https://doi.org/10.3201/eid1112.050533.

Navarro JC, Del Ventura F, Zorrilla A, Liria J (2010) Registros de mayor altitud para mosquitos (Diptera: Culicidae) en Venezuela. Rev Biol Trop 58: 245–254.

Navarro JC, Medina G, Vasquez C, *et al.* (2005b) Post-epizootic Persistence of Venezuelan Equine Encephalitis. Emerg Infect Dis 11: 1907–1915.

Navarrro JC, Zorrilla A, Moncada N, *et al.* (2009) Primer registro de *Aedes albopictus* (Skuse) en Venezuela. Importancia como vector de Dengue y acciones a desarrollar. Bol Mal Salud Amb XLIX: 864–866.

Osborn FR, Rubio-Palis Y, Herrera M, Figuera A, Moreno JE (2004) Caracterización Ecoregional de los Vectores de Malaria en Venezuela. Bol Mal Salud Amb 2: 77–92.

Pacheco MA, Forero-Peña DA, Schneider KA *et al.* (2020) Malaria in Venezuela: changes in the complexity of infection reflects the increment in transmission intensity. Malar J 19: 176. https://doi.org/https://doi.org/10.1186/s12936-020-03247-z.

Pagac BB, Spring AR, Stawicki JR, *et al.* (2021) Incursion and establishment of the Old-World arbovirus vector *Aedes* (*Fredwardsius*) *vittatus* (Bigot, 1861) in the Americas. Acta Trop 213: 105739. https://doi.org/10.1016/j.actatropica.2020.105739.

Rico-Hesse R, Weaver SC, de Siger J, *et al.* (1995) Emergence of a new epidemic/epizootic Venezuelan equine encephalitis virus in South America. Proc Natl Acad Sci U S A 92: 5278–5281. https://doi.org/10.1073/pnas.92.12.5278.

Rodríguez-Morales AJ, Bonilla-Aldana DK, Suárez JA, *et al.* (2021) Yellow fever reemergence in Venezuela – Implications for international travelers and Latin American countries during the COVID-19 pandemic. Travel Med Infect Dis 44: 102192. https://doi.org/10.1016/j.tmaid.2021.102192.

Rubio-Palis Y (2005) Situación actual de la taxonomía de la Subfamilia Anophelinae (Diptera:Culicidae) en Venezuela. Bol Mal Salud Amb 1: 1–10.

Rubio-Palis Y (2022) Anophelinae mosquitoes of Venezuela: species complex and epidemiological implications. Salus 26(1): 25–34.

Rubio-Palis Y, Wirtz RA, Curtis CF (1992) Malaria entomological inoculation rates in western Venezuela. Acta Trop 52(2–3): 167–74. https://doi.org/10.1016/0001-706x(92)90033-t.

Rubio-Palis Y, Bevilacqua M, Medina DA *et al.* (2013) Malaria entomological risk factors in relation to land cover in the Lower Caura River Basin, Venezuela. Mem Inst Oswaldo Cruz 108(2): 220–228. https://doi.org/10.1590/0074-0276108022013015.

Sunthorn S, Galindo P (1967) The Isolation of Eastern Equine Encephalitis from *Culex* (*Melanoconion*) *taeniopus* Dyar and Knab in Panama. Mosq News 27: 74–76.

Turell MJ, O'Guinn ML, Jones JW, *et al.* (2005) Isolation of viruses from mosquitoes (Diptera: Culicidae) collected in the Amazon Basin region of Peru. J Med Entomol 42(5): 891–898. https://doi.org/10.1603/0022-2585(2005)042[0891:IOVFMD]2.0.CO;2.

Vincenti-Gonzalez MF, Grillet ME, Velasco-Salas ZI, *et al.* (2017) Spatial Analysis of Dengue Seroprevalence and Modeling of Transmission Risk Factors in a Dengue Hyperendemic City of Venezuela. PLoS Negl Trop Dis 11: 1–21. https://doi.org/10.1371/journal.pntd.0005317.

Walder R, Calisher CH, Suarez OM (1984) Arbovirus Studies in the Guajira Region of Venezuela: Activities of Eastern Equine Encephalitis and Venezuelan Equine Encephalitis Viruses during an Interepizootic Period. Am J Trop Med Hyg 33: 699–707. https://doi.org/10.4269/ajtmh.1984.33.699.

Walder R, Suarez OM (1976) Studies of Arboviruses in Southwestern Venezuela: I. Isolations of Venezuelan and Eastern Equine Encephalitis Viruses from Sentinel Hamsters in the Catatumbo Region. Int J Epidemiol 5: 375–384. https://doi.org/10.1093/ije/5.4.375.

Weaver SC, Ferro C, Barrera R, *et al.* (2004) Venezuelan Equine Encephalitis. Annu Rev Entomol 49: 141–174. doi.org/10.1146/annurev.ento.49.061802.123422.

World malaria report 2021 (2021) Geneva: World Health Organization; 2021. Licence: CC BY-NC-SA 3.0 IGO. https://www.who.int/publications/i/item/9789240040496.

Wilk-da-Silva R, Mucci LF, Ceretti-Junior W, Duarte AMRC, Marrelli MT, Medeiros-Sousa AR (2020) Influence of landscape composition and configuration on the richness and abundance of potential sylvatic yellow fever vectors in a remnant of Atlantic Forest in the city of São Paulo, Brazil. Acta Trop. 204: 105385. https://doi.org/10.1016/j.actatropica.2020.105385.

Zúñiga MA, Rubio-Palis Y, Brochero H (2021) Updating the bionomy and geographical distribution of *Anopheles* (*Nyssorhynchus*) *albitarsis* F: A vector of malaria parasites in northern South America. PLoS One 16(6): e0253230. https://doi.org/10.1371/journal.pone.0253230.3. Malaria in the Amazon Basin: how climate change and natural disasters create new challenges for an old disease

CHAPTER 3

Malaria in the Amazon Basin: how climate change and natural disasters create new challenges for an old disease

Leonardo Suveges Moreira Chaves[1†], *Tatiane Moraes de Sousa*[2], *Luiz Carlos Ferreira Penha*[3] *and Sandra S. Hacon*[2*]

[1]Departamento de Epidemiologia, Faculdade de Saúde Pública, Universidade de São Paulo, Av. Dr. Arnaldo, 715 – Pacaembu, CEP 01246-904, São Paulo, SP, Brazil; [2]Departamento de Endemias Samuel Pessoa (DENSP), Sergio Arouca National School of Public Health (ENSP), Fundação Oswaldo Cruz – FIOCRUZ, Rua Leopoldo Bulhões 1480, Sala 601, Bairro Manguinhos, CEP 21041–210, Rio de Janeiro, RJ, Brazil; [3]Programa VigiFronteiras Brasil, Fundação Oswaldo Cruz – FIOCRUZ, Av. Brasil, 4365 – Manguinhos, CEP 21040–900, Rio de Janeiro, RJ, Brazil; [†]Dr Chaves passed away on January 20, 2023; *sandrahacon@gmail.com

Abstract

Amazon Basin has experienced intense forest degradation of its ecosystems, increasing environmental, social, and economic threats. Deforestation is the major threat to biodiversity as well as increasing pollution levels and their impacts, and the frequency of extreme hydrometeorological events. These natural disasters cause serious damage and losses to human social systems, impacting the ability of communities to keep their houses and altering their welfare, livelihood systems, health services capacity, and opportunities for social development. In addition, these forces disrupt natural systems through changing seasonal patterns and variable long-term trends in rainfall and temperature and increases in frequency and intensity of climate and weather extremes. Most natural disasters have been associated with floods, heatwaves, and tropical cyclones. These can have corresponding impacts on zoonotic and other infectious diseases, leading to emergence in new areas in the world and increased risks of epidemics. Flooding and other hydrometeorological hazards, storms, heat waves also can affect vector breeding sites and transmission of vector-borne diseases such as malaria, dengue and chikungunya. Open gold mining, fishponds, deforestation, and hydroelectric power plant in Amazon are some examples of drivers that can represent synergistic anthropogenically driven disasters, leading to events, such as mudslide, mosquito proliferation and vector-borne diseases. These events impact the most vulnerable populations, with people most impacted by floods, severe droughts, and loss of income at the highest risks of disease outbreaks. Malaria may not represent severe illness and deaths

 | DOI:10.3920/9789004688650_005

in Amazon Basin; however, the disease has strong impact in public health, with harmful effects in socio-economic and cultural development, with high morbidity, economic productivity losses, and severe negative impact on cognitive development of children, with anaemia, malnutrition, and saturating health services capacity. In this chapter, we present the main drivers and vulnerabilities associated with malaria incidence in Amazon Basin in time of extreme climatic events.

Keywords

natural disaster – extreme events – flood – land use change – deforestation – gold mining – tropical forest – vector-borne disease

1 Introduction

Tropical forests house the biggest hotspots of biodiversity of the world and are largely distributed between intertropical zone on the globe, composed by three major areas: the Congo-Gabonese block in Africa, the Greater Mekong in Southeast Asia, and the Amazon Basin in South America (Lambin and Geist 2008). These ecosystems were able to adapt to great climate changes in the past, such as glacial and interglacial events (Puig 2001). However, human growth activities to generate wealth on Anthropocene era have disrupting the micro and macroclimate dynamics of the forests, changing the wet and dry season period, breaking hydrologic patterns (WMO 2021) and biological cycles (Kingsolver *et al.* 2011). It has deteriorated refuges of core species (Nobre *et al.* 2016, Davidson *et al.* 2012), biodiversity stocks which enable the recolonization areas of lost forest after extreme events (Duminil *et al.* 2015, Boulton *et al.* 2022). In this context, high temperature, increase greenhouse gas concentrations, and changes in precipitation patterns are factors which put forests and their ecosystem services at risk (MEA 2005), increasing the frequency and intensity of extreme events (IPCC 2013). Predatory exploitation of natural resources, and people migration are threats to spread epidemics in many regions (Richards *et al.* 2014, Cohen *et al.* 2017), as Amazon Basin (see Chapters 5 and 6 of socioeconomic systems section for details).

Amazon Basin has an area covering approximately 7 million km^2, shared by nine countries (MapBiomas 2022): Brazil, with 60.7%, followed by Peru (11.3%), Bolivia (8.2%), Colombia (6.6%), Venezuela (5.7%), Guyana (3.1%), Suriname (2.1%), French Guiana (1.2%) and Ecuador (1.1%) (Figure 1). This biome includes high proportions of water bodies; notably, this includes the Amazon River, the largest river system in the world. This river system which contributes an estimated 15–20% of all freshwater discharged into oceans annually (Barthem *et al.* 2004), 10–15% of

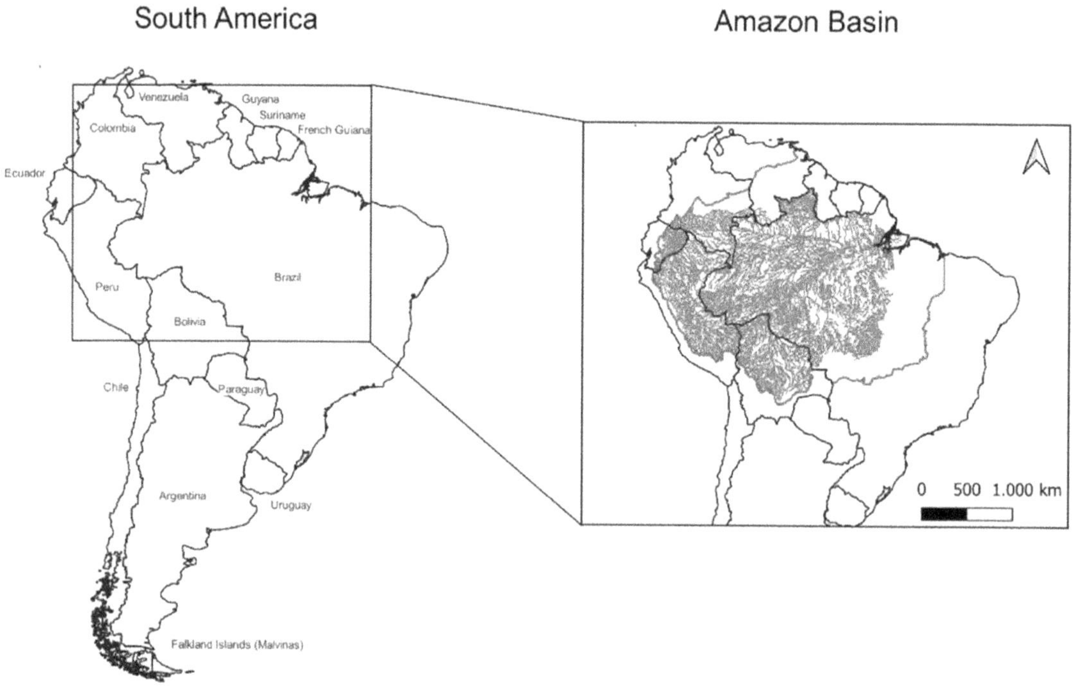

FIGURE 1 Limits of Amazon Basin (orange line) used by consortium of civil society organizations from the Amazon countries (RAISG 2022). Reprinted from QGIS version 3.22 without any changes, under a CC BY license

global land biodiversity (Hubbell *et al.* 2008, Nobre *et al.* 2016), and is a major global contributor to climate regulation (Li *et al.* 2015, Latrubesse *et al.* 2017, Metzger *et al.* 2019).

The region is currently under a process of biophysical transition, involving deforestation, changes in rainfall regime, and multiple anthropogenic activities such as timber, agriculture and mining (Gutierrez-Cori *et al.* 2021, Leite-Filho *et al.* 2019, Brando *et al.* 2020, Ruiz-Vásquez *et al.* 2020). Studies demonstrate that changes in land use and land cover can affect the biodiversity, climate change and the sustainability at local and global scales (Ferreira *et al.* 2014, Barlow *et al.* 2016, Abessa *et al.* 2019). Consequently, it can impact the provision of essential ecosystem services and has been repeatedly linked to the increased risk (and incidence) of emerging and re-emerging infectious diseases (Castro *et al.* 2019, MacDonald and Mordecai 2019). The Amazon Basin also plays an important role in regulating local and regional climate patterns, contributing as a buffer against global climate change (Nobre *et al.* 2016).

Climate change has been called the 'biggest global health threat of the 21st century' (Watts *et al.* 2019). The effects of climate change on ecosystem services and human health are wide and broad-ranging – from direct impacts of extreme weather such as hurricanes, drought and heatwaves, heavy rains with extensive areas of flooding, to indirect effects mediated through natural systems such as the rise and re-emergence of vector – and waterborne diseases, to tertiary effects such as undernutrition and mental health. The crisis has deep implications for human health and will affect the entire population, but vulnerable groups such as traditional communities, children, the elderly, and people with comorbidities are the most impacted due to structural and social vulnerabilities and their lifestyles. For example, the climate crisis has increasingly recognized implications for children's health and well-being (Helldén *et al.* 2021).

The Amazon Basin includes a diversity of native and anthropogenic environments that determine the sustainability of life of the local populations and the biodiversity of the Amazonian fauna and flora. Native tropical forest is divided into primary forest, with greater coverage, and secondary forest. This region also includes savannas such as the Cerrado on the eastern and southern limits of the Brazilian Amazon and in the Llanos de Mojos, in the Bolivian Amazon. In addition to natural water bodies, this area also includes artificial bodies of water, such as reservoirs, large dams, and areas dedicated to agropastoral production (Carreiras *et al.* 2006, Maezumi *et al.* 2022).

This diverse region is characterized by a range of weather patterns. Studies analysing rainfall trends in the Amazon for last four decades have showed average annual precipitation of 2,200 mm, ranging from 3,000 mm in west due to the influence of the Andes mountains, to values around 1,700 mm over southeast of the basin. There is a North-South opposite rainfall trend, with precipitation increase in the Northern and decrease in Southern of Amazon (SPA 2021). Long-term changes in precipitation trends in the basin can affect the continental water balance and the world's climate (Paca *et al.* 2020). This scenario results in environments conducive to expansion of populations of disease vectors associated with malaria and other vector-borne diseases, such as yellow fever, chikungunya, and dengue (Pan *et al.* 2014, Lowe *et al.* 2021). This can increase disease transmission, outbreaks, vector breeding sites, and change the distribution of vector-borne diseases (VBD). Although this encompasses a diverse group of mosquito species, the development of larvae and mosquitos are intrinsically associated to environmental factors, mainly due the link to aquatic breeding sites in climatic favourable conditions for their development. Because of this, all mosquito-borne diseases are impacted by land use changes (Norris 2004) and climate change (Reiter 2010).

Although the entire biome is characterized by the coverage of areas suitable to mosquitoes, specific areas and populations are more vulnerable to vector-borne diseases due to changes in land cover and resulting environmental consequences as well as the social and behavioural characteristics of highly vulnerable resident populations (Richards *et al.* 2014, Orellana *et al.* 2017). In this scenario of high sensitivity and vulnerability associated with the occurrence of vector-borne diseases, malaria has historically impacted the health of local populations driven largely by anthropogenic disasters (Howard *et al.* 1996, Kouadio *et al.* 2012). These anthropogenic disasters are directly and indirectly associated with human actions in the region and can intensify VBD occurrence, incidence and impacts on the population and the health system.

In the last decade, (2010–2020) natural disasters of extreme proportions have impacted different areas of the world, lead to infectious disease outbreaks when they result in substantial population displacement and exacerbate synergic risk factors for disease transmission. These disasters cause unparalleled destruction and loss of lives and property. In all cases, they increased the potential for acquisition of infectious diseases caused by bacteria, viruses, protozoans, mould, and mildew. This has highlighted how disasters represent a public health concern exacerbated by the fact that many factors may work synergistically to increase the risk of morbidity and mortality caused by communicable diseases (Kouadio *et al.* 2012).

Classifying the taxonomy of natural disasters is challenging as events can occur simultaneously or sequentially (Below *et al.* 2009). This difficulty is particularly pronounced for associated disasters or secondary disasters, as exemplified by The Centre for Research on the Epidemiology of Disasters (CRED): '*a flood which was a consequence of a windstorm may be recorded as one or the other; or a flood recorded as such in one database could be recorded as a cyclone in another*' (Below et al. 2009). One of the cores aims of CRED is to define a standard to improve the comparison of data sets, to find and assess associations between impacts and compare the cases, enabling development of mitigatory measures and policies to damage reduction. Therefore, extreme events are categorized into six disaster groups: biological (e.g. parasitic infectious diseases), geophysical (e.g. earthquake), meteorological (e.g. storms), hydrological (e.g. floods), climatological (e.g. droughts, heat weaves, etc.) and extra-terrestrial (e.g. meteorite) (Below *et al.* 2009). Hydrometeorological hazards are the most common natural hazards; these relate to the climate, or movement of wet mass such as floods, droughts, oceans. Other common hazards include heat waves, such as the 2010 Russian heat wave, which resulted in a disaster responsible for 56,000 deaths (Prasad and Francescutti 2017).

Hazards are defined as the potential occurrence of a natural or human-induced physical event or trend that may cause loss of life, injury, or other health impacts, as well as damage and loss to property, infrastructure, livelihoods, service provision, ecosystems and environmental resources (IPCC 2022a). They are grouped into three categories, technological, natural, and environmental degradation hazards (UNISDR 2004). Technological hazards are industrial (pollution), nuclear (nuclear leak), or structural (dam collapse), while environmental degradation hazards include events that disrupt the environment, ecosystem, or natural resources, i.e. deforestation, forest fires and climate change (Prasad and Francescutti 2017).

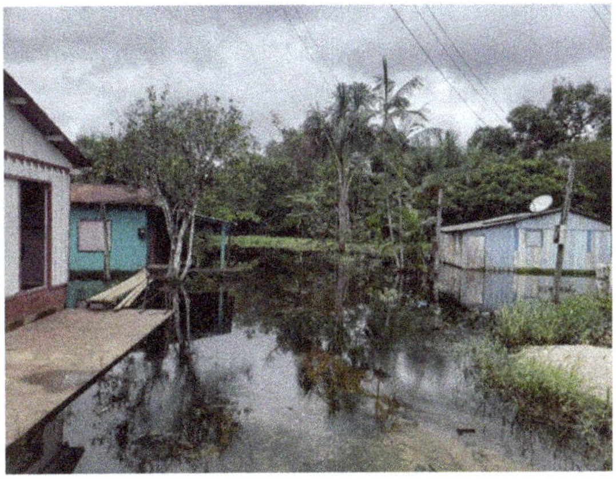

FIGURE 2
Flooded houses in Amazonian riverine community, Barcelos/Amazonas, Brazil
PHOTO FROM JUNE-2022; LEONARDO SUVEGES MOREIRA CHAVES

Biological hazards are included in environmental degradation hazards and are events that involve the rapid incidence of vector-driven diseases, toxins, or pathogens. These hazards can act synergistically to increase the impact of a disaster. For example, a technological hazard (dam collapse) and biological hazard (dengue fever) caused major human impacts when the rupture of a dam belonging to a mining company caused a 19% increase in the probability of dengue fever epidemic in Mariana municipality, Minas Gerais, Brazil. This occurred mainly due to water supply failures, reducing the amounts of water suitable for human consumption leading to incorrect water storage which increased mosquito proliferation and human migration (Nishijima and Rocha 2020, Parekh *et al.* 2020). Meteorological hazards such as flooding (Figure 2), storms, heat waves also can affect vector breeding sites and vector-borne disease transmission.

In this chapter, we present the complexity of drivers of malaria components such as effects from deforestation into directions linked to climate change, and other degradation factors that are increasing malaria transmission in Amazon Basin. There are explored the vulnerabilities associated to natural disaster scenarios, and how this impacts community exposure to the illness, considering the historic and structural patterns of land use and recent climate threats.

2 Disasters, extreme climate events and malaria outbreaks: synergistic forces

While the most attention has been given to hydrometeorological and geophysical disasters, whether they are driven by anthropogenic actions, or not, natural disasters cause synergistic human and environmental impacts, including serious damage and losses to human. This chapter contextualized these forces on environmental disturbance and wellbeing of human health. Affected populations are typically unable to live in their houses after a disaster, creating knock on effects to community welfare, livelihood systems, health services capacity, and social development (Munang *et al.* 2013). Globally, 44% of hydrologic disasters, and 17% have been associated with tropical cyclones (WMO 2021). Tropical cyclones and droughts were the most common hazards with respect to human loss of life, accounting for 38% and 34% of disaster related deaths from 1970 to 2019, respectively (WMO 2021). In terms of economic losses, 38% were associated with tropical cyclones, 3% of all of deaths from meteorological, climate and hydrological hazards (Zhongming and Wei 2021). The World Bank reports 82% of deaths associated with natural disasters occurred in low and lower-middle-income countries while most (88%) of the economic losses have occurred in upper-middle- and high-income countries (World Bank 2021). According to Georeferenced Emergency Events Database (EM-DAT) records from 1970 to 2019 (www.emdat.be), weather, climate and hydrological hazards accounted for 50% of all disasters, 45% of all reported deaths and 74% of all reported economic losses, translating to 2.06 million deaths and US$ 3.6 trillion in economic losses (WMO 2021). When outbreaks of disease, including epidemics and pandemics, and societal hazards are added, these figures grow substantially. People with higher levels of vulnerability and lower capacity to manage risks are disproportionately affected. Factors affecting vulnerability include poverty, gender, age, disability, poor health, and poor nutritional status. Poverty is therefore both a cause and consequence of disaster risk, particularly extensive risk, with drought being the hazard most closely associated with poverty (UNDRR 2022). The effects on populations include disabilities, disease outbreaks, death and longer-term health impacts (Leaning and Guha-Sapir 2013).

However, the increase of endemic diseases and the risk of outbreaks are dependent on many factors. In general, the risk of outbreaks is associated not only with the scale of the disaster but also with the underlying health status of the population, the capacity of health services and living conditions of the population displaced by the natural disaster (Charnley *et al.* 2021). In countries with large populations with high social vulnerabilities, low economic status and living under political instability, of disasters can have disproportionate impacts (Raju and Otto 2022, Seneviratne *et al.* 2021). While the mortality and financial cost of a natural disaster is certainly linked to the severity of the hazard, it is also highly dependent on how vulnerable a population is to potential disastrous effects (Prasad and Francescutti 2017). Managing risk may be a matter of not only identifying environmental dimensions of hazards but also understanding the nature of vulnerability and resilience, and how this relates to the social determinants of health (Wisner *et al.* 2012). Whereas resilience is defined as the capacity of social, economic and ecosystems to cope with a hazardous event or trend or disturbance, responding or reorganizing in ways that maintain their essential function, identity, and structure as well as biodiversity in case of ecosystems while also maintaining the capacity for adaptation, learning and transformation (IPCC 2022a).

3 Climate change in the Amazon Basin

Globally, the main impact of forest degradation is the increase in greenhouse gas (GHG) emissions due to carbon loss (Aguiar *et al.* 2016). The intensification of the global warming process represents numerous risks for natural ecosystems and consequently to human health. However, the most vulnerable natural systems are those that lose a significant portion of their life-supporting mechanisms such as biodiversity conservation, income, subsistence farms and agriculture for self-consumption, water security (IPCC 2014). In the Amazon Basin, traditional communities depend on natural systems for their survival and cultural life. Extreme events, such as heatwaves, extreme temperatures, and increased frequency of droughts, are causing regional abrupt changes and pushing ecosystems towards tipping points with severe impacts local and globally (Allan *et al.* 2021). While the ongoing COVID-19 crisis is causing unprecedented stress and disruptions to health systems, climate change will have even greater and more significant consequences (Mariana and Mashida 2020).

Brazilian Amazon has received considerable attention in relation to climate change as a large fraction of tropical forest clearing has occurred within this region (Ellwanger *et al.* 2020). Studies carried out in the Amazon basin have predicted a nearly 60% rainfall reduction and a 2 °C increase in the air temperature with possible scenarios of Amazonian deforestation (Lovejoy and Nobre 2019). This would convert forest to savannah areas, leading to major increases in heating. This elevated heat stress exposure is highly likely to increase morbidity and mortality in heat-vulnerable populations, including children, the elderly, pregnant women, and people with comorbidity (De Oliveira *et al.* 2020). Considering that exposure is here defined as the presence of people; livelihoods; species or ecosystems; environmental functions, services, and resources; infrastructure; or economic, social or cultural assets in places and settings that could be adversely affected (IPCC 2022a).

Extreme temperatures can be detrimental to the development of mosquitoes, and extreme weather events, such as droughts, can limit mosquito-breeding sites. However, deforestation and the increase in average temperature may favour the proliferation of disease vectors, such as *Aedes aegypti* and *Ae. albopictus* in different regions of Brazil, and other Amazonian countries (Ellwanger *et al.* 2020). Extreme events and deforestation can act synergistically through coupled mechanisms. Environmental changes such as land degradation have increased the destructive potential of extreme climatic events. Deforested areas can affect regional climate, and the regional climate can amplify the impact of deforestation, by increasing forest degradation far beyond the limits of the deforestation edges (Kruid *et al.* 2021). The increase in the frequency and intensity of extreme climate-related disasters in the recent decades highlights the need for global governance.

The Amazon rainforest is crucial for maintaining planetary health due to its role in regulating the Earth's climate (Nobre *et al.* 2016). Planetary health is a concept based on the understanding that human health and human civilization depend on ecosystem health and the wise stewardship of ecosystems. The term 'losses and damages' refer to adverse observed impacts and/or projected risks and can be economic and/or non-economic impacts and risks are expressed in terms of their damages, harms, economic, and noneconomic losses (IPCC 2022a). Therefore, in a broader perspective, protecting Amazon ecosystems is essential for biodiversity preservation, global climate regulation, energy production, food and water security and to maintain a resilient social-ecological system. It is also important for pollination, natural and biological control of pests, technological advances in the production of new medicines and new materials as well as the region's economy, human health, and culture. The biodiversity of the Amazon rainforest plays a role of local, regional and global importance for the structure, dynamics and control of zoonoses and vector-borne infections (Metzger *et al.* 2019, Moraes *et al.* 2019, Valli and Bolzani 2019).

Projections of environmental degradation in South America show that Amazon region is has the highest increase in wildfire throughout the present century (Pivello *et al.* 2021). Forest fires in the Amazon exemplify the immense problem of deforestation with profound implications on ecosystem services, changing water, air and soil quality, impoverishing habitats and biodiversity, and affecting carbon cycling (Pellegrini *et al.* 2018, Brando *et al.* 2020) and, consequently, the resilience of terrestrial and aquatic ecosystems (Pellegrini *et al.* 2021). In addition, changes in the atmospheric composition such as GHG, nitrogen oxides (NOx) and sulphur dioxide (SO_2), can alter climatic variables in several regions of the planet, among them the Brazilian Amazon Basin (Bonan *et al.* 2008, Houghton *et al.* 2015, Gomes *et al.* 2019). Air pollution from fires poses a serious health risk to the Amazon population in relation respiratory and cardiovascular diseases (Butt *et al.* 2020, Campanharo *et al.* 2021). Additionally, forest fires can trigger of infectious diseases outbreaks and/or disasters related to endemic diseases. All these impacts create health hazards for traditional people, indigenous and urban populations in the Amazon.

4 Drivers of land use change in the Amazon Basin

Anthropogenic land use change (LUC) is the major driver of global environmental change (Song *et al.* 2018). The process decreases biodiversity and carbon storage, shifting the local microclimate, affecting the burden, and distribution of infectious disease (Alkama and Cescatti 2016). Vector-borne diseases – pathogens transmitted by biting arthropods – are particularly linked to forest loss and fragmentation due to changes in host and vector communities, vector breeding habitat, microclimate suitability, and vector-human contact rates (Bonan and Doney 2018).

Changes in land use, involving deforestation, have been associated with the proliferation of *Ny. darlingi* (formerly *Anopheles darlingi*) species, the main vector of *Plasmodium* in Amazon Basin (Recht *et al.* 2017), illustrating how malaria emergence and deforestation are often linked in a web of causal mechanisms (Tucker *et al.* 2017). Deforestation creates stark transitions between forests and open areas with major impacts on ecosystems (Curtis *et al.* 2018), economies (Geist and Lambin 2002), and human health (Dobson *et al.* 2020). Forest disturbance is an important predictor for the emergence of arboviral and parasitic diseases (Laporta 2019). This process is associated with involves social, economic, and environmental factors. Tree cover loss is driven by anthropogenic land use changes that increase extreme climate events (IPCC 2012), and malaria incidence (Chaves *et al.* 2018, Laporta *et al.* 2021, MacDonald and Mordecai 2019, Garg 2019, Berazneva and Byker 2017).

In most cases, the ecological mechanisms that guide the emergence and persistence of human malaria in these areas result in favourable environmental conditions for mosquitoes, mainly by creating larval habitats (Barros *et al.* 2011, Barros and Honório 2015, Rufalco-Moutinho *et al.* 2016). Deforestation can cause physical changes linked to the formation of breeding sites, the chemical composition of water and soil due to pH conditions and microbiota, an important element for the trophic chain to larvae of these insects. These variables alter the composition of mosquito species (Chaves *et al.* 2021), increasing vector density and their distribution in certain landscapes (Hiwat and Bretas 2011). Other anopheline species also have this close ecological relationship with deforestation, such as *Anopheles gambiae* and *An. arabiensis* in Africa (Afrane *et al.* 2006, Afrane *et al.* 2007), and *An. dirus* and *An. minimus* s.l. in Southeast Asia (Manguin *et al.* 2002, Van Bortel *et al.* 2000). This highlights how extractive and farming practices, such as mining and fish farming, can increase risks of malaria outbreaks.

Open gold mining in the Amazon is characterized by formation of pits, the result of excavation of clay, mud, sand, and gravel left by flowing streams. The environmental liabilities left by mining, becoming water reservoirs and excellent breeding grounds for mosquitoes (Galardo *et al.* 2013, Oliveira-Ferreira *et al.* 2010). In addition to the pits, the morphology of rivers can be seriously altered by excavation and abandoned mining sites, impeding the flow of rivers, and forming backwaters favourable to mosquitoes (Sanchez-Ribas *et al.* 2012, Sánchez-Ribas *et al.* 2015). Other land-use impacts occur through fish farming for trade and consumption, with fishponds identified as important breeding sites of *Ny. darlingi* in Brazil (Dos Reis *et al.* 2015, Ferreira *et al.* 2015, Rufalco-Moutinho *et al.* 2021). In this context,

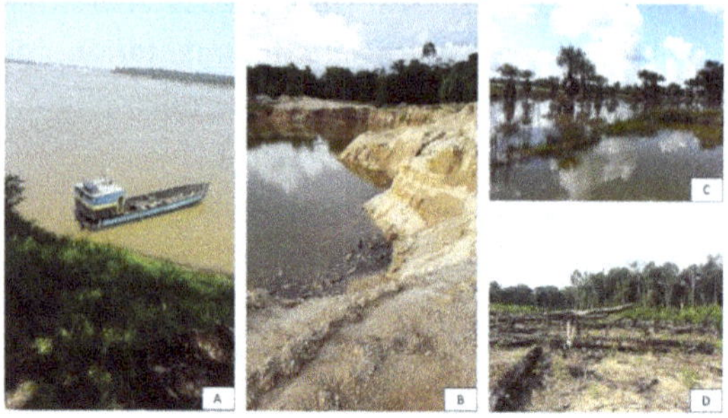

FIGURE 3
Examples of anthropogenic drivers that can increase malaria incidence in Amazon Basin areas. A) hydroelectric power plant, B) open gold mining, C) fishponds, and D) deforestation
PHOTOS: LEONARDO SUVEGES MOREIRA CHAVES

some local economic activities can cause anthropogenic disasters, either biological or geophysical types, driven by a global demand for primary commodities associated with deforestation for international trade of exports (Chaves *et al.* 2020).

Abandoned pits from gold mining, fishponds, deforestation or establishment of hydroelectric power plants in Amazon (Figure 3) exemplify synergistic effects of anthropogenic disaster forces; for example, with these changes leading to combined impacts of mudslide, mosquito proliferation and vector-borne diseases (Soares *et al.* 2021, Rufalco-Moutinho *et al.* 2021, dos Reis *et al.* 2015). There is a critical need to define regulations for activities such as mining, fish farming activities and the expansion of agropastoral activity as a driver of both human disease impacts and changes in land use in the Amazon Basin.

Characterizing land use changes in the Amazon requires understanding of temporal cycles of deforestation. These cycles are marked by a period of increased fires occurring illegally during the dry season in the biome. At the end of the fire season, areas of the soil without forest cover are largely occupied by pastures, mainly in areas close to the rivers (Dos Reis *et al.* 2021). These newly occupied areas create environments conducive to the development of malaria vectors, as well as an increase in human population flow and the intensification of local environmental degradation and inequalities (Castro *et al.* 2019).

Under 1985 to 2020, the agropastoral activity was the main cause of loss of forested area (~ 75,000 ha) in Amazon Basin (mapbiomas.org). Causes of expansion of water bodies include hydroelectric projects, as discussed in Box 1. In this period, Brazil was the country that lost the most forested area (15%), followed by Bolivia (13%), Colombia (7%), Ecuador (7%) and Peru (5%) (Figure 4). The countries with the lowest loss of forested area were Guyana, French Guiana and Suriname, with 1% each, and Venezuela with 3%. Most previously forested land was converted into agriculture except in countries where forest loss was comparatively much lower, such as Guyana, French Guiana and Suriname. This highlights the role of agricultural expansion in the deforestation of the Amazon Basin (MapBiomas 2022). The change of areas previously covered by native forest to land for agricultural production or pasture is one of the main drivers of deforestation in the Amazon (Fearnside 2001, MapBiomas 2022).

Box 1: Large and small dams in the Amazon Basin and impacts on the incidence of malaria

One of the main anthropogenic environmental changes in the Amazon Basin is the construction and operation of dams. These changes create environments conducive to malaria vector populations by permanently altering the water flow and the coverage of riverbanks. This additionally compromises the way of life of the riverside populations and may intensely increasing influxes of vulnerable human populations (Castro *et al.* 2019). Sanches *et al.* 2012 presented a review of the effects of dam construction on anopheline bionomics and malaria transmission. The authors found six different vector species with increased densities and identified increased malaria transmission in four of ten dams included in the study.

Not only can large dams result in increases in the density of vectors and the incidence of malaria, but small dams can also impact the distribution of the disease. In a study carried out in sub-Saharan Africa, Kibret *et al.* (2021) identified that the impact of small dams on the incidence of malaria was greater than that of large dams, due to the higher population density close to these dams and the fact that small dams can create an environment more conducive to malaria transmission.

A well-known example of the impact of dam construction on the diversity and density of malaria vectors is the Tucuruí Dam, in the state of Pará, in

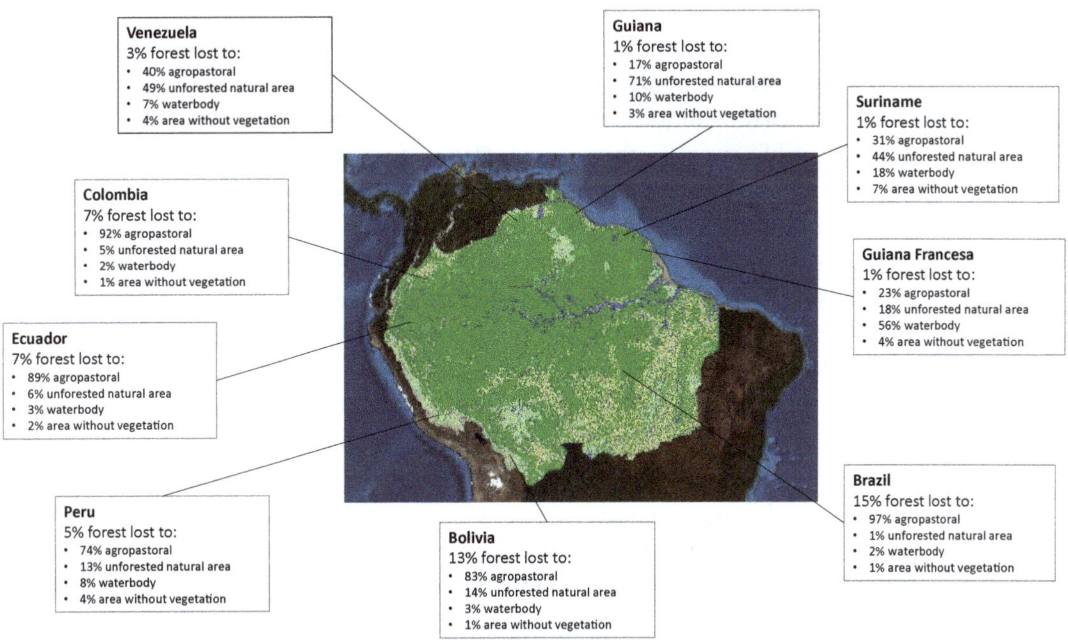

FIGURE 4 Area of native forest lost (%) and new land cover by country of Amazonian Basin between 1985 to 2020 (MapBiomas 2022)

the Brazilian Amazon. While *Ny. darlingi*, the main vector of malaria in the Brazilian Amazon, decreased in abundance after the construction of the dam, introductions of new species not previously recorded in the region, such as *Ny. braziliensis*, were reported. Additionally, there were other species detected with similar abundance before and after the reservoir was filled, including *Ny. oswaldi*, *Ny. argyritarsis*, *An. mediopunctatus*, *Ny. evansae*, *An. intermedius* and *Ny. rangeli*. This diversity of vectors, associated with the large increase in the human population in the area resulting from the presence of the hydroelectric plant, resulted in the persistence of malaria in the region and challenged existing vector control measures (Fearnside 2015).

Overall, it is reasonable to consider mosquito proliferation a biological disaster, often occurring after other natural disasters such as after tropical cyclones (typhoons, hurricanes, and cyclones) which are frequently associated with flooding (Barrera *et al.* 2019, Qualls and Breidenbaugh 2020).

5 Forest disturbance, influences on seasonality patterns and malaria incidence

Malaria has many drivers, causing dynamic and heterogeneous transmission patterns. These can be classified into three major components: entomological factors, parasite transmission, and human behaviour. These components interact in receptive environments. For example, malaria incidence is highly correlated with seasonal patterns of rainfall and dry season length (Chaves *et al.* 2018, Galardo *et al.* 2009), leading to increasing vector sources, decreases in the duration of the *Plasmodium* life cycle (Gething *et al.* 2011), or forced human migration (Barbieri and Carr 2005). Warming temperatures have nonlinear associations with malaria transmission; transmission may increase in warmer temperatures due to decreased of parasites sporogony duration but this trend is reversed with extremely temperatures causing thermal death of vector populations (Gething *et al.* 2011). These temperature trends can also impact mosquito populations by reducing the duration of the aquatic immature life stage (Chu *et al.* 2019).

In this context, climate phenomena such as El Niño-Southern Oscillation (ENSO) and La Niña-Southern Oscillation (LNSO) have great influence on precipitation regimes and temperature in Amazon region, causing extreme events (Marengo *et al.* 2011). The occurrence of LNSO is associated to increase the volume of precipitation, while ENSO can also increase the temperature within this region (Moura *et al.* 2019). Despite apparently random intervals of both phenomena, the Intergovernmental Panel on Climate Change (IPCC) have indicated that extreme ENSO and LNSO events are projected to increase in frequency in the 21st century, intensifying the hazards, causing drier or wetter responses in regions across the globe, including in the Amazon. These synergistic hazards threaten local people through weather-sensitive outbreaks of malaria, and other mosquito borne diseases. Flooding caused by ENSO has been associated with malaria epidemics in northern Peru, while conversely, droughts are associated with increased malaria cases in Colombia, Guyana, and Venezuela (Gagnon *et al.* 2002).

In ecological system of malaria, much of the natural environment of Amazon Basin has been exposed to radical changes and severe alterations of its ecosystems, (Pan *et al.* 2007, Ferreira and Castro 2016) with impacts on human health, especially for the traditional and indigenous communities (Da Cruz Franco 2019). The main environmental factors that can explain the spatial and temporal variations of the malaria transmission in the Amazon are the presence and characteristics of water bodies, climate change, economic activities, land use, urban-to-rural mobility and social conditions. These factors interact with individual based characteristics and behaviours of mosquitoes and humans to give rise to complex spatial and temporal patterns (Pizzitutti *et al.* 2013). The Amazon Basin contributes approximately 90% of the region's malaria burden (Ferreira and Castro 2019). In addition, vectors and parasites can be influenced by extent of daily temperature and precipitation variation.

The development of *P. falciparum* is highly dependent on temperature and ceases when the temperature is below 16 °C (Paaijmans *et al.* 2010). In addition, variation in climatic conditions such as temperature, rainfall patterns, and humidity, has a profound effect on the longevity of the mosquito and on the development of malaria parasites in the mosquito and, subsequently, on malaria transmission. Higher ambient temperatures increase the metabolic rate of the insect, increasing the number of bites. In addition, higher temperatures support faster development of the malaria parasite within the mosquito, increasing the probability that vectors will become infective before they die. As a result, human-vector contact – and the frequency of infective bites – are increased at higher temperatures. However, beyond temperatures of 35 °C, the survival of the vector declines. The transmission potential of the vector appears to have an optimal temperature of around 28–31 °C, however, recent findings show that this value could be as low as 25 °C (Blanford *et al.* 2013, Mordecai *et al.* 2013). Rainfall is also an important predictor of vector density, with commonly reported lag times of 1–2 weeks (Koenraadt *et al.* 2004). The onset of the rainy season has been associated with increasing incidence of malaria, leading to the development of seasonal forecasts and early warning systems in some regions (Ikeda *et al.* 2017). Humidity has been assessed as a relevant variable to lifespan of mosquitoes in some regions (Chaves and Koenraadt 2010).

However, we can ask: do extreme meteorological events have reciprocal responses in malaria transmission? Do rivers flooding, triggered by these events, flush out and wash away larvae breeding sites of vectors, and could decreasing malaria transmission? Do extreme temperatures increase mortality rate of adult females? What is the optimum temperature range for the dominant vector? There are so few fieldworks studies about bionomy of Amazonian malaria vectors on extreme events and their meteorological parameters in natural disasters scenario, but there are some clues that might help answer these questions. Studies have observed that adults of *Ny. darlingi* increase with the rise in temperature, within the range 16–34 °C, with results showing that approximately two months with consecutives days with a minimal temperature below 22.5 °C increase adult densities, while approximately two weeks consecutive days with a maximal temperature above 33.2 °C decrease *Ny. darlingi* densities, and a maximum number of consecutive days without rainfall during the 49 days decrease the densities (Vezenegho *et al.* 2015, Adde *et al.* 2016). Therefore, the perturbation represented by recent climate change scenario can shift ecological niches, turning it a suitable habitat to other species such as *Ny. marajoara* and *Ny. albitarsis* complex vectors or expand *Ny. darlingi* distribution together *Plasmodium* to other areas on Amazon Basin (Conn *et al.* 2002, Laporta *et al.* 2015).

6 Malaria in the Amazon Basin – complex interactions and endemic challenges

Countries of Amazon Basin reported an estimated 483,000 malaria cases in 2020 (WHO 2021). These countries have also experienced natural disasters such as flooding in 2020, leading to population displacements and public health service disruptions, increasing the risk of exposure to malaria infection (Rentschler and Salhab 2020, WHO 2021). With the increase of frequency of natural disasters due to climate change, the understanding epidemiological patterns of disease in relation to extreme events is crucial to surveillance and control of malaria cases in the Amazon basin.

Besides climate conditions, the dynamics of malaria transmission is also highly sensitive to anthropogenic activities (Castro *et al.* 2019, Parham and Michael 2010). This vector-borne disease is caused by Apicomplexa parasites, *Plasmodium falciparum, P. vivax, P. malariae, P. ovale,* and *P. knowlesi,* and is capable to drive out entire communities, some through death and others fleeing for a safe place to live (Williams *et al.* 2003). *Plasmodium falciparum* is more dangerous to human health than the *P. vivax*, as the parasites species reproduces at much higher rates in humans (Johansen *et al.* 2020). There is evidence that *P. falciparum* entered in Amazon Basin carried by Trans-Atlantic slave trade between the 16th and 17th centuries, and *P. vivax* lineages have originated from Melanesia and were carried to Amazon Basin by the Australasian migrants to native Americans in pre-Columbian times (Rodrigues *et al.* 2018). It is a tropical and subtropical endemic disease with incidence in Amazon basin and other tropical forests frontiers in the world, such as in sub-Saharan Africa, and Southeast Asia (WHO 2021). The process of European colonization of South American continent carried human malaria to native peoples through infected colonizers and competent vectors (Rodrigues *et al.* 2018). These vectors include species of mosquitoes that already present in the ecosystems of the colonies such as *Ny. darlingi*, capable of triggering epidemics resulting in many indigenous deaths.

In some areas of Amazon, malaria may not be a severe illness or cause of death, but it may have an extensive public health impact through harmful effects on socio-cultural and economic development, loss of work productivity, increased morbidity and causing children to have low levels of cognitive development, anaemia, and malnutrition (Tapajós *et al.* 2019, Castro *et al.* 2019). This also places a burden on health systems withing this region, leading to increased demand for hospitalization and outpatient care due to malaria cases, costs for malaria surveillance strategies and provision of resources for diagnosis and treatment. These costs are borne by the primary care facilities within the region, demanding increased financial and human resources. In addition to the impacts on human health, malaria is still responsible for absenteeism, including school absenteeism, resulting in the intensification of factors associated with socioeconomic vulnerability in the region (Braz and Barcellos 2016).

The incidence of malaria in the region varies spatially, that is, between and within countries, but also temporally, with varying incidence over time. Across all countries in the Amazon Basin, there was a reduction in the number of cases until 2014. In 2015 there was an increase in the registration of cases until 2019. However, the 2020 records should be interpreted with caution, as the region's epidemiological surveillance systems were overwhelmed by the COVID-19 pandemic. Thus, it is possible that the number of malaria cases in the region has increased, including cases in indigenous peoples.

Observing the evolution of the number of malaria cases between 2010 and 2020 in each country that makes up the Amazon Basin, it is possible observed that second half of decade is marked by an increase in cases in many countries: Bolivia, Brazil, Ecuador and Venezuela. Other countries show a certain stability, such as Colombia, or a moderate reduction in Peru.

The vulnerabilities associated with the incidence of malaria in the Amazon biome refer to biological, socioeconomic and environmental determinants. In relation to biological determinants, biophysical factors can increase not only the incidence of the disease, but its severity, by increasing the demand for care through hospitalization or treatment and increasing the number of deaths associated with severe malaria, a multi-syndromic disease with cerebral, anaemia and respiratory implications (WHO 2021). The population group most vulnerable to malaria are children under 5 years of age and pregnant women, mainly in Sub-Saharan Africa, (Barbieri and Soares-Filho 2005, WHO 2021), with highest burdens of disease mortality and morbidity (Meremikwu *et al.* 2009, Cohee and Laufer 2017). Furthermore, children under 5 years of age who survive malaria may remain with neurological sequelae due to *falciparum* malaria infection (Meremikwu *et al.* 2009, Kihara *et al.* 2006).

7 Vulnerabilities to malaria in disaster scenarios in the Amazon

The vulnerabilities to malaria in Amazon Basin are quite different of Africa and Southeast Asia. In general, the vulnerable groups in Africa are children and pregnant women, in Asia are forest workers, while in Amazon are males of working age with occupation activities such as artisanal mining (garimpo) workers, loggers for timber or hunters (Feged-Rivadeneira *et al.* 2019). These groups may be highly vulnerable to malaria due to socioeconomic factors. These include the level of socioeconomic development of the population, which should be understood not only as per capita income, but also in terms of access to urban infrastructure services, such as adequate sanitation, and access to health services. Among the main socioeconomic factors associated with malaria incidence are educational level of the population exposed, location and housing type, health services, nutritional level, income education and/or occupation (Worral *et al.* 2005). These factors have been demonstrated to be associated with the incidence of malaria in the Amazon Basin (Gomes *et al.* 2020).

It is important to note that, despite the strong associations between human development factors and *Plasmodium* infection, these factors do not occur in isolation, so that populations with less access to educational services and sanitary structure also tend to have lower nutritional levels and limited health service access. As highlighted by Worral *et al.* (2005), it is difficult to indicate that there is a direct link between malaria and individual or household poverty, but rather a complex manifestation of poverty in association with economic activity and health care. An example of interactions between social factors that increase malaria transmission in the Amazon Basin is the association between illegal gold mining and the increase in the number of malaria cases (Sanches *et al.* 2017, Ueno *et al.* 2021). In the Brazilian Amazon from 2010 to 2020, the areas invaded by illegal gold mining within indigenous lands grew by 495%; this change may explain a considerable increase in the spread of malaria in indigenous territories, mainly in recent years (Oliveira 2022).

The low level of education, combined with the lower availability of formal jobs and the high profitability of the activity, compared to other possible occupations in the region, means that there is no shortage of manpower for illegal mining activities. Associated with this is the maintenance and promotion of the activity by politicians or entrepreneurs with high regional and/or national power, the maintenance of international trade links and the absence of effective control policies that stop these activities (Siqueira-Gay and Sanchez 2021). Finally, illegal mining alters the forest environment so that, in addition to deforestation, soil and water bodies are contaminated and environments conducive to the proliferation of malaria vectors (Basta and Hacon 2020). Therefore, regions are found in the Amazon Basin where the local population, in some cases with high food insecurity and other vulnerabilities, live with frequent epidemics of malaria and other endemic diseases, in addition to exposure to pollutants such as mercury. This increases the burden of comorbidities in the population and results in preventable deaths. Such a scenario has been observed among the Yanomami indigenous population living in the state of Roraima, Brazil (Orellana *et al.* 2019).

Environmental vulnerabilities are understood as the environmental aspects that favour exposure to vectors, such as exposure to the drivers indicated above, but also to factors that intensify the flow of people and threats to the way of life of the native population. In this sense, populations residing in border areas are particularly more exposed, especially in the triple border formed by Brazil, Peru and Colombia (Castro *et al.* 2006, Peiter *et al.* 2013). Border regions are especially vulnerable due not only to the population flow, but also to the difficulties imposed on epidemiological and environmental surveillance due to the different actors responsible for assistance and surveillance in the region, which often act in a disjointed way (Peiter *et al.* 2013).

Another environmental factor that results in greater exposure to malaria vectors is proximity to roads in the Amazon Basin since these local populations are more exposed to the flow of people and the pressure of human actions that alter the land cover in the Amazon. In these scenarios, in addition to the intense forest fragmentation, which results in peri-urban environments conducive to the development of vectors, there is also an expansion of settlements without sanitary structures and generally less access to health services (Souza *et al.* 2019).

8 The first public actions to combat malaria in indigenous territories in Brazil: a brief history

Considering the relevance of malaria on public health into South America, and vulnerabilities of indigenous people to government policies (Conceição *et al.* 2021), the Brazilian fight against malaria on indigenous territories shows a good overview about strengths, weaknesses, opportunities, and threats in South America context.

With the formation of Brazilian State and the Federative Republic of Brazil, the Brazilian government created, in 1965, the Malaria Eradication Campaign (in Portuguese *Campanha de Erradicação da Malária* – CEM) and five years later the Superintendence of Public Health Campaigns (in Portuguese *Superintendência de Campanhas de Saúde Pública* – SUCAM), subordinated to the Secretary of Health Public, until 1991. In 1993 the malaria control began to be decentralized, transferring responsibilities to municipalities and states (Fiocruz 2009), with the establishment of the National Health Foundation (in Portuguese *Fundação Nacional de Saúde* – *FUNASA*). These political processes were responsible for malaria care among indigenous peoples and to development good practices to combating the vector carried out by 'Endemics Guards' also known as Endemic Combat Agents (in Portuguese *Agente de Combate a Endemias* – *ACE*). Nowadays, activities such as indoor residual spraying and thermal fog are routinely carried out. Some weaknesses of the program involve difficulties in rapid diagnosis because long journeys to the villages for several days and months, that represent a great obstacle to control.

Between 1960s and 1970s, Brazilian Amazon experienced an abrupt increase of, infrastructure implementation and economic development, with constructions of roads, railways, hydroelectric plants, mining, oil exploration and the formation of colonization centres, communities, and villages. These events helped to spread malaria cases by creating favourable environmental conditions for the development of the *Ny. darlingi*, known in the villages as carapanã or malaria mosquito.

In 1967 was created the National Indian Foundation (in Portuguese Fundação Nacional do Índio – FUNAI) responsible for guaranteeing the permanent possession of indigenous lands and the exclusive usufruct of the natural resources and all the utilities existing therein, and in 1988 Brazil's Federal Constitution (art. 231) established the responsibility of the Union to protect and ensure respect for indigenous rights. At end of 20th century, FUNASA took over health care actions for indigenous people, founding the Indigenous Health Care Subsystem of the Brazilian Unified Health System (In Portuguese Subsistema de Atenção à Saúde Indígena do SUS – SASI-SUS), which included the formation of Multidisciplinary Teams of Indigenous Health (in Portuguese *Equipe Multidisciplinares de Saúde Indígena* – *EMSI*) organized into 'health territories', or Special Indigenous Health Districts (in Portuguese *Distrito Sanitário Especial Indígena* – *DSEI*) (Brazil 2016). This reorganization provided ACEs contracts to compose the EMSIs to continue vector control activities in the villages, previously carried out by SUCAM. In this way, municipalities and DSEIs became responsible for malaria prevention actions in indigenous territories. For decades, the main actions carried out in the villages were solely vector control activities. At beginning of 21st century was created the National Program to Combat Malaria (in Portuguese *Programa Nacional de Combate à Malária* – *PNCM*), highlighted the relevance of surveillance and health education (Brasil 2003). Therefore, the DSEIs and municipalities are currently responsible for creating strategies for preventing and combating malaria based on diagnostics, treatment, and vector control (Brasil 2003, Brasil 2016).

Historically, indigenous populations associated malaria with something serious, as it decimated many indigenous people and was considered an incurable disease. This was traditionally treated by shamans. However, within the 21st century, malaria (*P. vivax* and *P. falciparum*) has been understood by indigenous populations as a health problem, highlighted in many speeches of indigenous leaders and activists. External factors such as illegal mining, invasions of territories, large enterprises, deforestation, are an even greater challenge for health care when overlaid anthropogenic disasters. Therefore, it is necessary to invest in the training of ACEs and in the inclusion of EMSI in health surveillance and education actions (in practice). This highlights the fundamental role of the AIS in translating activities into indigenous language to communicate treatment and control activities. This enables indigenous communities to contribute to the supervision and conduction of vector control activities, such as the environmental management of potential breeding sites in their territories. The implementation of new socioeconomic policies is necessary to decrease the mobility of indigenous populations to urban areas and to promote the sanitation of the villages with the supply of treated water, reducing the search for water in the igarapés, where they can receive mosquito bites.

9 Challenges of malaria control in indigenous territories: the case of Amazonian Brazil

Local communities and indigenous people have been invited to partnerships with scientists to respond to climate change and to find opportunities to minimize negative impacts, including malaria (Huntington *et al.* 2017, Ogar *et al.* 2020). In this context, the main challenges in the fight against malaria highlighted by indigenous from Brazilian Amazon is the organization of health surveillance is necessary to incorporate local realities and cultural and linguistic differences between indigenous ethnicities. In the Brazilian Legal Amazon, formed by states of Acre, Amapá, Amazonas, Maranhão, Mato Grosso, Pará, Rondônia, Roraima and Tocantins, there are 160 different languages distributed among at least 180 different groups of indigenous peoples. This includes groups considered isolated accounting for approximately 114 records of indigenous people who chose to live freely and autonomously, without contact with the surrounding society (COIAB 2020). Thus, it is necessary to implement methodologies, socio-educational materials in indigenous languages, considering the prevention and control of the vectors in these regions.

Malaria in indigenous territories has been a major health problem in the villages. The Brazilian department of indigenous health (in Portuguese *Secretaria Especial de Saúde Indígena – SESAI*), malaria is officially one of the main indicators for assessing the health status. So, what is happening? Why does this disease remain persistent for many decades and outbreaks and epidemics reported in these villages? Answering these questions is a challenge but we can share some important points for understanding the problem, as shown in the diagram below (Figure 5).

However, misconceptions have been created, both by the population and by the health professionals themselves, that the only way to stop malaria is through deployment of control measures. Thus, promoting actions such as immediate diagnosis, treatment supervision, health surveillance and health education is a challenge in health services. Experiences carried out in Alto Solimões river, in 2018, and Alto

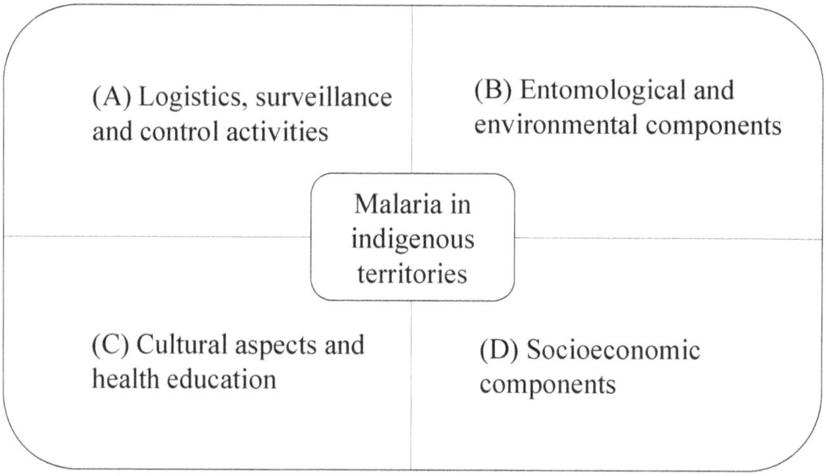

FIGURE 5 Main aspects that can influence malaria in indigenous territories

Rio Negro Basin, in 2019, which achieved significant reductions in malaria in their territories, demonstrate the importance of incorporating diagnostic, treatment, supervision and education actions to suppress malaria (SES-AM 2019). Surveillance must ensure timely diagnosis, especially in hard-to-reach villages, together with supervised treatment and even the establishment of new surveillance strategies that involve new drugs and local stratification.

Implementing new technologies such as larvicides, adulticides, as indoor residual spraying and thermal fogging, is limited by restrictions for application, as these can generate resistance in the vector to active insecticidal substances and risks to the health of professionals involved (Brasilia 2021). Indoor residual spraying has been an important strategy in indigenous villages and remains in use today. However, this is not appropriate for all situations; for example, some villages do not have walls in all houses, making the practice unfeasible. Vector control must also consider the larval phase of the vector, cleaning natural foci (igarapés) and artificial (fish farming ponds) to prevent proliferation of the anopheline vector. These actions must be encouraged and understood both by health professional agents and by indigenous village leaders.

Starting the treatment early, emphasizing the importance of completing treatment, and verifying parasite clearance are important steps to interrupting the cycle of the malaria parasite. These needs must be communicated to the patient through culturally appropriate methods. It is necessary for professionals to be able to transmit the necessary information in their language. The Indigenous Health Agents (in Portuguese *Agentes Indígenas de Saúde – AIS*) have been the main mediator in this part because they are residents of the villages, speak their languages and are integrated with malaria control technical teams. Despite recognition that indigenous health care policies need to be customized for local contexts, in practice it is difficult to obtain these differences.

To reclaim their rights and search for new opportunities, indigenous populations have increasingly moved to urban areas, sometimes closer other away to their villages. This constant mobility between villages and cities drive diseases transmission and challenge surveillance systems. In many cases, the villages with greater mobility are most vulnerable to malaria incidence; this is the case of Alto Rio Negro Basin, which had the highest records of malaria in the last few years (Brazil 2021). In other villages, illegal mining and territory invasions have been associated with an increase in malaria cases. This occurred in Yanomami territory, where high migratory flows, driven by socioeconomic factors, were associated with an increase of 100% of incidence of malaria caused by *P. falciparum* in 2021 (Ministério da Saúde 2022).

9.1 *Epidemiological and environmental surveillance in the control of malaria in disaster scenarios and extreme weather events*

As discussed throughout this chapter, malaria in the Amazon Basin is a historical problem, but it has increased in incidence and special distribution in recent years. Both the increase in the number of malaria cases and the persistence of the disease as endemic in the Amazon Basin can be explained by the natural and anthropogenic disasters that have intensified in the region. In this sense, health systems have encountered several challenges that act in a cumulative way. On the other hand, the increase in the intensity and frequency of environmental changes has demanded new strategies or the refinement of strategies already used, especially about the link between environmental surveillance and control, epidemiological surveillance, and health care. In this way, it is important that effective vector control measures are strengthened, but also it is essential that new strategies and approaches are implemented and monitored. Afterwards, we propose some suggestions to surveillance measures for malaria and disease vectors that should be promoted, especially in disaster scenarios and the intensification of their drivers.

9.2 *Strengthening community surveillance with indigenous peoples and other forest peoples*

Amazonian indigenous peoples and local communities has contributed with the mission of guardians of the forest but recently, with the increase in deforestation and, consequently, the increase in greenhouse gas emissions, the invasion and degradation within indigenous territories and protected natural areas remain under constant threat of forest unsustainability across the nine-nation region (Walker *et al.* 2020). In addition, often overlooked, indigenous and local communities are increasingly vulnerable to forest degradation and disturbance, which diminish the ecological integrity of their territories, affecting their health and well-being. The weakening of the national policy of environmental protection, indigenous land rights and the rule of law poses an existential threat to indigenous and local Amazonian peoples in their territories (Conceição *et al.* 2021). This scenario has implications on the distribution and intensity of transmission of malaria, that is expected to decrease in some areas due to high temperatures, however, increase in others, mainly along the current edges of its geographic distribution in endemic areas of South America (IPCC 2022b).

Different community surveillance strategies have been used to control malaria vectors, including in the Amazon Basin. Such strategies are based on the actions of residents of communities that historically reside in the region. The actions of health systems in partnership with local communities can take place in different ways, such as financing residents in the control, monitoring and reduction of environments favourable to the proliferation of vectors. The knowledge that forests peoples have of the environment where they live allows them to act on potential creators. Additionally, they play an essential role in environmental conservation, such as indigenous peoples, when residing on titled lands, especially in relation to maintaining environmental integrality and biodiversity, acting in the control of anthropogenic disaster drivers (Fernandez-Llamazares *et al.* 2021). However, for community surveillance to be effective, it is essential that partnerships are being established, and investments made, so that the use of adequate equipment is allowed, but guarantees the continuity of surveillance actions at different times of the year and not only during epidemic periods. The continuity of community actions is essential in mitigating the main drivers, but also in controlling vectors and monitoring the number of cases.

Unsustainable land-use and land cover change, deforestation, loss of biodiversity, pollution load, and their interactions, adversely affect the capacities support of ecosystems, communities, and individuals to adapt to climate change (Walker *et al.* 2020). Loss of ecosystems and their services has long-term impacts on people, especially for indigenous peoples and local communities (Conceiçao *et al.* 2021) who are directly dependent on ecosystems, to meet basic needs, such as food. Indigenous communities in Amazonian territories used to live with abundance and prosperity. In the last years, food security of these peoples is a reason for concern, because thousands of indigenous families depend on essential food aid or welfare programs like which is the most direct and visible effect of climate change in the life of indigenous peoples (Port Lourenço *et al.* 2008).

9.3 *Closer epidemiological and environmental surveillance and actions*

A large part of the environmental drivers that result in natural and anthropogenic disasters are monitored by environmental agencies, whether national, state or municipal, and not by the health sector. It is urgent to strengthen these sectors in the management, policies and implementation of surveillance actions. Commonly, the monitoring of activities with environmental impact and changes in land use are carried out by environmental agencies, such as the environmental agencies responsible for inspecting deforested areas or assessing the impact of large enterprises. Sometimes, the results of these actions and studies are under the knowledge and management of these agencies, without reaching health services. For example, monitoring of air and water quality with health outcomes highlights the need for coordinated planning and joint action between the sectors.

10 Conclusions

Changes in climate regimes associated with anthropogenic environmental in LUC in Amazon pose great pressing challenges to human society and natural ecosystems. The scenarios presented by the IPCC (2022b) for global climate change is predicted to disrupt seasonal periodicities and long-term trends in rainfall and temperature, altering natural climate cycles and variation with increases in the frequency and intensity of climate and weather extremes. Also, including hot extremes on land and in the ocean, heavy precipitation events, long term drought and fire weather causing widespread adverse impacts, losses and damages to natural ecosystems and human health, increasing human mortality and morbidity, decreased diet diversity and increased malnutrition in many communities, especially for traditional communities, such as indigenous peoples, with children, elderly people, and pregnant women particularly impacted. The incidence of vector-borne diseases has increased from range expansion and/or increased reproduction of disease vectors. Animal and human diseases, including zoonoses, are emerging in new areas, which include the risk of new epidemics (Ellwanger and Chies 2020). Increased exposure to wildfire smoke, atmospheric dust, and aeroallergens have been associated with climate-sensitive cardiovascular and respiratory distress, and health services have been disrupted by extreme events such as floods that have led to increases in vector-borne, such as malaria, dengue, chikungunya, and water-borne diseases and to disturbances of public health services (IPCC 2022b).

Regarding malaria, there is a need to align monitoring of deforested areas, as well as forest fires and other factors of environmental change, with vector surveillance measures and the response capacity of health systems. The preparation of the response of health systems to health emergencies, which includes the increase in malaria cases, must take place through the monitoring of environmental indicators, in addition to epidemiological ones. Therefore, it is essential to promote integrated environmental and health information systems, where it is possible to monitor health indicators, and threats associated with vulnerability and socio-environmental sensitivity. Therefore, a good example of opportunity to help malaria control in a natural disaster scenario, could be integrate the knowledge and good practices of the Brazilian health system to meteorological institutes such as the National Center for

Monitoring and Early Warning of Natural Disasters (In Portuguese Centro Nacional de Monitoramento e Alertas de Desastres Naturais – CEMADEN), that develops programs that works with environmental education living in cities with risk areas for socio-environmental disasters, project recognized by United Nations Framework Convention on Climate Changes (UNFCCC) as inspiring practice to contribute with creating a culture of disaster risk perception to construct sustainable and resilient societies (http://educacao.cemaden.gov.br/site/project/).

Across sectors and regions, the most vulnerable people and health systems are observed to be disproportionately affected by the climate change impacts. Furthermore, poverty can be both, a cause and consequence of disaster risk, particularly extensive risk, with drought and flood being the hazard most closely associated with poverty (UNDRR 2022). The linkage of impact of disasters and malaria in Amazon Basin is still constrained by limited quantitative and qualitative information about causal mechanisms linking climate with health impacts on a global and local scale. Meanwhile, these threats have a high impact on people at risk with human vulnerability determinants associated to colour, race, gender, ethnicity, and geography (IPCC 2022b), such as disability-adjusted life years (DALY) (Bezerra *et al.* 2020), a measure of health loss and disease burden estimated by the sum of years lived with disabilities, and years of life lost due to premature death (Hay *et al.* 2017).

Acknowledgements

LSMC (deceased) was funded by US National Institutes of Health grant 2R01AI110112. SH was supported by the National Council of Technological and Scientific Development (CNPq, Brazil, Process 312901/2021-6 and the Post-Graduate Program of Public Health and Environment at the National School of Public Health/FIOCRUZ. TCMS acknowledges support from the São Paulo Research Foundation (FAPESP), Grant 2022/10997-1.

Author contributions

LSMC, SSH and TMS designed the chapter. LCFP interpreted and wrote the indigenous perspectives. LSMC, TMS and SSH interpreted the data and wrote the text. TMS, LCFP and LSMC prepared the figures and tables. SSH reviewed and improved the text. LSMC, TMS, LCFP and SSH wrote the paper. All authors were involved in critical revision of the chapter. SSH supervised the chapter.

Competing interests

The authors declare no competing interests.

References

Adde A *et al.* (2016) Dynamical mapping of *Anopheles darlingi* densities in a residual malaria transmission area of French Guiana by using remote sensing and meteorological data.' PLoS One 11.10: e0164685.

Allan RP, Hawkin E, Bellouin N and Collins B (2021) IPCC, 2021: Summary for Policymakers. In: Masson-Delmotte V, Zhai P, Pirani A, Connors SL, Péan C, Berger S, Caud N, Chen Y, Goldfarb L, Gomis MI, Huang M, Leitzell K, Lonnoy E, Matthews JBR, Maycock TK, Waterfield T, Yelekçi O, Yu R and Zhou B. (eds) Climate Change 2021: the physical science basis. Contribution of Working Group I to the Sixth Assessment Report of the Intergovernmental Panel on Climate Change. Cambridge University Press. (In Press)

Alkama R and Cescatti A (2016) Biophysical climate impacts of recent changes in global forest cover. Science 351: 600–604.

Afrane YA, Zhou G, Lawson BW, Githeko AK and Yan G (2006) Effects of microclimatic changes caused by deforestation on the survivorship and reproductive fitness of *Anopheles gambiae* in western Kenya highlands. The American journal of tropical medicine and hygiene, 74, 772–778.

Afrane YA, Zhou G, Lawson BW, Githeko AK and Yan G (2007) Life-table analysis of *Anopheles arabiensis* in western Kenya highlands: effects of land covers on larval and adult survivorship. The American journal of tropical medicine and hygiene, 77, 660–666.

Aguiar APD, Vieira ICG, Assis TO, Dalla-Nora EL, Toledo PM, Oliveira Santos-Junior RA, Batistella M, Coelho AS, Savaget EK, Aragão LEOC and Nobre CA (2016) Land use change emission scenarios: anticipating a forest transition process in the Brazilian Amazon. Global change biology, 22(5), pp. 1821–1840.

Basta PC and Hacon SS (2020) Impacto do mercúrio em áreas protegidas e povos da floresta na Amazônia Oriental: Uma abordagem integrada saúde-ambiente. Aspectos Metodológicos e Resultados Preliminares.

Basta PC, Viana PVS, Vasconcellos ACS, *et al.* (2021) Mercury Exposure in Munduruku Indigenous Communities from Brazilian Amazon: Methodological Background and an Overview of the Principal Results. Int. J. Environ. Res. Public Health, 18: 9222. https://doi.org/10.3390/ijerph18179222.

Barbieri AF and Carr DL (2005) Gender-specific out-migration, deforestation and urbanization in the Ecuadorian Amazon. Global and Planetary Change, 47, 99–110.

Barbieri AF and Soares-Filho BS (2005) Population and land use effects on malaria prevalence in the southern Brazilian Amazon. Human Ecology, 33(6), 847–874.

Barrera R, Felix G, Acevedo V, Amador M, Rodriguez D, Rivera L, Gonzalez O, Nazario N, Ortiz M and Muñoz-Jordan JL (2019) Impacts of Hurricanes Irma and Maria on *Aedes aegypti* populations, aquatic habitats, and mosquito infections with dengue, chikungunya, and Zika viruses in Puerto Rico. The American journal of tropical medicine and hygiene, 100, 1413.

Barros F, Arruda M, Gurgel H and Honório N (2011) Spatial clustering and longitudinal variation of *Anopheles darlingi* (Diptera: Culicidae) larvae in a river of the Amazon: the importance of the forest fringe and of obstructions to flow in frontier malaria. Bulletin of entomological research, 101, 643–658.

Barros FS and Honório NA (2015) Deforestation and malaria on the amazon frontier: larval clustering of *Anopheles darlingi* (Diptera: Culicidae) determines focal distribution of malaria. The American journal of tropical medicine and hygiene, 93, 939–953.

Brando P. *et al.* (2020) Amazon wildfires: Scenes from a foreseeable disaster. Flora, v. 268, p. 151609.

Below R, Wirtz A and Guha-Sapir D (2009) Disaster category classification and peril terminology for operational purposes.

Berazneva J and Byker TS (2017) Does Forest Loss Increase Human Disease? Evidence from Nigeria. American Economic Review, 107, 516–521.

Bezerra JMT, Barbosa DS, Martins-Melo FR, Werneck GL, Braga ÉM, Tauil PL and Carneiro M (2020) Changes in malaria patterns in Brazil over 28 years (1990–2017): results from the Global Burden of Disease Study 2017. Population Health Metrics, 18(1), 1–15.

Blanford JI, Blanford S, Crane RG, Mann ME, Paaijmans KP, Schreiber KV, Thomas MB (2013) Implications of temperature variation for malaria parasite development across Africa. Sci Rep 3: 1300. https://doi.org/10.1038/srep01300.

Bonan GB (2008) Forests and climate change: forcings, feedbacks, and the climate benefits of forests. Science 320, 1444–1449.

Bonan GB and Doney SC (2018). Climate, ecosystems, and planetary futures: The challenge to predict life in Earth system models. Science 359, eaam8328.

Boulton CA, Lenton TM and Boers N (2022) Pronounced loss of Amazon rainforest resilience since the early 2000s. Nature Climate Change, p. 1–8.

Braz RM and Barcellos C (2018) Análise do processo de eliminação da transmissão da malária na Amazônia brasileira com abordagem espacial da variação da incidência da doença em 2016. Epidemiol Serv Saúde, 27(3): e2017253.

Brasil. Ministério da Saúde (2016) Secretaria de Gestão do Trabalho e da Educação na Saúde. Departamento de Gestão da Educação na Saúde. Programa de Qualificação de Agentes Indígenas de Saúde (AIS) e Agentes Indígenas de Saneamento (AISAN) / Ministério da Saúde, Secretaria de Gestão do Trabalho e da Educação na Saúde, Departamento de Gestão da Educação na Saúde. – Brasília-DF: Ministério da Saúde.

Brasil. Ministério da Saúde (2003) Secretaria de Vigilância em Saúde. Programa Nacional de Prevenção e Controle da Malária PNCM / Ministério da Saúde, Secretaria de Vigilância em Saúde. – Brasília: Ministério da Saúde.

Butt EW, Conibear L, Reddington CL, Darbyshire E, Morgan WT, Coe H, Artaxo P, Brito J, Knote C and Spracklen DV (2020). Large air quality and human health impacts due to Amazon forest and vegetation fires. Environmental Research Communications, 2, 095001. https://doi.org/10.1088/2515-7620/abbodb.

Brasil. Câmara dos Deputados (2021) Proposta determina indenização a ex-servidor contaminhado por DDT. Available at: https://www.camara.leg.br/noticias/756902-proposta-determina-indenizacao-a-ex-servidor-contaminado-por-ddt.

Campanharo WA, Morello T, Christofoletti MA, Anderson LO (2021) Hospitalization Due to Fire-Induced Pollution in the Brazilian Legal Amazon from 2005 to 2018. Remote Sensing. Dec 24;14(1):69.

Carreiras J, Pereira JMC and Shimabukuro YE (2006) A land cover map for the Brazilian Legal Amazon using SPOT-4 VEGETATION data and machine learning algorithms. Photogrammetric Engineering and Remote Sensing, 72, 97–910.

Castro MC, Baeza A, Codeço CT, Cucunubá ZM, Dal'asta AP, De Leo GA, Dobson AP, Carrasco-Escobar G, Lana, RM and Lowe R (2019) Development, environmental degradation, and disease spread in the Brazilian Amazon. PLoS biology, 17, e3000526.

Castro MC and Singer BH (2019) Malaria in the Brazilian Amazon: new understanding and directions for intervention. Water and Sanitation-Related Diseases and the Changing Environment: Challenges, Interventions, and Preventive Measures: 127–146.

Castro MC, Monte-Mór RL, Sawyer DO, Singer BH (2006) Malaria risk on the Amazon frontier. Proc Natl Acad Sci USA, 103: 2452–2457.

Charnley GEC, Kelman I, Gaythorpe KAM, Murray KA (2021) Traits and risk factors of post-disaster infectious disease outbreaks: a systematic review. Sci Rep, Mar 10;11(1): 5616. https://doi.org/10.1038/s41598-021-85146-0.

Chaves LF, Koenraadt CJ (2010) Climate change and highland malaria: fresh air for a hot debate. The Quarterly review of biology, 85(1), 27–55.

Chaves LSM, Bergo ES, Conn JE, Laporta GZ, Prist PR and Sallum MAM (2021) Anthropogenic landscape decreases mosquito biodiversity and drives malaria vector proliferation in the Amazon rainforest. PLoS One, 16, e0245087.

Chaves LSM, Conn JE, López RVM and Sallum MAM (2018) Abundance of impacted forest patches less than 5 km^2 is a key driver of the incidence of malaria in Amazonian Brazil. Scientific reports, 8, 7077.

Chaves LSM, Fry J, Malik A, Geschke A, Sallum MAM and Lenzen M (2020) Global consumption and international trade in deforestation-associated commodities could influence malaria risk. Nature Communications, 11, 1–10.

Chowell G, Mizumoto K, Banda JM, Poccia S, Perrings C (2019) Assessing the potential impact of vector-borne disease transmission following heavy rainfall events: a mathematical framework. Philosophical Transactions of the Royal Society B, 374(1775), 20180272.

Chu V, Sallum M, Moore T, Lainhart W, Schlichting C and Conn J (2019) Regional variation in life history traits and plastic responses to temperature of the major malaria vector Nyssorhynchus darlingi in Brazil. Scientific reports, 9, 5356.

Cohee LM, Laufer MK (2017) Malaria in children. Pediatr. Clin. N. Am., 64:851–866. https://doi.org/10.1016/j.pcl.2017.03.004.

Cohen JM, Le Menach A, Pothin E, Eisele TP, Gething PW, Eckhoff PA, Moonen B, Schapira A and Smith DL (2017) Mapping multiple components of malaria risk for improved targeting of elimination interventions. Malar J, 16, 459.

COIAB – Coordenação das Organizações Indígenas da Amazônia Brasileira (2022) História e missão. Available at https://coiab.org.br/quemsomos.

Conceição KV *et al.* (2021) Government policies endanger the indigenous peoples of the Brazilian Amazon. Land Use Policy, v. 108, p. 105663.

Conn JE *et al.* (2002) Emergence of a new neotropical malaria vector facilitated by human migration and changes in land use. Am. J. Trop. Med. Hyg. 66, 18–22.

Curtis PG, Slay CM, Harris NL, Tyukavina A and Hansen MC (2018) Classifying drivers of global forest loss. Science, 361, 1108–1111.

Da Cruz FV, Peiter PC, Carvajal-Cortés JJ, Dos Santos PR, Mendonça GMDS, Suárez-Mutis MC (2019) Complex malaria epidemiology in an international border area between Brazil and French Guiana: challenges for elimination. Tropical medicine and health, 47(1), 1–12.

Davidson EA, De Araújo AC, Artaxo P, Balch JK, Brown IF, Bustamante CMM, Coe MT, Defries RS, Keller M and Longo M (2012) The Amazon basin in transition. Nature, 481, 321–328, 2012.

De Oliveira BFA *et al.* (2020) Impacts of heat stress conditions on mortality from respiratory and cardiovascular diseases in Brazil. Sustain. Debate 11, 297–313, 2020.

Dobson AP, Pimm SL, Hannah L, Kaufman L, Ahumada JA, Ando AW, Bernstein A, Busch J, Daszak P and Engelmann J (2020) Ecology and economics for pandemic prevention. Science, 369, 379–381.

Dos Reis IC, Codeço CT, Degener CM, Keppeler EC, Muniz MM, De Oliveira FGS, Cortês JJC, De Freitas MA, De Souza CAA and Rodrigues FCM (2015) Contribution of fish farming ponds to the production of immature *Anopheles* spp. in a malaria-endemic Amazonian town. Malaria Journal, 14, 1–12.

Dos Reis M, Graça PMLA, Yanai AM, Ramos CJP and Fearnside PM (2021) Forest fires and deforestation in the central Amazon: Effects of landscape and climate on spatial and temporal dynamics. Journal of Environmental Management, 288, 112310. https://doi.org/10.1016/j.jenvman.2021.112310.

Duminil J, Mona S, Mardulyn P, Doumenge C, Walmacq F, Doucet JL and Hardy OJ (2015) Late Pleistocene molecular dating of past population fragmentation and demographic changes in African rain forest tree species supports the forest refuge hypothesis. Journal of biogeography, 42, 1443–1454.

Ellwanger JH, Kulmann-Leal B, Kaminski VL, *et al.* (2020) Beyond diversity loss and climate change: Impacts of Amazon deforestation on infectious diseases and public health. An Acad Bras Cienc Apr 17;92(1): e20191375. https://doi.org/10.1590/0001-3765202020191375. PMID: 32321030.

Fearnside PM (2001) Land-tenure issues as factors in environmental destruction in Brazilian Amazonia: the case of southern Pará. World Development 29(8): 1361–1372. https://doi.org/10.1016/S0305-750X(01)00039-0.

Fearnside PM (2015) Impactos Sociais da Barragem de Tucuruí. pp. 37–52. In: Hidrelétricas na Amazônia: Impactos Ambientais e Sociais na Tomada de Decisões sobre Grandes Obras. Vol. 1. Editora do Instituto Nacional de Pesquisas da Amazônia (INPA), Manaus, Amazonas. 296 pp.

Feged-Rivadeneira A and Evans S (2019) Ethnography of a parasite: A quantitative ethnographic observation of forest malaria in the Amazon basin. Scandinavian journal of public health 47.8: 820–831.

Fernández-Llamazares A, López-Baucells PM, Velazco A, Rocha GR, Terraube J and Cabeza M (2021) The Importance of indigenous territories for conserving bat diversity across the Amazon biome. Perspectives in Ecology and Conservation. https://doi.org/10.1016/j.pecon.2020.11.001.

Ferreira FADS, Arcos AN, Sampaio RTDM, Rodrigues IB and Tadei WP (2015) Effect of *Bacillus sphaericus* Neide on *Anopheles* (Diptera: Culicidae) and associated insect fauna in fish ponds in the Amazon. Revista Brasileira de Entomologia, 59, 234–239.

Ferreira MU, Castro MC (2019) Malaria situation in Latin America and the Caribbean: residual and resurgent transmission and challenges for control and elimination. In Malaria Control and Elimination (pp. 57–70). Humana, New York, NY.

Fiocruz (2022) Agentes de Combate a Endemias. Available at: https://www.epsjv.fiocruz.br/educacao-profissional-em-saude/profissoes/agente-de-combate-a-endemias.

Foster PG *et al.* (2017) Phylogeny of Anophelinae using mitochondrial protein coding genes. R. Soc. Open Sci. 4(11), 170758.

Gagnon AS, Smoyer-Tomic KE and Bush AB (2002) The El Niño southern oscillation and malaria epidemics in South America. International Journal of Biometeorology, 46, 81–89.

Galardo AKR, Zimmerman R and Galardo CD (2013) Larval control of *Anopheles* (*Nyssorhinchus*) *darlingi* using granular formulation of *Bacillus sphaericus* in abandoned gold-miners excavation pools in the Brazilian Amazon rainforest. Revista da Sociedade Brasileira de Medicina Tropical, 46, 172–177.

Galardo AKR, Zimmerman R, Lounibos LP, Young L, Galardo C, Arruda M and D'almeida C (2009) Seasonal abundance of Anopheline mosquitoes and their association with rainfall and malaria along the Matapi River, Amapi, Brazil. Medical and veterinary entomology, 23, 335–349.

Garg T (2019) Ecosystems and human health: The local benefits of forest cover in Indonesia. Journal of Environmental Economics and Management, 98, 102271.

Geist HJ and Lambin EF (2002) Proximate causes and underlying driving forces of tropical deforestation tropical forests are disappearing as the result of many pressures, both local and regional, acting in various combinations in different geographical locations. BioScience, 52, 143–150.

Gething PW, Van Boeckel TP, Smith DL, Guerra CA, Patil AP, Snow RW and Hay SI (2011) Modelling the global constraints of temperature on transmission of *Plasmodium falciparum* and *P. vivax*. Parasites and vectors, 4, 1–11.

Goddard J (2018) Mosquito-borne diseases. In: Infectious Diseases and Arthropods. Infectious Disease. Humana Press, Cham, Switzerland. https://doi.org/10.1007/978-3-319-75874-9_3.

Gomes VHF, Vieira ICG, Salomão RP *et al.* (2019) Amazonian tree species threatened by deforestation and climate change. Nat. Clim. Chang. 9, 547–553. https://doi.org/10.1038/s41558-019-0500-2.

Gomes MF, Codeço CT, Bastos LS, Lana RM (2020) Measuring the contribution of human mobility to malaria persistence. Malaria journal, 19(1), 1–12.

Gutierrez-Cori O, Espinoza JC, Li L, Wongchuig S, Arias P, Ronchail J and Segura H (2021) On the hydroclimate-vegetation relationship in the southwestern Amazon during the 2000–2019 period. Frontiers in Water, 3, 648499.

Hansen MC, Stehman SV, Potapov P, Loveland TR, Townshend JRG, *et al.* (2008) Humid tropical forest clearing from 2000 to 2005 quantified by using multitemporal and multiresolution remotely sensed data. Proc Natl Acad Sci 105: 9439–9444.

Hansen J, Ruedy R, Sato M and Lo K (2010) Global surface temperature change. Reviews of Geophysics, 48.

Hay SI *et al.* (2017) Global, regional, and national disability-adjusted life-years (DALYS) for 333 diseases and injuries and healthy life expectancy (HALE) for 195 countries and territories, 1990–2016: a systematic analysis for the Global Burden of Disease Study 2016. The Lancet, v. 390, n. 10100, p. 1260–1344.

Helldén D, Andersson C, Nilsson M, Ebi KL, Friberg P, Alfvén T (2021) Climate change and child health: a scoping review and an expanded conceptual framework. Lancet Planet Health; 5: e164–75.

Hiwat H and Bretas G (2011) Ecology of *Anopheles darlingi* Root with respect to vector importance: a review. Parasites and vectors, 4, 177.

Houghton RA, Byers B Nassikas AA (2015) A role for tropical forests in stabilizing atmospheric CO2. Nat. Clim. Change 5, 1022–1023.

Howard MJ, Brillman JC and Burkle FM (1996) Infectious disease emergencies in disasters. Emergency Medicine Clinics, 14(2), 413–428.

Huntington HP, Begossi A, Gearheard SF, Kersey B, Loring PA, Mustonen T, Paudel PK, Silvano RA and Vave R (2017) How small communities respond to environmental change: patterns from tropical to polar ecosystems. Ecology and Society, 22.

Ikeda T, Behera SK, Morioka Y, Minakawa N, Hashizume M, Tsuzuki A *et al.* (2017) Seasonally lagged effects of climatic factors on malaria incidence in South Africa. Scientific reports, 7(1), 1–9.

IPCC – Intergovernmental Panel on Climate Change (2013) Climate change 2013: The Physical Science Basis.

IPCC – Intergovernmental Panel on Climate Change (2012) Managing the risks of extreme events and disasters to advance climate change adaptation. A special report of working groups I and II of the Intergovernmental Panel on Climate Change., Cambridge University Press.

IPCC – Intergovernmental Panel on Climate Change (2014) Summary for policy makers In: Climate Change 2014: Impacts, Adaptation, and Vulnerability. Part A: Global and Sectoral Aspects. Contribution of Working Group II to the Fifth Assessment Report of the Intergovernmental Panel on Climate Change ed CB Field *et al.* (Cambridge) (Cambridge University Press) (Cambridge, United Kingdom and New York, NY, USA) pp. 1–32.

IPCC – Intergovernmental Panel on Climate Change (2022a) Working Group II Contribution to the Sixth Assessment Report of the Intergovernmental Panel on Climate Change. Summary for Policymakers. Climate Change 2022 Impacts, Adaptation and Vulnerability. Working Group II Technical Support Unit, Final Draft unpublished. Available at: https://www.ipcc.ch/report/ar6/wg2/downloads/report/IPCC_AR6_WGII_SummaryForPolicymakers.pdf.

IPCC – Intergovernmental Panel on Climate Change (2022b) Working Group II Contribution to the Sixth Assessment Report of the Intergovernmental Panel on Climate Change. Technical Summary, Final Draft unpublished. Available at: https://www.ipcc.ch/report/ar6/wg2/downloads/report/IPCC_AR6_WGII_FinalDraft_TechnicalSummary.pdf.

Kingsolver JG, Woods H, Buckley LB, Potter KA, Maclean HJ and Higgins JK (2011) Complex life cycles and the responses of insects to climate change. Oxford University Press.

Koenraadt CJM, Githeko AK, Takken W (2004) The effects of rainfall and evapotranspiration on the temporal dynamics of *Anopheles gambiae* ss and *Anopheles arabiensis* in a Kenyan village. Acta tropica, 90(2), 141–153.

Kouadio IK, Aljunid S, Kamigaki T, Hammad K, Oshitani H (2012) Infectious diseases following natural disasters: prevention and control measures. Expert Rev Anti Infect Ther 10(1): 95–104, https://doi.org/10.1586/eri.11.155.

Kruid S, Macedo MN., Gorelik SR., Walker W, Moutinho P, Brando PM., Castanho A, Alencar A, Baccini A, Coe MT (2021) Beyond deforestation: carbon emissions from land grabbing and forest degradation in the Brazilian Amazon. Frontiers in Forests and Global Change. Vol. 4.

Johansen IC, Rodrigues PT, Ferreira MU (2020) Human mobility and urban malaria risk in the main transmission hotspot of Amazonian Brazil. PloS one, 15(11), e0242357.

Lambin EF and Geist HJ (2008). Land-use and land-cover change: local processes and global impacts. Springer Science & Business Media.

Laporta GZ, Linton YM, Wilkerson RC, Bergo ES, Nagaki SS, Sant'Ana DC, Sallum MAM (2015). Malaria vectors in South America: current and future scenarios. Parasites & vectors, 8(1), 1–13.

Laporta GZ (2019) Amazonian rainforest loss and declining malaria burden in Brazil. The Lancet Planetary Health vol. 3 e4–e5.

Laporta GZ, Ilacqua RC, Bergo ES, Chaves LSM, Rodovalho SR, Moresco GG, Figueira EA, Massad E, De Oliveira TM and Bickersmith SA (2021) Malaria transmission in landscapes with varying deforestation levels and timelines in the Amazon: a longitudinal spatiotemporal study. Scientific Reports, 11, 1–14.

Latrubesse EM, Arima EY, Dunne T, Park E, Baker V, D'horta F, *et al.* (2017) Damming the rivers of the Amazon Basin. Nature, 546, 363–369. https://doi.org/10.1038/nature22333.

Leaning J and Guha-Sapir D (2013) Natural disasters, armed conflict, and public health. New England journal of medicine, 369, 1836–1842.

Liu EK, He WQ, Yan CR (2014) 'White revolution' to 'white pollution' – agricultural plastic film mulch in China. Environmental Research Letters, 9(9): 091001.

Lovejoy TE and Nobre C (2019) Amazon tipping point: last chance for action. Sci. Adv. 5, eaba2949.

Lowe R *et al.* (2021) Combined effects of hydrometeorological hazards and urbanisation on dengue risk in Brazil: a spatiotemporal modelling study. The Lancet Planetary Health, 5(4): e209–e219.

Maezumi SY *et al.* (2022) Legacies of Indigenous land use and cultural burning in the Bolivian Amazon rainforest ecotone. Phil. Trans. R. Soc. B 377, 20200499. https://doi.org/10.1098/rstb.2020.0499.

Macdonald AJ and Mordecai EA (2019) Amazon deforestation drives malaria transmission, and malaria burden reduces forest clearing. Proceedings of the National Academy of Sciences, 116, 22212–22218.

Manguin S, Kengne P, Sonnier L, Harbach RE, Baimai V, Trung HD and Coosemans M (2002) SCAR markers and multiplex PCR-based identification of isomorphic species in the *Anopheles dirus* complex in Southeast Asia. Medical and Veterinary Entomology, 16, 46–54.

Mapbiomas Amazonía (2022) Colección v3.0 de la Serie Anual de Mapas de Cobertura y Uso del Suelo de la Amazonía, adquirido en April 2022 a través del enlace: https://amazonia.mapbiomas.org/.

Mariana S and Mashida R (2020) Coinciding crises: how COVID-19 and climate change are putting pressure on health systems worldwide – and how we can prepare for the future. UNDP. November 2, 2020.

Marengo JA, Tomasella J, Alves LM, Soares WR and Rodriguez DA (2011) The drought of 2010 in the context of historical droughts in the Amazon region. Geophysical research letters, 38.

MEA (2005) Ecosystems and Human Well-being: Biodiversity Synthesis. World Resources Institute. Island Press, Washington D.C.

Meremikwu MM, Asindi AA and Ezedinachi E (1997) The patternof neurological sequelae of childhood cererbral malaria amongsurvivors in Calabar, Nigeria. The Central African Journal of Medicine 43, 231–234.

Metzger JP, Bustamante M, Ferreira J (2019) Por que o Brasil precisa de suas reservas legais. Perspectives in Ecology and Conservation. Rio de Janeiro, v. 17, n. 3, p. 104–116, Julho–Setembro.

Ministério da Saúde. Brasil. Sistema de Informação de Agravos de Notificação – fonte de dados do Sivep-Malária e do Sinan. Availablet at: https://public.tableau.com/app/profile/mal.ria.brasil/viz/Dadosparacidado_201925_03_2020/Incio.

Mordecai EA, Paaijmans KP, Johnson LR, Balzer C, Ben-Horin T, De Moor E, Mcnally A, Pawar S, Ryan SJ, Smith TC, Lafferty KD (2013) Optimal temperature for malaria transmission is dramatically lower than previously predicted. Ecol Lett, Jan;16(1): 22–30. https://doi.org/10.1111/ele.12015.

Moura MM, Dos Santos AR, Pezzopane JEM, Alexandre RS, Da Silva SF, Pimentel S M, De Andrade MSS, Silva FGR, Branco ERF and Moreira TR (2019) Relation of El Niño and La Niña phenomena to precipitation, evapotranspiration and temperature in the Amazon basin. Science of The Total Environment, 651, 1639–1651.

Munang R, Thiaw I, Alverson K, Liu J and Han Z (2013) The role of ecosystem services in climate change adaptation and disaster risk reduction. Current Opinion in Environmental Sustainability, 5, 47–52.

Nishijima M, Rocha FF (2020) An economic investigation of the dengue incidence as a result of a tailings dam accident in Brazil. J Environ Manage. Jan 1;253:109748. https://doi.org/10.1016/j.jenvman.2019.109748.

Nobre P, Malagutti M, Urbano DF, De Almeida RA and Giarolla E (2009) Amazon deforestation and climate change in a coupled model simulation. Journal of Climate 22.21: 5686–5697.

Nobre CA, Sampaio G, Borma LS, Castilla-Rubio JC, Silva JS and Cardoso M (2016) Land-use and climate change risks in the Amazon and the need of a novel sustainable development paradigm. Proceedings of the National Academy of Sciences, 113, 10759–10768.

Norris DE (2004) Mosquito-borne diseases as a consequence of land use change. EcoHealth, 1, 19–24.

Ogar E, Pecl G and Mustonen T (2020) Science must embrace traditional and indigenous knowledge to solve our biodiversity crisis. One Earth, 3, 162–165.

Oliveira PTM (2022) Violação das terras indígenas pelo aumento da mineração ilegal na Amazonia e a atuação do Ministério Público Federal. Conference presentation of the Public Prosecutor's Office at Pará, Brazil.

Oliveira-Ferreira J, Lacerda MV, Brasil P, Ladislau JL, Tauil PL and Daniel-Ribeiro CT (2010) Malaria in Brazil: an overview. Malaria journal, 9, 115.

Orellana JDY, Marrero L, Alves CM, Ruiz CM, De Hacon SS, Oliveira WO, Basta P (2017) Associação de Baixa Estatura Severa Em Crianças Indígenas Yanomami Com Baixa Estatura Materna: Indícios de Transmissão Intergeracional.

Paaijmans KP, Blanford S, Bell AS, Blanford JI, Read AF and Thomas MB (2010) Influence of climate on malaria transmission depends on daily temperature variation. Proceedings of the National Academy of Sciences, 107(34), 15135–15139.

Paca VHDM, Espinoza-Dávalos GE, Moreira DM, Comair G (2020) Variability of trends in precipitation across the Amazon River basin determined from the CHIRPS precipitation product and from station records. Water, 12(5), 1244.

Parekh FK *et al.* (2020) Infectious disease risks and vulnerabilities in the aftermath of an environmental disaster in Minas Gerais, Brazil. Vector-Borne and Zoonotic Diseases 20.5: 387–389.

Pan W, Carr D, Barbieri A, Bilsborrow R, Suchindran C (2007) Forest clearing in the Ecuadorian Amazon: a study of patterns over space and time. Population Research and Policy Review, 26(5), 635–659.

Pan W, Branch O and Zaitchik B (2014) Impact of climate change on vector-borne disease in the Amazon. Global Climate Change and Public Health, E.K. Pinkerton and N.W. Rom, (eds) Springer, pp. 193–210. https://doi.org/10.1007/978-1-4614-8417-2_11.

Parham PE and Michael E (2010) Modeling the effects of weather and climate change on malaria transmission. Environ. Health Perspect. 118, 620–626.

Peiter PC, Franco VC, Gracie R, Xavier DR, Suárez-Mutis MC (2013) Situação da malária na tríplice fronteira entre Brasil, Colômbia e Peru. Cad. Saúde Pública; 29(12): 24972512. https://doi.org/10.1590/0102-311X00042213.

Pellegrini AFA *et al.* (2018) Fire frequency drives decadal changes in soil carbon and nitrogen and ecosystem productivity. Nature, v. 553, n. 7687, p. 194–198.

Pellegrini AFA *et al.* (2021) Decadal changes in fire frequencies shift tree communities and functional traits. Nature Ecology and Evolution, v. 5, n. 4, p. 504–512.

Pivello VR, Vieira I, Christianini AV, Ribeiro DB, Da Silva Menezes L, Berlinck CN, Melo FP, Marengo JA, Tornquist CG, Tomas WM *et al.* (2021) Understanding Brazil's catastrophic fires: Causes, consequences and policy needed to prevent future tragedies. Perspect. Ecol. Conserv. 2021, 19, 233–255.

Port Lourenço AE, Santos VR, Orellana JD, Coimbra Jr CE (2008) Nutrition transition in Amazonia: obesity and socioeconomic change in the Suruí Indians from Brazil. American Journal of Human Biology: The Official Journal of the Human Biology Association, 20(5), 564–571.

Prasad AS and Francescutti LH (2017) Natural Disasters. International Encyclopedia of Public Health, 215–222. https://doi.org/10.1016/B978-0-12-803678-5.00519-1.

Puig H (2001) La forêt tropicale humide, Paris: Berlin.

Qualls WA and Breidenbaugh MS (2020) Texas mosquito control response following Hurricane Harvey. Journal of the American Mosquito Control Association, 36, 61–67.

RAISG – Rede Amazônica de Informação Socioambiental Georreferenciada (2022) Available at: https://www.amazoniasocioambiental.org/.

Raju E, Boyd E and Otto F (2022) Stop blaming the climate for disasters. Commun Earth Environ 3, 1. https://doi.org/10.1038/s43247-021-00332-2.

Recht J, Siqueira AM, Monteiro WM, Herrera SM, Herrera S and Lacerda MV (2017) Malaria in Brazil, Colombia, Peru and Venezuela: current challenges in malaria control and elimination. Malaria journal, 16(1), 1–18.

Rentschler J and Salhab M (2020) People in harm's way: Flood exposure and poverty in 189 countries, The World Bank.

Reiter P (2001) Climate change and mosquito-borne disease. Environmental Health Perspectives; 109:141–161.

Richards PD, Walker RT and Arima EY (2014) Spatially complex land change: The Indirect effect of Brazil's agricultural sector on land use in Amazonia. Glob Environ Change, 29, 1–9.

Rodrigues PT, Valdivia HO, De Oliveira TC, Alves JMP, Duarte AMR, Cerutti-Junior C, Buery JC, Brito CF, De Souza JC and Hirano Z (2018) Human migration and the spread of malaria parasites to the New World. Scientific reports, 8, 1–13.

Rufalco-Moutinho P, Moura KS, Peres AD, Moreno M, Carrasco-Escobar G, Prussing C, Gamboa D, Vinetz JM, Sallum MAM and Conn JE (2021) Ecology and larval population dynamics of the primary malaria vector *Nyssorhynchus darlingi* in a high transmission setting dominated by fish farming in western Amazonian Brazil. PloS one, 16, e0246215.

Rufalco-Moutinho P, Schweigmann N, Bergamaschi DP and Sallum MAM (2016) Larval habitats of *Anopheles* species in a rural settlement on the malaria frontier of southwest Amazon, Brazil. Acta tropica, 164, 243–258.

Sanchez JF, Carnero AM, Rivera E, Rosales LA, Baldeviano GC, Asencios JL, Edgel KA, Vinetz JM and Lescano AG (2017) Unstable malaria transmission in the southern Peruvian Amazon and its association with gold mining, Madre de Dios, 2001–2012. Am J Trop Med Hyg 96: 304–311.

Sanchez-Ribas J, Parra-Henao G and Guimarães AÉ (2012) Impact of dams and irrigation schemes in Anopheline (Diptera: Culicidae) bionomics and malaria epidemiology. Revista do Instituto de Medicina Tropical de São Paulo, 54, 179–191.

Seneviratne S *et al.* (2021) in Climate Change 2021: The Physical Science Basis. 48 Contribution of Working Group I to the Sixth Assessment Report of the Intergovernmental Panel on Climate 49 Change (eds Masson-Delmotte, V *et al.*) Ch. 11 (Cambridge University Press, 2021).

Song, XP, Hansen MC, Stehman SV *et al.* (2018) Global land change from 1982 to 2016. Nature 560, 639–643. https://doi.org/10.1038/s41586-018-0411-9.

Soares GLH, Mello CF, Silva JDS, Oliveira JDS, Silva FSO, Rodríguez-Planes L, Da Costa FM and Alencar J (2021) Evaluation of Mansonia spp. Infestation on Aquatic Plants in Lentic and Lotic Environments of the Madeira River Basin in Porto Velho, Rondônia, Brazil. Journal of the American Mosquito Control Association, 37, 143–151.

Souza PF, Xavier DR, Suarez Mutis MC, Da Mota JC, Peiter PC, De Matos VP, *et al.* (2019) Spatial spread of malaria and economic frontier expansion in the Brazilian Amazon. PLoS ONE 14 (6): e0217615. https://doi.org/10.1371/journal. pone.0217615.

SPA – Science Panel for the Amazon. Amaz (2021) Assess. Rep. 2021. U. Nations Sustain. Dev. Solut. Netw., N.Y., p. 48.

Sánchez-Ribas J, Oliveira-Ferreira J, Rosa-Freitas MG, Trilla L and Silva-Do-Nascimento TF (2015) New classification of natural breeding habitats for Neotropical anophelines in the Yanomami Indian Reserve, Amazon Region, Brazil and a new larval sampling methodology. Memórias do Instituto Oswaldo Cruz, 110, 760–770.

Sawyer DR (1999). Deforestation and malaria on the Amazon frontier. In Bilsborrow, R.E., and Hogan, D. (eds.), Population and Deforestation in the Humid Tropics, IUSSP, Liége, 1999, pp. 268–291.

Tapajós R, Castro D, Melo G, Balogun S, James M, Pessoa R, Almeida A, Costa M, Pinto R and Albuquerque B (2019) Malaria impact on cognitive function of children in a peri-urban community in the Brazilian Amazon. Malaria Journal, 18, 1–12.

Tucker Lima JM, Vittor A, RIFAI S, Valle D (2017) Does deforestation promote or inhibit malaria transmission in the Amazon? A systematic literature review and critical appraisal of current evidence. Philos Trans R Soc Lond B Biol Sci; 372: 20160125.

Ueno TMRL, Lima LNGC, Sardinha DM, Rodrigues YC, Souza HUS, Teixeira PR, *et al.* (2021) Socio-epidemiological features and spatial distribution of malaria in an area under mining activity in the Brazilian Amazon Region. Int J Environ Res Public Health;18:10384.

UNISDR – United Nations International Strategy for Disaster Reduction (2004) Living with Risk: A Global Review of Disaster Reduction Initiatives. United Nations, Geneva, Switzerland.

UNISDR – United Nations International Strategy for Disaster Reduction (2011) Killer year caps deadly decade – reducing disaster impact is 'Critical' says top UN disaster official. United Nations, Geneva, Switzerland.

UNDRR – United Nations Office for Disaster Risk Reduction (2022) Available at: https://www.preventionweb.net/understanding-disaster-risk.

Van Bortel W, Trung H, Roelants P, Harbach R, Backeljau T and Coosemans M (2000) Molecular identification of *Anopheles minimus* sl beyond distinguishing the members of the species complex. Insect Molecular Biology, 9, 335–340.

Van Lieshout M, Kovats RS, Livermore MTJ, Martens P (2004) Climate change and malaria: analysis of the SRES climate and socio-economic scenarios. Global environmental change, 14(1), 87–99.

Vittor AY *et al.* (2006) The effect of deforestation on the human-biting rate of *Anopheles darlingi*, the primary vector of *falciparum* malaria in the Peruvian Amazon. Am. J. Trop. Med. Hyg. 74, 3–11.

Walker WS, *et al.* (2020) The role of forest conversion, degradation, and disturbance in the carbon dynamics of Amazon indigenous territories and protected areas. Proceedings of the National Academy of Sciences, v. 117, n. 6, p. 3015–3025.

Watts N, Amann M, Arnell N, *et al.* (2019) The 2019 report of The Lancet. Countdown on health and climate change: ensuring that the health of a child born today is not defined by a changing climate. Lancet 394: 1836–78.

Vezenegho SB, Carinci R, Gaborit P, Issaly J, Dusfour I, Briolant S, Girod R (2015) *Anopheles darlingi* (Diptera: Culicidae) dynamics in relation to meteorological data in a cattle farm located in the coastal region of French Guiana: advantage of Mosquito Magnet trap. Environmental entomology, 44(3), 454–462.

WHO – World Health Organization (2014) Quantitative risk assessment of the effects of climate change on selected causes of death, 2030s and 2050s.

WHO – World Health Organization (2021) World malaria report 2021. Geneva: World Health Organization; 2021. Licence: CC BY-NC-SA 3.0 IGO. Available at: https://www.who.int/teams/global-malaria-programme/reports/world-malaria-report-2021.

WHO – World Health Organization (2021) State of the global climate 2020. World Meteorological Organization Geneva, Switzerland.

Williams HA, Bloland PB, Council NR and Population CO (2003) Malaria control during mass population movements and natural disasters.

Wisner B, Gaillard JC and Kelman I (2012) Framing disaster: theories and storiesseeking to understand Hazards, vulnerability and risk. Handbook Hazards Disaster Risk Reduct, 1st ed., 18–34, Routledge, London.

WMO – World Meteorological Organization. State of the global climate 2020. World Meteorological Organization Geneva, Switzerland, 2021.

WMO – World Meteorological Organziation. WMO atlas of mortality and economic losses from weather, climate and water extremes (1970–2019), 2021.

World Bank (2021) World development report 2021: Data for better lives. The World Bank.

Worrall E, Basu S, Hanson K (2005) Is malaria a disease of poverty? A review of the literature. Trop Med Int Health 10(1): 1047–1059. 10.1111/j.1365-3156.2005.01476.x.

Zhongming Z, Wei L (2021) Climate and weather related disasters surge five-fold over 50 years, but early warnings save lives – WMO report.

CHAPTER 4

Relationship between environmental factors and arboviruses in urban areas

Thiago Salomão de Azevedo[1,2*] *and Rafael Piovezan*[1,3]

[1]Department of Epidemiology, School of Public Health, University of Sao Paulo, Av. Dr Arnaldo, 715, São Paulo, 05509–300, Brazil; [2]Secretary of Health of Santa Barbara d'Oeste, Rua Fernando de Noronha, 707, Santa Barbara d'Oeste, 13451–155, Brazil; [3]Secretary of Environmental of Santa Barbara d'Oeste, Avenida Sábato Ronsini, 905, Santa Barbara d'Oeste, 13450–075, Brazil; *azevedots@gmail.com

Abstract

Arboviruses are a major challenge for Public Health in the world. A relationship established between society such climate change and the ecological capacity for occupy different niches by vectors, particularly mosquitoes, make arboviruses increasingly objects of study that seek to minimize the impact of these diseases on society. Among the main aspects observed, the unplanned urbanization, the demographic growth, the environmental degradation, the low effectiveness and the discontinuity public policies are fundamental issues to face this serious public health problem. The arboviruses outbreaks that occurred in the last decade related to the geographic expansion of the occurrence of mosquitoes, the existence of etiological agents and susceptible vertebrate hosts. Some of these arboviruses are more relevant due to the impact on the health of communities, as well as the indirect, social and economic costs that result from infections. Among these arboviruses, we can highlight Dengue, Zika, Chikungunya, Yellow fever and West Nile fever. Understand the factors that determine the transmission of these arboviruses requires the use of spatial analysis tools and the monitoring the existing environmental variables. That way, the continuous study of the bioecology of the vectors produces the essential knowledge to map areas risk, contributing to the construction of effective surveillance and control programs.

Keywords

arboviruses – climate change – epidemiology – Dengue – Zika – Chikungunya – *Aedes aegypti*

 | DOI:10.3920/9789004688650_006

1 Introduction

The most relevant human factors that change landscape characteristics include unplanned urbanization, demographic increases, consumption habits, irregular disposal of unusable materials, lack of effluent treatment, international mobility, and social inequalities.

A lack of urban planning combined with other human behaviors has increased the number of areas susceptible to infectious disease epidemics associated with insect vectors of infectious agents. The urban environment is artificial and intrinsically dependent on imports of food produced in rural areas. The modifications necessary for the establishment of human populations in urban areas allow synanthropic species to use these spaces to develop their biological cycles (Telle *et al.* 2021).

In this context, different types of artificial habitats that are efficiently exploited by mosquitoes frequently occur in urban environments (Lafferty 2009). The association between vector infestation and human factors results in zoonotic cycles, which are becoming increasingly important to public health. These cycles can be established by the transmission of urban arboviruses or the overflow of etiological agents that circulate in wild and rural regions, especially when they have an interface with urban environments.

Owing to the importance of mosquitoes in the transmission of pathogens, entomological surveillance has been used to elucidate the biological and ecological characteristics of vectors (Wilke *et al.* 2021a). Understanding these characteristics is even more important when we consider that climate change may affect global mosquito distribution, favoring the invasion and establishment of these vector species in non-infested places, or even increasing the infestation density in areas where mosquito vectors are established.

The objective of this chapter is to address some relevant environmental factors in the urban landscape that impact the distribution of mosquito species and present the bioecological aspects of these vectors. The arboviruses covered in this approach are dengue, Zika, Chikungunya, and West Nile viruses, and the vectors are those mosquito species involved in the transmission of these diseases. Proposals for spatial analyses that can contribute to the development of public policies to deal with the aforementioned arboviruses are included.

2 The relationship between mosquitoes and arboviruses

Insects are the dominant class of animals on Earth, surpassing one million described species (Ruppert *et al.* 2005; Brusca and Brusca 2007). This group has diversified, occupying practically all environments on the planet (Triplehorn and Johnson 2011), including anthropized environments, and developing a great diversity of behaviors, including feeding on the blood of several vertebrates for development and/or reproduction (Gullan and Craston 2007).

Applied entomology focuses on studies of the usefulness or harmfulness of insects, including mosquitoes, given their socioeconomic and public health impacts. Every year, billion dollars are spent on the mitigation and control of mosquito vectors and the pathogens that they transmit (Forattini 2002; Marcondes 2011). Arboviruses are arthropod-borne viruses that cause human diseases globally. They are not a distinct taxonomic group, but all arboviruses have an arthropod vector and this mode of transmission defines and guides preventive and control actions (Jones *et al.* 2020).

Currently, the family Culicidae is divided into the subfamilies Anophelinae and Culicinae. The number of species described in this group is approximately 3,500, of which approximately 450 are in the subfamily Anophelinae and 3,100 are in the subfamily Culicinae (Consoli and Lourenço-de-Oliveira 1994; Sallum *et al.* 2000; Harbach 2016). Mosquitoes have a global distribution and are responsible for the transmission of numerous important etiological agents, mainly owing to the blood feeding behavior of females, which facilitates the transmission and, in certain situations, spread of pathogens (Forattini 2002).

The adaptive ability of mosquitoes, together with the current global conjuncture of unplanned urbanization, expands favorable environments for the establishment of vector species. In addition, the macro- and micro-actions of environmental degradation are influenced by climate issues, such as an increase in the global average temperature, which contributes to the proliferation and establishment of mosquito species of medical importance for public health (Liu-Helmersson *et al.* 2014; Misslin *et al.* 2016; Ochida *et al.* 2022).

Mosquito surveillance and control have the fundamental function of estimating the diversity and abundance of these insects. Understand the ecological characteristics of mosquitos is fundamental to developing effective control measures. Given the significant epidemiological relevance of mosquitoes, it is essential that research be conducted to aid control agencies (Gomes 2002). Knowledge of the distribution and abundance of Culicidae species in a given territory, as well as the dynamics between mosquitoes and anthropic environments, is an important focus of entomological surveillance (Donalísio and Glasser 2002).

Approximately 4,000 arboviruses have been isolated from mosquitoes (Powell 2018), of which 500 are known and approximately 100 have the ability to cause diseases in humans (Artsob *et al.* 2017). The best-known arboviruses that have recently had an impact on public health are dengue, Zika, Chikungunya, Mayaro, Venezuelan equine encephalitis, eastern equine encephalitis, western equine encephalitis, yellow fever, Rocio, Oropouche, West Nile, and Saint Louis encephalitis viruses (Forattini 2002).

The occurrence of any arbovirus depends on vector and human host presence, and the availability of a suitable environment (Reisen 2010). The global scenario of climate change, globalization, unplanned urban areas, and adaptation by vectors to human environments has raised concerns about the emergence and intensification of arbovirus outbreaks (Weaver and Reisen 2010; Weaver 2013). Recently, Jones *et al.* (2020) presented a review of the vector status of several mosquito species and the main urban arboviruses, such as dengue, Zika, and Chikungunya viruses. Many studies seek to better understand the impact of the environment and landscape on the epidemiological dynamics of these diseases, which have increased their occurrences worldwide.

3 *Aedes* (Stegomyia) *aegypti* (Linnaeus, 1762) and *Aedes* (Stegomyia) *albopictus* (Skuse, 1894): perspectives and occurrence risks of these species at Americas

It is estimated that mosquitoes transmit arboviruses to 350 million people worldwide annually (WHO 2017). *Aedes* (*Stegomyia*) *aegypti* (Linnaeus, 1762) and *Aedes* (*Stegomyia*) *albopictus* (Skuse, 1894) are the main species involved in the transmission of these viruses in urban areas. For example, approximately 2.5 billion people are at risk of dengue virus infection annually (Liu-Helmersson *et al.* 2014; Segura *et al.* 2021), and thousands more are affected by Zika, Chikungunya, and yellow fever viruses, especially in Latin American and Caribbean countries.

Aedes aegypti aegypti is a subspecies that has adapted to urban environments and is the main urban vector of these arboviruses (Tauil 2002; Catão 2012). The subspecies *Aedes aegypti formosus* has maintained more wild characteristics, reproducing in forests without a human presence. Both subspecies originated in continental Africa. Recent genetic evidence suggests that the ancestral origin of these species occurred approximately 16 million years ago in Madagascar (Soghigian *et al.* 2020). According to this hypothesis, *Ae. aegypti* invaded the nearby African continent approximately 85,000 years ago, and later specialized in the forms *Ae. aegypti formosus* and *Ae. aegypti aegypti.*

Favorable environmental factors, socioeconomic conditions, inadequate urban planning, discontinuity of control actions, and the incredible ability of this vector to adapt to man-made breeding sites have challenged the control of this species worldwide (Lwande *et al.* 2020; Souza *et al.* 2021).

Brazil exhibits an example of vector introduction and persistence despite efforts to eliminate them. *Aedes aegypti* was introduced during the colonial period in the 15th century, eradicated from much of the Americas in the 1950s, and then re-introduced during the following decade. Subsequently, it became the target of one of the largest public health campaigns in the history of Brazil (Câmara *et al.* 2007).

From 2015 to 2021, more than 12.4 million people in the Americas were infected with dengue, resulting in 6,155 deaths (PAHO-WHO 2022). Since 2015, more than

6.7 million people in Brazil have been affected by dengue and 3,707 deaths have been reported (Brasil 2016; 2017; 2018; 2019; 2020; 2021a,b; 2022a,b). These data demonstrate the importance of this arbovirus in Brazil. Over the last seven years, Brazil has registered more than half of the total number of dengue cases and deaths in the Americas.

The Chikungunya virus was first isolated in Tanzania in 1952 (Yactavo *et al.* 2016). Since its most recent resurgence in 2000, this disease has affected more than 2.5 million people and is present in more than 45 countries and territories in the Americas. Brazil has been challenged by successive epidemics of this arbovirus, with more than 900,000 infected people in the last seven years (Yactavo *et al.* 2016; Zeller *et al.* 2016). In 2021, the east Atlantic coast of São Paulo state faced an outbreak of this disease, with more than 14,000 confirmed autochthonous positive cases (São Paulo 2022).

The first record of Zika infection in humans was detected in Uganda (Dick *et al.* 1952). The first case of Zika infection in Latin America was detected in 2015. Subsequently, the number of registered cases have been frequent. Currently, 86 countries have reported Zika virus infections (Weaver *et al.* 2016). Over the past seven years, there were 267,118 confirmed cases in Brazil (Brasil 2016; 2017; 2018; 2019; 2020; 2021a,b; 2022a,b). Tragically, Brazil has recorded approximately 3,600 cases of congenital syndrome and microcephaly due to Zika virus infection (Brasil 2022b).

The arbovirus scenarios associated with climatic variables, particularly temperature, are a factor of concern in disease control programs. It is known that the effects of temperature on the mosquito life cycle influence the development rate in species such *Ae. aegypti*. At the highest temperatures, the development times of immature forms decreases (Lambrechts *et al.* 2011; Islam *et al.* 2021). By contrast, urban heat islands and climate change may have an effect on the thermal behavior of sites, affecting the viral susceptibility of organisms (mosquitos) and influencing public health in the infested localities (Lambrechts *et al.* 2011; Misslin *et al.* 2016; Azevedo *et al.* 2018).

As a domestic subspecies, *Ae. aegypti aegypti* met three fundamental citeria to become one of the most important mosquito species that threatens public health in human population centers: (1) it is highly anthropophilic; (2) it lives in close association with humans and has become an anthropogenic habitat specialist; and (3) it allows replication of the dengue virus and other viruses in its hemolymph, which infects the salivary glands and is reserved with saliva (Craford *et al.* 2017).

Another important species of *Stegomyia* is *Ae. albopictus*, a relevant vector of dengue and Chikungunya transmission in Europe and Asia. In the Americas, this vector plays a less important role in arbovirus transmission but has great potential for arbovirus transmission (Jones *et al.* 2020). *Aedes aegypti* and *Ae. albopictus* are sympatric species. Ecological competition between these species under normal environmental conditions or in situations where feeding is restricted results in the displacement of *Ae. aegypti* by *Ae. albopictus*. In addition, sterilization through copulation between these two species, known as satyrization, has a negative effect on *Ae. aegypti* populations (Yang *et al.* 2021).

However, *Ae. aegypti* has the ability to better withstand long periods of drought and egg desiccation, prefers highly urbanized environments with a wide variety and availability of artificial breeding sites, and can develop satyrization resistance (Yang *et al.* 2021). The ability of *Ae. aegypti* to adapt to unfavorable environmental conditions caused by human activities is superior to that of other mosquito species, enabling it to expand its geographic distribution, reinfest localities, and increase its abundance because it can utilize many kinds of breeding sites for oviposition and development of immature forms (Lounibos *et al.* 2016; Brennan *et al.* 2021).

The coexistence and segregation between two mosquito species have been considered in several studies. These studies recognized the importance of determining the factors that enable the sympatric coexistence of these species. In this way, factors such as the urban landscape (presence/absence of green areas, size and distribution of wooded areas, spatial distribution of neighborhoods based on socioeconomic categories, education, access to public services, etc.) generate the appropriate conditions for mosquito survival (Crespo *et al.* 2022).

The occurrence of *Ae. aegypti*, for example, is more abundant in neighborhoods with a high population density, which often have less wooded green areas, lower socioeconomic populations, and less access to public services (Crespo *et al.* 2022). Therefore, different variables often present a positive spatial correlation with the occurrence of *Ae. aegypti*; however, a detailed analysis demonstrated that many of these variables are related to larger concepts, such as poorly planned urbanization and different levels of social inequalities.

In addition to changes in urban areas, it is critical to recognize how environmental changes and their effects on mosquito species can be defined as important features of an infestation landscape. Brenan *et al.* (2021) demonstrated that *Ae. aegypti* re-established its occurrence in Florida (USA) after 26 years without entomological surveillance monitoring.

Piovezan *et al.* (2012; 2017) observed the displacement of *Ae. albopictus* by *Ae. aegypti* in an area with rural characteristics in the interior of São Paulo State, Brazil, after the largest drought in 100 years occurred in 2014 (Coelho *et al.* 2015; 2016). These findings reinforce what has been presented in other studies, where climatic effects influence the diversity and abundance of mosquito species, and *Ae. aegypti* is more resistant and adapted to prolonged drought conditions than other anthropophilic mosquito species of the *Aedes* genus.

The geographical distribution expansion of *Ae. aegypti* is dangerous owing to the transmission of arboviruses. This species is a more efficient vector for transmission of dengue as it has favorable characteristics for spreading this pathogen among human populations (Lambrechts *et al.* 2011; Liu-Helmersson *et al.* 2014).

Drought events, other climatic events, and urban landscapes that reflect unplanned social inequalities in São Paulo State, Brazil, are alarm signals for a possible expansion of the distribution of arboviruses in regions where they did not occur before (Crespo *et al.* 2022; Misslin *et al.* 2016).

Understanding how climatic phenomena can expand the distribution of *Ae. aegypti* appears to be something that is already consolidated in mosquito vector research. The fact that this species specializes in environments and breeding sites made by anthropic areas is something to be recognized and valued. Control actions often collide with the cultural behavior of communities, making entomological control even more difficult.

People collect water for consumption, owing to interruptions in the piped supply, and cultivate aquatic plants in plant vases, accumulating water in these containers. These human behaviors maintain mosquito breeding site availability without the need for rain to fill these sites. The collection and storage of recyclable materials without rain protection results in favorable and relevant environments for infestation by *Ae. aegypti* in neighboring areas, posing an important challenge to be overcome (Piovezan *et al.* 2019).

The dynamics of these vectors in the urban environment require daily infestation. Rate monitoring, as well as research that makes it possible to understand the relevant actions to be carried out by control agencies to reduce outbreaks and epidemic occurrence risks. Brazil is a country that must be viewed as an example of action for *Ae. aegypti* control, given the importance of this species in the transmission of dengue; thus, a control procedure was established at the federal level. The National Dengue Control Program (Brasil 2002) established specific procedures for the states of the federation, including São Paulo State, and has control actions under the supervision of the Superintendence for Control of Endemic Diseases (São Paulo 2001; 2010).

The fact that this state governmental agency exists makes it important to recognize more effective actions for mosquito control. Under all the aspects mentioned at the local scale (urban landscape) or in global dimensions (climate change), the converging factor is that mosquitoes use breeding sites for the development of immature forms, and this is the point that must be effectively controlled. Furthermore, nebulization and chemical control of adults should be performed whenever necessary, meeting all the inherent technical criteria and blocking the transmission of the virus by contaminated females. In addition, active searching and caring for infected patients is necessary to avoid underreporting and ensure that patients are isolated, making it difficult for mosquitoes to be exposed to viremic people.

Thus, entomological surveillance is increasingly necessary to combat arboviruses as it is an effective tool for guiding different types of mosquito control. Therefore, methods that allow for the optimization of control, directing interventions to places of greatest epidemiological importance (Beatty *et al.* 2011; Carrasco *et al.* 2011; Constenla *et al.* 2015; Abe *et al.* 2018), and reducing the impacts of dengue, Zika, and Chikungunya infections on urban populations are extremely important for these diseases (Morrison *et al.* 2008). Moreover, promoting a societal commitment to eliminate breeding site issues through educational campaigns and legal considerations (creation of specific regulations on arboviruses) must be addressed in a multifactorial manner by government agencies.

4 *Culex pipiens* complex and West Nile Fever

The two main species of Culicinae are *Culex* (*Culex*) *pipiens* (Linnaeus) and *Culex* (*Culex*) *quinquefasciatus* (Say). The distinction between these two species has been the focus of several studies (Forattini 2002). Both species were considered cosmopolitan and favored by anthropic changes, with a high degree of anthropophilia and domiciliation (Gomes and Forattini 1990). Immature forms can develop in different types of breeding sites, including highly polluted aquatic environments (Clements 1999; Reisen 2013).

The species *Cx. quinquefasciatus* and *Cx. pipiens* have been present in large urban centers for decades, colonizing artificial and natural breeding sites and playing important roles in the transmission of arboviruses, such as West Nile virus (WNV) (Reisen 2013). The geographical distribution of *Cx. quinquefasciatus* is commonly in tropical and subtropical regions, whereas *Cx. pipiens* is found in temperate regions. In some South American and Central American countries, and the United States, it is possible to identify coexisting species. In addition to arboviruses, it is important to emphasize the role of *Cx. quinquefasciatus* as the main vector of the *Wuchereria bancrofti* filarial nematode in South America (Consoli *et al.* 1984).

The *pipiens* complex apparently emerged in the Ethiopian region and has adapted to different climates around the world (Ruybal *et al.* 2016). This adaptive capacity allows these species to be distributed both in urban environments, mainly using artificial breeding sites, and in rural areas, colonizing wetlands and ponds used to irrigate agricultural crops (Farajollahi *et al.* 2011).

An example of this ability of this species group were colonized urban centers. In these locations, *Cx. quinquefasciatus* colonizes small-volume artificial breeding sites, such as cans and pots improperly stored in homes, and also uses large bodies of water, such as polluted streams and lakes (Piovezan *et al.* 2012). In rural and peri-urban areas, this species can colonize the drinking fountains of farm animals, including horses and cattle.

Larval research carried out by Piovezan *et al.* 2012, in the municipalities of São Paulo State, Brazil, showed that *Cx quinquefasciatus* was the third most abundant species found alone after *Ae. aegypti* and *Ae. albopictus*, and the second most common found sharing breeding sites in cohabitation with *Ae. aegypti*. These results indicate a complex ecological relationship between *Cx quinquefasciatus* and other Culicidae species found in urban areas, and an intimate relationship with artificial breeding sites provided by humans.

The *pipiens* complex is highly important for the transmission of WNV. Originally identified in 1937 in Uganda, WNV gained great media attention in the late 1990s when it reached New York, USA, causing a large number of human infections and deaths in addition to the death of farm animals (equines) and wild birds (Reisen 2013). It is an avian zoonosis that is maintained in nature after cycles of contamination by birds and ornithophilous mosquitoes.

Urbanization processes result in interventions that typically produce urban spaces surrounded by fragments of vegetation that invariably became strongholds of wild diversity. These locations play an important role in the epidemiology of arboviruses because they connect reservoirs, vectors, and susceptible human hosts. Resisen (2013) described the conjuncture of factors that were fundamental for the WNV epidemic in New York in 1999. This study demonstrated that the migratory bird routes, presence of susceptible farm animals, high temperatures, and urban structure that allowed the great proliferation of mosquitoes were fundamental points in the process of transmission of WNV in that season.

The proximity and connection between wild areas and urban centers were the result of past human actions, often the construction of cities without proper urban planning. However, the current scenario presents another challenge. Societies seek to reduce the impacts of climate change by recovering degraded areas, implementing green areas, and building ecological corridors, which are important public policy processes for the environment and sustainability; however, these processes increase the entropy of urban ecosystems and intensify epidemiological arbovirus risks.

It is important to consider that the species of the *pipiens* complex use waters rich in organic matter, such as wastewater and water bodies containing sewage discharge. This area of basic sanitation has been an important object of public policies, especially in developing countries, with the objective of reducing inappropriate dumping of waste on the ground, and in rivers and streams.

These actions are important for fighting diseases transmitted by contaminated water or etiological agents transmitted by mosquito species that use polluted water to develop their immature forms. However, it is important to note that species such as *Cx. quinquefasciatus* breed in small artificial breeding sites containing clean water, demonstrating that surveillance and entomological control actions are necessary to reduce the occurrence of these mosquitoes in households.

WNV fever has been an important public health problem in North America since the 1999 epidemic, causing approximately 2.8 million infections, 20,000 of which were neuroinvasive, and approximately 1,902 deaths. Important studies have determined the main characteristics of this arbovirus in North America. The transmission of this arbovirus in North America is correlated with a rise in temperature, which increases the vector infestation rate in areas where the human population and domestic animals have not been pre-exposed to the virus (Ruybal *et al.* 2016).

Ruybal *et al.* 2016 modeled the impact of temperature rise on the life history of mosquitoes in the *pipiens* complex. They found that these environmental changes could affect the distribution of WNV cases, increasing the occurrence of this arbovirus in cooler temperate areas and potentially reducing the risk of cases in tropical areas owing to the negative impacts of temperature increase on mosquito survival. These simulations demonstrated that the effects of climate change on the epidemiological dynamics of arboviruses may be more diverse than expected.

Vector monitoring and epidemiological follow-up of the WNV are essential in South America. Mosquitoes of the *Culex* genus, particularly *Cx. quinquefasciatus*, exhibit very fast population growth as these species are able to colonize unstable habitats, have a short biological cycle, and produce more than ten generations per year (Brasil 2011).

Sharper peaks in the frequency of these mosquitoes, with explosive development between generations, occur after the summer rains (Moraes *et al.* 2006). Moreover, numerous studies have shown an association between climatic factors and the abundance of these mosquitoes with outbreaks of East Nile fever (Damos and Caballero 2021).

Mosquitos are referred to as bridging vectors, infection reservoirs, and incidental hosts of WNV because they blood feed on birds and mammals. The epidemiology of WNV circulation depends on the cycle of enzootic transmission between birds and mosquitoes (Kilpatrick *et al.* 2005). Lorenz *et al.* (2022) demonstrated that the areas most susceptible to outbreaks of WNV in South America were precisely conditioned by the migration routes of birds.

This scenario provides a favorable environment for the transmission of WNV in South America because it is precisely in the summer season that the migration of birds from North America occurs, coinciding with the highest frequency of occurrence of the *Culex* mosquito (Fischer and Schweigmann 2004).

5 Environmental variables, urban areas and some proposals for applied studies

Processes involving urbanization, which often influence the epidemiology of vector-borne diseases, have increased the number of outbreaks of various arboviruses (Souza 2021). In urban areas, anthropogenic changes influence Culicidae species dynamics. Considering the complexity inherent to the epidemiology of arboviruses, in addition to this spatial heterogeneity, there is a need for urban landscape studies to focus on vector bioecology while also addressing the social, behavioral,

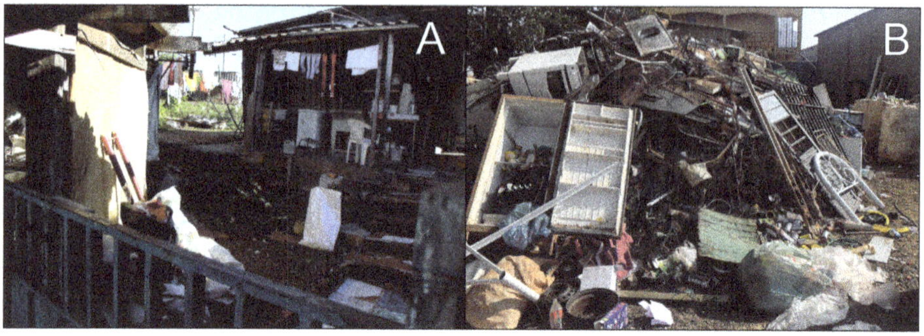

FIGURE 1 (A) House with different kinds of breeding sites in Santa Bárbara d'Oeste, SP, Brazil; (B) Local used for storage of recyclable materials and scrap in Santa Bárbara d'Oeste, SP, Brazil
PHOTO CREDITS: THIAGO SALOMÃO DE AZEVEDO

economic, and environmental conditions of urban landscapes (Maccormack-Gelles *et al.* 2018).

Different types of urban land use allow a range of niches to be exploited by different mosquito species (Crespo *et al.* 2022). Identifying the ovipositional sites of these vectors in urban landscapes is relevant for control programs. Physical, functional, and locational characteristics; type of container; and purpose of use produce differences in the abundance of immature mosquito forms (Flaibani *et al.* 2020; Wilke *et al.* 2021b).

Aedes aegypti has a preference for artificial and shaded breeding sites with clean water. Domestic containers that store water, such as plant pots and dishes, water tanks, and waste materials, are typically used for female oviposition (Figure 1A). Furthermore, in the urban landscape, sustainable recycling policies and the storage of recyclable materials have become increasingly important considerations in vector infestation control (Figure 1B). This situation is occurring in different places within Brazilian municipalities (Piovezan *et al.* 2019), and it is a problem that goes beyond health-related issues because it is closely related to environmental, social, and economic conditions.

Knowledge of Culicidae ecology in urban centers and use of domestic breeding sites for their development is very important in the current scenario of concern regarding the expansion of arboviruses. Understanding the environmental characteristics and urban structure of breeding sites is necessary to identify the spatial patterns of microenvironments that favor, for example, the occurrence of *Ae. aegypti* and *Ae. albopictus*. (Wimberly *et al.* 2020).

Admittedly, *Ae. albopictus* has an ecological preference for green areas within urban landscapes and are most often found near parks, gardens, and green squares (Heinisch *et al.* 2019). *Aedes aegypti* is already more abundant in neighborhoods with higher population densities, more built-up areas, and less vegetation cover (Wilke *et al.* 2021b).

Thus, the presence of this species often overlaps with issues related to socioeconomic variables. In a multifactorial analysis, there were environmental condition vulnerabilities with high rates of *Ae. aegypti* infestation. These places usually have unplanned urbanization resulting in landscape issues that are, as a rule, associated with the most vulnerable territories without adequate public services (Crespo *et al.* 2022).

The plasticity of the ecological niche of *Ae. aegypti* allows the expansion of its geographic distribution, re-infesting localities and increasing its abundance in places where it already exists (Brennan *et al.* 2021). In this context, the landscape structure can appropriately describe spatial variations in disease incidence and/or vector abundance (Acharya *et al.* 2018; Vanwmbeke *et al.* 2007).

In urban landscapes, vegetation dynamics may be a good indicator of mosquito habitats and the presence of breeding sites. Studies have shown a positive association between vector abundance and vegetation indices (Acharya *et al.* 2018). Vegetation provides the optimal moisture conditions necessary for mosquito proliferation and larval development sites. There are several types of vegetation indices, but the normalized difference vegetation index (NDVI) is the most commonly used in studies that correlate urban landscapes with diseases (Estallo *et al.* 2012).

The NDVI describes the difference between the visible and near-infrared reflectance of vegetation and is used to estimate the density of 'green' in a land cover area (Weier and Herring 2000). This index varies from −1.0 to 1.0; negative values represent urban areas and positive values represent vegetated areas (Cunha *et al.* 2021). Very small NDVI function values (≤ 0.1) correspond to areas of rocks, sand, or snow. Values between 0.2 and 0.3 represent areas with sparse vegetation and shrubs. Moderate vegetation tends to vary between values of 0.4 and 0.6, whereas large values (0.6–0.8) indicate the highest possible density of green leaves (i.e. temperate and tropical forests).

Figure 2 shows the spatial association between the positive breeding sites for *Ae. aegypti*, *Ae. albopictus*, and *Cx. quinquefasciatus* in the landscape structure gradient measured for the NDVI. This gradient ranged from preserved environments, composed of complex natural structures and high levels of vegetation cover, to urban environments with less vegetation cover. The patterns of association between species and habitats are well-defined. In more urbanized areas with less arboreal vegetation, *Ae. aegypti* was the most frequently observed species. In contrast, *Ae. albopictus* and *Cx. quinquefasciatus* were more frequent in areas with higher vegetation density. These results corroborate with those of Benitez *et al.* (2019), Acharya *et al.* (2018) and Estallo *et al.* (2018), who reported that urban areas with less arboreal vegetation promoted the establishment of *Ae. aegypti*. This also adds to the

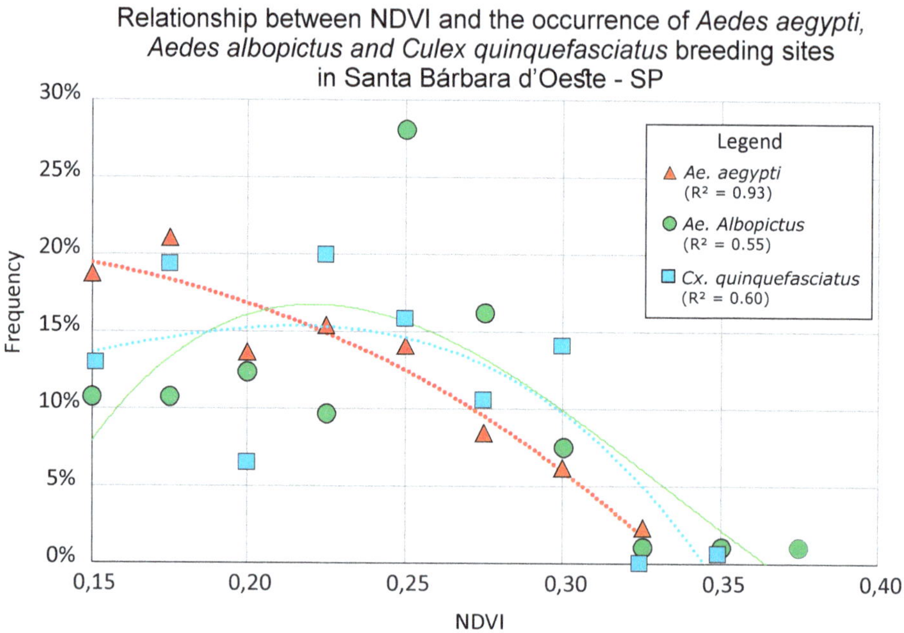

FIGURE 2 Structure of urban landscape and occurrence of different types of Culicidae breeding site

concepts presented by Crespo *et al.* (2022), in which more socioeconomically vulnerable neighborhoods generally have less vegetation cover.

In addition, understanding the response of vectors to climatic conditions in urban landscapes is essential for characterization of the geographic distribution of arboviruses. It is also important to know how the effects of climate on mosquito populations allow the expansion of vector infestations in favorable environments (Iwamura *et al.* 2020).

The effects of climate on vector-borne diseases are not linear; however, they are considered an important factor in the ecological cycle (Caldweel *et al.* 2021). Understanding these factors requires anticipating possible changes in the risk of arbovirus incidence (Iwamura *et al.* 2020).

Humidity and precipitation can trigger different ecological responses. Rain is necessary for the hatching of mosquito eggs and the colonization and infestation of new areas through the use of abandoned containers as breeding sites (Higa 2011). In contrast, heavy rains that occur in the summer can eliminate dormant eggs and expel larvae from these receptacles (Fischer and Schweigmann 2004).

One of the great challenges for infestation control methods is that *Ae. aegypti* can adapt to available breeding sites. For example, this mosquito species takes advantage of the containers that communities in certain regions use to store water for human or animal consumption because of interruptions in the regular piped supply (Huang *et al.* 2018). In other situations, aquatic plants and their dishes and vases, which serve ornamental and scenic purposes, provide places (habitats) for the development of these culicids. These human behaviors ensure that vector populations have access to water resources. These locations are regularly flooded, accumulating water regardless of rainfall. These situations are difficult to control as they fit into established cultural needs and behaviors; thus, they are difficult to eliminate (Piovezan *et al.* 2019).

In addition to precipitation, temperature also has a considerable influence on many aspects of the mosquito life cycle. Temperature influences the epidemiology of arboviruses (Huang *et al.* 2018). The ideal temperature ranges for the viral transmission of arboviruses by *Ae. aegypti*, *Ae. albopictus* (Ryan *et al.* 2019), and *Culex* spp. are 21.3–34 °C, 19.9–29.4 °C, and 16–24 °C (Ciota *et al.* 2014), respectively.

In addition to its effects on viral replication, temperature affects the development of mosquitoes. Tsai *et al.* (2018) determined that the critical temperature required to limit the occurrence of *Ae. aegypti* is 13.8 °C. In another study, *Ae. albopictus* eggs were able to survive at temperatures below −5 °C for 30 days, and larval emergence could occur at very low temperatures (Tippelt *et al.* 2020).

Marinho *et al.* (2016) demonstrated that temperature extremes of 16 and 36 °C considerably decreased the female fecundity and adult longevity of *Ae. aegypti*. Reinhold *et al.* (2018) demonstrated that *Ae. aegypti* mortality rates increased with prolonged exposure to temperatures below 0 and above 40 °C. In relation to *Ae. albopictus* it was concluded that this species was more tolerant to low temperatures than *Ae. aegypti*.

Liu-Helmersson (2014) and Lambrechts *et al.* (2011) tested temperature vs extrinsic incubation period and found that the vectorial transmission capacity for dengue virus decreased with temperatures below 12 and above 36 °C. Shocket *et al.* (2020) showed that the vectorial capacity for WNV transmission in *Culex* mosquitoes is between 23 and 26 °C.

In urban areas, heterogeneous land use generates a mosaic of temperatures that varies temporally and spatially throughout the day (Wimberly *et al.* 2020; Landsberg 1981). The patterns of dengue transmission in Brazil generally follow seasonal variations, with greater risks of transmission and outbreaks in the hottest seasons of the year. This is owing to the fact that with higher temperatures and relative humidity, the development time from egg to adult forms decreases, the longevity of females increases, and the time required for the virus to replicate and infect a host is reduced (Islam *et al.* 2021; Wilke *et al.* 2021b; Zapletal *et al.* 2018).

According to Huber *et al.* (2018), daily temperature variations are important because they affect vector competence. The authors observed that in winter, when the amplitude of daily temperature variation was greater, factors such as viral infection in the midgut, as well as mosquito survival, were negatively impacted, whereas in summer, when the daily temperature amplitude was smaller, the mosquitoes survived longer and became infected with the dengue virus more efficiently. Maintaining elevated temperatures also has a considerable impact on the extrinsic cycle of the dengue virus. Studies have demonstrated that when temperatures are maintained above 30 °C, this cycle is reduced from > 12 days to 7 days (Powell 2018).

Although transmission of the dengue virus is concentrated in the hottest periods of the year, there are environmental conditions that suggest that dengue occurs even at lower temperatures in tropical areas. Azevedo *et al.* (2018) found that dengue transmission remained uninterrupted for several years in the interior of São Paulo State, Brazil.

The findings of these studies show that the occurrence of urban heat islands is the main factor in the maintenance of viral transmission. This meteorological aspect reduces the daily temperature amplitude and provides suitable conditions, even in winter, for mosquito vectors of the dengue virus (Azevedo *et al.* al., 2018; Huber *et al.* 2018).

The association between vector infestation, climatic variables, and anthropic factors results in zoonotic cycles that have become increasingly important for public health. These scenarios are expected to increase the frequency of dengue outbreaks (Azevedo *et al.* 2020). Thus, in epidemiological studies, it is important to distinguish the probability of transmission from the risk of disease (arbovirus). Therefore, elaboration of transmission probability maps as a function of larval habitat occurrence, surface temperature, and the extrinsic incubation period of the virus provides an essential tool for the identification of epidemic outbreak areas (Figure 3).

The occurrence risk map is a function of dengue case history and transmission probability and predicts areas at risk of harboring the dengue virus (Figure 4).

There is congruence between the two maps (Figure 3 and 4) as they show that the northeast and southwest portions of the study area have a high probability of transmission and risk of occurrence of dengue fever. This situation appears to be associated with the socioeconomic conditions of the urban population.

Mapping areas at risk for the occurrence of dengue is a particularly important epidemiological tool to aid in vector control. Piovezan *et al.* (2012) studied the spatial correlation between *Ae. aegypti* breeding sites. The researchers noted that are an influence between is around 270 m of these habitats.

This pattern establishes that a spatial parameter should be considered in vector control. This will be superimposed over risk of transmission areas, with the aim of ensuring that decisions for combating mosquitoes have spatially solid subsidies, which may reflect better practices for outbreak disease control.

The studies presented in this chapter corroborate that temperature heterogeneity in urban areas should provide a mosaic for risk occurrences of diseases transmitted by vectors. The spatiotemporal analysis tools used proved to be highly informative

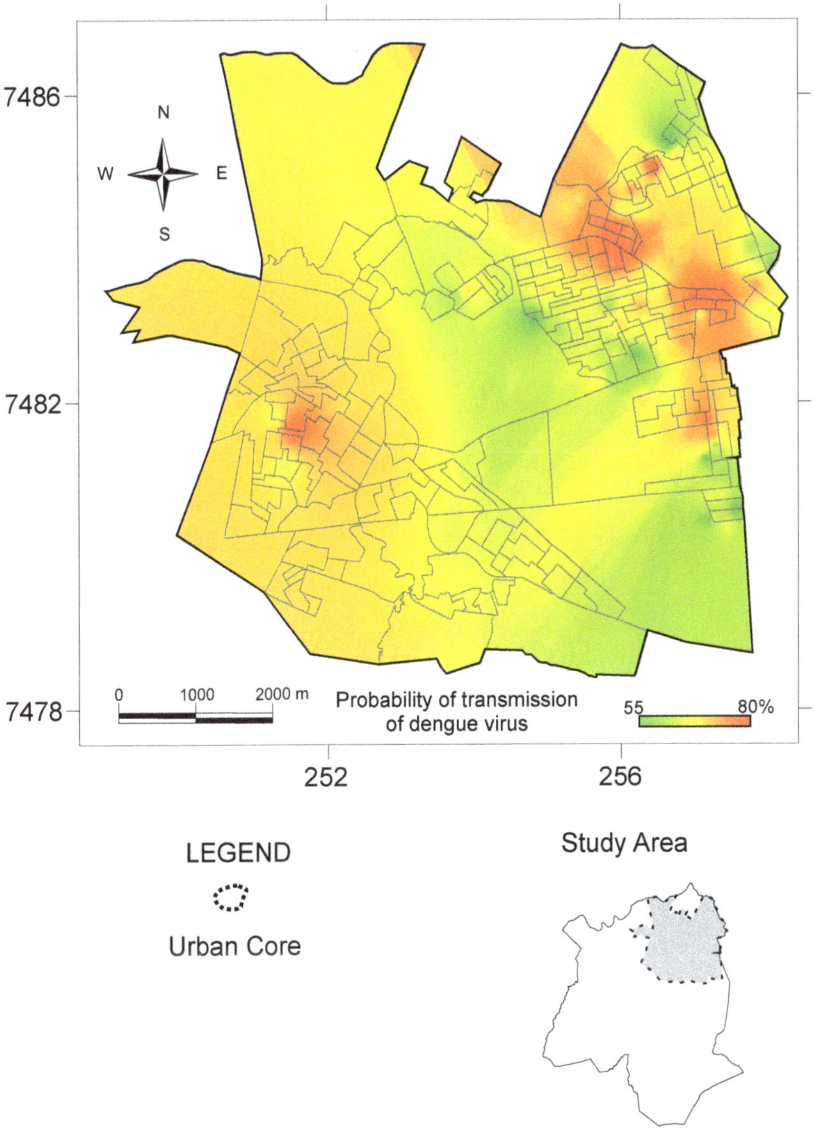

FIGURE 3 Map showing the probability of transmission of dengue virus in urban area of Santa Barbara d'Oeste, Sao Paulo, Brazil

and important in the development of activities for future vector control programs. They will help to provide integrated solutions for problems caused by unplanned urban areas that affect public health. New practices in the management and control of vector-borne diseases are of paramount importance given the adverse impacts that arboviruses have on vulnerable and poor communities.

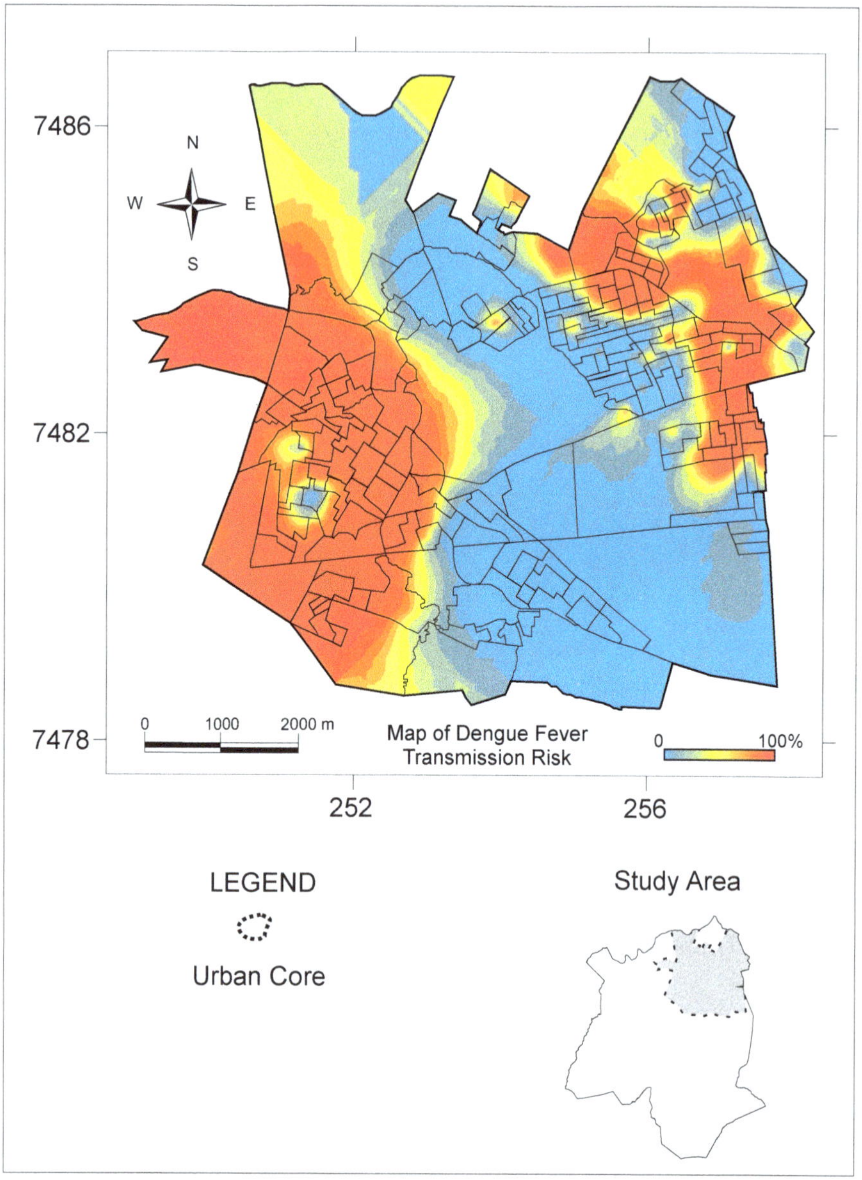

FIGURE 4 Risk map of dengue virus transmission in urban area of Santa Barbara d'Oeste, São Paulo, Brazil

The Pan American Health Organization recommends the daily monitoring of vector infestation rates as a way to protect populations at risk of infectious diseases, such as dengue, Zika, Chikungunya, yellow, and West Nile fevers.

The requirements for daily monitoring should contemplate new studies that consider how urban microclimate variables influence vector ecology and the risk of disease transmission. Understanding how these factors potentiate the occurrence of arboviruses in urban environments is essential for the development of more efficient environmental surveillance and disease control strategies.

Brazil has particularly extensive experience with disease control strategies, such as those for dengue (Brasil 2002, 2009; São Paulo 2001, 2010). However, continuous public policy and intersectional governmental support is essential for addressing this issue.

The effects of climate change will also alter the distribution of vectors and, consequently, arboviruses. It is very important to consider the entomological and ecological data for mosquito vector occurrence at local and regional geographical scales when predicting the consequences of climate change. This dynamic knowledge can also inform the decisions made by public managers regarding the mitigation of human impacts.

Acknowledgements

The authors wish to thank William K. Reisen, University of California, for helpful suggestions that greatly improved this chapter.

References

Abe KC, Georges S and Miraglia EK (2018) Incidência de dengue e custos associados, nos períodos anterior (2000–2008) e posterior (2009–2013) à construção das usinas hidrelétricas em Rondônia. Epidemiologia e Serviços em Saúde. 27(2): e2017232. https://doi.org/10.5123/S1679-49742018000200012.

Artsob H, Lindsay R and Drebot M (2017) Arboviruses, International Encyclopedia of Public Health. Editor(s): STELLA R. QUAH, Academic Press. 2nd Edit. p: 154–160. https://doi.org/10.1016/B978-0-12-803678-5.00023-0, 2017.

Acharya BK, Cao C, Xu M, Khanal L, Naeem S and Pandit S (2018) Temporal variations and associated remotely sensed environmental variables of dengue fever in Chitwan District, Nepal. International Journal of Geo-Information. 7(7): e275. https://doi.org/10.3390/ijgi7070275.

Azevedo TS, Lorenz C and Chiaravalloti-Neto F (2020) Spatiotemporal evolution of dengue outbreaks in Brazil. Royal Society of Tropical Medicine and Hygiene. 114(8): 593–602. https://doi.org/10.1093/trstmh/tra030.

Azevedo TS, Bourke BP, Piovezan R and Sallum MAM (2018) The influence of urban heat islands and socioeconomic factors on the spatial distribution of *Aedes aegypti* larval habitats. Geospatial Health. 13: 179–187. https://doi.org/10.4081/gh.2018.623.

Beatty ME, Beutels P, Meltzer MI, Shepard DS, Hombach J, Hutubessy R, Dessis D, Coudeville L, Dervaux B, Wichmann O, Margolis HS and Kuritsky JN (2011) Health Economics of Dengue: A systematic literature review and expert panel's assessment. American Journal of Tropical Medicine and Hygiene. 84(3): 473–488. https://doi.org/10.4269/ajtmh.2011.10-0521.

Benitez EM, Ludueña-Almeida F, Frías-Céspedes M, Almirón WR and Estallo EL (2019) Could land cover influence *Aedes aegypti* mosquito populations? Medical and Veterinary Entomology. 34: 138–144. https://doi.org/10.1111/mve.12422.

Brasil (2002) Ministério da Saúde, Fundação Nacional de Saúde (FUNASA). Programa Nacional de Controle da Dengue (PNCD). Brasília: FUNASA.

Brasil (2011) Guia de Vigilância do *Culex quinquefasciatus*. Brasília: Ministério da Saúde: Secretaria de Vigilância em Saúde. 1st edit. 76p.

Brasil (2016) Boletim Epidemiológico. Secretaria de Vigilância em Saúde – Ministério da Saúde. Volume 47 no. 3. Monitoramento dos casos de dengue, febre de chikungunya e febre pelo vírus Zika até a Semana Epidemiológica 52, 2015. Available at: https://antigo.saude.gov.br/images/pdf/2016/janeiro/15/svs2016-be003-dengue-se52.pdf.

Brasil (2017) Boletim Epidemiológico. Secretaria de Vigilância em Saúde – Ministério da Saúde. Volume 48 no. 3. Monitoramento dos casos de dengue, febre de chikungunya e febre pelo vírus Zika até a Semana Epidemiológica 52, 2016. Available at: https://antigo.saude.gov.br/images/pdf/2017/abril/06/2017-002-Monitoramento-dos-casos-de-dengue--febre-de-chikungunya-e-febre-pelo-v--rus-Zika-ate-a-Semana-Epidemiologica-52--2016.pdf.

Brasil (2018) Boletim Epidemiológico. Secretaria de Vigilância em Saúde – Ministério da Saúde. Volume 49 no. 2. Monitoramento dos casos de dengue, febre de chikungunya e febre pelo vírus Zika até a Semana Epidemiológica 52, 2017. Available: at https://antigo.saude.gov.br/images/pdf/2018/janeiro/23/Boletim-2018-001-Dengue.pdf.

Brasil (2019) Boletim Epidemiológico. Secretaria de Vigilância em Saúde – Ministério da Saúde. Volume 50 no. 4. Monitoramento dos casos de dengue, febre de chikungunya e febre pelo vírus Zika até a Semana Epidemiológica 52, 2018. Available at: https://antigo.saude.gov.br/images/pdf/2019/janeiro/28/2019-002.pdf.

Brasil (2020) Boletim Epidemiológico. Secretaria de Vigilância em Saúde – Ministério da Saúde. Volume 51 no. 2. Monitoramento dos casos de dengue, febre de chikungunya e febre pelo vírus Zika até a Semana Epidemiológica 52, 2019. Available at: https://antigo.saude.gov.br/images/pdf/2020/janeiro/20/Boletim-epidemiologico-SVS-02-1-.pdf.

Brasil (2021a) Boletim Epidemiológico. Secretaria de Vigilância em Saúde – Ministério da Saúde. Volume 51 no. 33. Óbito por arboviroses no Brasil de 2008–2019. Available at: https://antigo.saude.gov.br/images/pdf/2020/August/21/Boletim-epidemiologico-SVS-33.pdf.

Brasil (2021b) Boletim Epidemiológico. Secretaria de Vigilância em Saúde – Ministério da Saúde. Volume 52 no. 3. Monitoramento dos casos de dengue, febre de chikungunya e febre pelo vírus Zika até a Semana Epidemiológica 52, 2020. Available at: https://www.gov.br/saude/pt-br/assuntos/media/pdf/2021/fevereiro/01/boletim_epidemiologico_svs_3.pdf.

Brasil (2022a) Boletim Epidemiológico. Secretaria de Vigilância em Saúde – Ministério da Saúde. Volume 53 no. 1. Monitoramento dos casos de dengue, febre de chikungunya e febre pelo vírus Zika até a Semana Epidemiológica 23, 2021. Available at: https://www.gov.br/saude/pt-br/media/pdf/2021/junho/21/boletim_epidemiologico_svs_23.pdf.

Brasil (2022b) Boletim Epidemiológico. Secretaria de Vigilância em Saúde – Ministério da Saúde. Volume 52 no. 4. Situação epidemiológica da síndrome congênita associada à infecção pelo vírus Zika: Brasil, 2015 a 2021. Available at: https://www.gov.br/saude/pt-br/centrais-de-conteudo/publicacoes/boletins/boletins-epidemiologicos/edicoes/2021/boletim_epidemiologico_svs_4.pdf.

Brennan SA, Grob IC, Bartz CE, Baker JK and Jiang Y (2021) Displacement of *Aedes albopictus* by *Aedes aegypti* in gainesville, Florida. Journal of the American Mosquito Control Association. 37(2):93–97. https://doi.org/10.2987/20-6992.1.

Brusca RC and Brusca GJ (2007) Invertebrados. Rio de Janeiro: Guanabara Hoogan 2nd edit. 968 p.

Caldwell JM, Labeaud AD, Lambin EF, Stewart-Ibarra AM, Ndenga BA, Mutuku FM, Amy R, Krystosik AR, Ayala EB, Anyamba A, Borbor-Cordova MJ, Damoah R, Grossi-Soyster EM, Heras FH, Ngugi HN, Ryan SJ, Shah MM, Sippy R and Mordecai EA (2021) Climate predicts geographic and temporal variation in mosquito-borne disease dynamics on two continents. Nature Communications. 12: e1233. https://doi.org/10.1038/s41467-021-21496-7.

Câmara FP, Theophilo RLG, Santos GT, Pereira SRFG, Camara DC and Matos RRC (2007) Estudo retrospectivo (histórico) da dengue no Brasil: características regionais e dinâmicas. Revista da Sociedade Brasileira de Medicina Tropical. 40 (2): 92–96.

Catão RC (2012) Dengue no Brasil: abordagem na escala nacional. São Paulo: Cultura Acadêmica. 1st edit. 75p.

Carrasco LR, Lee LK, Lee VJ, Ooi EE, Shepard DS, Thein TL, Gan V, Cook AR, Lye D, Ching N and Leo YS (2011) Economic Impact of Dengue Illness and the Cost-Effectiveness of Future Vaccination Programs in Singapore. Plos Neglected Tropical Diseases. 5(12): e1426. https://doi.org/0.37/journal.pntd.000426.

Ciota AT, Matachiero AC, Kilpatrick AM and Kramer LD (2014) The effect of temperature on life history traits of *Culex* mosquitoes. Journal of Medical Entomological. 51(1): 55–62. https://doi.org/10.1603/me13003.

Clements AN (1999) The biology of mosquitoes. Volume 2: sensory reception and behaviour. ISBN: 9780851993133, CABI Publishing, Wallingford, UK, 740p.

Coelho CAS, Cardoso DHF and Firpo MAF (2015) Precipitation diagnostics of a exceptionally dry event in São Paulo, Brazil. Theoretical and Applied Climatology. 125:769–778. https://doi.org/10.1007/s00704-015-1540-9.

Coelho CAS, Oliveira CP, Ambrizzi T, Reboita MS, Carpenedo CB, Campos JLPS, Tomaziello CAN, Pampuch LA, Custódio MS, Dutra LMM and Da Roocha RP (2016) The 2014 southeast Brazil austral summer drought: regional scale mechanisms and teleconnections. Climate Dynamics. 46: 3737–3752. https://doi.org/10.1007/s00382-015-2800-1.

Consoli RAGB and Lourenço-De-Oliveira R (1994) Principais mosquitos de importância sanitária no Brasil. Rio de Janeiro, FIOCRUZ, Rio de Janeiro: FIOCRUZ. 1st edit. 228p.

Consoli RAGB, Guimarães CT, Souza CP and Santos BS (1984) Atividade predatória de Helobdella triserialis lineata (Hirudinea: Glossiphonidae) sobre formas imaturas de *Aedes fluviatilis* e *Culex quinquefasciatus* (Diptera: Culicidae) em laboratório. Revista de Saúde Pública. 18 (5): 359–366.

Constenla D, Garcia C and Lefcourt N (2015) Assessing the Economics of Dengue: Results from a systematic review of the literature and expert survey. Pharmaco Economic. 33: 1107–1135. https://doi.org/0.007/s40273-05-0294-7.

Crawford JE, Alves JM, Palmer WJ, Day JP, Sylla M, Ramasamy R, Surendran SN, Black WC, Pain A and Jiggins FM (2017) Population genomics reveals that an anthropophilic population of *Aedes aegypti* mosquitoes in West Africa recently gave rise to American and Asian populations of this major disease vector. BMC Biology. 15(1): e16. https://doi.org/0.86/s295-07-035-0.

Crespo RJ and Rogers RE (2022) Habitat segregation patterns of container breeding mosquitos: the role of urban heat island, vegetation cover, and income disparity in cemeteries of New Orleans. International Journal of Environmental Research and Public Health. 19(1): e245. https://doi.org/0.3390/ijerph900245.

Cunha MC, Ju Y, Morais MHF, Dronova I, Ribeiro SP, Bruhn RP, Lima LL, Sales DM, Schultes OL, Rodriguez DA and Caiaffa WT (2021) Disentangling associations between vegetation greenness and dengue in a Latin American city: Findings and challenges. Landscape and Urban Planning. 216: 104255. https://doi.org/0.06/j.landurbplan.202.04255.

Damos P and Caballero P (2021) Detecting seasonal transient correlations between populations of the West Nile virus vector *Culex* sp. and temperatures with wavelet coherence analysis. Ecological Informatics 61: e101216. https://doi.org/10.1016/j.ecoinf.2021.101216.

Dick WA, Kitchen SF and Haddow AJ (1952) Zika Virus (I). Isolations and serological specificity. Transactions of The Royal Society of Tropical Medicine and Hygiene. 46 (5): 509–520. https://doi.org/10.1016/0035-9203(52)90042-4.

Donalísio MR and Glasser CM (2002) Vigilância Entomológica e controle de vetores do dengue. Revista Brasileira de Epidemiologia. 5 (3): 259–272.

Estallo EL, Sangermani F, Grech M, Ludueña-Almeida FM, Frías-Cespedes M, Ainete M, Almirón W and Livdahl T (2018) Modelling the distribution of the vector *Aedes aegypti* in a central Argentine city. Journal of Medical Entomology. 32 (4): 451–461. https://doi.org/0./mve.2323.

Farajollahi A, Fonseca DM, Kramer LD and Kilpatrick AM (2011) 'Bird biting' mosquitoes and human disease: a review of the role of *Culex pipiens* complex mosquitoes in epidemiology. Infection, Genetics and Evolution. 11 (7): 1577–1585. https://doi.org/10.1016/j.meegid.2011.08.013.

Fischer S and Schweigmann N (2004) *Culex* mosquitoes in temporary urban rain pools: seasonal dynamics and relation to environmental variables. Journal of Vector Ecology. 29 (2): 365–373.

Flaibani N, Pérez AA, Barbero IM and Burroni NE (2020) Different approaches to characterize artificial breeding sites of *Aedes aegypti* using generalized linear mixed models. Infectious Diseases of Poverty. 9 (1): 107. https://doi.org/0.86/s40249-020-00705-3.

Forattini OP (2002) Culicidologia Médica. Vol 2, São Paulo, Edusp. 864.

Gomes AC (2002) Vigilância Entomológica. Informe Epidemiológico do SUS. 11 (2): 79–90.

Gomes AC and Forattini OP (1990) Abrigos de mosquitos *Culex* (*Culex*) em zona Rural (Diptera: Culicidae). Revista de Saúde Pública. 24 (5): 394–397. https://doi.org/10.1590/S0034-89101990000500007.

Gullan PJ and Cranston PS (2007) Os insetos: um resumo de entomologia. São Paulo: Roca. 1st edit. 456p.

Harbch RE (2016) Mosquitoes Taxonomic Inventory. Valid Species List. Available at http://mosquito-taxonomic-inventory.info/valid-species-list.

Heinisch MRS, Diaz-Quijano FA, Chiaravalloti-Neto F, Pancetti FGM, Coelho RR, Andrade PS, Urbinatti PR, Almeida RMMS and Lima-Camara TN (2019) Seasonal and spatial distribution of *Aedes aegypti* and *Aedes albopictus* in a municipal urban park in São Paulo, SP, Brazil. Acta Tropica. 189: 104–111. https://doi.org/0.06/j.actatropica.208.09.0.

Higa Y (2011) Dengue vectors and their spatial distribution. Tropical Medicine and Health. 39 (4 Suppl): 17–27. https://doi.org/0.249/tmh.20-S04.

Huang C, Tam TYT, Chern Y, Lung SC, Chen N and Wu C (2018) Spatial Clustering of Dengue Fever Incidence and Its Association with Surrounding Greenness. International Journal of environmental Research and Public Health. 15(9): 1869. https://doi.org/0.3390/ijerph509869.

Huber JH, Childs ML, Caldwell JM and Mordecai EA (2018) Seasonal temperature variation influences climate suitability for dengue, chikungunya, and Zika transmission. Plos Neglected Tropical Diseases. 12 (5): e0006451. https://doi.org/0.37/journal.pntd.000645.

Islam S, Haque CE, Hossain S and Hanesiak J (2021) Climate variability, dengue vector abundance and dengue fever cases in Dhaka, Bangladesh: a time-series study. Atmos. 12 (7): e905. https://doi.org/0.3390/atmos2070905.

Iwamura T, Guzman-Holst A and Murray KA (2020) Accelerating invasion potential of disease vector *Aedes aegypti* under climate change. Nature Communications. 11(1): e2130 https://doi.org/10.1038/s41467-020-16010-4.

Jones R, Kulkarni MA and Davidson TMV (2020) Arbovirus vectors of epidemiological concern in the Americas: A scoping review of entomological studies on Zika, dengue and chikungunya virus vectors. PLoS One. 15(2): e0220753. https://doi.org/0.37/journal.pone.0220753, 2020.

Kilpatrick AM, Kramer LD, Campbell SR, Alleyne O, Dobson AP and Daszak P (2005) West Nile virus risk assessment and the bridge vector paradigm. Emerging Infectious Diseases. 11(3): 425–429. https://doi.org/10.3201/eid1103.040364.

Lafferty KD (2009) The ecology of climate change and infectious diseases. Ecology. 90 (4): 888–900.

Landsberg HE (1981) The urban climate. Academic Press. New York. 1st edit. 275 p.

Lambrechts L, Paaijmans KP, Fansiri T, Carrington LB, Kramer LD, Thomas MB *et al.* (2011) Impact of daily temperature fluctuations on dengue virus transmission by *Aedes aegypti*. Proceedings of the National Academy of Sciences of the United States of America. 108 (18): 7460–7465. https://doi.org/0.073/pnas.037708.

Liu-Helmersson J, Stenlund H, Wilder-Smith A and Rocklov J (2014) Vectorial capacity of *Aedes aegypti*: effects of temperature and implications for global dengue epidemic potential. PLoS One. 9 (3): e89783. https://doi.org/0.37/journal.pone.0089783.

Lorenz C, Azevedo TS and Chiaravalloti-Neto F (2022) Impact of climate change on West Nile virus distribution in South America. Transactions of the Royal Society of Tropical Medicine and Hygiene. 116 (11): 1043–1053. https://doi.org/10.1093/trstmh/trac044.

Lounibos LP, Bargielowski I, Carrasquilla C and Nishimura N (2016) Coexistence of *Aedes aegypti* and *Aedes albopictus* (Diptera: Culicidae) in Peninsular Florida two decades after competitive displacements. Journal of Medical Entomology. 53 (6): 1385–1390. https://doi.org/0.093/jme/tjw22.

Lwande OW, Obanda V, Lindstro A, Ahlm C, Evander M, Na Slund J and Bucht G (2020) Globe-Trotting *Aedes aegypti* and *Aedes albopictus*: Risk Factors for Arbovirus Pandemics. Vector-Borne and Zoonotic Diseases. 20 (2): 71–81. https://doi.org/0.089/vbz.209.2486.

Maccormack-Gelles B, Lima Neto AS, Sousa GS, Nascimento OJ, Machado MMT, Wilson ME and Castro MC (2018) Epidemiological characteristics and determinants of dengue transmission during epidemic and non-epidemic years in Fortaleza, Brazil: 2011–2015. Plos Neglected Tropical Diseases. 12 (12): e0006990. https://doi.org/0.37/journal.pntd.0006990.

Marcondes CB (2001) Entomologia médica e veterinária. Rio de Janeiro: Atheneu. 2nd edit. 544p.

Marinho, R.A.; Beserra, E.B.; Bezerra-Gusmão, M.A.; Porto, V.S.; Olinda, R.A.; Santos, CAC (2016) Effects of temperature on the life cycle, expansion, and dispersion of *Aedes aegypti* (Diptera: Culicidae) in three cities in Paraiba, Brazil. Jounal of Vector Ecology. 41 (1): 1–10. https://doi.org/0./jvec.287.

Misslin R, Telle O, Daudé E, Vaguet A and Paul RE (2016) Urban climate versus global climate change-what makes the difference for dengue? Annals of the New York Academy of Sciences. 1382 (1): 56–72. https://doi.org/0./nyas.3084.

Moraes SA, Marrelli MT and Natal Delsio (2006) Aspectos da distrobuição de *Culex* (*Culex*) *quinquefasciatus* Say (Diptera: Culicidae) na região do Pinheiros, na cidade de São Paulo, Estado de São Paulo, Brasil. Revista Brasileira de Entomologia 50 (3): 413–418. https://doi.org/10.1590/S0085-56262006000300012.

Morrison AC, Zielinski-Gutierrez E, Scott TW and Rosenberg R (2008) Defining Challenges and Proposing Solutions for Control of the Virus Vector *Aedes aegypti*. PLoS Medicine. 5 (3): e68. https://doi.org/0.37/journal.pmed.0050068.

Ochida N, Mangeas M, Dupont-Rouzeyrol M, Dutheil C, Forfait C, Peltier A, Descloux E and Menkes C (2022) Modeling present and future climate risk of dengue outbreak, a case study in New Caledonia. Environmental Health. 21: e22. https://doi.org/10.1186/s12940-022-00829-z.

PAHO-WHO (2022) Pan American Health – World Health Organization. Dengue: PAHO/WHO data, Maps and Statistics. https://www3.paho.org/data/index.php/es/temas/indicadores-dengue/dengue-regional/506-dengue-reg-ano-es.html.

Piovezan R, Azevedo TS and Von Zuben CJ (2012) Spatial evaluation of larvae of Culicidae (Diptera) from different breeding sites: application of a geospatial method and implications for vector control. Revista Brasileira de Entomologia. 56 (3): 368–376. https://doi.org/0.590/S0085-56262020050000037.

Piovezan R, Acorinthe JPO, Souza JHT, Visockas A, Azevedo TS and Von Zuben CJ (2017) Spatial distribution of culicidae (diptera) larvae, and its implications for public health, in five areas of the Atlantic Forest biome, state of São Paulo, Brazil. 61 (2): 123–135. Revista Brasileira de Entomologia. https://doi.org/0.06/j.rbe.206.2.

Piovezan R, Visockas A, Azevedo TS, Zuben CJ and Sallum MAM (2019) Spatial-temporal distribution of *Aedes* (*Stegomyia*) *aegypti* and locations of recycling unitis in southeastern Brazil. Parasite & Vectors. 12 (1): 541. https://doi.org/0.86/s307-09-3794-z.

Powell JR (2018) Mosquito-Borne Human Viral Diseases: Why *Aedes aegypti*? American Journal of Tropical Medicine and Hygiene. 98 (6): 1563–1565. https://doi.org/0.4269/ajtmh.7-0866.

Reinhold JM, Lazzari CR and Lahondère C (2018) Effects of the Environmental Temperature on *Aedes aegypti* and *Aedes albopictus* Mosquitoes: A Review. Insects. 9 (4):158. https://doi.org/10.3390/insects9040158.

Reisen WK (2013) Ecology of West Nile Virus in North America. Viruses. 5 (9): 2079–2105. https://doi.org/10.3390/v5092079.

Reisen WK (2010) Landscape epidemiology of vector-borne diseases. Annual Review of Entomology. 55: 461–483.

Ruppert EE, Fox RS and Barnes RD (2005) Zoologia dos Invertebrados. São Paulo: Roca. 4th edit. 1046p.

Ruybal JE, Kramer LD and Kilpatrick M (2016) Geographic variation in the response of *Culex pipiens* life history traits to temperature. Parasites & Vectors. 9: e116. https://doi.org/10.1186/s13071-016-1402-z. 2016.

Ryan SJ, Carlson CJ, Mordecai EA and Johnson LR (2019) Global expansion and redistribution of *Aedes*-borne virues transmission risk with climate change. Plos Neglected Tropical Diseases. 13 (3): e0007213. https://doi.org/10.1371/journal.pntd.0007213.

Sallum MAM, Schutz TR and Wilkerson RC (2000) Phylogeny of Anophelinae (Diptera: Culicidae) based on morphological characters. Annals of the Entomological Society of America. 93(4): 745–775.

Segura NA, Muñoz AL, Losada-Barragán M, Torres O, Rodríguez AK, Rangel H and Bello F (2021) Minireview: Epidemiological impact of arboviral diseases in Latin American countries, arbovirus-vector interactions and control strategies. Pathogens and Disease. 79 (7): eftab043. https://doi.org/10.1093/femspd/ftab043.

Soghigian J, Gloria-Soria A, Robert V, Le Goff G, Failloux AB and Powell JR (2020) Genetic evidence for the origin of *Aedes aegypti*, the yellow fever mosquito, in the southwestern Indian Ocean. Molecular Ecology. 29 (19): 3593–3606.

São Paulo (2001) Superintendência de Controle de Endemias. Vigilância e controle do *Aedes aegypti*: Normas, orientações e recomendações técnicas. Plano de Intensificação das ações de controle de dengue no Estado de São Paulo. Secretaria de Estado da Saúde de São Paulo, Governo do Estado de São Paulo. 71 p.

São Paulo (2010) Superintendência de Controle de Endemias. Coordenadoria de Controle de Doenças: Programa de Vigilância e Controle da Dengue. Secretaria de Estado da Saúde de São Paulo Governo do Estado de São Paulo. Available at: http://www.cve.saude.sp.gov.br/htm/zoo/pdf/Programa10_Estadual_dengue.pdf.

São Paulo (2022) CVE – Centro de Vigilância Epidemiológica 'Prof. Alexandre Vranjac'. Distribuição dos casos confirmados de Chikungunya importado, autoctone, lpi, semana epidemiológica ESP, 202. Available at: https://www.saude.sp.gov.br/ resources/cve-centro-de-vigilancia-epidemiologica/areas-de-vigilancia/doencas-de-ransmissao-por-vetores-e-zoonoses/dados/chikung/202/chikung2_import_autoc_res.htm.

Shocket MS, Verwillow AB, Numazu MG, Slamani H, Cohen JM, Moustaid FE, Rohr J, Johnson LR and Mordecai EA (2020) Transmission of West Nile and five other temperate mosquitos-borne viruses peaks at temperatures between 23 °C and 26 °C. eLife. 9: e58511. https://doi.org/10.7554/eLife.58511.

Souza SC, Carneira M, Eiras AE, Bezerra JMT and Barbosa DS (2021) Factors associated with the occurrence of dengue epidemics in Brazil: a systematic review. Revista Panamericana de Salud Publica. 45: e84. https://doi.org/0.26633/RPSP.202.84.

Tauil PL (2002) Aspectos críticos do controle do dengue no Brasil. Cadernos de Saúde Pública. 18 (3): 867–87.

Telle O, Nikolay B, Kumar V, Benkimoun S, Pal S, Nagpal BN and Paul RR (2021) Social and environmental risk factors for dengue in Delhi city: A retrospective study. Plos Neglected Tropical Diseases. 15 (2): e0009024. https://doi.org/0.37/journal.pntd.0009024.

Tippelt L, Werner D and Kampen H (2020) Low temperature tolerance of three *Aedes albopictus* strains (Diptera: Culicide) under constant and fluctuating temperature scenarios. Parasite & Vectors. 13 (1): 587. https://doi.org/10.1186/s13071-020-04386-7.

Triplehorn CA and Jonnson NF (2011) Estudo dos insetos. São Paulo: Cengage Learning. 7th edit. 776p.

Tsai PJ, Lin TH, Teng HJ and Yeh HC (2018) Critical low temperature for the survival of *Aedes aegypti* in Taiwan. Parasite & Vectors. 11: e22. https://doi.org/10.1186/s13071-020-04386-7.

Vanwambeke SO, Somboon P, Harbach R, Isenstadt M, Lambin EF, Walton C and Butlin RK (2007) Landscape and land cover factors influence the presence of *Aedes* and *Anopheles* larvae. Journal of Medical Entomology. 44 (1): 133–144. https://doi.org/0.603/0022-2585.

Yactavo S, Staples JE, Millot V, Cibrelus L and Ramon-Pardo P (2016) Epidemiology of Chikungunya in the Americas. The Journal of Infectious Diseases. 214 (Suppl 5): 441–445. https://doi.org/0.093/infdis/jiw390.

Yang B, Borget BA, Alto BW, Boohene CK, Brew J, Deutsch K, *et al.* (2021) Modelling distributions of *Aedes aegypti* and *Aedes albopictus* using climate, host density and interspecies competition. Plos Neglected Tropical Diseases. 15(3): e0009063. https://doi.org/0.37/journal.pntd.0009063.

Weier J and Herring D (2000) Measuring vegetation (NDVI & EVI). NASA. Available at: https://earthobservatory.nasa.gov/features/MeasuringVegetation.

Weaver SC and Reisen W (2010) Present and future arboviral threats. Antiviral Research. 85 (2): 328–345. https://doi.org/10.1016/j.antiviral.2009.10.008.

Weaver SC (2013) Urbanization and geographic expansion of zoonotic arboviral diseases: mechanisms and potential strategies for prevention. Trends in Microbiology. 21 (8): 360–363. https://doi.org/10.1016/j.tim.2013.03.003.

Weaver SC, Costa F, Garcia-Blanco MA, Ko AI, Ribeiro GS, Saade G, Yongshi P and Vasilakis N (2016) Zika vírus: History, emergence, biology and prospects for control. Antiviral Research. 130: 69–80. https://doi.org/10.1016/j.antiviral.2016.03.010. 2016.

Wilke ABB, Benelli G and Beier JC (2021a) Urbanization and the rise of vector mosquitoes and arbovirus transmission. Proceedings. 1st International Electronic Conference on Entomology. https://doi.org/0.3390IECE-050.

Wilke ABB, Vasquez C, Carvajal A, Moreno M, Fuller DO, Cardenas G, Petrie WD and Beier JC (2021b) Urbanization favors the proliferation of *Aedes aegypti* and *Culex quinquefasciatus* in urban areas of Miami-Dade County, Florida. Scientific Reports. 11: e 22989. https://doi.org/10.1038/s41598-021-02061-0.

WHO (2017) Global vector control response 207–2030. Geneva: World Health Organization; Document A70/26 Rev.1. 5p. Available at: https://apps.who.int/gb/ebwha/pdf_files/WHA70/A70_R16-en.pdf?ua=1.

Wimberly MC, Davis JK, Evans MV, Hess A, Newberry PM, Solano-Asamoah N and Murdock CC (2020) Land cover affects microclimate and temperature suitability for arbovirus transmission in an urban landscape. Plos Neglected Tropical Diseases. 14 (9): e0008614. https://doi.org/10.1371/journal.pntd.0008614.

Zapletal J, Erraguntla M, Adelman ZN, Myles KM and Lawley MA (2018) Impacts of diurnal temperature and larval density on aquatic development of *Aedes aegypti*. Plos One. 13 (3): e0194025. https://doi.org/0.37/journal.pone.094025.

Zeller H, Bortel WV and Sudre B (2016). Chikungunya: its history in Africa and Asia and its spread to new regions in 203–204. The Journal of Infectious Diseases. 214 (suppl 5): 436–440. https://doi.org/https://doi.org/0.093/infdis/jiw39.

PART 2

Coupled human and natural systems

CHAPTER 5

A conceptual framework for understanding extractive settlements and disease: demography, environment, and epidemiology

Natasha Glendening[1], *Werissaw Haileselassie*[2] *and Daniel M. Parker*[1*]

[1]Program in Public Health, College of Health Sciences, University of California at Irvine, Irvine, CA 92697, USA; [2]School of Public Health, College of Health Sciences, Addis Ababa University, Addis Ababa, Ethiopia; *dparker1@hs.uci.edu

Abstract

Health services are normally focused on communities that already exist. Communities that fall outside of this situation (short-term migrant communities, refugee camps, new settlements) often fall outside of the normal healthcare system. Here we describe a framework for conceptualising and understanding the environmental, demographic, and epidemiologic dynamics of settlements based on extractive endeavours. We argue that this type of settlement is sufficiently common that it warrants attention, and that a planetary health perspective is optimal for addressing the needs of such settlement communities. We then provide a case study from a gold mining settlement in a malarious region of Western Ethiopia. We close with some suggestions for provision of health services for such settlements. Namely, any aggregation of humans should have access to basic healthcare services; special consideration should be made to ensure that health services are steadily available to the community; employing members of the community for healthcare services may be optimal; and the health considerations should include environmental considerations beyond what is normally included in public health practices (i.e. vector control, basic hygiene).

Keywords

forests – settlements – extractive – demography – environment – epidemiology

1 Health services considerations for atypical communities

Health services are most commonly geared toward pre-existing communities, with efforts at establishing services where they are absent or improving services in places

 | DOI:10.3920/9789004688650_007

where they already exist (Wright *et al.* 1998). Researchers might focus on catchment areas and their respective population size or demographic attributes, or on the capacity of health facilities to adequately address the needs of the catchment area (Bureau of Primary Health Care, n.d.; Grad 2002; Macharia *et al.* 2021). How many beds are available, how many physicians per unit of population are there, how far must a community member travel in order to receive care (Blanford *et al.* 2012; Macharia *et al.* 2021; McGrail 2012; Ouma *et al.* 2018)?

Occasionally there are special circumstances that require approaches that differ from this norm. For example, migrant communities may be more ephemeral. Seasonal migrants reside in one geographic location for a period of time and then move along to another geographic location depending on, for example, the agricultural calendar. Oftentimes such special, atypical communities are missed in national and regional healthcare systems, partially because of political contexts, but also because of nationality, language, and socio-cultural attributes or because of the ephemeral nature of the 'community' (Adhikary *et al.* 2020; Arcury and Quandt 2007; Hansen and Donohoe 2003; Rural Health Information Hub n.d.).

Another related situation is one in which a community has only recently been established. For example, during disasters and conflicts populations may be displaced, with groups of people moving to new locations and establishing settlements which last for varying amounts of time (Guha-Sapir 1991). Some of these settlements will last for short periods of time, with community members returning to the place of origin when it is safe to do so. Sometimes these settlements last for long periods of time as well. Refugee camps in Kenya, India, and Thailand have now existed for decades – over half a century in the case of Cooper's Camp of West Bengal (Finch 2015).

There are organisations that are devoted to working with such displaced populations and increasingly migrant communities as well. International non-governmental organisations (NGOs) such as the International Organisation for Migration (IOM), Doctors Without Borders (MSF), the International Rescue Committee (IRC), as well as numerous local NGOs and community based organisations (CBOs) focus on the needs of these types of communities. These NGOs and CBOs often provide invaluable, life-sustaining services for migrant and displaced communities. However, there is also a chaotic nature to these settings that can hinder the sustained provision of quality services (Moss *et al.* 2006; Srikanok *et al.* 2017; World Health Organization (WHO), n.d.).

A related type of settlement, with unique characteristics, are those which have been formed by migrants or settlers primarily for the goal of making a living from extracting resources in that new geographic location. We will refer to this type of migrant as a 'settler' and the space and place which they occupy as a 'settlement'. Extractive based settlements are common, and specifically in relation to artisanal and small scale mining (ASM), the World Bank (2020) has recently estimated that

44.75 million people are engaged in this sector, rising from 13 million in 2002, across 80 countries (Hentschel *et al.* 2002). Whilst much of this chapter focuses on settlements centred around mining as the extractive sector of focus, there are many other types of extractive industry around which settlements form (i.e. logging and agriculture). As such, the total number of people living in settlements that are based on small-scale and informal extractive industries is likely to be much higher.

Settlers living in extractive orientated settlements often have unique health needs and experiences. Such health needs can include above average exposure to mercury poisoning (Bose-O'Reilly *et al.* 2010; Calao-Ramos *et al.* 2021; Esdaile and Chalker 2018; Gibb and O'Leary 2014; Hentschel *et al.* 2002) and lead poisoning (Bartrem *et al.* 2014; Landrigan *et al.* 2022; Nriagu 1992) in ASM based settlements – even affecting people not directly engaged in mining itself. Communities living close to mines have also been shown to experience higher odds of respiratory infections (Saha *et al.* 2011). Sexually transmitted infections (STIs), including HIV, are also often highly prevalent in such extractive based settlements as well (Baltazar *et al.* 2015; Clift *et al.* 2003; Nigussie *et al.* 2021; Sagaon-Teyssier *et al.* 2017). Other communicable diseases can also be high, such as malaria or tuberculosis (Hentschel *et al.* 2002; Moyo *et al.* 2021; Smith *et al.* 2016).

Additionally, health interventions to address the health needs of these communities tend to be limited because of poor communal access to health services, in part because of the often geographically remote locations, or the legally ambiguous nature of the work and settlements (Hentschel *et al.* 2002; Schwartz *et al.* 2021). The health needs of such populations may be thus 'hidden' from government agencies or NGOs who could be in a position to implement health resources in these settlements.

The perceived temporality of extractive based settlements can also hinder official investment in health services for these communities, even when population size increases rapidly, and it can take extended periods of time (often decades) for the settlement to gain the prerequisite official recognition in order to qualify for health investment (Hentschel *et al.* 2002). Where health interventions are conducted, they often focus exclusively on mercury poisoning or mine-related occupational safety, potentially neglecting other health needs (Gottesfeld and Khoza 2022; Smith *et al.* 2016; Spiegel and Veiga 2005; Tsang *et al.* 2019) even when key stakeholders state other pressing health needs in their communities, such as infectious disease (Smith *et al.* 2016).

In this chapter we describe the processes that lead to the formation of such settlements and how the dynamics of such settlements, their surroundings and health needs evolve. We describe a conceptual framework (Figure 1) for understanding and describing a common process through which: new settlements are formed by settlers (Figure 1A); there are associated changes to the environment from the act of settlement (Figure 1B); the demography of that community changes over time

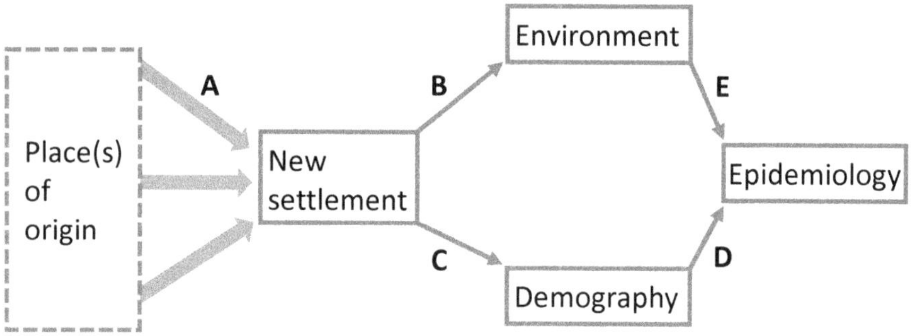

FIGURE 1 Conceptual diagram, indicating: (A) formation of a new settlement; (B) migration/settlement induced environmental changes; (C) demographic changes as the community evolves over time; (D) epidemiological changes that result from demographic changes; (E) epidemiological changes that result from environmental changes. The following chapter sections correspond to each element of this diagram

(Figure 1C); and these changes in demography and environment impact the epidemiological dynamics of the community (Figure 1E and 1D). We will explain each of these components in the following sections, followed by a case study from an informal gold mining site in Western Ethiopia, and closing with recommendations for public health systems that incorporate a planetary health framework.

2 Establishment of a new settlement

Migrant destinations are not random. A broad array of complex socio-cultural, political, economic, and even epidemiological factors influence migration decisions (Fields 1976; Portes and Sensenbrenner 1993; Stark and Bloom 1985; Todaro 1980). Migrants often move to places that offer increased economic realisations and improved (or perceived improved) quality of life. Negative environments (from socio-cultural, political, economic, or epidemiological) may encourage individuals to out-migrate, whereas perceived positive environments might act as a 'pull' for migrants.

Following the establishment of a settlement by pioneer migrants, the population of the settlement often expands through fertility and continued migration into the settlement. Whilst these secondary migrants may have similar reasons for moving to the settlement (i.e. economic opportunity) other aspects of the decision-making process may differ. For example, once the settlement has been established, the ongoing flow of movement to the settlement may be influenced by social networks (Banerjee 1983; Boyd 1989; Ryan 2011).

Having personal ties to the new settlement can help reduce the social and economic costs of moving as there is more information known about the opportunities and conditions in the new settlement and aid with other assistance as well (Boyd 1989). When more people within a particular social network move to the new settlement that others in their network have already moved to, this creates favourable conditions to facilitate further migration of network members from origin communities to the new settlement. These flows can grow larger and can become self-sustaining, creating a chain within a social network to a new settlement (Boyd 1989).

Here we focus on a particular kind of migration: that of migrants who have moved to a new location with environmental characteristics that are sufficient (or perceived to be sufficient) for extractive economic enterprises. Examples could include informal logging, mining, farming, or ranching. Such examples span history.

We acknowledge that while economics often plays a major role in migration decisions, the choice to change geographies is also often complex, multifactorial, and multi-level (i.e. some decisions might be made at the household or community level rather than at the individual level (Boyd 1989; De Jong and Gardner 1981)). We do not focus on this aspect of migration here, but rather in a generalized process through which settlements emerge and exist, with an overarching focus on epidemiology and planetary health.

We also recognize settler colonialism as one variant of the type of migration we describe here, whereby settlers begin a new settlement, displace local and indigenous populations (often violently), and establish a new political system (Veracini 2016). While we do not focus explicitly on settler colonialism in this chapter, this type of settlement establishment also has similar ecological and epidemiological implications for a particular geographic space and for the people that both settle there and who originally inhabited the space. The environmental, demographic, and epidemiologic impacts of settler colonialism are well-documented, particularly with regards to frontier expansion in the USA, in the Amazon (e.g. Barros and Honório 2015; Singer and de Castro 2001) and elsewhere (see Regassa and Korf 2018 for an example from Ethiopia). We also recognize the assaults on human rights that accompany settler colonialism.

3 Settler-induced environmental change

Settlers alter the environments of their new settlements. The frontiers to which people migrate are often explicitly defined in terms of their potential for change induced by such movements, from initially undeveloped space to large land transformation (Baeza *et al.* 2017).

The introduction of extractive industry, even at a small artisan scale, in newly settled places, will have particularly stark implications for the local environment. Mining activities and other extractive enterprises are often associated with negative externalities, including: deforestation, water pollution (from sewage, waste or chemicals, and mining activities), soil erosion and threats of extinction to plants, insects and animals (Singer and de Castro 2001; Sonter *et al.* 2017). Gold mining specifically is estimated to release more mercury into the environment than any other sector – an estimate of 1,400 tonnes of mercury were released from ASM in 2011 (Intergovernmental Forum on Mining, Minerals, Metals and Sustainable Development (IGF), 2014) – and overall is estimated to contribute 37.7% of global mercury pollution (World Bank 2020). CO_2 levels have also been shown to rapidly increase as a result of extractive industries, particularly those present in previously forested areas (Csillik and Asner 2020). For example, using remote sensing Csillik and Asner (2020) estimated that 1.12 Tg C emissions was created by gold mining activities in a 750,000 hectare area of the Peruvian Amazon between 2017–18.

These environmental changes from extractive industry, and wider global climate changes, can make settlers and the settlements they inhabit vulnerable. For example. extractive industries set up along rivers and coastlines (e.g. for extractive fishing enterprises) are prone to flooding from rising sea levels – a global climate change phenomena (Adelekan and Fregene 2014). Heat exposure risk from outdoor extractive work is also increasing because of climate change-induced temperature rises, in extractive orientated settlements (Nunfam *et al.* 2019). That such settlements are often geographically isolated, and lack sustained access to health services and infrastructure investment, can exacerbate the problem.

The impact of local environmental degradation can, at least in some cases, extend far beyond the community. Localised environmental degradation as a result of mining in the Amazon, for example, has also been suggested to be a major contributor to global climate change (Ellwanger *et al.* 2020; Kahhat *et al.* 2019). Nonetheless, the relationship between informal and small-scale mining with climate change has been under-studied, with most work focusing on large-scale mining communities instead.

Conversely, climate change may also be a driver of extractive settlement establishment and expansion, because of the precariousness of other economic activities and climate change-related disruptions to those endeavors (Bartrem *et al.* 2022; Fisher *et al.* 2019; Odell *et al.* 2018). For example, agricultural work is becoming less secure in some areas because of changing environments, which in turn fuels demand for non-farm work such as mining, especially among subsistence workers (Fisher *et al.* 2019). This can draw people to then establish or join settlements where other extractive-industry work is possible.

When people then begin to inhabit a new settlement, there is often a need to clear and alter the landscape for suitable living spaces and basic services. This may also include accompanying agricultural development for sustenance and additional economic opportunity and can result in a built-environment, previously unknown to the space the settlement now occupies. Potent environmental changes include establishment of building structures, drainage and alteration of natural water bodies, and establishment of irrigation and waste management facilities using varying degrees of technology.

The need for access to and within the settlement will also lead to the creation, widening or formalisation of tracks and roads across previously undeveloped landscapes. In terms of extractive industries such as mining, pollution of waterways may be an immediate byproduct of industry establishment, along with severe landscape changes such as soil erosion and deforestation. Similarly, land clearing for agricultural use, both at a small-scale and larger-scale, can lead to changes in soil quality and composition as well as disruption to animal, insect and plant dynamics and their habitats. All of these things involve altering the physical landscape of the space the settlement forms on, and can lead to resulting changes in the overlap between humans, pathogens, and vectors of pathogens (Gottdenker *et al.* 2014).

Over time, as the demographic composition of the community changes, because of increasing inward movement of migrants or changes to the fertility rate of the settled population, this too can stress space and resources, leading to expansion of the settlement (Sonter *et al.* 2017). For example, there may be a need to construct housing for the settler population, or to transform land for further productive potential, such as mine expansion or for the establishment of industries and supply chains to support the community and its constituents. In turn, this expansion further alters the landscape and characteristics of the environment.

4 Settlement demography: the life cycle of a new community

The demographic composition of a new community is driven by the demographic characteristics of its founders, as well as ongoing in- and out-migration (Castro and Rogers 1984). There are strong age patterns in migration, with most migrants being young adults ('independent' migrants), and occasionally their offspring ('dependent' migrants in the sense that they are linked to independent migrants) (Castro and Rogers 1983). A newly established settlement is therefore likely to reflect this pattern.

One metric that is used to quantify the age structure of a population is the dependency ratio (Hadley *et al.* 2011; Wachs *et al.* 2020): the ratio of persons in non-working age groups to those in working age groups (for example, a ratio of those in the 0–14 and 66 + age group to those in the 15–65 age group). A population with a high dependency ratio may experience difficulties in providing sustenance, as well as social, economic, and healthcare needs for the population. Conversely, a low dependency ratio might be considered desirable.

A variant of the dependency ratio (a ratio of consumers to producers, or the 'C/P ratio' (Chayanov 1966)) has often been used often in agricultural studies. C/P ratios differ from dependency ratios in that they weight consumers and producers by their relative contributions (production) and use (consumption), which likewise vary across the life-cycle of individuals (Han and Cheng 2017). For example, a 20-year-old adult might have a heavier production weight than a 2 year old or an 80 year old. A 2-year-old would consume food, but would contribute (produce) little for their respective population. Chayanov was interested in understanding and quantifying peasant farming household agricultural and economic outputs with regard to a society that was shifting toward socialism. More recently C/P ratios have been used in micro-level studies to measure general wellbeing and to predict out-migration from households, kin groups, and communities (Hammel 2005; Lee and Kramer 2002; Parker *et al.* 2014; Tomita *et al.* 2015).

The dependency, or C/P, ratio of a single population can shift over time, as the age and sex structure of the population evolves (Simon *et al.* 2012; Wachs *et al.* 2020). We refer to this shift in the demographic structure of the community as the 'life cycle of the community'. Whereas high fertility populations have large proportions of young age groups, populations that have undergone a shift from high to low fertility will, over time, experience a shift toward a higher mean age of the population. Migrant communities (including the types of settlements that are the focus of this chapter) are often skewed toward young adults and their offspring. If there are no in-migrants to the community, and if the community members survive and don't out-migrate, the mean age of the community will consistently increase over time. Conversely, in a system with in- and out-migration, the evolution of the age and sex structure of the population will be dependent both on the population dynamics of original inhabitants and of those who move in and out of the community.

A generalised process for a community without in- and out-migration could be one whereby: A.) the original founders were young adults, some with children and others soon to have children (a relatively low dependency ratio, depending on the proportion of children); B.) as those young adults and children age, the dependency ratio decreases (as children move out of dependency age or increase their productive abilities); C.) as the entire community reaches older ages, and if many of the community member survive, the dependency ratio could increase (as community members move into dependency ages and their productive abilities decrease). The fertility of individuals who have recently entered reproductive ages will influence the dependency ratio as well.

The age structure dynamics and progression within this process also depends on the duration of the settlement. Policymakers have for a long time viewed extractive settlements as temporary entities, with much of the literature now citing this perception of short temporality as often misguided and at the very least a hindrance to adequate healthcare and infrastructure support. These types of extractive industrial settlements have reoccurred across space and time and whilst some have been temporary – (Bryceson 2018) estimates that artisanal mining settlements during the California Gold rush in the 1800s lasted roughly six years – other settlements persist, even when the original extractive commodity is depleted (Bryceson 2018; Bryceson *et al.* 2020; Carson *et al.* 2020; Hentschel *et al.* 2002). The settlement's persistence may in turn be influenced by the demography of the place at the time of commodity depletion. If people have established families and strong social networks in the community then it may be harder to move elsewhere, even if there is no longer as much economic opportunity in the present settlement (Bryceson 2018). More work is warranted in analysing and studying the lifespans of these types of settlements.

Furthermore, while we have focused on the age structure of communities, other demographic and socio-cultural characteristics may also shift. For example, the gender and ethnic composition of a community can evolve over periods of time. Given socio-cultural and economic implications of things like age, gender, and ethnicity, these factors too have importance for understanding the epidemiology (and epidemiological dynamics) of a community.

5 Epidemiological shifts following the life cycle of the settlement

The demographic characteristics of a community or settlement can have a profound impact on epidemiology and general healthcare needs. Since risk of morbidity or mortality for many diseases varies by age (and sometimes gender), the age and gender structure of a population can influence the overall burden of morbidity or mortality. This is the impetus behind age and gender standardization in calculating morbidity and mortality statistics at aggregate scales (Anderson and Rosenberg 1998).

For example, in recent years, we've experienced a pandemic of a novel coronavirus (SARS-CoV-2), which as of January 2022 has touched almost every population on the planet. In the early waves of the disease, it was clear that the heaviest burden of mortality fell on older age groups (e.g. in the Lombardi region of Italy (Boccia *et al.* 2020) or in New York City (Thompson *et al.* 2020)). Populations with larger compositions of older age groups experienced some of the greatest burdens of mortality (pre-existing morbidities and socio-economic factors were also important drivers of morbidity and mortality).

Shifts in demographic characteristics can likewise lead to shifts in epidemiological characteristics of a community or settlement. Communities with younger populations (i.e. low mean ages) will experience diseases that are most common among young age groups (i.e. diarrheal and respiratory diseases) and with reproductive health (i.e. neonatal diseases). An ageing community, whereby the mean age of the population has increased (often following a decrease in fertility and/or a decrease in overall mortality) might be expected to experience heavier burdens of non-communicable and chronic disease – which tend to be the leading causes of death for older age groups. Many populations have experienced shifts towards higher mean ages, with attributable shifts in the most important causes of morbidity and mortality. During such transitions, it is common to experience a combined burden of both infectious and non-communicable diseases, sometimes referred to as 'the double burden of disease' (Boutayeb 2006; Bygbjerg 2012; Ciccacci *et al.* 2020). In this scenario, a population may still be characterised by a somewhat moderate to high mortality and fertility rate and experiencing an accompanying burden of communicable and acute infections, but at the same time also experiencing a substantial disease burden from non-communicable and chronic diseases. These shifts can present a substantial burden for health care systems, which may be unable to easily shift focus and priorities as the demography and health needs of a population evolve (Colwill *et al.* 2008; Haddad *et al.* 2022).

For example, globally, there has been a demographic shift from high to low mortality and fertility over time and the average age of the global population is increasing. The number of people aged 65 years or older increased by 105% between 1990–2017 and is predicted to rise to 1.5 billion people by 2050 (Cheng *et al.* 2020). Meanwhile, the percentage of children in the global population has decreased gradually over the same time period. This change in global demographics has had consequential effects on the state of health (Colwill *et al.* 2008; Haddad *et al.* 2022). Until recently, there was a global increase in chronic and degenerative non-communicable diseases as major burdens of morbidity and mortality (World Health Organization (WHO), 2011). As fertility rates decline at a global level, and as populations age, morbidity and mortality from maternal and neonatal diseases have decreased (Cheng *et al.* 2020).

Similar patterns are seen at national scales (Figure 2). Japan is an example of an extremely low fertility nation, and the top five diseases contributing to disability-adjusted life years (DALYs) in Japan include four non-communicable diseases (cancers as the top contributor) and the fifth related to injury (Global Burden of Disease (GBD), 2019). In high fertility nations such as Nigeria, infectious diseases (especially maternal and neonatal diseases, and enteric diseases) remain high contributors to the overall disease burden (GBD 2019). The United Arab Emirates (UAE) has a particularly stark and skewed population pyramid, towards young men of working age due in part to its status as a hub for expatriate workers (Blair and Sharif 2012). The fertility rate of the country is also low, with a small proportion of young children. The country has likewise experienced a shift towards non-communicable diseases being the dominated cause of disability adjusted life years per 100,000 people in the country. Four of the top five diseases that contribute to the disease burden are non-communicable as of 2019, with transport injuries being the third cause of DALYs in the country (GBD 2019).

Epidemiological shifts in the burden of disease as the demographic makeup of a population changes are not restricted to aggregate (national or global level) populations. Similar patterns have been described at smaller scales (camps, communities,

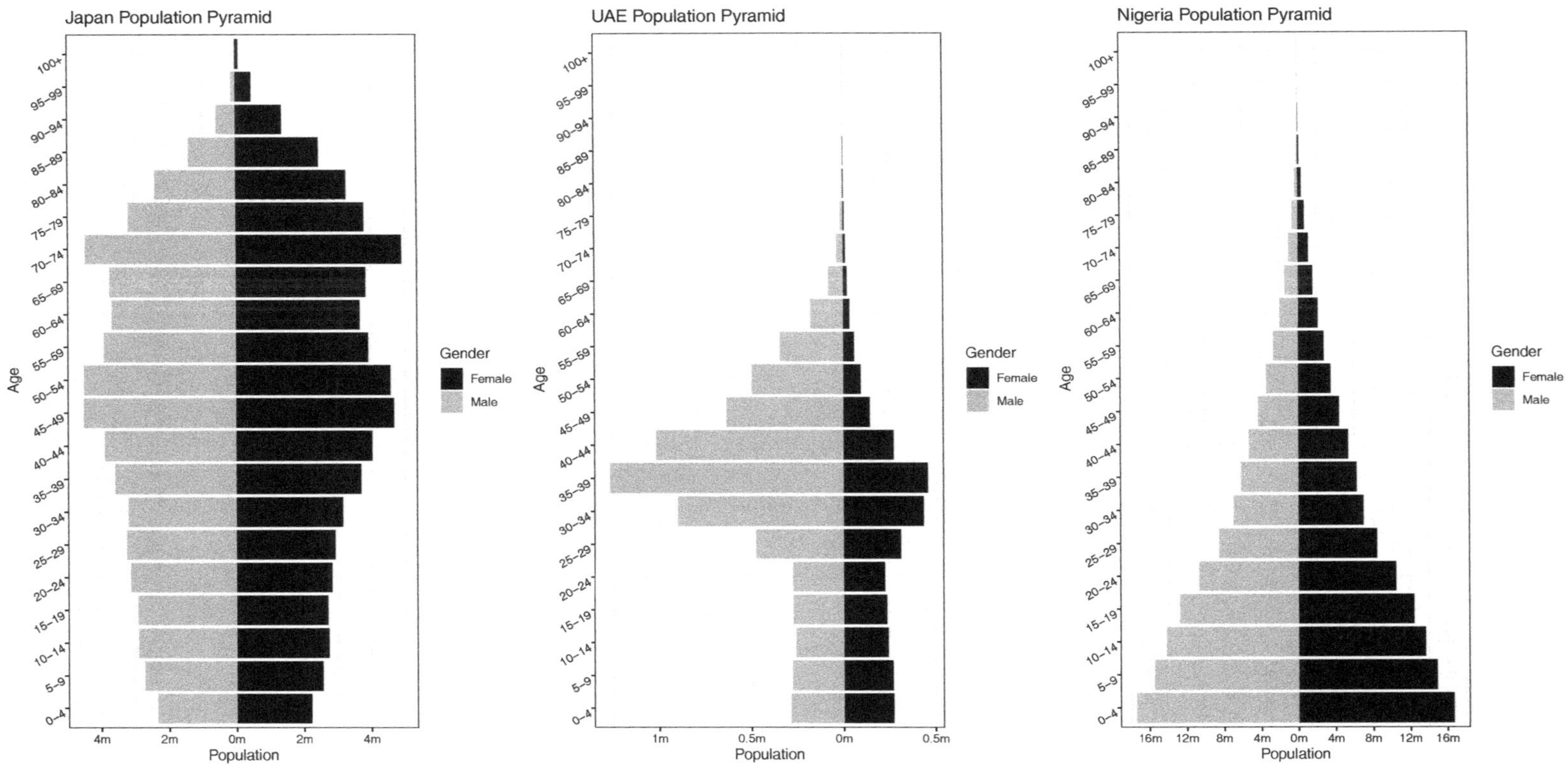

FIGURE 2 Population pyramids for three different population types: (A) Low fertility, older mean age (Japan); (B) Low fertility and skewed toward working age males (UAE); and (C) high fertility and therefore skewed toward younger ages (Nigeria)

and even at a household level) (Holck and Cates 1982; Parker *et al.* 2018; Srikanok *et al.* 2017; Tomita *et al.* 2015). For example, at a community level, in a study of pioneer settlements at Machadinho in the Brazilian Amazon, Singer and de Castro, (2001) found the mean age of the settlement population to increase over time and the percentage of the population aged 0–14 to decrease by 7.2% in the first ten years. Sellers *et al.* (2017) found similar results in new pioneer settlements in the Ecuadorian Amazon between 1990–2014, with the mean age of the settlement increasing over time whilst simultaneously, the fertility rate and dependency ratio of the population decreased. They also found in their case study that the sex ratio of the settlement became more balanced over time, a change from the initial imbalance of mostly young men. Also in the Amazon, Feged-Rivadeneira *et al.* (2018) studied the changing demographic and epidemiological profiles of community populations in Colombia and argued that the demographic changes are influential in shaping the epidemiology of the population. For example, they found incidence of malaria infections to be higher in settlements with higher proportions of children. Meanwhile, at a household level, a study by Geard *et al.* (2015) modelled demographic changes for the spread and control of diseases and found that a decline in household fertility was associated with a decrease in disease incidence and increase in mean age of infection at the household level.

6 Patterns and pathways to epidemiological changes resulting from environmental transformation

Anthropogenic environmental change is a significant factor in infectious disease epidemiology (Gottdenker *et al.* 2014; Patz *et al.* 2004). Human encroachment into new environments can expose individuals to pathogens that they have not previously encountered. Likewise, anthropogenic environmental changes can shift the distributions of flora and fauna of landscapes. Such alterations can lead to changes to epidemiology through shifts in contact patterns between humans, non-human hosts or environmental sources of pathogens, and vectors of disease (e.g. ticks, mites, sandflies, mosquitoes). This can result in increased disease incidence of emerging and re-emerging infections, occasionally of pandemic proportions (Baeza *et al.* 2017; Ellwanger *et al.* 2020; Plowright *et al.* 2021; Quick and Fry 2018; Rogalski *et al.* 2017; Snowden 2019).

Focusing on settlements and *Plasmodium* infections in the Amazon, Castro and colleagues (Castro *et al.* 2019; de Castro *et al.* 2006; Singer and de Castro 2001) described a general epidemiologic pattern following the establishment of new settlements. Initially there is an epidemic stage, where malaria incidence rapidly increases following the onset of a new settlement. Over time (approximately 5 years) Castro and colleagues describe a shift toward stable malaria incidence.

Castro and colleagues attribute the initial epidemic stage to novel environmental exposures among the settlers. If the settlers are immunologically naïve (having come from non-malarious landscapes) they may likewise have higher proclivity for development of symptomatic infections (which will be more obvious in the data than asymptomatic infections which are rarely detected).

The first housing structures of a new Amazonian settlement may be in or near forested areas, requiring some clearance of the forest for construction (both for space and for materials) (Barros and Honório 2015; Macdonald and Mordecai 2019). Barros and Honório (2015) found that new settlers to the Amazon tended to be concentrated closest to forested areas. Deforested areas near these settlements exhibited clustering of *Anopheles darlingi* (an important vector of malaria) larva, and settlers who lived closest to those larval clusters had greater risk of malaria infection than those who lived farther (> 400 m) away. Roadways and other land-clearing exercises lead to further fragmentation of the landscape, potentially increasing habitats that are suitable for some arthropod vectors and/or increasing human-vector contact (Conn *et al.* 2002; Cuenca *et al.* 2021; Norris 2004; Silbergeld *et al.* 2002; Singer and de Castro 2001; Walsh *et al.* 1993). In particular, dengue fever cases have been associated with population expansion and land-clearing, including roadway expansion, in Acre, Brazil 2000–2015 (Lana *et al.* 2017). Additionally, one of the most important vectors of malaria in the Americas (*An. darlingi*) is thought to preferentially inhabit deforested areas (Vittor *et al.* 2006).

Land clearance may also lead to less-permeable grounds, resulting in pools of water that can act as habitats for arthropod vectors. In settlements centred around extractive industries such as mining, the work itself can directly cultivate new breeding grounds for vector habitats and provide a prime disease transmission environment between humans and the vector (Conn *et al.* 2002; Silbergeld *et al.* 2002; Singer and de Castro 2001). In particular, run-off pits used in mining can collect rain and run-off water.

Some recent studies have found an association between stagnant water collected in mining work and incidence of Buruli ulcer in Ghana. This association is likely the result of the metal-laced water found in mining acting as a fertile breeding ground for *Mycobacterium ulcerans* – the bacteria causing Buruli ulcer (Hagarty *et al.* 2015; Wu *et al.* 2015). Meanwhile other occupational disease risks from land use change include Rift Valley fever, which has associated with livestock and forestry work in Africa, fuelled by exposure to *Aedes* mosquito vectors and infected livestock (LaBeaud *et al.* 2015; Olaleye *et al.* 1996).

Anthropogenic driven environmental change such as deforestation, from increasing urbanisation, have also resulted in disturbances in the forest fringe and increasing vector-human interactions in other contexts, such as Malaysia (Brock *et al.* 2019; Byrne *et al.* 2021; Cuenca *et al.* 2021; Davidson *et al.* 2019; Fornace *et al.* 2016; William *et al.* 2013). Such environmental transformation of land has been associated with a rise in *P. knowlesi* malaria cases in Malaysia, particularly through the landscape fragmentation/change and the resulting increase in the suitability of larval habitats in close proximity to human settlements (Byrne *et al.* 2021; Fornace *et al.* 2016).

Importantly, associations between landscapes, human populations, and infectious diseases can exhibit a large amount of spatial and temporal heterogeneity. While studies have documented associations between deforestation and increases of a given disease in one location, the pattern may differ widely in other locations or over time (Gottdenker *et al.* 2014). Likewise, environmental changes can simultaneously lead to decreases in the burden of one disease and increases in another. For example, in much of Southeast Asia malaria is considered a disease of rural, forested areas (Prothero 1999; Rosenberg and Maheswary 1982). As deforestation and urbanisation have drastically changed the landscape over the last half century or more, there has been a general decrease in malaria and an increase in *Aedes* borne diseases with important *Aedes* mosquito vectors thriving in urban environments (Kolimenakis *et al.* 2021; Li *et al.* 2014)).

Environmental changes are not the only drivers of epidemiological shifts. Initial migrant populations to pioneer settlements are often characterised by limited socio-economic means, with settlers often having limited education and knowledge of prevalent diseases in the settlement environment (Douine *et al.* 2020; Singer and de Castro 2001). Migrants to pioneer settlements frequently live in housing that offers little protection from arthropod vectors, and with poor overall sanitary conditions (Argaw *et al.* 2021; Guyant *et al.* 2015; Tadesse *et al.* 2021). They may need to bathe and collect water in river ways that are host to extensive mosquito populations.

On top of increased opportunity for human-vector interactions from environmental change in new settlements, apparent disease incidence may be further facilitated by the immunological naivety of the migrants that populate the settlement. In much of the world, malaria is now overwhelmingly concentrated in rural or remote areas (in Southeast Asia and in the Americas this is often in forested areas). Many settlers originate from high population centres located far from malarious regions and have little or no pre-existing immunity (Alemu *et al.* 2014; Castro *et al.* 2019; Deressa *et al.* 2006; Malede *et al.* 2018; Martens and Hall 2000; Nega and Meskal 1991; Singer and de Castro 2001; Tadesse *et al.* 2021). Alongside the previously mentioned socio-economic problems (living in poor housing conditions) and little or no biological defence (being immunologically naïve), individuals who are encountering new disease systems may not have socio-cultural or behavioural defences against the new disease. Bednet use, skin protections (clothing or topical chemicals), and other behavioural factors can influence risk of infection but often must be learned either through experience or education (Pooseesod *et al.* 2021).

Finally, long-term changes in the environment continue to impact disease ecology. As a population grows or expands, there will likely be continued alterations to the environment. In some cases, this can lead to improvements of overall health of the settlement – especially if changes lead to improved access to diagnosis and treatment, public health programmes, and improvements in living conditions and hygiene (Singer and de Castro 2001). Conversely, some settlements in rural and remote areas exist on the margins of society and never receive such structural improvements. Even for those that do eventually achieve such improvements, the timing in between original settlement and acquiring needed structural improvements can be fraught with heavy burdens of disease.

7 Case study: Malaria concerns and perceptions in a newly-established informal gold mining settlement in Gambella Region of Western Ethiopia

7.1 *Malaria and migration in Ethiopia*

In 2019 there were approximately 900,000 confirmed cases, and an estimated total of 5.5 million cases, of malaria in Ethiopia (Ministry of Health Ethiopia 2020). The impact of malaria on Ethiopia is stark, with the economic cost of malaria recently estimated at 102.8 million US Dollars per annum and an estimation that malaria accounts for 30% of all DALYs in the country (Ministry of Health Ethiopia 2020). However, there have been significant decreases in reported malaria incidence and malaria-related deaths in the country, with a 47% reduction in malaria cases and a 58% reduction in deaths, between 2016 and 2019 (Ministry of Health Ethiopia 2010, 2020). Nonetheless, recent estimates are that 52% of the total population in Ethiopia is at risk of malaria as of 2020 (Ministry of Health Ethiopia 2020). The Ethiopian government has made malaria control a key public health policy, and has expressed determination for malaria elimination in some of its regions, along with near-zero malaria cases in other areas of the country (Ministry of Health Ethiopia 2010, 2020).

Nonetheless, there are many barriers to actualising this goal. While *Plasmodium falciparum* is the most common malaria species in most of Africa, Ethiopia is endemic to both *P. falciparum* and *P. vivax* (Ministry of Health Ethiopia 2020; Taffese *et al.* 2018). Ethiopia also exhibits extreme heterogeneity in malaria endemicity across the nation (Ministry of Health Ethiopia 2020; Nega and Meskal 1991; Taffese *et al.* 2018; Tulu 1993). Large population centres are primarily clustered in high elevation areas and have little-to-no malaria transmission, in comparison to lower elevation regions with high malaria endemicity (Ministry of Health Ethiopia 2010, 2020; Nega and Meskal 1991; Taffese *et al.* 2018; Tulu 1993). Malaria cases remain high along the low-elevation western border regions (Taffese *et al.* 2018). Gambella Region, along the international border with South Sudan, has the highest annual incidence of malaria in Ethiopia – 6% of all total malaria cases in the country and 21% of malaria cases among under 5s in 2015 (Tadesse *et al.* 2021).

7.2 *Highland-to-lowland migration in Ethiopia*

Whilst historically Ethiopia's population has mostly been concentrated in the central highlands of the country, there have been increasing movements of people from high-elevation areas to low-elevation areas since the 1950s (Deressa *et al.* 2006; Hailemariam and Kloos 1993; Meskal and Kloos 1989; Nega and Meskal 1991). An array of factors have led to the increasing stream of people to relocate, temporarily or permanently, from highland areas to malaria endemic lowlands. These include: effective malaria control strategies making low-land areas more hospitable, increasing population density and resulting pressures on environmental resources and economic opportunities in highland areas (Deressa *et al.* 2006; Nega and Meskal 1991; Tulu 1993). These factors have led to some directed government policies to invest in developmental projects, with related schemes to resettle parts of the highland-located population in lowland areas (Deressa *et al.* 2006; Hailemariam and Kloos 1993; McCann 2014; Meskal and Kloos 1989; Tadesse *et al.* 2021; Tulu 1993). Aside from these formal streams of population movement, individuals and groups of migrants likewise move to lowland areas for economic purposes on their own, outside of official government or corporate sponsored projects.

The interaction between internal migration from highland areas of Ethiopia to lowland areas, and its corresponding effects on malaria incidence has often been highlighted as a potent public health concern, dating back to at least the 1980s e.g. Meskal and Kloos (1989). There are two overarching themes in the literature concerning this interaction between internal migration and malaria in Ethiopia: Migrants having heightened risk for malaria, and migrants' origin communities also having increased risk for increasing malaria incidence (from importation when migrants return home).

7.3 *Migrants' increased risk of malaria*

Several studies have shown that migrants have increased risk of malaria in Ethiopia (Argaw *et al.* 2021; Aschale *et al.* 2018; Demissie *et al.* 2021; Haile *et al.* 2017; Malede *et al.* 2018; Tadesse *et al.* 2021; Tesfahunegn *et al.* 2019). Many of these studies have taken place in highland settings, with migrants to lowland areas having larger malaria burdens as a result of their exposure to malarious environments. Fewer studies have explored the risk of migrants and 'locals' within malarious environments (but do see Degefa *et al.* 2015).

There are several dominant explanations for the heightened risk of malaria among migrants (Argaw *et al.* 2021; Deressa *et al.* 2006; Nega and Meskal 1991; Tadesse *et al.* 2021). Migrants from highland areas of the country are immunologically naive to malaria and are therefore at increased risk of experiencing symptomatic infections when infected (Alemu *et al.* 2014; Deressa *et al.* 2006; Malede *et al.* 2018; Martens and Hall 2000; Tadesse *et al.* 2021). Supporting this explanation are similar findings regarding malaria acquisition in migrant settings elsewhere, in Colombia (Castellanos *et al.* 2016) and Brazil (Souza *et al.* 2019).

Migrants are also at increased risk for malaria acquisition because of the risky environments in which they work (Argaw *et al.* 2021; Tadesse *et al.* 2021) and because of their often low socio-economic status (Argaw *et al.* 2021; Haile *et al.* 2017; Tadesse *et al.* 2021). In particular, poor housing options for migrants exacerbate exposure to malaria vectors and increases risk of malaria infection (Haile *et al.* 2017; Tadesse *et al.* 2021). This problem may be particularly acute for independent migrants, who will not have companies that provide bed nets, sleeping quarters, or access to diagnosis and treatment (which occurs in some large scale agricultural projects). Migrants or settlers in a new location might also not have the same level of malaria knowledge as those who have spent long periods of time living in malarious environments, either through lived experiences or through public health education campaigns that understandably target malarious areas. Importantly, knowledge about malaria and malaria prevention does not always lead to malaria preventive behaviours (Demissie *et al.* 2021).

7.4 *Study objectives*

Here we report results from a pilot study at a remote gold mining settlement in Gambella Region, Ethiopia that has been recently settled. The recent establishment of the settlement means that the ecological impact of migration to the area and the resulting anthropogenic change is only just beginning to be seen and we know of no prior research on either the environmental change or the health situation of this settlement. We focused specifically on understanding the places of origin of settlers in this location, their current occupations in the settlement, and on the general healthcare and malaria situation in the settlement during our pilot study.

7.5 *Study location*

Lunga is a settlement in Gambella Region of Western Ethiopia. The settlement is centred around an informal gold mining site and is the product of recent pioneer migration, only being established in 2017–2018 when discovery of gold in the area prompted word-of-mouth, informal migration to the site. Mining in this location is of the artisan and small-scale mining variety (ASM). Due to the small-scale nature of this type of mining, the industry's contribution to Ethiopia's GDP has historically been low (Ethiopian Extractive Industries Transparency Initiative (EEITI), 2016) and such settlements have not been a national priority (for public health or otherwise). Nonetheless, mining is viewed as a viable occupation for many Ethiopians and mining prospects have started to attract more and more people from across Ethiopia, particularly among those who are traditionally disadvantaged in the labour market. In the wider Gambella Region, mining has attracted migrants from across the country due the potential economic opportunities it can provide and as a result the mining industry in Gambella dominated by migrants from other regions in Ethiopia – over 95% of all mining operations estimated to be conducted by migrants (EEITI 2016).

Malaria is endemic to the region and Gambella regularly has one of the highest burdens of the disease in Ethiopia (Haileselassie *et al.* 2022). *Plasmodium falciparum* is the most common causative agent of malaria in the area, though *P. vivax* is also prevalent. Malaria cases in the area peak at coinciding times with land-use changes, such as developmental agricultural project investments including rice intensification and irrigation projects in 2012 and 2013 (Haileselassie *et al.* 2022). Furthermore, whilst data on land use change is not officially collected at a local level, Haileselassie *et al.* (2022) note that Abobo district health officials have indicated that there is ongoing and extensive land use change in the local area.

8 Data and Methods

We conducted a pilot household survey (n = 51) in March of 2020 in Lunga settlement in Gambella Region of Ethiopia using a household registry and by selecting households at random.

We interviewed heads of households using a questionnaire that was developed to assess the knowledge, attitudes, and practices (KAP) of community members with regard to malaria; access to health services; and places of origin. The survey also included questions about housing materials, the duration of time in which a settler had lived in Lunga, occupations, and educational attainment. The settler places of origin were geocoded using a registry of Woredas and regions (Ethiopian administrative units). We then calculated the Euclidean distance and mapped the migration trajectories between a settler's Woreda of origin and the study location in Gambella. We then generated scores (proportion of correct answers) across four main question types related to malaria KAP. We used simple descriptive statistical analyses to assess the general KAP of the setting with regards to malaria.

We also downloaded a raster layer for forest loss to visualize potential changes in forest coverage in and around the settlement. The raster came from the Global Forest Change dataset which was generated from Landsat images from 2000 through 2020 (Hansen *et al.* 2013). The raster layer indicates areas (pixels) which shift from being forested to non-forested, by year, from 2001–2020. Maps were created using QGIS version 3.4.9 and R statistical software version 4.0.3.

9 Results

In the several years since the discovery of gold in Lunga, migration to the site has rapidly expanded the population and led to the creation of the settlement. The estimated population size of the settlement in 2021 was estimated at around 12,000 people (though the population remains in flux). There are official plans to make the settlement into a Kebele administrative area (an administrative title for areas populated with around 3,000–5,000 people) in the near future (source: word of mouth information from public health officials in Gambella).

Just over half of the interviewed participants at the Gambella gold mining settlement (total of 51) were female (54.9%, n = 28). The median age of participants was 27 years (range of 19–45 years) and women had a lower median age (25 vs 28). Protestantism was the most common religion reported by the participants (47.06%, n = 24), followed by Ethiopian Orthodox Christianity (37.25%, n = 19) and then Islam (15.69%, n = 8). There were eight different self-reported ethnicities: the most common was Agnauk (31.37%, n = 16), followed by Amhara (27.45%, n = 14), and Oromo (27.45%, n = 14).

One third (n = 17) of the participants could read and write, but had no formal education. Approximately 13.73% (n = 7) could not read and write, while only 9.8% (n = 5) had 10 cumulative years of education. Most interviewed participants (n = 43) were married and living together whereas 5.88% (n = 3) were divorced, 1.96% (n = 1) were married but not living together, 1.96% (n = 1) were not married but were living together, 1.96% (n = 1) were widowed and 3.92% (n = 2) were single. The mean household size in the sample was 3.67 people and 18 participants (35%) lived in households with at least one child under five years.

Alongside gold mining, farming, merchants, and running a private business were other professions that participants reported as their primary occupation. The median age was lowest for farmers, whilst joint-highest for merchants and private business. The most common profession among men was gold mining (43.48%, n = 22) and the least common profession was farming (8.7%, n = 4). Comparatively, the joint-most common profession among women was merchant and private business (35.71%, n = 18 each).

Among the study participants, men tended to have lived at the settlement for longer periods of time than women. The mean length of time lived in the gold mining settlement for men was 26.8 months, compared with 16.6 months for women. Male farmers tended to have lived in the settlement for longer than men or women employed in other occupations.

Household construction was generally poor. The most common wall type was plastic (n = 31) then wood (n = 20). The most common roof type for houses in the sample was plastic (n = 38), followed by grass (n = 11), then iron sheet (n = 2). One household in the sample had a toilet. No households in the sample had electricity, a TV or a radio and 45 households had a mobile phone.

While most people surveyed at the study site had moved there from nearby Woredas with low-elevation topography, there was a proportion of migrants who had moved to the study site from high elevation areas much further away (Figure 3). Three quarters (75%, n = 38) of the participants reported moving to the new settlement from elsewhere in the region, whilst 25% (n = 13) came from outside of

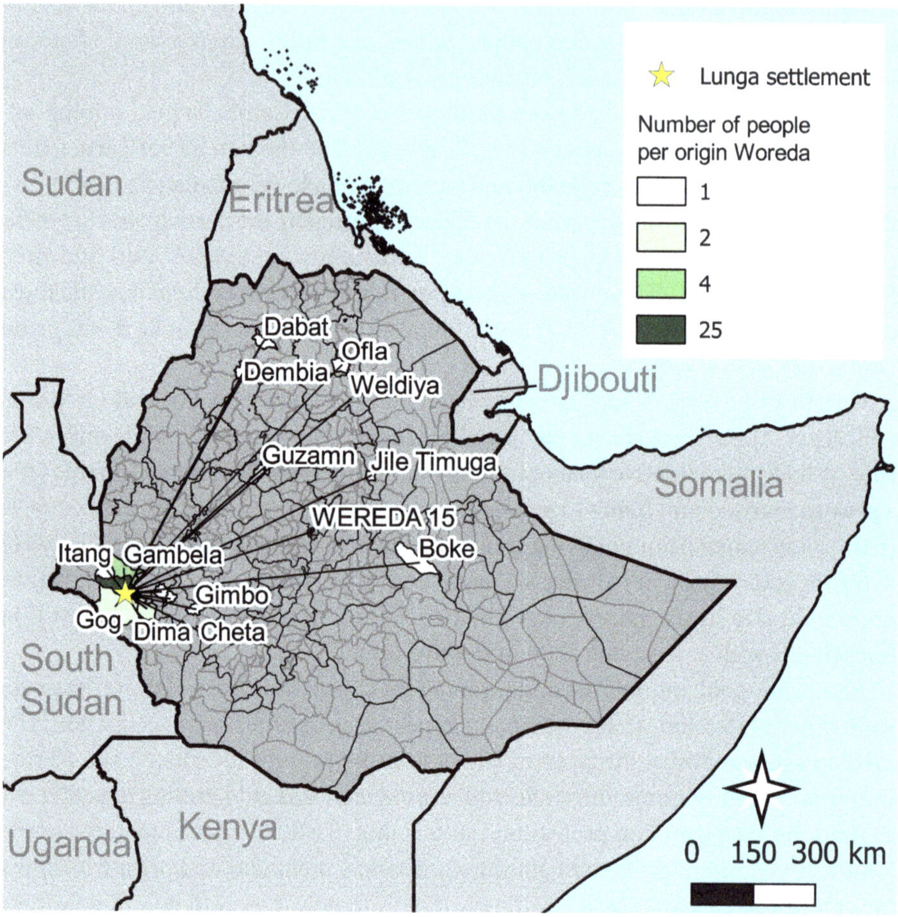

FIGURE 3 Locations of origin woredas for migrants at Lunga settlement, Gambella Region, Ethiopia, by number of people per origin woreda

Gambella Region. Approximately half (49%, n = 25) of all participants reported moving to the new settlement from the same woreda in Gambella Region, as the new settlement.

With regards to the KAP survey, the median proportion of correct scores in the population sample regarding malaria symptoms was 0.25 and the median proportion of correct answers regarding knowledge about protection against malaria was 0.40. Meanwhile the median proportion of correct answers regarding knowledge of the causes of malaria was 1.00. The median proportion of correct answers among the population sample for beliefs about who was at risk for serious cases of malaria was 0.60. However, only 17.65% (n = 9) of respondents correctly believed that pregnant women were at risk of a serious case of malaria and 88.24% (n = 45) of

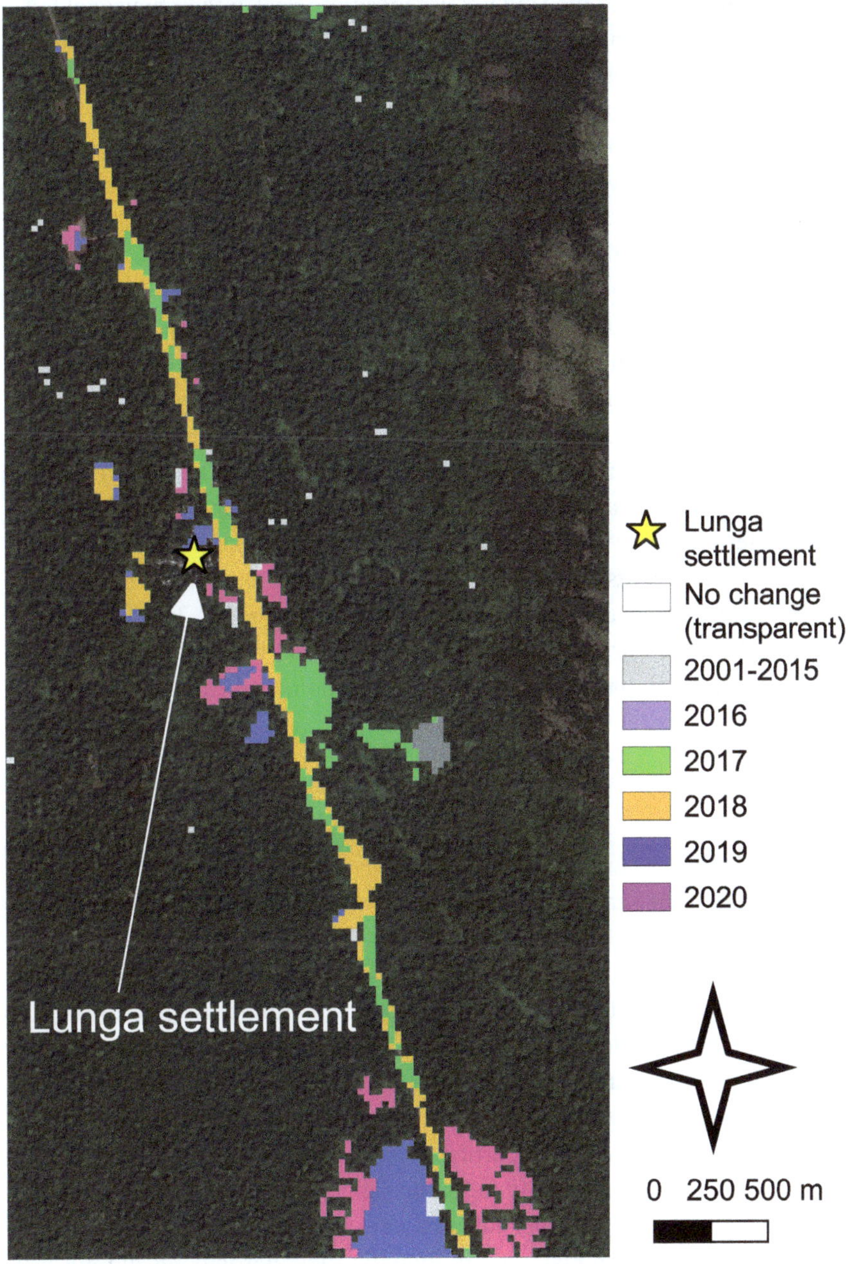

FIGURE 4 Forest loss by year (2001–2020) around Lunga settlement (Hansen *et al.* 2013). Forest loss is defined as the change from forest to non-forest state (when all trees in a stand are eliminated). Forest loss is represented by a colour pixel that indicates the year in which the loss took place in that pixel (2001–2020)

migrants interviewed stated they did not use mosquito nets in their household. The dominant reported explanation for not using mosquito nets was because they did not own them. Among those who did report owning mosquito nets, 83.33% (n = 37) reported using one the night prior to the interview.

Of the 13.71% (n = 7) of households that reported a household member being sick with fever in the past two weeks, 100% of them reported seeking treatment at a formal health facility, mostly at a health centre but also at private clinics. The nearest health facility was approximately a 2 hour walk from the settlement.

Figure 4 displays changes in forest coverage before and after the settlement at Lunga. There was minimal forest loss prior to 2016, and a rapid increase in forest loss post settlement (from 2017 to 2020). This aligns with the discovery of gold in the area and the resulting increased movement of people to the area to establish a settlement at Lunga, in around 2017–2018. The coloured pixels showing forest loss indicate a diagonal pattern from north-west to south-west of the settlement; this represents the clearing of a section of the forest for the creation of a road that runs by the settlement in 2017/18, around the same time that the settlement started to be established. This highlights the start of anthropogenic environmental change in the area of, and surrounding, the new settlement, Lunga (Figure 1B). Further research will be needed to monitor the environmental changes to the space over time and to evaluate potential impacts of this on the epidemiological situation of the area (Figure 1E).

10 Discussion

The composition of the settlement was diverse, with community members coming from both proximal and distal geographic regions, from different ethnic groups and religions (Figure 1A and 1C). While gold mining is the major draw from most to this settlement, other occupations exist and have built up around the gold mining. As expected, most study participants were young adults (Figure 1C). The demographic characteristics of the community, in age and gender makeup but also in ethnicity, religion, and other characteristics, may shift over time.

While a majority of the study participants correctly identified the causes of malaria, most could not correctly identify the signs of, nor methods of protection against, malaria (Figure 1D). Few participants were also aware that pregnant women were at significant risk from malaria. Additionally, most participants did not have access to mosquito nets, but showed willingness to use them if they were made available. Similarly, individuals that reported experiencing a recent fever in their households all reported seeking treatment at formal health facilities, even though the nearest health facility is roughly 2 hours walk away from the settlement. These findings indicate that public health outreach and material investment is needed in this area and that such outreach could be effective among the local population if made available.

Presumably, the continued population expansion at this settlement will also alter the epidemiology of the place (Figure 1D and 1E). Due to their oft remote geographic location, along with their informal and small-scale nature, mining communities in Ethiopia experience limited health coverage and access to health facilities (EEITI 2016). Limited access to healthcare facilities and resources is expected to contribute to worse health outcomes for the population (Carrara *et al.* 2006; Desai *et al.* 2014; Landier *et al.* 2018; Zurovac *et al.* 2014) and an increase in disease prevalence (Figure 1D).

Part of this limited access to healthcare is a result of the informal nature of this migration flow (Figure 1A). Whilst informal migration across the country is common, in other circumstances where official economic migration flows are planned there are often concomitant government or business led investments. For example, formalisation can give visibility of the population to local and national decision makers, which may lead to a dispersion of funds for health services and interventions. While formal migration may not always lead to investment in health services for migrants, it is arguably more likely to occur in a situation of planned migrations than in informal, hidden migration streams (Tadesse *et al.* 2021).

There has been some recognition of the current unmet needs and gaps in health service provision for migrant communities by the Ethiopian government (Ministry of Health Ethiopia 2020; Nega and Meskal 1991) and there have been attempts to rectify this gap in service provision by increasing health facility provision across the country (Taffese *et al.* 2018) and establishing some health infrastructure in migrant communities. However, this is often limited to migrant populations involved in major developmental projects with formalised migration support and promoted by government actors and policy. Overall, this study illustrates some of the planetary health-related problems associated with new settlements, especially given the rural and remote setting, in an already strained healthcare system.

11 Conclusions and recommendations

In this chapter we've presented a conceptual framework for understanding and describing co-incident shifts in demographic, environmental, and epidemiological patterns following settlement of a new community for extractive purposes (Figure 1). While there is a wealth of literature describing similar situations from other settings, we argue that there are commonalities that exist across most of these settings that are worth describing and worth considering specifically with regard to health services and public health interventions, within a holistic Planetary Health framework. This type of community is widespread, as is the neglect of public health resources for such communities.

Importantly, such settlements often exist outside of the realm of normal healthcare delivery, for a wide variety of reasons. Migrants are often missed in official government health delivery, and the type of settlement we describe here would have the same problems (Riza *et al.* 2020; World Health Organization (WHO), 2019). Furthermore, the unofficial (sometimes illegal) nature of this type of settlement community often leads the population to be under the radar or hidden from normal healthcare delivery. The precarious legal nature of such settlements is often exacerbated by tensions with other established or indigenous communities in surrounding areas, who may resent and view the new settlement as imposing on their own livelihoods and resources. This can make implementing new, or expanding existing local health services, difficult. Special, locally tailored considerations are often needed to reach such populations (Bonevski *et al.* 2014; Crawley *et al.* 2013; Elgabry and Camilleri 2021; Krabbe *et al.* 2021). Finally, many such settlements are in remote, rural areas or in regions that are deemed unsafe (conflict zones, contested regions) – further complicating access for normal services (Chatham House 2019; Druce *et al.* 2019; Footer and Rubenstein 2013; Nickerson 2015; Sousa and Hagopian 2011). Regardless, it is crucial that health services are provided for such communities, both from a humanitarian perspective and because they are often linked to other communities (to which they could transfer disease, etc.).

We have three main recommendations for such settlements. If an aggregation of humans exists, it needs access to basic healthcare services. First, if the settlement has only recently been established, healthcare provision may be possible through travelling community workers (Lee *et al.* 2006; McGowan *et al.* 2020; Omam *et al.* 2021). However, this is only a short-term fix as ready access to diagnosis and treatment of illnesses needs to be steady, so that access is not delayed (Prentice and Pizer 2007), and this is not achieved through periodic visits by outside healthcare workers.

Second, once it is clear that the settlement will be long-term, efforts should be made toward establishing a community health system within the settlement (Lee and Kim 2018; Mullany *et al.* 2010; National Heart Lungs Blood Institute (NHLBI), 2022; Riza *et al.* 2020). This will necessitate either having a healthcare worker relocate to the community, or training a member of the community, to do the healthcare work. Again, it is imperative that the healthcare worker be a regular resident of the community. Frequent travel out of the community will mean that health services are irregular and could lead to disruptions in early diagnosis and treatment, which can lead to onward transmission of infectious diseases or delayed treatment of diseases which often lead to worse health outcomes. Ensuring such constant availability may necessitate a salary and budget for the community health worker.

There are ongoing efforts to fund and expand community health worker programs already, in low resource and remote settings. Examples include Last Mile Health in Liberia and a recent philanthropic project in Africa, aided by The Global Fund (The Global Fund 2022). However, there is a need to ensure that people living within atypical settlements – such as extractive based settlements – receive benefits from these programs and are not ignored because of their often remote or politically precarious situation. Indeed, creating community health programs within these extractive communities may also alleviate tensions between different communities within the same locality, that may otherwise resent sharing resources with 'newcomers' or 'outsiders'.

Third, health considerations should go beyond a human-centred approach, and should include the built environment (healthy housing and access to clean water) and other inhabitants of the environment (other species that coexist in the location). Inherently, there are questions about environmental sustainability with regard to this type of settlement, and examples of environmental degradation are common (Barraclough and Ghimere 1995). Conversely, forests (and other environs) are a home to a significant number of people worldwide, who depend on forests for their homes and livelihoods (Cheng *et al.* 2017; Pokharel *et al.* 2007; World Bank 2013). Frontier areas and their environments can potentially be pathways to economic gains. For example, forests can provide a safety net for its users and inhibitors, to help provide supplementary income, and opportunities for foraging and nourishment, as well as long term opportunities for subsistence activities and economic gain. Rather than bar individuals, often with low socio-economic standing, from access to natural resources, sustainable use of such resources should be encouraged. Oftentimes for indigenous peoples, sustainability is already well-understood and advocacy of their traditional practices may be needed (Johnson *et al.* 2016; McGregor *et al.* 2020; Sherpa 2015). In other circumstances, as when the settlers are not local or indigenous, educational efforts may be warranted. To ensure such methods are incorporated within the extractive industry of a particular settlement, a community-focused approach and community participation should be encouraged to overcome many of the barriers identified to sustainable extractive work. Community and cooperative groups may in turn be more successful at promoting sustainable methods, when using the available knowledge and technology resources within their own community (Hilson *et al.* 2007; Massaro and de Theije 2018).

In conclusion, we have described a general settlement process that is sufficiently common as to warrant a conceptual framework, and planetary health approaches to addressing the health of settler communities. Arguably, such an approach could lead to development of improved health for the communities and their environments. Oftentimes such settlements are viewed with disdain and the community members are hidden from official government provisions. The legal and political circumstances under which such settlements and communities exist complicates provision of health services. Regardless, basic public health services should be provided to all despite legal status, nationality, or indigeneity. We do recognize the need to balance environmental concerns against population health, but the current status quo is one whereby these communities are ignored and neglected, leading to both widespread environmental degradation and poor population health – both of which then impact the wider landscape. While environmental degradation is certainly a concern, we believe that a formalized process for dealing with this very human process would be optimal.

Acknowledgements

DMP was partially supported by a grant from the Bill & Melinda Gates Foundation (INV-028123).

References

Adelekan I and Fregene B (2014) Vulnerability of artisanal fishing communities to flood risks in coastal southwest Nigeria. *Climate and Development*, 7(4), 322–338.

Adhikary P, Aryal N, Dhungana RR, Kc, RK, Regmi PR, Wickramage KP, Duigan P, Inkochasan M, Sharma GN, Devkota B, Van Teijlingen E and Simkhada P (2020) Accessing health services in India: experiences of seasonal migrants returning to Nepal. *BMC Health Services Research*, 20(1). https://doi.org/10.1186/s12913-020-05846-7.

Alemu K, Worku A, Berhane Y and Kumie A (2014) Men traveling away from home are more likely to bring malaria into high altitude villages, Northwest Ethiopia. PLoS ONE, 9(4): e95341. https://doi.org/10.1371/journal.pone.0095341.

Anderson RN and Rosenberg H (1998) Age standardization of death rates: implementation of the year 2000 standard. *National Vital Statistics Reports*, 47(3), 1–20.

Arcury TA and Quandt SA (2007) Delivery of health services to migrant and seasonal farmworkers. *Annual Review of Public Health*, 28(1), 345–363. https://doi.org/10.1146/annurev.publhealth.27.021405.102106.

Argaw MD, Woldegiorgis AG, Workineh HA, Akelom BA, Abebe ME, Abate DT and Ashenafi EG (2021) Access to malaria prevention and control interventions among seasonal migrant workers: a multi-region formative assessment in Ethiopia. PLOS ONE, 16(2), e0246251. https://doi.org/10.1371/journal.pone.0246251.

Aschale Y, Mengist A, Bitew A, Kassie B and Talie A (2018) Prevalence of malaria and associated risk factors among asymptomatic migrant laborers in West Armachiho District, Northwest Ethiopia. *Research and Reports in Tropical Medicine*, 9, 95–101. https://doi.org/10.2147/RRTM.S165260.

Baeza A, Santos-Vega M, Dobson AP and Pascual M (2017) The rise and fall of malaria under land-use change in frontier regions. *Nature Ecology & Evolution*, 1(5), 1–7. https://doi.org/10.1038/s41559-017-0108.

Baltazar CS, Horth R, Inguane C, Sathane I, César F, Ricardo H, Botão C, Augusto Â, Cooley L, Cummings B, Raymond HF and Young PW (2015) HIV prevalence and risk behaviors among Mozambicans working in South African mines. *AIDS and Behavior*, 19(1), 59–67. https://doi.org/10.1007/s10461-014-0941-6.

Banerjee B (1983) Social networks in the migration process: empirical evidence on chain migration in India. *The Journal of Developing Areas*, 17(2), 185–196.

Barraclough SI and Ghimere K (1995) Forests and livelihoods: the social dynamics of deforestation in developing countries. Palgrave Macmillan. https://doi.org/10.1057/9780230375802.

Barros FSM and Honório NA (2015) Deforestation and malaria on the Amazon frontier: larval clustering of *Anopheles darlingi* (Diptera: Culicidae) determines focal distribution of malaria. *The American Journal of Tropical Medicine and Hygiene*, 93(5), 939–953. https://doi.org/10.4269/ajtmh.15-0042.

Bartrem C, Lindern I von, Braun M von and Tirima S (2022) Climate change, conflict, and resource extraction: analyses of Nigerian artisanal mining communities and ominous global trends. *Annals of Global Health*, 88(1), 17. https://doi.org/10.5334/aogh.3547.

Bartrem C, Tirima S, von Lindern I, von Braun M, Worrell MC, Mohammad Anka S, Abdullahi A and Moller G (2014) Unknown risk: co-exposure to lead and other heavy metals among children living in small-scale mining communities in Zamfara State, Nigeria. *International Journal of Environmental Health Research*, 24(4), 304–319. https://doi.org/10.1080/09603123.2013.835028.

Blair I and Sharif AA (2012) Population structure and the burden of disease in the United Arab Emirates. *Journal of Epidemiology and Global Health*, 2(2), 61–71. https://doi.org/10.1016/j.jegh.2012.04.002.

Blanford JI, Kumar S, Luo W and MacEachren AM (2012) It's a long, long walk: accessibility to hospitals, maternity and integrated health centers in Niger. *International Journal of Health Geographics*, 11(1), 24. https://doi.org/10.1186/1476-072X-11-24.

Boccia S, Ricciardi W and Ioannidis JPA (2020) What other countries can learn from Italy during the COVID-19 pandemic. *JAMA Internal Medicine*, 180(7), 927–928. https://doi.org/10.1001/jamainternmed.2020.1447.

Bonevski B, Randell M, Paul C, Chapman K, Twyman L, Bryant J, Brozek I and Hughes C (2014) Reaching the hard-to-reach: a systematic review of strategies for improving health and medical research with socially disadvantaged groups. *BMC Medical Research Methodology*, 14(1), 42. https://doi.org/10.1186/1471-2288-14-42.

Bose-O'Reilly S, McCarty KM, Steckling N and Lettmeier B (2010) Mercury exposure and children's health. *Current Problems in Pediatric and Adolescent Health Care*, 40(8), 186–215. https://doi.org/10.1016/j.cppeds.2010.07.002.

Boutayeb A (2006) The double burden of communicable and non-communicable diseases in developing countries. *Transactions of the Royal Society of Tropical Medicine and Hygiene*, 100(3), 191–199. https://doi.org/10.1016/j.trstmh.2005.07.021.

Boyd M (1989) Family and personal networks in international migration: recent developments and new agendas. *The International Migration Review*, 23(3), 638–670. https://doi.org/10.2307/2546433.

Brock PM, Fornace KM, Grigg MJ, Anstey NM, William T, Cox J, Drakeley CJ, Ferguson HM and Kao RR (2019) Predictive analysis across spatial scales links zoonotic malaria to deforestation. *Proceedings of the Royal Society B: Biological Sciences*, 286(1894), 20182351. https://doi.org/10.1098/rspb.2018.2351.

Bryceson D (2018) Artisanal gold-rush mining and frontier democracy: juxtaposing experiences in America, Australia, Africa and Asia. In Between the plough and the pick: informal mining in the contemporary world. (pp. 31–61). ANU Press.

Bryceson D, Jonsson JB and Clarke Shand M (2020) Mining mobility and settlement during an East African gold boom: seeking fortune and accommodating fate. *Mobilities*, *15*(3), 446–463. https://doi.org/10.1080/17450101.2020.1723879.

Bureau of Primary Health Care (n.d.) Chapter 3: Needs Assessment 2018. Bureau of Primary Health Care. Retrieved 28 February 2022, from https://bphc.hrsa.gov/program requirements/compliancemanual/chapter-3.

Bygbjerg, I.C. (2012). Double Burden of Noncommunicable and Infectious Diseases in Developing Countries. Science, 337(6101), 1499–1501. https://doi.org/10.1126/science.1223466.

Byrne I, Aure W, Manin BO, Vythilingam I, Ferguson HM, Drakeley CJ, Chua TH and Fornace KM (2021) Environmental and spatial risk factors for the larval habitats of *Plasmodium knowlesi* vectors in Sabah, Malaysian Borneo. *Scientific Reports*, 11(1), 11810. https://doi.org/10.1038/s41598-021-90893-1.

Calao-Ramos C, Bravo AG, Paternina-Uribe R, Marrugo-Negrete J and Díez S (2021) Occupational human exposure to mercury in artisanal small-scale gold mining communities of Colombia. *Environment International*, 146, 106216. https://doi.org/10.1016/j.envint.2020.106216.

Carrara VI, Sirilak S, Thonglairuam J, Rojanawatsirivet C, Proux S, Gilbos V, Brockman A, Ashley EA, McGready R, Krudsood S, Leemingsawat S, Looareesuwan S, Singhasivanon P, White N and Nosten F (2006) Deployment of early diagnosis and mefloquine-artesunate treatment of *falciparum* malaria in Thailand: the Tak Malaria Initiative. *PLOS Medicine*, 3(6), e183. https://doi.org/10.1371/journal.pmed.0030183.

Carson DB, Nilsson LM and Carson DA (2020) The mining resource cycle and settlement demography in Malå, Northern Sweden. Polar Record, 56:e10. https://doi.org/10.1017/S0032247420000200.

Castellanos A, Chaparro-Narváez P, Morales-Plaza CD, Alzate A, Padilla J, Arévalo M and Herrera S (2016) Malaria in gold-mining areas in Colombia. Memórias Do Instituto Oswaldo Cruz, 111, 59–66. https://doi.org/10.1590/0074-02760150382.

Castro LJ and Rogers A (1983) What the age composition of migrants can tell us. *Population Bulletin of the United Nations*, 15, 63–79.

Castro L and Rogers A (1984) What the age composition of migrants can tell us (p. 24). International Institute for Applied Systems Analysis.

Castro MC, Baeza A, Codeço CT, Cucunubá ZM, Dal'Asta AP, De Leo GA, Dobson AP, Carrasco-Escobar G, Lana RM, Lowe R, Monteiro AMV, Pascual M and Santos-Vega M (2019) Development, environmental degradation, and disease spread in the Brazilian Amazon. *PLOS Biology*, 17(11), e3000526. https://doi.org/10.1371/journal.pbio.3000526.

Chatham House (2019) Getting serious about protecting health care in conflict. Chatham House. Available at: https://www.chathamhouse.org/2019/05/getting-serious-about-protecting-health-care-conflict.

Chayanov A (1966) A.V. Chayanov on the theory of the peasant economy. University of Wisconsin Press.

Cheng SH, Ahlroth S, Onder S, Shyamsundar P, Garside R, Kristjanson P, McKinnon MC and Miller DC (2017) What is the evidence for the contribution of forests to poverty alleviation? A systematic map protocol. *Environmental Evidence*, 6(1), 10. https://doi.org/10.1186/s13750-017-0088-9.

Cheng X, Yang Y, Schwebel DC, Liu Z, Li L, Cheng P, Ning P and Hu G (2020) Population ageing and mortality during 1990–2017: a global decomposition analysis. *PLOS Medicine*, 17(6), e1003138. https://doi.org/10.1371/journal.pmed.1003138.

Ciccacci F, Orlando S, Majid N and Marazzi C (2020) Epidemiological transition and double burden of diseases in low-income countries: the case of Mozambique. *The Pan African Medical Journal*, 37(49), Article 49. https://doi.org/10.11604/pamj.2020.37.49.23310.

Clift S, Anemona A, Watson-Jones D, Kanga Z, Ndeki L, Changalucha J, Gavyole A and Ross D (2003) Variations of HIV and STI prevalences within communities neighbouring new goldmines in Tanzania: importance for intervention design. *Sexually Transmitted Infections*, 79(4), 307–312. https://doi.org/10.1136/sti.79.4.307.

Colwill J, Cultice J and Kruse R (2008) Will generalist physician supply meet demands of an increasing and aging population? Health Affairs. *Health Affairs*, 27(1). https://doi.org/10.1377/hlthaff.27.3.w232.

Conn JE, Wilkerson RC, Segura MNO, Souza RTL de, Schlichting CD, Wirtz RA and Póvoa MM (2002) Emergence of a new neotropical malaria vector facilitated by human migration and changes in land use. *The American Journal of Tropical Medicine and Hygiene*, 66(1), 18–22. https://doi.org/10.4269/ajtmh.2002.66.18.

Crawley J, Kane D, Atkinson-Plato L, Hamilton M, Dobson K and Watson J (2013) Needs of the hidden homeless – no longer hidden: a pilot study. *Public Health*, 127(7), 674–680. https://doi.org/10.1016/j.puhe.2013.04.006.

Csillik O and Asner GP (2020) Aboveground carbon emissions from gold mining in the Peruvian Amazon. *Environmental Research Letters*, 15(1), 014006. https://doi.org/10.1088/1748-9326/ab639c.

Cuenca PR, Key S, Jumail A, Surendra H, Ferguson HM, Drakeley CJ and Fornace K (2021) Chapter Six – Epidemiology of the zoonotic malaria *Plasmodium knowlesi* in changing landscapes. In C. Drakeley (ed.), Advances in Parasitology (Vol. 113, pp. 225–286). Academic Press. https://doi.org/10.1016/bs.apar.2021.08.006.

Davidson G, Chua TH, Cook A, Speldewinde P and Weinstein P (2019) The role of ecological linkage mechanisms in *Plasmodium knowlesi* transmission and spread. *EcoHealth*, 16(4), 594–610. https://doi.org/10.1007/s10393-019-01395-6.

de Castro M, Monte-Mor R, Sawyer D and Singer B (2006) Malaria risk on the Amazon frontier. *PNAS*, 103(7), 2452–2457. https://doi.org/10.1073/pnas.0510576103.

de Jong G and Gardner R (1981) Migration decision making: multidisciplinary approaches to microlevel studies in developed and developing countries. Pergamon. https://www.elsevier.com/books/migration-decision-making/de-jong/978-0-08-026305-2.

Degefa T, Zeynudin A, Godesso A, Michael YH, Eba K, Zemene E, Emana D, Birlie B, Tushune K and Yewhalaw D (2015) Malaria incidence and assessment of entomological indices among resettled communities in Ethiopia: A longitudinal study. *Malaria Journal*, 14(1), 24. https://doi.org/10.1186/s12936-014-0532-z.

Demissie GD, Ayele TA, Wami SD, Sisay MM, Fetene D, Wolde HF, Akalu TY and Gelaye KA (2021) Low practice of malaria prevention among migrants and seasonal farmworkers in Metema and west Armacheho districts, Northwest Ethiopia. *BMC Infectious Diseases*, 21(1), 145. https://doi.org/10.1186/s12879-021-05853-x.

Deressa W, Ali A and Berhane Y (2006) Review of the interplay between population dynamics and malaria transmission in Ethiopia. *The Ethiopian Journal of Health Development*, 20(3), Article 3. https://ejhd.org/index.php/ejhd/article/view/604.

Desai M, Buff AM, Khagayi S, Byass P, Amek N, Van Eijk A, Slutsker L, Vulule J, Odhiambo FO, Phillips-Howard PA, Lindblade KA, Laserson KF and Hamel MJ (2014) Age-specific malaria mortality rates in the KEMRI/CDC health and demographic surveillance system in Western Kenya, 2003–2010. *PLOS ONE*, 9(9), e106197. https://doi.org/10.1371/journal.pone.0106197.

Douine M, Lambert Y, Musset L, Hiwat H, Blume LR, Marchesini P, Moresco GG, Cox H, Sanchez JF, Villegas L, de Santi VP, Sanna A, Vreden S and Suarez-Mutis M (2020) Malaria in gold miners in the Guianas and the Amazon: current knowledge and challenges. *Current Tropical Medicine Reports*, 7(2), 37–47. https://doi.org/10.1007/s40475-020-00202-5.

Druce P, Bogatyreva E, Siem FF, Gates S, Kaade H, Sundby J, Rostrup M, Andersen C, Rustad SCA, Tchie A, Mood R, Nygård HM, Urdal H and Winkler AS (2019) Approaches to protect and maintain health care services in armed conflict – meeting SDGs 3 and 16. *Conflict and Health*, 13(1), 2. https://doi.org/10.1186/s13031-019-0186-0.

Elgabry M and Camilleri J (2021) Conducting hidden populations research: a reflective case study on researching the biohacking community. Futures, 132, 102769. https://doi.org/10.1016/j.futures.2021.102769.

Ellwanger JH, Kulmann-Leal B, Kaminski VL, Valverde-Villegas JM, Veiga ABGD, Spilki FR, Fearnside PM, Caesar L, Giatti LL, Wallau GL, Almeida SEM, Borba MR, Hora VPD and

Chies JAB (2020) Beyond diversity loss and climate change: impacts of Amazon deforestation on infectious diseases and public health. *Anais Da Academia Brasileira de Ciências*, 92(1), e20191375. https://doi.org/10.1590/0001-3765202020191375.

Esdaile LJ and Chalker JM (2018) The mercury problem in artisanal and small-scale gold mining. *Chemistry – A European Journal*, 24(27), 6905–6916. https://doi.org/10.1002/chem.201704840.

Ethiopian Extractive Industries Transparency Initiative (EEITI) (2016) Artisanal mining operation and its economic values, Ethiopia. EEiTI. https://eiti.org/files/documents/artisana_mining_3_0.pdf.

Feged-Rivadeneira A, Del Cairo C and Vargas W (2018) Demographic and epidemic transitions in peri-urban areas of Colombia: a multilevel study of malaria in the Amazonian city of San José del Guaviare. *Environment and Urbanization*. 31(1). https://doi.org/10.1177/0956247818808207.

Fields GS (1976) Labor force migration, unemployment and job turnover. *The Review of Economics and Statistics*, 58(4), 407–415. https://doi.org/10.2307/1935872.

Finch T (2015) In limbo in world's oldest refugee camps: where 10 million people can spend years, or even decades. *Index on Censorship*, 44(1), 53–56. https://doi.org/10.1177/0306422015569438.

Fisher R, Ling H, Natonis R, Hobgen S, Kaho NR, Mudita W, Markus J, Bunga W and Nampa W (2019) Artisanal and small-scale mining and rural livelihood diversification: the case of manganese extraction in West Timor, Indonesia. *The Extractive Industries and Society*, 6(1), 229–240. https://doi.org/10.1016/j.exis.2018.08.004.

Footer KHA and Rubenstein LS (2013) A human rights approach to health care in conflict. *International Review of the Red Cross*, 95(889), 167–187. https://doi.org/10.1017/S1816383113000349.

Fornace KM, Abidin TR, Alexander N, Brock P, Grigg MJ, Murphy A, William T, Menon J, Drakeley CJ and Cox J (2016) Association between landscape factors and spatial patterns of *Plasmodium knowlesi* infections in Sabah, Malaysia Volume 22, Number 2 February 2016 – Emerging Infectious Diseases journal – CDC. *Emerging Infectious Diseases*, 22(2). https://doi.org/10.3201/eid2202.150656.

Geard N, Glass K, McCaw J, McBryde E, Korb K, Keeling M and McVernon J (2015) The effects of demographic change on disease transmission and vaccine impact in a household structured population. *Epidemics*. 13: 56–64. https://doi.org/10.1016/j.epidem.2015.08.002.

Gibb H and O'Leary KG (2014) Mercury exposure and health impacts among individuals in the artisanal and small-scale gold mining community: a comprehensive review. *Environmental Health Perspectives*, 122(7), 667–672. https://doi.org/10.1289/ehp.1307864.

Global Burden of Disease (GBD) (2019) Global burden of disease compare. Global Burden of Disease. https://vizhub.healthdata.org/gbd-compare/.

Gottdenker NL, Streicker DG, Faust CL and Carroll CR (2014) Anthropogenic land use change and infectious diseases: a review of the evidence. *EcoHealth*, 11(4), 619–632. https://doi.org/10.1007/s10393-014-0941-z.

Gottesfeld P and Khoza NN (2022) Urgent need for a comprehensive public health response to artisanal small-scale mining. *Annals of Work Exposures and Health*, 66(1), 1–4. https://doi.org/10.1093/annweh/wxab058.

Grad FP (2002) The preamble of the constitution of the World Health Organization. *Bulletin of the World Health Organization*, 80(12), 981–984.

Guha-Sapir D (1991) Rapid assessment of health needs in mass emergencies: review of current concepts and methods. World Health Statistics Quarterly. *Rapport Trimestriel De Statistiques Sanitaires Mondiales*, 44(3), 171–181.

Guyant P, Canavati SE, Chea N, Ly P, Whittaker MA, Roca-Feltrer A and Yeung S (2015) Malaria and the mobile and migrant population in Cambodia: a population movement framework to inform strategies for malaria control and elimination. *Malaria Journal*, 14(1), 252. https://doi.org/10.1186/s12936-015-0773-5.

Haddad LM, Annamaraju P and Toney-Butler TJ (2022) Nursing shortage. In StatPearls. StatPearls Publishing. http://www.ncbi.nlm.nih.gov/books/NBK493175/.

Hadley C, Belachew T, Lindstrom D and Tessema F (2011) The shape of things to come? Household dependency ratio and adolescent nutritional status in rural and urban Ethiopia. *American Journal of Physical Anthropology*, 144(4), 643–652. https://doi.org/10.1002/ajpa.21463.

Hagarty J, Azanu D, Atosona B, Voegborlo R, Smithwick EAH and Singha K (2015) Chemistry of natural waters and its relation to Buruli ulcer in Ghana. *Journal of Hydrology: Regional Studies*, 3, 457–472. https://doi.org/10.1016/j.ejrh.2015.03.006.

Haile M, Lemma H and Weldu Y (2017) Population movement as a risk factor for malaria infection in high-altitude villages of Tahtay-Maychew District, Tigray, Northern Ethiopia: a case-control study. *The American Journal of Tropical Medicine and Hygiene*, 97(3), 726–732. https://doi.org/10.4269/ajtmh.17-0129.

Hailemariam A and Kloos H (1993) Population. In: The ecology of health and disease in Ethiopia. Westview Press.

Haileselassie W, Parker DM, Taye B, David RE, Zemene E, Lee MC, Zhong D, Zhou G, Alemu T, Tadele G, Kazura JW, Koepfli C, Deressa W, Yewhalaw D and Yan G (2022) Burden of malaria, impact of interventions and climate variability in Western Ethiopia: an area with large irrigation based farming. *BMC Public Health*, 22(1), 196. https://doi.org/10.1186/s12889-022-12571-9.

Hammel EA (2005) Chayanov revisited: a model for the economics of complex kin units. *Proceedings of the National Academy of Sciences*, 102(19), 7043–7046. https://doi.org/10.1073/pnas.0501987102.

Han X and Cheng Y (2017) Consumption- and productivity-adjusted dependency ratio with household structure heterogeneity (ADB Economics Working Paper Series) [ADB Economics Working Paper Series]. Asian Development Bank. https://doi.org/10.22617/WPS179182-2.

Hansen E and Donohoe M (2003) Health issues of migrant and seasonal farmworkers. *Journal of Health Care for the Poor and Underserved*, 14(2), 153–164. https://doi.org/10.1353/hpu.2010.0790.

Hansen MC, Potapov PV, Moore R, Hancher M, Turubanova SA, Tyukavina A, Thau D, Stehman SV, Goetz SJ, Loveland TR, Kommareddy A, Egorov A, Chini L, Justice CO and Townshend JRG (2013) High-resolution global maps of 21st-century forest cover change. *Science*, 342(6160), 850–853. https://doi.org/10.1126/science.1244693.

Hentschel T, Hruschka F and Priester M (2002) Global report on artisanal & small-scale mining (No. 70; p. 67). IIED.

Hilson G, Hilson CJ and Pardie S (2007) Improving awareness of mercury pollution in small-scale gold mining communities: challenges and ways forward in rural Ghana. *Environmental Research*, 103(2), 275–287. https://doi.org/10.1016/j.envres.2006.09.010.

Holck SE and Cates W (1982) Fertility and population dynamics in two Kampuchean refugee camps. *Studies in Family Planning*, 13(4), 118–124. https://doi.org/10.2307/1965707.

Intergovernmental Forum on Mining, Minerals, Metals and Sustainable Development (IGF) (2017) Global Trends in Artisanal and Small-Scale Mining (ASM): A review of key numbers and issues (p. 91). IISD.

Johnson JT, Howitt R, Cajete G, Berkes F, Louis RP and Kliskey A (2016) Weaving indigenous and sustainability sciences to diversify our methods. *Sustainability Science*, 11(1), 1–11. https://doi.org/10.1007/s11625-015-0349-x.

Kahhat R, Parodi E, Larrea-Gallegos G, Mesta C and Vázquez-Rowe I (2019) Environmental impacts of the life cycle of alluvial gold mining in the Peruvian Amazon rainforest. *Science of The Total Environment*, 662, 940–951. https://doi.org/10.1016/j.scitotenv.2019.01.246.

Kolimenakis A, Heinz S, Wilson ML, Winkler V, Yakob L, Michaelakis A, Papachristos D, Richardson C and Horstick O (2021) The role of urbanisation in the spread of Aedes mosquitoes and the diseases they transmit – a systematic review. *PLOS Neglected Tropical Diseases*, 15(9), e0009631. https://doi.org/10.1371/journal.pntd.0009631.

Krabbe J, Jiao S, Guta A, Slemon A, Cameron AA and Bungay V (2021) Exploring the operationalisation and implementation of outreach in community settings with hard-to-reach and hidden populations: protocol for a scoping review. *BMJ Open*, 11(2), e039451. https://doi.org/10.1136/bmjopen-2020-039451.

LaBeaud A, Pfeil S, Muiruri S, Dahir S, Sutherland L, Traylor Z, Gildengorin G, Muchuri E, Morrill J, Peters CJ, Hise AG, Kazura J and King C (2015) Factors associated with severe human Rift Valley Fever in Sangailu, Garissa County, Kenya. *PLOS Neglected Tropical Diseases*. 9(3): e0003548. https://doi.org/10.1371/journal.pntd.0003548.

Lana RM, Gomes MF da C, Lima TFM de, Honório NA and Codeço CT (2017) The introduction of dengue follows transportation infrastructure changes in the state of Acre, Brazil: a network-based analysis. *PLOS Neglected Tropical Diseases*, 11(11), e0006070. https://doi.org/10.1371/journal.pntd.0006070.

Landier J, Parker DM, Thu AM, Lwin KM, Delmas G, Nosten FH, Andolina C, Aguas R, Ang SM, Aung EP, Baw NB, Be SA, B'Let S, Bluh H, Bonnington CA, Chaumeau V, Chirakiratinant M, Cho WC, Christensen P, Yuwapan D (2018) Effect of generalised access to early diagnosis and treatment and targeted mass drug administration on *Plasmodium falciparum* malaria in Eastern Myanmar: an observational study of a regional elimination programme. *The Lancet*, *391*(10133), 1916–1926. https://doi.org/10.1016/S0140-6736(18)30792-X.

Landrigan P, Bose-O'Reilly S, Elbel J, Nordberg G, Lucchini R, Bartrem C, Grandjean P, Mergler D, Moyo D, Nemery B, von Braun M, Nowak D and on behalf of the Collegium Ramazzini (2022) Reducing disease and death from Artisanal and Small-Scale Mining (ASM) – the urgent need for responsible mining in the context of growing global demand for minerals and metals for climate change mitigation. *Environmental Health*, 21(1), 78. https://doi.org/10.1186/s12940-022-00877-5.

Lee RD and Kramer KL (2002) Children's economic roles in the Maya family life cycle: Cain, Caldwell, and Chayanov revisited. *Population and Development Review*, 28(3), 475–499.

Lee TJ, Mullany LC, Richards AK, Kuiper HK, Maung C and Beyrer C (2006) Mortality rates in conflict zones in Karen, Karenni, and Mon states in eastern Burma. *Tropical Medicine & International Health*, 11(7), 1119–1127. https://doi.org/10.1111/j.1365-3156.2006.01651.x.

Lee Y and Kim H (2018) The turning point of China's rural public health during the Cultural revolution period: barefoot doctors: a narrative. *Iranian Journal of Public Health*, 47(Suppl 1), 1–8.

Li Y, Kamara F, Zhou G, Puthiyakunnon S, Li C, Liu Y, Zhou Y, Yao L, Yan G and Chen XG (2014) Urbanization increases *Aedes albopictus* larval habitats and accelerates mosquito development and survivorship. *PLOS Neglected Tropical Diseases*, 8(11), e3301. https://doi.org/10.1371/journal.pntd.0003301.

Macdonald A and Mordecai E (2019) Amazon deforestation drives malaria transmission, and malaria burden reduces forest clearing. *PNAS*, 116(44), 22212–22218. https://doi.org/www.pnas.org/cgi/doi/10.1073/pnas.1905315116.

Macharia PM, Ray N, Giorgi E, Okiro EA and Snow RW (2021) Defining service catchment areas in low-resource settings. *BMJ Global Health*, 6(7), e006381. https://doi.org/10.1136/bmjgh-2021-006381.

Malede A, Alemu K, Aemero M, Robele S and Kloos H (2018) Travel to farms in the lowlands and inadequate malaria information significantly predict malaria in villages around Lake Tana, northwest Ethiopia: a matched case-control study. *Malaria Journal*, 17(1), 290. https://doi.org/10.1186/s12936-018-2434-y.

Martens P and Hall L (2000) Malaria on the move: human population movement and malaria transmission. *Emerging Infectious Diseases*, 6(2), 103–109. https://doi.org/10.3201/eid0602.000202.

Massaro L and de Theije M (2018) Understanding small-scale gold mining practices: an anthropological study on technological innovation in the Vale do Rio Peixoto (Mato Grosso, Brazil). *Journal of Cleaner Production*, 204, 618–635. https://doi.org/10.1016/j.jclepro.2018.08.153.

McCann J (2014) The historical ecology of malaria in Ethiopia. Ohio University Press.

McGowan CR, Baxter L, Deola C, Gayford M, Marston C, Cummings R and Checchi F (2020) Mobile clinics in humanitarian emergencies: a systematic review. *Conflict and Health*, 14(1), 4. https://doi.org/10.1186/s13031-020-0251-8.

McGrail MR (2012) Spatial accessibility of primary health care utilising the two step floating catchment area method: an assessment of recent improvements. *International Journal of Health Geographics*, 11(1), 50. https://doi.org/10.1186/1476-072X-11-50.

McGregor D, Whitaker S and Sritharan M (2020) Indigenous environmental justice and sustainability. *Current Opinion in Environmental Sustainability*, 43, 35–40. https://doi.org/10.1016/j.cosust.2020.01.007.

Meskal F and Kloos H (1989) Vector-borne disease occurrence and spread as affected by labor migrations to irrigation schemes in Ethiopia. In Demography and Vector Borne Disease (pp. 225–236). CRC Press.

Ministry of Health Ethiopia (2010) National strategic plan for malaria prevention control and elimination in Ethiopia 2011–2015 (p. 76). Ministry of Health, Ethiopia. https://extranet.who.int/countryplanningcycles/sites/default/files/country_docs/Ethiopia/ethiopia_malaria_national_strategic_plan_2011-2015_130810.pdf.

Ministry of Health Ethiopia (2020) Ethiopia malaria elimination strategic plan: 2021–2025 (p. 90). Ministry of Health, Ethiopia. https://govshop.com/media/opportunities/documents/02f2d44a21f5000fb133215b3973e35fethiopia-malaria-elimination-strategic-plan-2021-2025-final.pdf.

Moss WJ, Ramakrishnan M, Storms D, Henderson Siegle A, Weiss WM, Lejnev I and Muhe L (2006) Child health in complex emergencies. *Bulletin of the World Health Organization*, 84(1), 58–64. https://doi.org/10.2471/blt.04.019570.

Moyo D, Zishiri C, Ncube R, Madziva G, Sandy C, Mhene R, Siziba N, Kavenga F, Moyo F, Muzvidziwa O, Ncube P, Chigaraza B, Nyambo A and Timire C (2021) Tuberculosis and silicosis burden in artisanal and small-scale gold miners in a large occupational health outreach programme in Zimbabwe. *International Journal of Environmental Research and Public Health*, 18(21), 11031. https://doi.org/10.3390/ijerph182111031.

Mullany LC, Lee TJ, Yone L, Lee CI, Teela KC, Paw P, Oo EKS, Maung C, Kuiper H, Masenior NF and Beyrer C (2010) Impact of community-based maternal health workers on coverage of essential maternal health interventions among internally displaced communities in Eastern Burma: the MOM project. *PLOS Medicine*, 7(8), e1000317. https://doi.org/10.1371/journal.pmed.1000317.

National Heart Lungs Blood Institute (NHLBI) (2022) Role of community health workers. NHLBI. Available at: https://www.nhlbi.nih.gov/health/educational/healthdisp/role-of-community-health-workers.htm.

Nega A and Meskal F (1991) Malaria and development in Africa: a cross-sectional approach. (p. 220). American Association for the Advancement of Science Sub-Saharan Africa Program. https://pdf.usaid.gov/pdf_docs/PNABM357.pdf.

Nickerson JW (2015) Ensuring the security of health care in conflict settings: an urgent global health concern. *Canadian Medical Association Journal*, 187(11), E347–E348. https://doi.org/10.1503/cmaj.140410.

Nigussie T, Mamo Y, Qanche Q, Yosef T, Wondimu W and Asefa A (2021) HIV preventive behaviors and associated factors among gold mining workers in Dima District, Southwest Ethiopia, 2019: community-based cross-sectional study. *BioMed Research International*, 2021, 4797590. https://doi.org/10.1155/2021/4797590.

Norris D (2004) Mosquito-borne diseases as a consequence of land use change. *EcoHealth*, 1(1), 19–24. https://doi.org/10.1007/s10393-004-0008-7.

Nriagu J (1992) Toxic metal pollution in Africa. *The Science of The Total Environment*, 121, 1–37. https://doi.org/10.1016/0048-9697(92)90304-B.

Nunfam VF, Oosthuizen J, Adusei-Asante K, Van Etten EJ and Frimpong K (2019) Perceptions of climate change and occupational heat stress risks and adaptation strategies of mining workers in Ghana. *Science of The Total Environment*, 657, 365–378. https://doi.org/10.1016/j.scitotenv.2018.11.480.

Odell SD, Bebbington A and Frey KE (2018) Mining and climate change: a review and framework for analysis. *The Extractive Industries and Society*, 5(1), 201–214. https://doi.org/10.1016/j.exis.2017.12.004.

Olaleye OD, Tomori O, Ladipo MA and Schmitz H (1996) Rift Valley fever in Nigeria: infection in humans. *Rev Sci Tech.* 15(3): 923–35. 10.20506/rst.15.3.967.

Omam LA, Jarman E, Ekokobe W, Evon A and Omam EN (2021) Mobile clinics in conflict-affected communities of North West and South West regions of Cameroon: an alternative option for differentiated delivery service for internally displaced persons during COVID-19. *Conflict and Health*, 15(1), 90. https://doi.org/10.1186/s13031-021-00427-9.

Ouma PO, Maina J, Thuranira PN, Macharia PM, Alegana VA, English M, Okiro EA and Snow RW (2018) Access to emergency hospital care provided by the public sector in sub-Saharan Africa in 2015: a geocoded inventory and spatial analysis. *The Lancet Global Health*, 6(3), e342–e350. https://doi.org/10.1016/S2214-109X(17)30488-6.

Parker AL, Parker DM, Zan BN, Min AM, Gilder ME, Ringringulu M, Win E, Wiladphaingern J, Charunwatthana P, Nosten F, Lee SJ and McGready R (2018) Trends and birth outcomes in adolescent refugees and migrants on the Thailand-Myanmar border, 1986–2016: an observational study. *Wellcome Open Research*, 3, 62. https://doi.org/10.12688/wellcomeopenres.14613.1.

Parker DM, Wood JW, Tomita S, DeWitte S, Jennings J and Cui L (2014) Household ecology and out-migration among ethnic Karen along the Thai-Myanmar border. *Demographic Research*, 30, 1129–1156. https://doi.org/10.4054/DemRes.2014.30.39.

Patz JA, Daszak P, Tabor GM, Aguirre AA, Pearl M, Epstein J, Wolfe ND, Kilpatrick AM, Foufopoulos J, Molyneux D and Bradley DJ (2004). Unhealthy landscapes: policy recommendations on land use change and infectious disease emergence. *Environmental Health Perspectives*, 112(10), 1092–1098. https://doi.org/10.1289/ehp.6877.

Plowright RK, Reaser JK, Locke H, Woodley SJ, Patz JA, Becker DJ, Oppler G, Hudson PJ and Tabor GM (2021) Land use-induced spillover: a call to action to safeguard environmental, animal, and human health. *The Lancet Planetary Health*, 5(4), e237–e245. https://doi.org/10.1016/S2542-5196(21)00031-0.

Pokharel BK, Branney P, Nurse M and Malla YB (2007) Community forestry: conserving forests, sustaining livelihoods and strengthening democracy. *Journal of Forest and Livelihood*, 12.

Pooseesod K, Parker DM, Meemon N, Lawpoolsri S, Singhasivanon P, Sattabongkot J, Cui L and Phuanukoonnon S (2021) Ownership and utilization of bed nets and reasons for use or non-use of bed nets among community members at risk of malaria along the Thai-Myanmar border. *Malaria Journal*, 20(1), 305. https://doi.org/10.1186/s12936-021-03837-5.

Portes A and Sensenbrenner J (1993) Embeddedness and immigration: notes on the social determinants of economic action. *American Journal of Sociology*, 98(6), 1320–1350.

Prentice JC and Pizer SD (2007) Delayed access to health care and mortality. *Health Services Research*, 42(2), 644–662. https://doi.org/10.1111/j.1475-6773.2006.00626.x.

Prothero RM (1999) Malaria, forests and people in Southeast Asia. *Singapore Journal of Tropical Geography*, 20(1), 76–85. https://doi.org/10.1111/1467-9493.00044.

Quick J and Fry B (2018) The end of epidemics: the looming threat to humanity and how to stop it. St Martins Press.

Regassa A and Korf B (2018) Post-imperial statecraft: High modernism and the politics of land dispossession in Ethiopia's pastoral frontier. *Journal of Eastern African Studies*, 12(4), 613–631. https://doi.org/10.1080/17531055.2018.1517854.

Riza E, Kalkman S, Coritsidis A, Koubardas S, Vassiliu S, Lazarou D, Karnaki P, Zota D, Kantzanou M, Psaltopoulou T and Linos A (2020) Community-based healthcare for migrants and refugees: a scoping literature review of best practices. *Healthcare*, 8(2), 115. https://doi.org/10.3390/healthcare8020115.

Rogalski MA, Gowler CD, Shaw CL, Hufbauer RA and Duffy MA (2017) Human drivers of ecological and evolutionary dynamics in emerging and disappearing infectious disease systems. *Philosophical Transactions of the Royal Society B: Biological Sciences*, 372(1712), 20160043. https://doi.org/10.1098/rstb.2016.0043.

Rosenberg R and Maheswary NP (1982) Forest malaria in Bangladesh. II. Transmission by Anopheles dirus. *The American Journal of Tropical Medicine and Hygiene*, 31(2), 183–191. https://doi.org/10.4269/ajtmh.1982.31.183.

Rural Health Information Hub (n.d.) Rural migrant health overview – rural health information hub. https://www.ruralhealthinfo.org/topics/migrant-health.

Ryan L (2011) Migrants' social networks and weak ties: accessing resources and constructing relationships post-migration. *The Sociological Review*, 59(4), 707–724. https://doi.org/10.1111/j.1467-954X.2011.02030.x.

Sagaon-Teyssier L, Balique H, Diallo F, Kalampalikis N, Mora M, Bourrelly M, Suzan-Monti M, Spire B and Dembélé Keita B (2017) Prevalence of HIV at the Kokoyo informal gold mining site: what lies behind the glitter of gold with regard to HIV epidemics in Mali? A community-based approach (the ANRS-12339 Sanu Gundo cross-sectional survey). *BMJ Open*, 7(8), e016558. https://doi.org/10.1136/bmjopen-2017-016558.

Saha S, Pattanayak SK, Sills EO and Singha AK (2011) Under-mining health: environmental justice and mining in India. *Health & Place*, 17(1), 140–148. https://doi.org/10.1016/j.healthplace.2010.09.007.

Schwartz FW, Lee S and Darrah TH (2021) A review of the scope of artisanal and small-scale mining worldwide, poverty, and the associated health impacts. *GeoHealth*, 5(1), e2020GH000325. https://doi.org/10.1029/2020GH000325.

Sellers S, Bilsbarrow R, Salinas V and Mena C (2017) Population and development in the Amazon: a longitudinal study of migrant settlers in the Northern Ecuadorian Amazon. *Acta Amazônica*. 47(4). https://doi.org/10.1590/1809-4392201602663.

Sherpa PY (2015) Institutional climate change adaptation efforts among the sherpas of the Mount Everest region, Nepal. In Climate Change, Culture, and Economics: Anthropological Investigations (Vol. 35, pp. 1–23). Emerald Group Publishing Limited. https://doi.org/10.1108/S0190-128120150000035001.

Silbergeld EK, Nash D, Trevant C, Strickland GT, de Souza JM and da Silva RSU (2002) Mercury exposure and malaria prevalence among gold miners in Pará, Brazil. *Revista Da Sociedade Brasileira De Medicina Tropical*, 35(5), 421–429. https://doi.org/10.1590/s0037-86822002000500001.

Simon C, Belyakov AO and Feichtinger G (2012) Minimizing the dependency ratio in a population with below-replacement fertility through immigration. *Theoretical Population Biology*, 82(3), 158–169. https://doi.org/10.1016/j.tpb.2012.06.009.

Singer BH and de Castro MC (2001) Agricultural colonization and malaria on the Amazon frontier. *Annals of the New York Academy of Sciences*, 954, 184–222. https://doi.org/10.1111/j.1749-6632.2001.tb02753.x.

Smith N, Ali S, Bofinger C and Collins N (2016) Human health and safety in artisanal and small-scale mining: an integrated approach to risk mitigation. *Journal of Cleaner Production*, 129. https://doi.org/10.1016/j.jclepro.2016.04.124.

Snowden F (2019) Epidemics and society: from the Black death to the present. Yale University Press.

Sonter L, Herrera D, Barrett DJ, Galford G, Moran C and Soares-Filho B (2017) Mining drives extensive deforestation in the Brazilian Amazon | Nature Communications. *Nature Communications*, 8(1013). https://www.nature.com/articles/s41467-017-00557-w.

Sousa C and Hagopian A (2011) Conflict, health care and professional perseverance: a qualitative study in the West Bank. *Global Public Health*, 6(5), 520–533. https://doi.org/10.1080/17441692.2011.574146.

Souza PF, Xavier DR, Mutis MCS, Mota JC da, Peiter PC, Matos VP de, Magalhães M de AFM and Barcellos C (2019) Spatial spread of malaria and economic frontier expansion in the Brazilian Amazon. *PLOS ONE*, 14(6), e0217615. https://doi.org/10.1371/journal.pone.0217615.

Spiegel SJ and Veiga MM (2005) Building capacity in small-scale mining communities: health, ecosystem sustainability, and the global mercury project. *EcoHealth*, 2(4), 361–369. https://doi.org/10.1007/s10393-005-8389-9.

Srikanok S, Parker DM, Parker AL, Lee T, Min AM, Ontuwong P, Oo Tan S, Sirinonthachai S and McGready R (2017) Empirical lessons regarding contraception in a protracted refugee setting: a descriptive study from Maela camp on the Thai-Myanmar border 1996–2015. *PLOS ONE*, 12(2), e0172007. https://doi.org/10.1371/journal.pone.0172007.

Stark O and Bloom DE (1985) The new economics of labor migration. *The American Economic Review*, 75(2), 173–178.

Tadesse Y, Irish SR, Chibsa S, Dugassa S, Lorenz LM, Gebreyohannes A, Teka H, Solomon H, Gezahegn E, Petros Y, Haile M, Eshetu M and Murphy M (2021) Malaria prevention and treatment in migrant agricultural workers in Dangur district, Benishangul-Gumuz, Ethiopia: social and behavioural aspects. *Malaria Journal*, 20(1), 224. https://doi.org/10.1186/s12936-021-03766-3.

Taffese HS, Hemming-Schroeder E, Koepfli C, Tesfaye G, Lee M, Kazura J, Yan GY and Zhou GF (2018) Malaria epidemiology and interventions in Ethiopia from 2001 to 2016. *Infectious Diseases of Poverty*, 7(1), 103. https://doi.org/10.1186/s40249-018-0487-3.

Tesfahunegn A, Berhe G and Gebregziabher E (2019) Risk factors associated with malaria outbreak in Laelay Adyabo district northern Ethiopia, 2017: case-control study design. *BMC Public Health*, 19(1), 484. https://doi.org/10.1186/s12889-019-6798-x.

The Global Fund (2022) Catalytic investment to improve community health care for millions across Africa. Available at: https://www.theglobalfund.org/en/news/2022/2022-08-08-catalytic-investment-to-improve-community-health-care-for-millions-across-africa/.

Thompson CN (2020) COVID-19 outbreak – New York City, February 29–June 1, 2020. *MMWR. Morbidity and Mortality Weekly Report*, 69. https://doi.org/10.15585/mmwr.mm6946a2.

Todaro M (1980) Internal migration in developing countries: a survey. In: R.A. Easterlin (ed.) Population and economic change in developing countries (Midway reprint edition 1987). The University of Chicago Press.

Tomita S, Parker DM, Jennings JA and Wood J (2015) Household demography and early childhood mortality in a rice-farming village in Northern Laos. *PLOS ONE*, 10(3), e0119191. https://doi.org/10.1371/journal.pone.0119191.

Tsang VWL, Lockhart K, Spiegel SJ and Yassi A (2019) Occupational health programs for artisanal and small-scale gold mining: a systematic review for the WHO global plan of action for workers' health. *Annals of Global Health*, 85(1), 128. https://doi.org/10.5334/aogh.2592.

Tulu A (1993) Malaria. In: H. Kloos and Z. Zein (eds) The ecology of health and disease in Ethiopia. Westview Press.

Veracini L (2016) Introduction: settler colonialism as a distinct mode of domination. In: E. Cavanaugh and L. Veracini (eds) The Routledge Handbook of the History of Settler Colonialism. Routledge.

Vittor AY, Gilman RH, Tielsch J, Glass G, Shields T, Lozano WS, Pinedo-Cancino V and Patz JA (2006) The effect of deforestation on the human-biting rate of anopheles darlingi, the primary vector of falciparum malaria in the Peruvian Amazon. *The American Journal of Tropical Medicine and Hygiene*, 74(1), 3–11. https://doi.org/10.4269/ajtmh.2006.74.3.

Wachs D, Roman-Urrestarazu A, Brayne C and Onrubia-Fernández J (2020) Dependency ratios in healthy ageing. *BMJ Global Health*, 5(4), e002117. https://doi.org/10.1136/bmjgh-2019-002117.

Walsh JF, Molyneux DH and Birley MH (1993) Deforestation: effects on vector-borne disease. *Parasitology*, 106 Suppl, S55–75. https://doi.org/10.1017/s0031182000086121.

William T, Rahman HA, Jelip J, Ibrahim MY, Menon J, Grigg MJ, Yeo TW, Anstey NM and Barber BE (2013) Increasing incidence of *Plasmodium knowlesi* malaria following control of *P. falciparum* and *P. vivax* malaria in Sabah, Malaysia. *PLOS Neglected Tropical Diseases*, 7(1), e2026. https://doi.org/10.1371/journal.pntd.0002026.

World Bank (2013) Sustaining forests and livelihoods in a changing world. World Bank. Available at: https://www.worldbank.org/en/news/feature/2013/01/29/sustaining-forests-livelihoods-changing-world.

World Bank (2020) 2020 State of the artisanal and small-scale mining sector. World Bank. Available at: https://www.trafigura.com/media/3127/2020_trafigura_state_of_artisanal_and_small_scale_mining_sector_report.pdf.

World Health Organization (WHO). (2011). Global health and aging. Available at: https://www.who.int/ageing/publications/global_health.pdf.

World Health Organization (WHO). (2019). Promoting the health of refugees and migrants: draft global action plan, 2019–2023. Available at: https://www.who.int/publications-detail-redirect/promoting-the-health-of-refugees-and-migrants-draft-global-action-plan-2019-2023.

Wright J, Williams R and Wilkinson JR (1998) Development and importance of health needs assessment. *BMJ* (*Clinical Research Ed.*), 316(7140), 1310–1313. https://doi.org/10.1136/bmj.316.7140.1310.

Wu J, Tschakert P, Klutse E, Ferring D, Ricciardi V, Hausermann H, Oppong J and Smithwick EAH (2015) Buruli ulcer disease and its association with land cover in southwestern Ghana. *PLOS Neglected Tropical Diseases*, 9(6), e0003840. https://doi.org/10.1371/journal.pntd.0003840.

Zurovac D, Githinji S, Memusi D, Kigen S, Machini B, Muturi A, Otieno G, Snow RW and Nyandigisi A (2014) Major improvements in the quality of malaria case-management under the 'Test and Treat' policy in Kenya. *PLOS One*, 9(3), e92782. https://doi.org/10.1371/journal.pone.0092782.

CHAPTER 6

The economic impacts of malaria: past, present, and future

Nikolas Kuschnig and Lukas Vashold*

Vienna University of Economics and Business, Welthandelsplatz 1, 1020 Vienna, Austria; *nikolas.kuschnig@wu.ac.at

Abstract

Malaria places a great burden on the health and prosperity of many and occupies a great number of scientists and policymakers. The dynamics of the disease are tightly interwoven with economics – incidence is both tied to economic circumstances and impacts them. Economic research plays an important role in understanding and supporting the fight against malaria. The economic literature, however, features a number of peculiarities that can hamper accessibility and has been slow to approach interdisciplinary issues. In this chapter, we explain the economic perspective and summarise the literature on the economic impacts of malaria. Malaria has severe impacts on individual and aggregate economic outcomes, including mortality and morbidity, but also indirect burdens that materialise with a delay. The fight against malaria is not an economic policy per se, but may provide beneficial economic spillovers and can be vital in establishing an environment that allows for prosperity. Economic insights can make a difference in the design and implementation of effective and efficient eradication and control strategies. This is critical in the light of increasing disease (re-)exposure due to climate change and the emergence of resistant vectors and pathogens.

Keywords

malaria – development – economic growth – education – health

1 Introduction

Vector-based diseases place a great burden upon affected populations. Among them, malaria is the most prevalent, with about 241 million cases and 627,000 deaths in 2020 (Global Malaria Programme 2021). Today, the disease is endemic to tropical and subtropical regions, home to some of the poorest countries on earth. Whether

 | DOI:10.3920/9789004688650_008

and how these facts are related continues to occupy many scientists. Disease and economics interweave tightly in many dimensions that prove hard to disentangle. Research questions are complex and of a fundamentally interdisciplinary nature, making reliable analysis challenging. Insights into the economic impacts of malaria can only be obtained with a broad understanding of the disease and its interrelations. Similarly, economic circumstances play an important role in the spread, control, and eradication of malaria; evidenced by considerable interest from the wider literature.

The importance of economics for malaria is reflected in a large body of research. However, the relation is not as clear as it may seem and insights are not as accessible as one would like. The strong link between malaria, development, and poverty noted in macroeconomic studies (e.g. Gallup and Sachs 2000) caught considerable attention. The same is true for the widespread backlash (e.g. Acemoglu and Johnson 2007), pointing out a lack of causality. More nuanced economic studies do not command as much attention, but offer, e.g. robust evidence of malaria impacting human capital accumulation, labour productivity and a range of other important socioeconomic factors (see Kuecken *et al.* 2021, for a recent example). Meanwhile, more generalist approaches could benefit from an economic perspective (see Duflo 2017, for an argument why this may be the case), but collaborations are rare, which is partly due to a lack of incentives. Knowledge of the economic impacts of malaria and a comprehensive understanding of the disease are vital for interdisciplinary research, but also for selecting efficient adaptation and mitigation measures (Sicuri *et al.* 2022).

Malaria has a wide range of economic impacts, ranging from immediate ones, due to mortality and morbidity, to indirect ones. Among many other impacts, the disease lowers cognitive skills (Venkataramani 2012), educational attainment (Lucas 2010), labour market participation (Hong 2013), and affects fertility choices (Lucas 2013), civil unrest (Cervellati *et al.* 2022a), as well as foreign direct investment (Cervellati *et al.* 2022b). Studies have found pronounced links between malaria and economic circumstances at large (Gallup and Sachs 2000), although the strength of these links, and whether a causal relationship exists, remains debated (Acemoglu and Johnson 2007; Cervellati and Sunde 2011). Insights into the effects of control and eradication campaigns, like the one by Kuecken *et al.* (2021) for the recent 'Roll Back Malaria' campaign in sub-Saharan Africa, can help with the efficient and effective use of sparse resources for the design, implementation, and funding of malaria control and eradication strategies.

However, insights are only useful when they are accessible, and both the languages of economics and malaria itself can be particular. With this in mind, we provide some background for the disease, and introduce essential features of the economic literature – most prominently its focus on identifying causal effects from non-experimental data. We review the literature on the economic impacts of malaria, both in micro- and macroeconomic terms. Topics include impacts at the individual-level, such as health and educational outcomes, at aggregate levels, such as economic development, and the economics of malaria eradication and control. The goal of this chapter is to summarize and reconcile the economic literature, paving the way for future interdisciplinary research efforts. The fight against malaria will pose many known and unknown challenges – including climate change – and well-informed strategies are needed, as are knowledge spillovers across disciplines.

2 Malaria

Human malaria is caused by six *Plasmodium* parasite species – most notably *P. falciparum* and *P. vivax* – that are transmitted primarily via the bite of female *Anopheles* mosquitoes. Incidence is tied to the spread and activity of these vectors and depends on environments that are suitable in terms of climate, altitude, vegetation, and control measures (Ashley *et al.* 2018). This enabled the elimination of malaria from many temperate regions in the past (see Feachem *et al.* 2010, and c.f. Figure 1), and highlights the importance of human settlement and migration patterns (Carrasco-Escobar *et al.* 2022; Kounnavong *et al.* 2017). In recent years, however, gains against malaria have been stalling (Global Malaria Programme 2021), which may be exacerbated by land use change and climate change in the future (Caminade *et al.* 2014; Patz and Olson 2006).[1]

The disease is routinely separated into uncomplicated cases, with relatively mild symptoms like headache and fever, and severe malaria, which may cause anemia, respiratory distress, renal failure, and neurological symptoms (Ashley *et al.* 2018). The severity of the disease relates to the species of the pathogen, with *P. falciparum* causing most acute cases and almost all deaths globally (Global Malaria Programme 2021). The most severe neurological complication of an infection with *P. falciparum* is cerebral malaria, which invariably leads to death when untreated (Idro *et al.* 2010). Even when treated, its case-fatality rate is usually 10–20% (Ashley *et al.* 2018). Children, pregnant women, and patients with co-morbidities are most affected by cerebral malaria in endemic areas. Repeated exposure in adults leads to infection-immunity that protects against the effects of the disease to a degree, but not against infection. In addition, there are a number of inherited and acquired factors that affect chance of infection and severity (Ashley *et al.* 2018), which are most prevalent on the African continent. Infection rates that dictate mortality and

1 The environmental suitability for malaria and, relatedly, the population at risk are likely to increase in the face of climate change (also see Ferguson and Govella, 2023; Shocket, 2023, in Chapters 15 and 11). Due to climate change, malaria may decline in relative importance compared to arboviruses with *Aedes* mosquitoes as vectors (see de Azevedo *et al.* 2023, in Chapter 3).

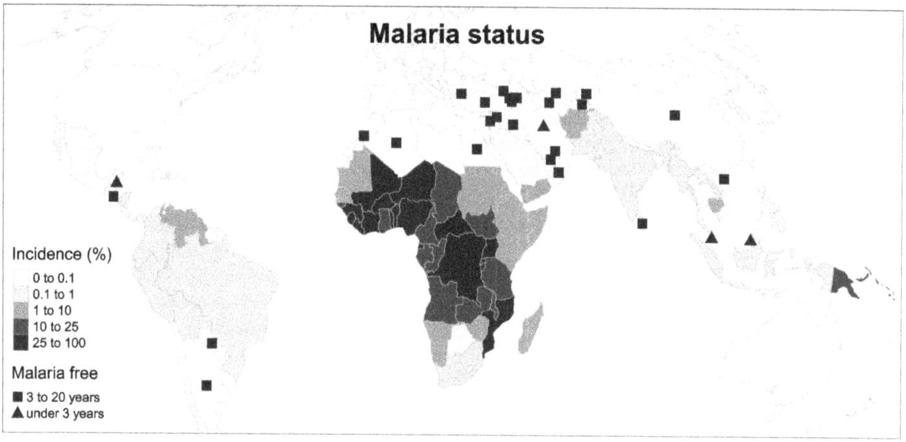

FIGURE 1 Global malaria status. Global malaria status as indicated by the incidence in percent of the population at risk in 2018 or the time since the last indigenous case was recorded
SOURCES: WORLD HEALTH ORGANIZATION, GLOBAL HEALTH OBSERVATORY DATA REPOSITORY/WORLD HEALTH STATISTICS AND GLOBAL MALARIA PROGRAMME 2021

morbidity also depend heavily on vectors and their capacity to transmit malaria; some members of the African *A. Gambiae* complex are particularly efficient at human transmission.

Malaria is treated using one of a number of antimalarial medications (Ashley *et al.* 2018). The most prominent antimalarials are derived from: (1) chloroquine, the most widespread compound until recently; and (2) artemisinin, which revolutionized treatment starting in the 1990s. Resistance against established antimalarials is common, and artemisinin-resistant lines of *P. falciparum* are emerging in Southeast Asia (Ménard *et al.* 2016). Combination therapy, where antimalarials are combined with partner drugs, offers the best treatment outcomes (Alven and Aderibigbe 2019) and is effective at avoiding the emergence of resistance. However, combination therapy is more costly and – even more importantly – demanding in terms of expertise, logistics, and adherence.

The World Heath Organisation (WHO) recognises three main strategies for the control and potential elimination of malaria. First is vector control, with insecticide-treated bednets and indoor residual spraying with insecticides as the main interventions. These interventions have been highly effective and efficient where they are applicable,[2] but are under threat by emerging insecticide-resistance

2 The efficacy and efficiency of such measures depends (inter alia) on the feeding behavior of predominant vectors. Species in Africa tend to feed and rest indoors (Sherrard-Smith *et al.* 2019); in Latin America and South-East Asia, bites occur more frequently in the outdoors (e.g. Saavedra *et al.* 2019).

and changing bionomic traits among mosquitoes (Global Malaria Programme 2021). Climate change and local land use changes are also likely to have impacts on vector types and abundance (see e.g. Gottdenker *et al.* 2014; Rocklöv and Dubrow 2020). Second is chemoprophylaxis for susceptible populations, such as children, pregnant women, or travellers. This strategy may reduce morbidity, prevent infection, and decrease the rate of transmission (Global Malaria Programme 2021). Third, new malaria vaccines can play an important role in reducing malaria incidence and severity in children (Datoo *et al.* 2022), although many open questions remain (see e.g. Olotu *et al.* 2016; Doshi 2020). These strategies can differ considerably in effectiveness, efficiency, and requirements for implementation. As laid out later in this chapter, economics and thus economic research plays a crucial for these considerations.

3 The economics of malaria

Millions of malaria cases globally impose an exceptionally high burden of disease on affected populations. This burden is concentrated in some of the world's poorest countries (Global Malaria Programme 2021, and c.f. Figure 1). Control and treatment of the disease and, as a result, the burden it imposes are heavily reliant on socioeconomic circumstances, leading to the notion of malaria being a 'disease of poverty' (see e.g. Worrall *et al.* 2005). Effective vector control, efficient prophylaxis, vaccination programmes, and successful therapy require ample financial resources, structure, and know-how. Beyond the impacts of economic structures on malaria, there are also considerable vice versa impacts – i.e. economic impacts of malaria. The existence of these impacts is relatively uncontroversial, but their scale and the mechanisms behind them remain the subject of a large and diverse body of literature.

The economic impacts of malaria manifest in several ways. For one, there is an enormous direct burden in terms of premature mortality and morbidity. A way to quantify this burden are disability-adjusted life years,[3] which can be economised, e.g. using yearly average per capita income. Bloom *et al.* (2022) use this approach and attribute direct costs in the hundreds of billions to malaria. They place the direct cost of malaria as the third largest among all infectious diseases, topped only by HIV/AIDS and tuberculosis. This approach may still underestimate the impacts of morbidity – infections with malaria may 'result in recurrent debilitating bouts of illness, which prevents individuals from supplying their labour productively' (Cole

3 The measure takes into account both mortality (via years of life lost) and morbidity (via years lived with disability) effects. Life expectancy is another popular measure of overall health, but does not adequately reflect the burden implied by morbidity.

and Neumayer 2006, p.919). In another study, Cervellati *et al.* (2022a) put the number of workdays that are directly lost to malaria in affected agrarian households at 20–60 per year. Such estimates of the direct economic cost of malaria cover one important dimension, but are by no means comprehensive. The total economic impacts of malaria may be considerably larger.

Indirect and long-term economic impacts of disease are likely to be decisive elements, but are considerably harder to trace and quantify. One problem is the long time period until impacts on economic outcomes materialize and fully manifest, which may mask causal links. For example, Barreca (2010) finds increased poverty rates after high in-utero and postnatal exposure to malaria, while Hong (2013) documents increased occurrence of chronic diseases in old age – both using US data. Another prominent argument concerns even longer-term development impacts of malaria (Sachs and Malaney 2002; Malaney *et al.* 2004). Evolutionary pressure gave rise to genetic dispositions, such as the sickle cell trait or the lack of the Duffy antigen receptor, that offer some protection against malaria, but can themselves be harmful or even fatal.[4] This would suggest that the long-term development impacts of the disease are roughly comparable to the drawbacks from these dispositions. A more immediate type of long-term impact concerns economic growth and poverty, which may reflect aggregate direct and indirect impacts on smaller, individual scales.

The crux of much economic research on malaria is related to this multiplicity of connections and possible pathways – the causal identification of impacts. Generally, estimated effects are correlations that may occur for many reasons, but they are not causal relations. For example, in a well-known study, Gallup and Sachs (2000) report strong correlations of economic growth and poverty with malaria. Their findings cannot be interpreted causally, i.e. they suggest a connection, but not a cause and effect relationship, due to a series of limitations. To unveil a causal effect, we would ideally compare hypothetical outcomes with and without the cause (see e.g. Imbens 2020).[5] Since we can only ever observe one outcome, we need to infer causal differences using an *identification strategy* (see e.g. Athey and Imbens 2017). A classic example for such a strategy is a randomised experiment that enables control over known and unknown confounding factors that could influence

4 Variants of the haemoglobin beta gene offer protection against severe malaria. They give rise to the sickle cell trait in heterozygous form, but cause deadly sickle cell disease when both parents are affected. The Duffy antigen acts as a receptor for *P. vivax*, offering Duffy-negative individuals some protection (Ashley *et al.* 2018). Infections with *P. vivax* are extremely rare in sub-Saharan Africa, where the population is almost entirely Duffy-negative.

5 An example for a potential causal effect and outcome is the days of schooling received with and without a malaria infection. These could, e.g. be confounded by social status – less affluent children might be more likely to experience an infection and, unrelated to their health status, have fewer opportunities to attend school.

results. Good experimental data can get us closer to true causal effects, but often we have to rely on observational data instead (e.g. due to budgetary, ethical, or operative constraints). In order to identify any causal effect using observational data, additional care and the right setting are required. In very simple settings, we can argue for some causality when the right variables are controlled for. However, this is not possible when any important factors are unobservable, effects occur simultaneously, the selection process of observations is relevant, or in the presence of many other complications. In such cases, specialised methods and elaborate identification strategies, such as instrumental variables or quasi-experimental research designs, can help distil causal effects.

For these reasons, the economic literature lays much emphasis on strong identification strategies. As a result, findings are generally very reliable and estimated effects reflect what they ought to – causal relations. However, further challenges for insightful and practical research remain, and there are certain trade-offs for identification. Strong identification strategies often need tightly focused research questions or specific settings. If studies are specific, e.g. in terms of region or time, even reliable findings can be limited in their applicability – i.e. how well they generalise – and thus in their practical utility.

This issue is exacerbated by the heterogeneity of malaria and its interaction with other factors. Pathogens vary in regional spread and severity (Ashley *et al.* 2018); vectors are arguably even more heterogeneous. Impacts are moderated by socioeconomic circumstances, health status, and available interventions, all of which are highly variable over time, space, and individuals. As a result, studies like Bleakley (2010)'s analysis of childhood exposure to malaria during eradication campaigns in the early to mid 1900s Americas, must primarily be understood within their specific contexts – generally applicable insights are rare.

Heterogeneities can also be problematic in terms of conclusions drawn – even within a narrow context. Most studies investigate average effects, and do not delve deeper into how they arise. However, averages may mask vital insights, e.g. when different strata of society are afflicted differently, that would allow for much more effective, targeted interventions.

This issue is also pronounced at an aggregate level – while malaria may hamper economic development in Nigeria, it could have no effect in Vietnam. The analysis of heterogeneous effects has seen a lot of progress in recent years, and many new specialised methods are available (e.g. Athey and Imbens 2016; Hahn *et al.* 2020). However, any statistical method is limited by data – and more flexible ones even more so. The availability and quality of data is particularly disadvantageous in poorer regions, which are also hit the hardest by malaria (c.f. Figure 2).

Hence, accurate and detailed insights into the economic impacts of malaria are of great importance, but difficult to obtain. The intensive interplay of malaria

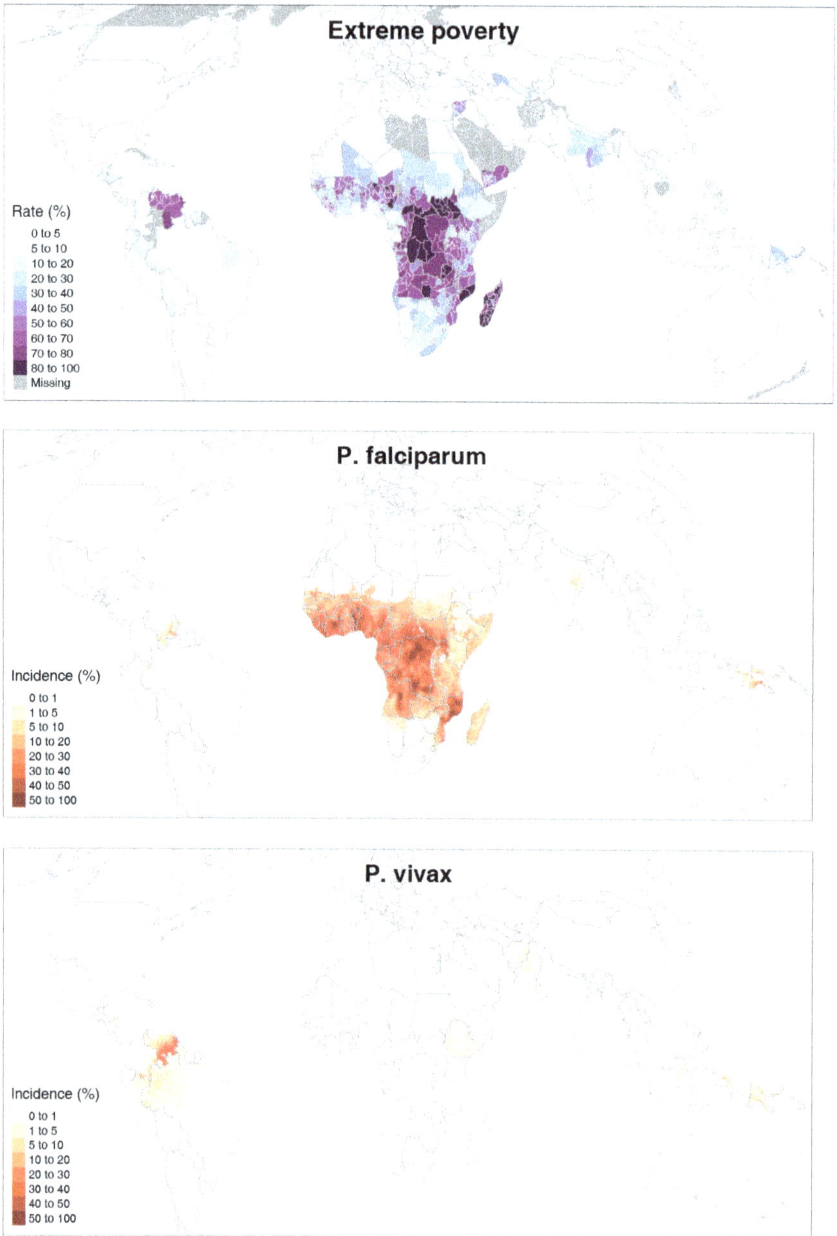

FIGURE 2 Poverty and the incidence of malaria. Subnational measures of recent extreme poverty rates, i.e. population living with less than $1.9 per day (A), incidence rates from 2019 of *P. falciparum* (B), and *P. vivax* (C)

SOURCES: WORLD BANK (2022) AND UNIVERSIDAD CATÓLICA ANDRÉS BELLO (2022) FOR POVERTY RATES, AND BATTLE *ET AL.* (2019) AND WEISS *ET AL.* (2019) FOR *PLASMODIUM* INCIDENCE RATES

and economics as well as the countless connections to other relevant factors can confound estimates, and thus, insights. Clever research design can prevail against these issues, but further challenges must be overcome. Ideally, insights translate into improved real-life circumstances (e.g. by informing policy to reduce education losses due to malaria). This requires results to be applicable to relevant situations, somewhat generalisable, and sufficiently in-depth.

With this background information in mind, we can now provide an overview of the economic impacts of malaria. In the following subsections, we review the current state of the economic literature on malaria, both on a microeconomic level and a macroeconomic level, and the economics of its eradication.

3.1 *The microeconomic impacts of malaria*

Microeconomic studies of malaria focus on its impacts at an individual level, and are typically confined to certain countries and narrow causal pathways. This allows them to obtain strong causal evidence, but their generalisability can often be lacking. Results may not have direct implications for current efforts at controlling or eliminating malaria. However, they illuminate certain mechanisms behind impacts, guide theory and provide a foundation for further studies. Notably, there are few results for contemporaneously most affected regions (e.g. sub-Saharan Africa) from these studies, in part due to data issues. An important exception is the study by Kuecken *et al.* (2021) that analyses the effects of the recent 'Roll Back Malaria' campaign on a broad set of demographic and economic indicators for 27 Sub-Saharan countries.

A common identification strategy of microeconomic studies is a quasi-experimental research design. One popular example is induced by the emergence of historical malaria eradication programmes. Differences in pre-eradication exposure, inter alia due to ecological conditions favouring spread of vectors and parasites, are used to assign quasi-randomised control and treatment groups from observational data. Eradication programmes can have considerable impacts on malaria exposure that are arguably unrelated to other important factors. These programmes are usually driven by independent advances in the understanding of malaria transmission and prevention methods that stem from outside the region where they apply.[6] There are only few experimental studies, due to their cost and ethical concerns. A recent exception is Dillon *et al.* (2021), who estimate that an infection reduces workers' weekly earnings by around 10%, primarily driven by reduced labour supply. In their randomised control trial, sugarcane plantations

6 For example, Bleakley (2010) argues that eradication programmes in the US South were not primarily driven by developments inherent to the area and its residents. Instead, the knowledge US Army doctors gained in Cuba and the Panama Canal zone spurred advancements and enabled the programmes. Several smaller projects in rural Southern towns were followed by large-scale efforts of the federal government at the start of World War I, primarily to reduce the number of troops unfit for service.

workers in Nigeria were offered malaria testing and treatment, with the week of the offer being randomised. Dillon *et al.* (2021) also find that news of a negative test increases daily productivity due to selection to more challenging and hence more rewarding tasks. Despite some limitations, microeconomic studies and their strong identification strategies have produced several important findings.

A recurrent finding is that early-life exposure to malaria is likely to impact future economic outcomes through various channels beyond contemporaneous morbidity and mortality. One prevalent channel is the ability to accumulate human capital in the form of education. Malaria affects children's educational capacity directly by leading to poorer nutritional status, impairing brain development, lowering cognitive performance (Kihara *et al.* 2006), and increasing school absenteeism (Thuilliez *et al.* 2010). Antimalarial campaigns in turn have positive effects on schooling performance in the form of increases in test scores (inter alia in Mexico, see Venkataramani 2012), providing further evidence for the adverse effects of malaria on cognition. Various studies in the microeconomic literature have found positive effects of malaria eradication on educational outcomes and human capital accumulation in terms of years spent in school – for example in the US (Barreca 2010), Paraguay and Sri Lanka (Lucas 2010), India (Cutler *et al.* 2010), and 27 sub-Saharan countries (Kuecken *et al.* 2021).

High infant and child mortality rates due to malaria may affect the fertility choices of parents. The 'child-survivor hypothesis' postulates that parents base their choices on the number of surviving children; e.g. as a guarantee of a suitable heir or as a kind of old-age insurance (Sachs and Malaney 2002). The empirical evidence on direct fertility impacts is somewhat mixed. Lucas (2013) finds that malaria eradication increased fertility and led to a younger maternal age Sri Lanka, while Wilde *et al.* (2020) document a recent rise in total fertility in sub-Saharan Africa. Conversely, Kuecken *et al.* (2021) provide empirical support for reduced fertility in recent sub-Saharan Africa. Higher exposure to malaria campaigns (in terms of proportion of lifetime in their post-period) showed no discernible impact on the probability of the first birth, but reduced the probability of a second birth by around two percentage points. The overall probability of a woman giving birth in a given year was reduced by 0.4 percentage points. These findings lend some support to the 'child-survivor hypothesis'.

Fertility choices, in turn, play an important role in the investment in education of children. A higher number of dependants in the household implies that average education investments are reduced, leading to a quantity-quality trade-off in children's education (Sachs and Malaney 2002). Hence, besides reducing the capacity of children to receive an education, exposure to malaria may also decrease the resources available for their education; in part also by diverting some of them on spending for the treatment of the disease. This impact on education can be particularly pronounced for females – high fertility rates imply that women spend much of their working years with child-related activities, constraining employment choices and their time in labour markets. This is exacerbated by frequent and severe infections of children, which increase care needs (Asenso-Okyere *et al.* 2011). As a result, the opportunity cost of female education is raised and educational investment is biased towards males. These impacts on gender disparities are still under-explored in the empirical literature, warranting further research. Generally speaking, however, empirical assessments of antimalarial campaigns almost unequivocally showed higher educational attainment and better educational outcomes, including improvements in literacy rates in adulthood.

By depressing human capital accumulation over the lifetime, childhood exposure to malaria has adverse effects on future labour productivity in adulthood and resulting economic outcomes. Spending on the treatment of the disease can also divert resources from other forms of consumption or investment. A number of empirical studies establish such effects at a microeconomic level. Reductions in early childhood exposure to malaria led to greater incomes and consumption in adulthood in the US, Brazil, Colombia, and Mexico (Bleakley 2010); India (Cutler *et al.* 2010); Uganda (Barofsky *et al.* 2015); and Vietnam (Laxminarayan 2004). In another study on the US, Barreca (2010) finds that high in-utero and postnatal exposure to malaria is linked to higher poverty rates later in life. The recent antimalarial campaign in 27 sub-Saharan countries increased the probability of being employed in adulthood, with a marginal increase in treatment intensity raising the probability by 6 percentage points (Kuecken *et al.* 2021). Hong (2013) finds that early exposure to malaria in US veterans (prior to the eradication of malaria) is associated with more frequent chronic diseases in old age (specifically rheumatism/musculoskeletal, rectum/haemorrhoids, and eye diseases) and less frequent labour force participation.

A different strand of the literature focuses on the impacts of economic conditions on malaria. Pan and Singhal (2019), for example, find that a large-scale agricultural extension programme in Uganda reduced the proportion of household members with malaria by 8.9 percentage points. Their results suggest that these reductions were primarily driven by income gains and a resulting increase in ownership and usage of bednets. This highlights the interdependencies between malaria exposure, access and affordability of protective equipment, and economic outcomes. From a researcher's point of view, entangled effects make obtaining robust and accurate insights challenging. This is particularly the case for analyses of aggregate impacts that account for spillovers, as is the focus of macroeconomic studies. Policy-wise however, interdependencies may be an opportunity, allowing for beneficial spillover effects.

3.2 *The macroeconomic impacts of malaria*

Macroeconomic research questions related to disease focus on the impacts on economic growth and development at large, as well as the related impacts on poverty. These studies deal with aggregated units of observations, be it countries or sub-national administrative units, and generally have a broader concept of potential impacts and how they may manifest. This holistic approach makes strong identification strategies elusive, since factors of interest often cannot be disentangled from others. Instead, macroeconomic studies rely more heavily on theory than microeconomic ones, with the latter offering an important impetus to guide this theory. Nonetheless, good insights into the macroeconomic effects of malaria (or disease in general) are essential in delivering a bigger picture and can play a deciding role for policymakers (see e.g. Sicuri *et al.* 2022).

One of the main challenges for the assessment of macroeconomic effects of malaria and other diseases lies in disentangling the potential pathways. One of the earliest studies on the economic effects of malaria, by Barlow (1967), acknowledges counteracting impacts along four axes: (1) increasing population growth, leading to lower per capita income; (2) rising quantity and quality of labour inputs for production, leading to higher per capita income; (3) lowered household saving and capital inputs for production (larger households tend to consume more), leading to lower per capita income; and (4) potential additional effects on output, including the exploitation of new, malaria-free territories. Studies without strong enough identification strategies and theoretical grounding run the risk of conflating impacts of interest (e.g. of malaria eradication on income) with counteracting (e.g. increasing population) and confounding factors (e.g. reverse causality from income being spent on malaria prevention).

Empirical macro-level studies often build on the theoretical notion of conditional convergence (Barro 1991), where economies converge to similar levels of prosperity, governed by structural features of specific countries – such as the prevalence of malaria. A prominent example is the work of Gallup and Sachs (2000), who find strong correlations between economic growth rates and a malaria index. Specifically, they found that a ten percent reduction in malaria intensity (an index that combines information about the population at risk and the share of cases with *P. falciparum*) was associated with 0.3% higher growth. Contemporaneous work by McCarthy *et al.* (2000) reports somewhat smaller, but still significantly positive effects. These figures are likely excessive due to the confounding of effects mentioned above. One concrete example is the omission of other important structural features like the health status (e.g. the burden of HIV or the age structure), such that malaria-related variables may include their effects. These omitted features complicate the identification of causal effects of individual diseases on macroeconomic quantities.

More generally, the impacts of health improvements on macroeconomic outcomes are still debated in the economic literature. Acemoglu and Johnson (2007) set out to identify the causal effects of health improvements on demographic and macroeconomic variables, in part as a response to the complications faced by studies like Gallup and Sachs (2000). They posit that increases in life expectancy following what they call the 'international epidemiological transition' – referring to the wide-spread expansion of health interventions, introduction of novel drugs and chemicals, and more effective public health measures in the 1940s – led to increases in population growth, but was not accompanied by significant increases of aggregate economic growth. Specifically, they find that reductions in mortality at the time – also induced by a reduction of malaria exposure – did not increase the average economic output growth per capita. One important caveat of this finding by Acemoglu and Johnson (2007) is that impacts are likely to vary across developmental stages of countries.

The notion of different types and drivers of growth at certain developmental stages – a feature of *unified growth theory* – has strong implications for the impacts of infectious diseases. Increased life expectancy, i.e. lower mortality, will make it more worthwhile for individuals to invest in education, raising the opportunity costs (in terms of lost income) of having children. The result are reduced fertility rates in the medium-term. At the same time, the higher human capital stock increases economic output, leading to a sustained increase in average incomes. This process in the interplay of reduced mortality rates and the lagged reaction of fertility rates is referred to as the 'demographic transition' (Galor and Weil 2000). The burden of infectious diseases may inhibit this demographic transition, inducing a form of poverty trap (Cervellati and Sunde 2005). For countries that have undergone this transition, increased life expectancy raises income per capita, as shown empirically by Cervellati and Sunde (2011).[7] It is likely that rising average income per capita does not occur in the short term – the productivity and education gains from reduced malaria exposure take time to manifest (also see Lucas 2013).

Still, the effects of malaria on economic development remain disputed. Depetris-Chauvin and Weil (2018) find a lack of effects in the very long run, using the prevalence of the sickle cell trait as an indicator of high historical exposure to malaria. They argue that, historically, the 'disease was not very important, primarily because the vast majority of deaths that it caused were among the very young, in whom society had invested few resources' (p.1232 Depetris-Chauvin and Weil 2018).[8] Other recent work on the macroeconomic impacts of malaria using cross-country comparisons confirms positive economic effects of malaria eradication (Berthélemy

7 Cervellati and Sunde (2011) use the same data as Acemoglu and Johnson (2007) to show that the effects of increased life expectancy hinge crucially on whether countries have gone through the demographic transition. For countries that have not, higher life expectancy had either no or a negative effect on per capita income. In contrast, in countries that had already transitioned, increases in life expectancy were accompanied by substantive increases in average incomes.

8 Notably, their model does not incorporate microeconomic evidence of impacts on human capital and labour productivity. They follow Ashraf *et al.* (2008) instead, who report small impacts from morbidity.

and Thuilliez 2015; Datta and Reimer 2013; Sarma *et al.* 2019), albeit of a considerably smaller magnitude than the results of Gallup and Sachs (2000) imply. Most of these studies employ a form of panel (also called longitudinal) regression setting, where the inclusion of unit-specific effects purges unobserved time-invariant differences (see e.g. Sarma *et al.* 2019). This alleviates some concerns compared to a purely cross-sectional approach, but confounders and contemporaneous relationships remain problematic.

Recent macroeconomic work generally pursues one of two directions. First, there is less focus on malaria-specific impacts, as opposed to general health impacts on larger scales. Identifying disease-specific impacts is considerably more challenging at this scale – especially considering the importance of comorbidities. This can be challenging, since the combination of various diseases into a single index as a measure of health is 'likely to be a source of misspecification' (footnote 1 in Bleakley 2010) and may thus have only limited informative value. Second, there are more targeted macroeconomic studies using within-country variations as identification strategies. Geo-referenced data, which is often derived from remote sensing sources, is used commonly to identify unconfounded variation of malaria exposure and outcome variables. These studies arguably bridge a gap to more micro-level ones, putting more emphasis on identification, while operating at a (focused) macro-level (see Bloom *et al.* 2019, for an in-depth discussion of the reconciliation of micro- and macroeconomic evidence).

Among the more targeted studies, Cervellati *et al.* (2017) use different indices of malaria incidence and exposure in combination with a satellite-derived proxy for economic activity in Africa. They document a negative association between them that is robust to a number of different specifications. Cervellati *et al.* (2022b) use geo-referenced data on Chinese investments and the social media posts of Chinese workers to investigate the potential effects of malaria exposure on foreign investments and worker settlement. They show that African regions with higher malaria exposure attract fewer Chinese investments. Highly exposed regions show lower levels of Chinese economic activity and a lower density of Chinese workers. In yet another study, Cervellati *et al.* (2022a) document an increase in civil violence for regions prone to epidemic outbreaks. This effect is particularly strong during short harvesting seasons of high-calorie subsistence crops. Higher prevalence of immunity (either by the sickle cell trait or acquired through previous infection) or anti-malarial policies attenuate this effect.

Overall – even though there remains some disagreement on the specific effects of malaria and other infectious diseases on macroeconomic outcomes – there are clear impacts on the individual level that have at least some repercussions for the economy at large. In this sense, Bleakley (2009) stresses the importance of eradicating tropical diseases for economic development, but acknowledges that it is not a panacea that can fix everything.

3.3 *The economics of eradication*

The eradication or control of malaria is a forefront issue for many international organizations and governments, motivated by the tremendous human and economic burden of malaria. An important question is whether to pursue eradication or control. So far, successful eradication has mostly been limited to temperate regions (c.f. Figure 1).[9] Countries in the tropical zones, however, have been much less successful in either achieving sustained reductions of malaria cases, or eliminating the disease altogether. Beside possible regional factors, these countries are among the poorest ones in the world and suffer from economic constraints (c.f. Figure 2).

Cost and cost-benefits are obvious factors in the decision of whether to opt for controlling or eliminating the disease. Eradication efforts are generally more expensive in the short-run, and it should be no surprise that spending per case is higher in countries that strive for elimination (see Haakenstad *et al.* 2019, and c.f. Figure 3). Moreover, the marginal cost per reduced case increases as the burden of malaria decreases. The benefits of eliminating malaria still greatly outweigh the costs (Shretta *et al.* 2016), and simple cost-benefit analysis cannot reflect either the true cost or benefit of one approach. For one, eradication leads to a much lower risk for resurgence. The increase of malaria cases in the 1930–2000 period can largely be attributed to weakening control programmes. A decrease in cases saw reduced recurrent expenditure and aid, leading to resource constraints (Cohen *et al.* 2012). Furthermore, benefits of full eradication may also extend to other countries that benefit from fewer imported cases (Shretta *et al.* 2016).

The ecological integrity of biospheres also has to be considered in the fight against malaria. Land-use changes like deforestation may exacerbate malaria transmission, undermining control and elimination efforts (Berazneva and Byker 2017; MacDonald and Mordecai 2019; Santos and Almeida 2018). Other types of land-use change, such as agricultural expansion, as well as urbanization and related land management, on the other hand underpin the success of many eradication programmes (Fornace *et al.* 2021). The effects of land-use change are vital, but cumbersome to pursue – they are often location-specific and global scale analyses may suffer from conceptual and methodological issues (see e.g. Kuschnig 2021). Eradication programmes also have the potential to threaten natural ecosystems. Swamps are commonly drained during these programmes, which removes their ecosystem services (e.g. their roles as carbon sinks and biodiversity hotspots).

---

9 The WHO considers a country to be malaria-free if zero indigenous cases have been reported for more than three consecutive years. The latest countries to achieve this and be certified as malaria-free were El Salvador and China in 2021 (Global Malaria Programme, 2021). The Islamic Republic of Iran and Malaysia reported zero indigenous cases for the third consecutive year, while Cabo Verde and Belize reported zero indigenous cases for the second year in a row (Global Malaria Programme, 2021).

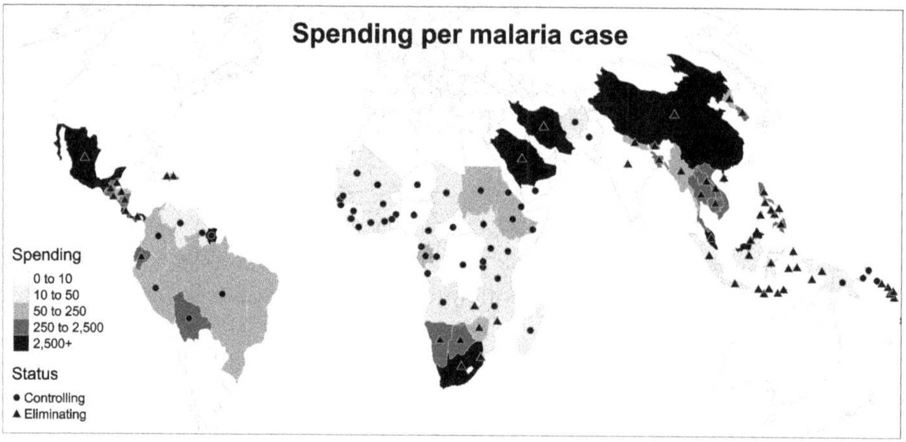

FIGURE 3 Spending on malaria control and eradication. Total spending per malaria case in 2016, separated by strategy – countries looking to control malaria in orange (mostly in South America and sub-Saharan Africa) and ones that target eradication (mostly in Central America, Southern Africa, the Middle East, and East Asia). All values in 2018 US$
SOURCE: HAAKENSTAD *ET AL.* 2019

While such interventions are recognized to reduce the risks of malaria transmission substantially (Keiser *et al.* 2005), the environmental impacts of malaria eradication programmes arguably remain underexplored.

Another important aspect is that the fight against malaria may become more tenuous in the future. Climate change is likely to increase vector and parasite suitability (Pascual *et al.* 2006; Patz and Olson 2006), potentially making present control measures less effective (see also Ferguson and Govella 2022, in Chapter 15). Similarly, the resistance of vectors and parasites to commonly used control methods is increasing, presenting another major ecological obstacle (Ferguson *et al.* 2010). Concerted efforts to effectively control or eradicate malaria hinge on the provision of sufficient funds. In 2016, US$4.3 billion was spent on malaria worldwide increasing by an annual rate of 8.5% from 2000 to 2016, with the bulk stemming from development assistance for health (Haakenstad *et al.* 2019). Despite these increases in spending, total resources spent on malaria control and eradication efforts in 2020 fell short of the US$6.8 billion funding target of the WHO (Global Malaria Programme 2021). The full impact of the COVID-19 pandemic and the associated economic crisis on international and domestic funding for malaria remains to be unraveled. 2020 marked the first year with a rise in malaria deaths after almost two decades of falling numbers, increasing by roughly 12% compared to 2019. Around two thirds of this increase were attributed to service disruptions during the pandemic (Global Malaria Programme 2021). Ongoing restrictions have and will likely impede eradication and control measures (Sicuri *et al.* 2022). However, the resumption and continuation of such efforts is of utmost importance. The impacts of climate change and environmental degradation on these funding targets is still uncertain and deserves further evaluation.

4 Concluding remarks

In this chapter, we reviewed the literature on the economic impacts of malaria. We put the focal points and crucial issues of economic studies into context – most prominently causal identification – and discussed how they guide research. We documented clear evidence of adverse effects on individuals, including impacts on health, productivity, fertility choices, and education. These microeconomic effects generally varied with disease severity and prevalence, socioeconomic status, location, and time horizon. Evidence for macroeconomic effects was not as clear-cut, in part due to the number and variety of channels through which impacts can potentially unfold, complicating the identification of aggregate causal effects. However, most evidence points towards non-negligible macroeconomic impacts of malaria, particularly in sub-Saharan Africa.

It is clear that malaria hampers development and economic prosperity, but there remains much room for research in the realm of malaria and its interactions with the human and natural environment. The link between economics and the disease – while established in numerous studies – still warrants further research, both on the micro- and macroeconomic levels, as does the reconciliation of empirical evidence across these levels. Particular blind spots that deserve a better understanding include the heterogeneity of effects, e.g. across socioeconomic status and location, and spillover effects. The economics of eradication strategies, and their wider impacts, remain under-explored. Climate change makes the adjustment of interventions to effectively control or eliminate malaria a pressing issue. Increased potential for resurgence means that malaria-free countries must be prepared to maintain this status. A better understanding of the interplay of natural environments and vector-borne diseases, as well as repercussions for health and economics, is urgently needed. More and improved new insights can help in the fight against malaria; economic research can play an important part in overcoming future challenges.

Acknowledgements

NK and LV acknowledge financial support from the Austrian national bank, OeNB anniversary fund, project No. 18799.

References

Acemoglu D and Johnson S (2007) Disease and development: the effect of life expectancy on economic growth. Journal of Political Economy 115: 6. https://doi.org/10.1086/529000.

Alven S and Aderibigbe B (2019) Combination therapy strategies for the treatment of malaria. Molecules 24: 3601.

Asenso-Okyere K, Chiang C, Thangata PH and Andam KS (2011) Interactions between health and farm-labor productivity. International Food Policy Research Institute (IFPRI). https://doi.org/10.2499/9780896295421.

Ashley EA, Pyae Phyo A and Woodrow CJ (2018) Malaria. Lancet 391: 1608–1621.

Athey S and Imbens G (2016) Recursive partitioning for heterogeneous causal effects. Proceedings of the National Academy of Sciences 113: 7353–7360.

Athey S and Imbens GW (2017) The state of applied econometrics: causality and policy evaluation. Journal of Economic Perspectives 31: 3–32.

Azevedo TS de and Piovezan R (2023) Relationship between environmental factors and arboviruses in urban areas. In: Fornace K, Conn J, Sallum MAM, Moreira Chaves LS and Logan J (eds) Planetary health approaches to understand and control vector-borne diseases. Brill | Wageningen Academic, pp. 92–117.

Barlow R (1967) The economic effects of malaria eradication. American Economic Review 57: 130–148.

Barofsky J, Anekwe TD and Chase C (2015) Malaria eradication and economic outcomes in sub-saharan Africa: evidence from Uganda. Journal of Health Economics 44: 118–136.

Barreca AI (2010) The long-term economic impact of in utero and postnatal exposure to malaria. Journal of Human Resources 45: 865–892.

Barro RJ (1991) Economic growth in a cross section of countries. Quarterly Journal of Economics 106: 407–443.

Berazneva J and Byker TS (2017) Does forest loss increase human disease? Evidence from Nigeria. American Economic Review 107: 516–21.

Berthélemy JC and Thuilliez J (2015) The economics of malaria in Africa. In: Lin JY and Monga C (eds) The oxford handbook of Africa and economics. Oxford University Press, Oxford, UK.

Bleakley H (2009) Economic effects of childhood exposure to tropical disease. American Economic Review 99: 218.

Bleakley H (2010) Malaria eradication in the Americas: a retrospective analysis of childhood exposure. American Economic Journal: Applied Economics 2: 1–45.

Bloom DE, Canning D, Kotschy R, Prettner K and Schünemann JJ (2019) Health and economic growth: Reconciling the micro and macro evidence. NBER Working Paper. https://doi.org/10.3386/w26003.

Bloom DE, Kuhn M and Prettner K (2022) Modern infectious diseases: macroeconomic impacts and policy responses. Journal of Economic Literature 60(1): 85–131. https://doi.org/10.1257/jel.20201642.

Caminade C, Kovats S, Rocklov J, Tompkins AM, Morse AP, Colón-González FJ, Stenlund H, Martens P and Lloyd SJ (2014) Impact of climate change on global malaria distribution. Proceedings of the National Academy of Sciences 111: 3286–3291.

Carrasco-Escobar G, Matta-Chuquisapon J, Manrique E, Ruiz-Cabrejos J, Barboza JL, Wong D, Henostroza G, Llanos-Cuentas A and Benmarhnia T (2022) Quantifying the effect of human population mobility on malaria risk in the Peruvian Amazon. Royal Society Open Science 9: 211611.

Cervellati M, Esposito E and Sunde U (2022) Epidemic shocks and civil violence: evidence from malaria outbreaks in Africa. Review of Economics and Statistics 104(4): 780–796. https://doi.org/10.1162/rest_a_01050.

Cervellati M, Esposito E and Sunde U (2017) Long term exposure to malaria and development: disaggregate evidence for contemporaneous Africa. Journal of Demographic Economics 83: 129–148.

Cervellati M, Esposito E, Sunde U and Yuan S (2022) Malaria and Chinese economic activities in Africa. Journal of Development Economics 154: 102739.

Cervellati M and Sunde U (2005) Human capital formation, life expectancy, and the process of development. American Economic Review 95: 1653–1672.

Cervellati M and Sunde U (2011) Life expectancy and economic growth: the role of the demographic transition. Journal of Economic Growth 16: 99–133.

Cohen JM, Smith DL, Cotter C, Ward A, Yamey G, Sabot OJ and Moonen B (2012) Malaria resurgence: a systematic review and assessment of its causes. Malaria Journal 11: 1–17.

Cole MA and Neumayer E (2006) The impact of poor health on total factor productivity. Journal of Development Studies 42: 918–938.

Cutler D, Fung W, Kremer M, Singhal M and Vogl T (2010) Early-life malaria exposure and adult outcomes: evidence from malaria eradication in India. American Economic Journal: Applied Economics 2: 72–94.

Datoo MS, Natama HM, Somé A, Bellamy D, Traoré O, Rouamba T, Tahita MC, *et al.* (2022) Efficacy and immunogenicity of R21/Matrix-M vaccine against clinical malaria after 2 years' follow-up in children in Burkina Faso: a phase 1/2b randomised controlled trial. Lancet Infectious Diseases 22(12): 1728–1736. https://doi.org/10.1016/S1473-3099(22)00442-X.

Depetris-Chauvin E and Weil DN (2018) Malaria and early African development: evidence from the sickle cell trait. Economic Journal 128: 1207–1234.

Dillon A, Friedman J and Serneels P (2021) Health information, treatment, and worker productivity. Journal of the European Economic Association 19: 1077–1115.

Duflo E (2017) The economist as plumber. American Economic Review 107: 1–26.

Feachem RGA, Phillips AA, Targett GA and Snow RW (2010) Call to action: priorities for malaria elimination. Lancet 376: 1517–1521.

Ferguson HM, Dornhaus A, Beeche A, Borgemeister C, Gottlieb M, Mulla MS, Gimnig JE, Fish D and Killeen GF (2010) Ecology: a prerequisite for malaria elimination and eradication. PLOS Medicine 7: e1000303.

Ferguson HM and Govella NJ (2023) Impacts of climate change on malaria vector control in Africa. In: Fornace K, Conn J, Sallum MAM, Moreira Chaves LS and Logan J (eds) Planetary health approaches to understand and control vector-borne diseases. Brill | Wageningen Academic, pp. 387–421.

Fornace KM, Diaz AV, Lines J and Drakeley CJ (2021) Achieving global malaria eradication in changing landscapes. Malaria Journal 20: 69. https://doi.org/10.1186/s12936-021-03599-0.

Gallup JL and Sachs JD (2000) The economic burden of malaria. American Journal of Tropical Medicine and Hygiene 64: 85–96.

Galor O and Weil DN (2000) Population, technology, and growth: from Malthusian stagnation to the demographic transition and beyond. American Economic Review 90: 806–828.

Global Malaria Programme (2021) World malaria report 2021, World Health Organization.

Gottdenker NL, Streicker DG, Faust CL and Carroll CR (2014) Anthropogenic land use change and infectious diseases: A review of the evidence. EcoHealth 11: 619–632.

Haakenstad A, Harle AC, Tsakalos G, Micah AE, Tao T, Anjomshoa M, Cohen J, Fullman N, Hay SI, Mestrovic T, Mohammed S, Mousavi SM, Nixon MR, Pigott D, Tran K, Murray CJL and Dieleman JL (2019) Tracking spending on malaria by source in 106 countries, 2000–16: an economic modelling study. Lancet Infectious Diseases 19: 703–716.

Hahn PR, Murray JS and Carvalho CM (2020) Bayesian regression tree models for causal inference: regularization, confounding, and heterogeneous effects. Bayesian Analysis 15: 965–1056.

Hong SC (2013) Malaria: An early indicator of later disease and work level. Journal of Health Economics 32: 612–632.

Idro R, Marsh K, John CC and Newton CRJ (2010) Cerebral malaria: Mechanisms of brain injury and strategies for improved neuro-cognitive outcome. Pediatric research 68: 267.

Imbens GW (2020) Potential outcome and directed acyclic graph approaches to causality: Relevance for empirical practice in economics. Journal of Economic Literature 58: 1129–79.

Keiser J, Singer BH and Utzinger J (2005) Reducing the burden of malaria in different eco-epidemiological settings with environmental management: A systematic review. Lancet Infectious Diseases 5: 695–708.

Kihara M, Carter JA and Newton CRJC (2006) The effect of *Plasmodium falciparum* on cognition: a systematic review. Tropical Medicine & International Health 11: 386–397.

Kounnavong S, Gopinath D, Hongvanthong B, Khamkong C and Sichanthongthip O (2017) Malaria elimination in Lao PDR: the challenges associated with population mobility. Infectious Diseases of Poverty 6: 1–9, BioMed Central.

Kuecken M, Thuilliez J and Valfort M-A (2021) Disease and human capital accumulation: evidence from the roll back malaria partnership in Africa. Economic Journal 131: 2171–2202.

Kuschnig N (2021) Inadequate methods undermine a study of malaria, deforestation and trade. Nature Communications 12.

Laxminarayan R (2004) Does reducing malaria improve household living standards? Tropical Medicine & International Health 9: 267–272.

Lucas AM (2010) Malaria eradication and educational attainment: evidence from Paraguay and Sri Lanka. American Economic Journal: Applied Economics 2: 46–71.

Lucas AM (2013) The impact of malaria eradication on fertility. Economic Development and Cultural Change 61(3). https://doi.org/10.1086/669261.

Malaney P, Spielman A and Sachs J (2004) The malaria gap. American Journal of Tropical Medicine and Hygiene 71: 141–146.

McCarthy D, Wolf HC and Wu Y (2000) The growth costs of malaria. NBER Working Papers, https://doi.org/10.3386/w7541.

Ménard D, Khim N, Beghain J, Adegnika AA, Shafiul-Alam M, Amodu O, Rahim-Awab G, *et al.* (2016) A worldwide map of *Plasmodium falciparum* K13-propeller polymorphisms. New England Journal of Medicine 374: 2453–2464.

Olotu A, Fegan G, Wambua J, Nyangweso G, Leach A, Lievens M, Kaslow DC, Njuguna P, Marsh K and Bejon P (2016) Seven-year efficacy of RTS,S/AS01 malaria vaccine among young African children. New England Journal of Medicine 374: 2519–2529.

Pan Y and Singhal S (2019) Agricultural extension, intra-household allocation and malaria. Journal of Development Economics 139: 157–170.

Pascual M, Ahumada JA, Chaves LF, Rodó X and Bouma M (2006) Malaria resurgence in the east African highlands: Temperature trends revisited. Proceedings of the National Academy of Sciences 103: 5829–5834.

Rocklöv J and Dubrow R (2020) Climate change: an enduring challenge for vector-borne disease prevention and control. Nature Immunology 21: 479–483.

Saavedra MP, Conn JE, Alava F, Carrasco-Escobar G, Prussing C, Bickersmith SA, Sangama JL, Fernandez-Miñope C, Guzman M, Tong C, Valderrama C, Vinetz JM, Gamboa D and Moreno M (2019) Higher risk of malaria transmission outdoors than indoors by *Nyssorhynchus darlingi* in riverine communities in the Peruvian Amazon. Parasites & Vectors 12: 374. https://doi.org/10.1186/s13071-019-3619-0.

Sachs J and Malaney P (2002) The economic and social burden of malaria. Nature 415: 680–685.

Sala-i-Martin X, Doppelhofer G and Miller RI (2004) Determinants of long-term growth: a Bayesian averaging of classical estimates (BACE) approach. American Economic Review 813–835.

Sarma N, Patouillard E, Cibulskis RE and Arcand J-L (2019) The economic burden of malaria: revisiting the evidence. American Journal of Tropical Medicine and Hygiene 101: 1405–1415.

Shocket MS, Caldwell JM, Huxley PJ, Lippi CA, Windram FA and Keyel AC (2023) Modelling the effects of climate and climate change on transmission of vector-borne disease. In: Fornace K, Conn J, Sallum MAM, Moreira Chaves LS and Logan J (eds) Planetary health approaches to understand and control vector-borne diseases. Brill | Wageningen Academic, pp. 253–318.

Shretta R, Avanceña ALV and Hatefi A (2016) The economics of malaria control and elimination: a systematic review. Malaria Journal 15: 593. https://doi.org/10.1186/s12936-016-1635-5.

Sicuri E, Ramponi F, Lopes-Rafegas I and Saúte F (2022) A broader perspective on the economics of malaria prevention and the potential impact of SARS-CoV-2. Nature Communications 13: 2676. https://doi.org/10.1038/s41467-022-30273-z.

Thuilliez J, Sissoko MS, Toure OB, Kamate P, Berthélemy J-C and Doumbo OK (2010) Malaria and primary education in Mali: a longitudinal study in the village of Donéguébougou. Social Science & Medicine 71: 324–334.

Venkataramani AS (2012) Early life exposure to malaria and cognition in adulthood: evidence from Mexico. Journal of Health Economics 31: 767–780.

Worrall E, Basu S and Hanson K (2005) Is malaria a disease of poverty? A review of the literature. Tropical Medicine & International Health 10: 1047–1059.

CHAPTER 7

Mapping patchy malaria: the role of drone technologies in depicting particular environments and contingent risk

*Jacob Brockmann and Dalia Iskander**

Department of Anthropology, University College London, 14 Taviton St, London WC1H 0BW, UK; *dalia.iskander@ucl.ac.uk

Abstract

This chapter is based on an anthropological study of a global, multidisciplinary network of researchers (MACONDO) that use drone technologies to support malaria vector control programmes. The purpose of this study was to investigate the ways in which drone technology for malaria control is deployed by various researchers and the implications the different applications had for the way malaria was conceived of and dealt with. It reports two key findings. First, that drone technologies reflected and mediated a shift towards thinking about malaria as multiple and emergent within heterogenous landscapes. Second, that in the hands of various researchers, malaria 'environments' were rendered 'partial' and 'particular' and risk equally fragmented. As a result, we highlight the 'patchy' character of malaria landscapes that drone technologies mediate and the challenge this poses to global health narratives based on 'concrete' and 'neutral' scientific ways of knowing.

1 Background

Malaria is a life-threatening vector-borne disease caused by parasites and spread to humans through the bites of infected female *Anopheles* mosquitoes (WHO 2021). While there are over 400 different species of *Anopheles* mosquito that can transmit the disease to humans, around 30 are characterised as malaria vectors of major importance (ibid.). Five species of *Plasmodium* parasite are thought to cause illness in humans (*Plasmodium falciparum, Plasmodium vivax, Plasmodium ovale, Plasmodium malariae* and *Plasmodium knowlesi*) and people who contract malaria may experience a range of symptoms including fever, headache, muscle aches and tiredness (CDC 2021). Infection can also lead to severe illness and death if not treated (WHO 2021). Although malaria is treatable and preventable there were an estimated 229 million cases and 409,000 deaths in 2019, of which children under

 | DOI:10.3920/9789004688650_009

five accounted for 67% (ibid.). Malaria is found mostly in poor, tropical and subtropical areas of the world and is heavily concentrated in the African region which recorded 94% of global deaths in 2019 (CDC 2021). The disease is considered both a consequence and driver of poverty, with an estimated economic impact of US$ 12 billion per year (ibid.).

While these numbers indicate the epidemic proportions of the disease, they also obscure its multiplicity (Kelly and Beisel 2012). Malaria is a complex phenomenon that cannot be understood separately from the diverse contexts across which it is differentially situated and enacted. Not only is this term a 'simplification of several parasite-mosquito constellations that vary both locally and seasonally' (Eckl 2017, 424), it also captures 'a range of clinical manifestations, vector pathways and biological entities' (Kelly and Beisel 2012, 72). Due to the contingent and relational character of the disease, circulating across human, mosquito and host species, it is highly sensitive to social and ecological changes at the landscape level ranging from deforestation to armed conflict (Fornace *et al.* 2021, Ruckstuhl *et al.* 2017). For this reason, recent anthropological scholarship (e.g. Chandler and Beisel 2017; Hausmann-Muela and Eckl 2015) has pushed back against the assumption that malaria is a fixed natural entity and called for attention to 'malaria multiple' (Chandler and Beisel 2017, 413). Such a move entails a focus not simply on how malaria is variably represented or interpreted across different cultures or academic disciplines, but on the myriad ontological enactments of disease (Mol 2002). This chapter will explore practices of malaria making in the MACONDO network and the varied constructions of landscape and risk that come to the surface as a result.

On a global policy level, efforts to combat malaria are largely focused on prevention, case detection and treatment. Many prevention strategies are centred around indoor-based interventions which target the mosquitoes that transmit disease through insecticide treated nets (ITNs) and indoor residual spraying (IRS) (WHO 2020). Although there has long been recognition that environmental conditions (e.g. climatic conditions such as temperature and rainfall, as well as macroenvironmental factors such as local topography, human land-use and management) play an important role in malaria transmission (Randell *et al.* 2010), following the Second World War, environmental management strategies such as maintaining drains, removing pools of stagnant water, managing vegetation, irrigating intermittently, altering rivers to create faster flowing water and improving housing (Randell *et al.* 2010; Okumu 2020) 'fell off the malaria control agenda' (Lindsay *et al.* 2004:2). As Lindsay *et al.* (2004) explain, the perceived promise of Dichlorodiphenyltrichloroethane (DDT) for house spraying as the main tool for the World Health Organisation's (WHO) malaria eradication programme from 1956–67 spurred a neglect of wider environmental management techniques and coincided with a move towards vertical programmes lodged firmly in the health sector. Alongside the increased use of insecticide on bed nets and jungle hammocks that became widely available in the mid-1980's (Okumu 2020), the use of insecticides and chemicals in IRS has been a major feature of vector control strategies over the last three decades (Najera *et al.* 2011). Together with targeting parasites directly through drugs and more recently vaccines, these interventions have had a significant impact. According to the WHO World Malaria Report 2020, 7.6 million malaria related deaths have been averted since 2000 (WHO 2020). However, more recently, the WHO's progress towards malaria elimination has reached a plateau with 2020 targets for reduction in disease and death missed by 37% and 22% respectively (ibid.).

The introduction of drones to malaria research is largely motivated by a growing awareness of the need for additional environmentally-focused approaches and tools to complement existing efforts, namely indoor-based interventions for vector management (Hardy *et al.* 2017). In recent years, worrying trends of insecticide resistance have weakened the impact of IRS and ITNs, contributing to a recent slowing of progress in controlling malaria (Okumu 2020). Furthermore, these interventions have proved ineffective in areas where transmission is driven by exophagic mosquito species that bite outdoors (Fornace *et al.* 2021; Hardy *et al.* 2017). One complimentary control strategy being employed to combat this is larval source management (LSM). LSM refers to the targeted management of mosquito breeding sites, with the objective of reducing the number of mosquito larvae and pupae as they mature in aquatic habitats in the environment (WHO 2013; Tusting *et al.* 2013). LSM includes prevention strategies such as habitat modification (e.g. permanent land reclamation), habitat manipulation (e.g. flushing of streams, the shading or exposure of habitats), larviciding (e.g. the regular application of a biological or chemical insecticide to water bodies), and biological control (e.g. introducing natural predators into water bodies) (WHO 2013).

The effectiveness of LSM is determined largely by the capacity to map and identify aquatic mosquito habitats (Hardy *et al.* 2017). As such, drones have been advocated by some as a valuable asset to LSM campaigns in particular because they provide precise, high resolution spatial data in real-time that can be used to support this mapping process (Fornace *et al.* 2014). Drones also offer insights into the landscape (its classification and use) more broadly. The notion that 'malaria eradication will be the indirect outcome of a combination of targeted malaria control on the one hand and broader social and environmental change on the other hand' (Eckl 2017, 431) is evidenced by the historical success in areas such as Italy where the disease was eliminated through large scale hydrological and agricultural modifications (Fornace *et al.* 2021). Now, with factors such as climate change, population growth and deforestation driving accelerated environmental change, some scholars are asking whether we need to return to the pre-war focus on landscape and expand the present paradigm of vector control (ibid.; Tusting *et al.* 2013) While the labour intensive character of environmental management strategies (stream clearing, cutting branches, that shade larval habitats, etc.) has in the past placed a burden on communities and control programme staff, drone imagery opens up new opportunities for more precise and analytically driven interventions in malarial landscapes. As Lindsay *et al.* (2004, 2) suggest 'Environmental management needs to be considered a central pillar of malaria control that all other activities are linked to in an integrated fashion, informed by accurate ecosystem analyses' (ibid., 2).

2 Introduction

MACONDO was a multidisciplinary research network which used drone technology to support malaria vector control programmes. The network was brought together in 2019 through a Global Grand Challenges Research Fund for an 'International collaborative network for the Integration, Standardization and Assessment of the use of drones in malaria vector control strategies' (GGCRF 2019, 1). It was led jointly by the London School of Hygiene and Tropical Medicine, UK (LSHTM) and Universidad Peruana Cayetano Heredia, Peru (UPCH) and its remit was to assemble researchers from Southeast Asia, Sub-Saharan Africa and South America employing drones for malaria control and risk mapping. It aimed to elaborate guidelines for integrating drone technology into malaria control for use by researchers, ministries of health and national malaria control programmes. Specifically, the network intended to produce guidance on technical requirements, analysis methods and the usability of data; frameworks for assessing community engagement with drones; and guidance on technical and institutional limitations for incorporating drones into malaria control programmes. It comprised 29 researchers ranging from entomologists and epidemiologists to electronic engineers, and remote sensing specialists operating in multiple sites including Peru, Côte d'Ivoire, Burkina Faso, Tanzania, Zanzibar, the Philippines, and Malaysian Borneo (MACONDO 2021). The data presented in this chapter was collected as part of a masters project conducted by Jacob Brockmann (supervised by Dalia Iskander) in 2021. Jacob conducted semi-structured interviews with 10 MACONDO researchers and participated in two online webinars in order to elucidate the way in which they incorporated drones into their work and the implications of how malaria was conceived of and dealt with by each of them. Interviewees also pointed Jacob towards news and academic journal articles that had been published about their work, which provided more detailed insight into methodology and findings. A thematic analysis was applied to data to inductively identify themes that arose from the data. The study received ethics approval from UCL, LSHTM and UPCH. All participants were asked for their written, free, informed and prior consent to be interviewed and were provided with a written information and consent form to sign prior to data collection. Anonymity was optional for this research and pseudonyms used only when participants requested this. This was because there was a strong chance that participants would be identifiable due to the fact the network is relatively small and the nature of their work is quite specific.

3 Section 1 – Malaria as emergent within patchy landscapes

In the context of the aforementioned shift towards environmental management in malaria control, we argue that MACONDO researchers employed drones to effectively visualise some of the links between malaria and landscape and in doing so, revealed the heterogenous nature of such 'hotspots' (Brown and Kelly 2014). As Brown and Kelly (2014) suggest, this heuristic, borrowed from epidemiology, refers to the potential spatial and temporal sites where different kinds of human-animal-nonhuman entanglements may facilitate the exchange of pathogens and particularly speaks to the micro and macro interactions that create such 'conditions of pathogenic possibility' (ibid.: 282). Due to the different disciplinary perspectives adopted by various researchers, as they each zoomed out and in on different dimensions, features and relations within landscapes, they rendered them fluid, layered, dynamic and animated in nature at times as much as they rendered them static, flattened, immobile and inert. As such, we argue that the use of drones by multidisciplinary teams rather than reveal neutral and unmediated 'views from nowhere' (Haraway 1998), actively constructed 'particular' views from 'somewhere' (Haraway 1998), that were altogether 'patchy' (Tsing *et al.* 2019) in nature, challenging notions of 'neutral' and 'objective' and transmission dynamics that are sometimes presented in scientific accounts of malaria.

3.1 *Drones and heterogenous malaria landscapes*

As mentioned in the introduction, the use of drones for malaria research is closely related to a renewed interest in environmental management strategies such as LSM. Such interventions entail a shift away from a biomedical focus on mechanisms of pathogenic transfer towards a broader outlook on how multispecies encounters across temporally and spatially heterogenous landscapes give rise to varying patterns of malaria transmission. In interviews with MACONDO members, it was clear drone technology mediated a shift towards thinking about malaria as emergent within local landscapes. Many stressed that the 'visually striking character' of drone imagery, as Andy, a lecturer in Remote Sensing put it, offered a new perspective on how uneven interactions in the landscape shape patterns of disease transmission. Researchers such as Kim (a Spatial Statistician and Epidemiologist) articulated the significance of getting people 'quite excited about landscapes' that was felt to be instrumental for effective malaria management. As a result, drones facilitated researchers to explore a broad range of questions that they felt were important such as: how animal host habitats were impacted by land use change; how mosquito abundance related to different land types; and how human movement patterns intersected with vector biting behaviours. With their capacity to generate high resolution imagery at 'user-defined time points', drones offered new opportunities to explore these relationships and better understand the habitats in which diseases circulate. Through a focus on the mechanism of pathogenic transfer, dominant biomedical renderings of malaria tend to reify a singular version of the disease which obscures the multiple malaria realities that emerge across diverse social, historical and environmental contexts (Iskander 2015). Instead, through the gaze of the drone, malaria was transformed into a thoroughly visual, spatial, temporal and dynamic phenomenon that could be traced across particular 'hotspots' of interaction.

3.2 *Zooming out – macro-level features of the landscape*

As Brown and Kelly (2014) articulate, a great conceptual challenge is to do justice to the characteristics of the hotspot that defy scalar logics including social, economic and political drivers of environmental transformation. On a macro level, drones gave access to views of landscapes as they changed in space and time as well as the factors mediating such change. For example, in Kim's work with the MONKEYBAR project, she used drones to map the spatial epidemiology of *Plasmodium knowlesi* in Malaysian Borneo and the Philippines (Fornace *et al.* 2014). *Plasmodium knowlesi* is a primate malaria that afflicts long-tailed and pig-tailed macaques but also has the potential to infect humans (William *et al.* 2013). The purpose of the MONKEYBAR project was to explore the hypothesis that changes in the landscape, particularly exacerbated by deforestation, were driving an increase in *Plasmodium knowlesi* transmission by bringing human, mosquito and macaque habitats into closer proximity. In a public webinar, Kim explained that 'to test this hypothesis and really explore these dynamics, we needed to actually map land cover change [over time]'. Drones were invaluable in this sense because they 'really gave the ability to monitor land cover and change at these very … fine spatial and temporal resolutions'. To illustrate this, Kim showed two images of the same geographical area in February 2014 and May 2014. The first displayed a densely forested area, the second showed a scarred landscape that had been cleared for a rubber plantation. By integrating this spatial data with GPS information from collared macaques, Kim and her colleagues were able to create maps illustrating how deforestation had directly influenced macaque behaviour. Kim explained in her webinar that from these maps, the MONKEYBAR team were able to depict the increasing unpredictability of macaque habitats in deforested areas that was being driven by agricultural expansion of irrigated rice paddies as well as plantation industries such as palm oil, pulpwood, timber and rubber and illegal logging. Consequently, as macaques moved closer to villages, the risk of *Plasmodium knowlesi* transmission to human inhabitants increased particularly in increased forest edges. By using drones to specifically look for the movement of landscapes over time, in their analysis, malaria was not depicted as a static entity, but instead conceived of as a fluid process (Latour 1988; Law 2008) that unfolded unevenly across transforming patchworks making up the landscape.

As well as display the fluid nature of landscapes, drones were also used to highlight their layered and dynamic nature across multiple scales. Under the umbrella of the same MONKEYBAR project that Kim worked on, a Research Assistant in Vector Biology, Emma investigated factors that were associated with larval sites at different spatial scales in Malaysian Borneo. Using drone and satellite imagery, she extracted data about the land cover of 11 different areas at 50 to 500 m intervals surrounding multiple larval collection points (water bodies). Consequently, she was able to assess whether high amounts of particular land classes at specific distances from water bodies influenced the statistical probability that mosquito larvae were present at specific locales. Explaining her methodology, Emma said, 'I think it's really important ... to take [account of] the environment surrounding the water body and not just the exact pinpointed spot of the water body when you're looking at why mosquitoes choose breeding sites'. She explained that this was because different actors involved in malaria transmission such as monkeys, humans and mosquitoes operated and interacted across different sites and at different scales. For example, Emma found that being 'near to rubber plantations but not inside rubber plantations was a risk factor for *Anopheles* mosquitoes'. She hypothesized that, while insecticides might make water bodies within the plantation unsuitable habitats for mosquitoes to lay their eggs, the insects could breed nearby and travel to the plantation in search of a bloodmeal from a human or monkey. In this account, the landscape was constructed not as a flat and inert surface, but as a layered and mobile space where species interacted across multiple sites and scales. Together, Kim and Emma's work highlighted 'morphological patterns in which humans and non-humans [were] arranged' (Tsing *et al.* 2019, 188). In this rendering, malaria emerged out of a dynamic set of processes that intersected, yet extended beyond, the specific 'relevant' moments of pathogenic transfer.

3.3 *Zooming in – micro level features of the landscape*

At a micro level, drones provided new information on the fine-grained interactions of vectors, animal hosts and human populations which researchers linked to epidemiological heterogeneity in specific contexts. As described in the introduction, the interest in using drones reflected a shift in malaria control techniques towards broader environmental management. In line with this, Andy explained that from his perspective, the use of drones was motivated by a growing awareness of the need for new methods to supplement conventional indoor based interventions which were becoming ineffective against resistant strains of mosquitoes that have evolved to bite outdoors (Hardy *et al.* 2017). Working with the Zanzibar Malaria Elimination Campaign (ZAMEP), Andy used drones to support larval source management (LSM) campaigns on the ground, identifying potential mosquito breeding sites for precision larviciding. Compared to Kim's research, this project had a very fine-grained local applicability as the aim was to direct attention to real-time, micro-level features of specific places rather than highlight broad changes over time. The imagery captured by drones was shared with fieldworkers via a mobile application called Zzap which created a map of water bodies and access routes. This enabled users to treat potential mosquito habitats with larvicide and track their progress as they did so. Andy explained that 'when the fieldworkers are walking around, what they're seeing (on the app) is a big bunch of potential breeding sites that they need to go and visit and tick them off and say, 'I visited it'. Additionally, if the fieldworkers encountered any water bodies that the drone did not pick up, for example those under the canopy cover, they could take a photo and add it to the map. As the fieldworkers visited each of these sites, Andy explained that their manager could track this progress via an 'online dashboard' which showed 'hundreds if not 1000s' of these points and the percentage of them that had been treated with larvicide.

This precision focus on water bodies represents a much more focal view on malaria than the macro level processes of land use change that were observed in Kim's work. In their paper on neglected malarias in urban Dar es Salaam, Kelly and Beisel (2011, 73) contrast the Gates Foundation's approach to malaria as a 'global enemy' with the small-scale maps that fieldworkers produce of water bodies in the back streets of Tanzania's capital. They argue that global malaria control strategies often fail to recognise how malaria is 'multiply implicated in the environments we inhabit' (ibid., 71) and tend to leave out the malaria that 'begins where the pavement ends' (ibid., 73) which fieldworkers locate in blocked drains and discarded plastic cups. This 'discrepancy between malaria control as an arduous everyday practice and the targeting of malaria as a global enemy' (ibid.,73) is also visible within the MACONDO network. Whereas Kim's project focused on macro level environmental processes that shaped malaria distribution across large scales and time periods, the fieldworkers in Andy's study, as well as those who Kelly and Beisel (2011) observed in Tanzania, attended to the gritty, fine-scale, real-time details of the specific places (water bodies) from which malaria emerges. In contrast to Kim's work which emphasised landscape dynamism, this focal view of malaria rendered the landscape momentarily static. By virtue of the drone's ability to provide imagery in real time, the fieldworker was presented with a snapshot of the quite literally 'fluid' distribution of water bodies across the terrain. The shifting landscape was immobilised as a map of water bodies that could be visited, treated and then checked off on an online dashboard. In this way the complex landscape from which malaria emerges was briefly contained as a stable object of scientific knowledge and intervention as researchers 'necessarily simplify and provisionally freeze what entities they will notice and count' (Tsing *et al.* 2019, 190). In the hands of different researchers, malaria landscapes were thus constructed as variably dynamic and static across different spatial and temporal scales. The drone images MACONDO's members produced both elucidated large-scale dynamics shifting environments over time and froze the landscape on a small scale to render it an object of knowledge and intervention.

3.4 *Bringing mosquito behaviour into view – animating the landscape*

When analysing drone imagery, some MACONDO researchers animated certain areas of the landscapes by integrating the movements of mosquitoes into analyses. This was evidenced in the work of Marta (a Research Fellow in Vector Biology) and Gabriel (Associate Researcher in Epidemiology). Paying specific attention to vector behaviour, they attempted to define a distinctive spectral signature for water bodies that were favoured by *Nyssorynchus darlingi* mosquitoes – the main malaria vector in the Peruvian Amazon (Carrasco-Escobar *et al.* 2019). This project differed from Andy's work in that it was motivated by the aim of mapping not just *potential* breeding sites, but ones that were also *positive* for mosquito larvae. Marta explained to me that one of the challenges of larval source management 'is to find not only the aquatic habitats, but where the mosquitoes [actually] breed, because they use some [very] specific places'. Elaborating on the implications of this, she said that in places such as the Amazon rainforest where 'the water reservoir is huge', it is not possible to treat all water bodies with larvicide. For this reason, 'the idea is to identify *only* the ones that we want to target that are going to produce mosquitoes'. Similarly, to Kim and Andy's studies, this project was closely tied to an interest in vector ecology. Gabriel explained that the project was motivated in part by a desire to learn more about the behaviour of *Nyssorhynchus darlingi*, a vector that is 'behaviourally very plastic' and can select suitable breeding sites according to visual and olfactory cues. Through integrating drone imagery of aquatic habitats with entomological data from the same locations, Gabriel and Marta attempted to map these behaviours. In the process, they transformed the landscape from a patchwork of potential breeding spaces into a mosaic of risky places, animated by the agency of insects. This focus on the vector as an actor (Latour 2005), rather than a passive object of scientific knowledge, facilitated a more animated view of malaria transmission.

3.5 *Obscuring the complexities of mosquito behaviour – flattening the landscape*

While such attention to the behavioural choices of the vector enlivened the landscape, other researchers intentionally obscured certain complexities rendering it flattened. As Edwards (2010, 15), points out, models are data infrastructures which both 'enable and deaden observation'. This point was exemplified in Edgar's (an environmental engineering student) research, which was supported by Marta and Gabriel under the umbrella of the same project, coordinated by the International Centres of Excellence for Malaria Research (ICEMR) in the Loreto department of

Peru. Edgar's work investigated the abundance and distribution of *Nyssorynhcus darlingi* across different land cover types. He explained that previous studies in this region had discovered that there were more *Nyssorynhcus darlingi* located outside household structures than inside. Building on this information, he was interested in how far away from the household area mosquito presence extended. Edgar noted that, surrounding the village there were many different land types including crops, secondary forest and more densely forested areas. Consequently, he wanted to explore 'what types of landscapes or what types of vegetation we find more or less mosquitoes'. To do this, he adopted a 'stratified sampling strategy'. Using drone and Sentinel 2 satellite imagery and a 'clustering' algorithm, he constructed a regular hexagonal grid which classified the landscape into five land cover categories: households, forest, crops, degraded patches and flooded areas. In this way, the 500 m study area around Santa Rita village was broken down into what looked like a honeycomb mosaic of hexagonal landscape clusters. Each month, 20 of these hexagons were sampled at random, allowing Edgar to determine the relative abundance and distribution of *Nyssorynhcus darlingi* across the different land types.

When asked why he chose this hexagonal sampling strategy, Edgar explained that it was related to the 'human landing catch' method where researchers sit in a single location and count the mosquitoes that land on them over a given time period. The hexagonal sampling grid was well suited to this method because it created a 'symmetrical area of influence' around each catchment point, thus providing 'a way to simplify the landscape'. This classificatory scheme rendered the drone and satellite imagery intelligible to researchers and amenable to sampling, but it also arguably entailed applying a reductive violence. Edgar alluded to this when he said, 'these artificial boundaries tell us information about the general behaviour inside that area, but we have to understand that it is a continuous surface [between them]'. While the clusters were useful to his study purposes, he stressed that 'there are no [actual] boundaries between them that you cannot trespass'. In other words, while drone use animated specific aspects of the landscape for the purposes of research (such as mosquito preferences for breeding sites), it also dulled others (such as their presence and movement across different land cover types). In seeking to determine the distribution of *Nyssorynhcus Darlingi*, Edgar rendered the mosquito visible by simplifying the complex terrain it inhabited according to a classificatory scheme. This model simultaneously illuminated certain features of the landscape and excluded other ways of seeing. The hexagonal grid of land type clusters that he presented was at once a recognition and denial of the landscape's complexity and was another example of the 'partial' and 'particular' landscapes that were constructed as a result of intentional choices made in the use of drone technology.

3.6 *Patchy landscapes*

The landscapes that MACONDO members constructed through drones were therefore fluid, layered, dynamic and animated as well as static, flattened, immobile and inert. Somewhat ironically, given science's preference for the objective and panoptic view from above or 'conquering gaze from nowhere' (Haraway 1998, 581), it is precisely through the very 'patchiness' created that researchers were able to comprehend the 'whole'. The pictures captured by the drone were so rich and multifaceted that only by drawing attention to specific features, by painting an incomplete picture so to speak, could MACONDO researchers generate knowledge that was 'useful' to malaria research and control. This idea was expressed well in Maz's (Senior Research Officer in Primatology) work with the MONKEYBAR project in which she used a drone with a thermal camera to conduct rapid estimates of macaque populations (Jumail *et al.* 2020) to inform understanding of zoonotic malaria transmission. Maz explained that in the conditions of high canopy cover in Sabah's Lower Kinabatangan Wildlife Sanctuary, standard drone imagery and traditional visual counting methods along the riverbank were ineffective for primate censuses. In this context, the advantage of the thermal camera was that it could identify animals by the body heat that they emitted in the form of infrared rays (Jumail *et al.* 2020). Interestingly, Maz noted that this technique worked best at night-time or early morning when the contrast between the macaques' body heat and the surrounding environment was highest. In other words, this process of mapping landscapes involved cutting through the visual 'noise' of the drone image to highlight a specific aspect of it that was relevant to malaria transmission. Instead of offering a transparent and unmediated 'view from nowhere' (Haraway 1998), Maz's complex visual work with the drone generated a partial perspective on the landscape that suited her needs. As Haraway (1998, 590) points out, 'the only way to find a larger vision is to be somewhere in particular'. Although Maz aspired to see the full picture of malaria transmission, it was only by accentuating the incomplete and 'patchy' nature of her imagery that she was able to comprehend it.

3.7 *Summary*

Thus far in this chapter, we have argued that MACONDO researchers employed drones to elucidate links between malaria and landscape in different ways. In the process of mapping these interactions in partial and particular ways, 'patchy' landscapes emerged in the resultant drone images that were used to guide malaria control. However, rather than present an obstacle to the pursuit of scientific knowledge, this patchiness was a necessary feature of it, rendering complex contexts 'visible', 'comprehendible' and therefore arguably more 'manageable.'

4 Section 2 – The patchy character of risk

In the remainder of this chapter, we argue that the patchy character of malaria landscapes trickled down to frame equally fragmented and incomplete accounts of disease risk and manifested in many different ways. First, it was clear that drones could only map small areas of the landscape at a time, requiring researchers to make calculated choices about where to conduct surveys and consequently where they 'looked' for risk. Second, in classifying and categorizing features of drone images, researchers engaged in a process of compartmentalisation denying the 'blurriness' of the landscape where malaria risk was arguably highest. Third, MACONDO members presented a simplified notion of risk as they encountered many difficulties in analysing the relationships and connections between different factors. Fourth, multiple dimensions of incertitude influenced the 'accuracy' of risk assessments. Lastly, we describe how the multidisciplinary character of the MACONDO network evoked multiple constructions of malaria. Pushing back against the notion that scientific risk assessment is distinctively comprehensive and robust, we argue that just as malaria landscapes are 'patchy', risk as a consequence and the way malaria is advised to be dealt with is equally 'patchy'. This patchiness is not random but emerges from a series of strategic and political manoeuvres made by researchers.

4.1 *Deciding where to map*

The images that drones capture of malaria landscapes are limited in scope, meaning that researchers had to make deliberate choices about where to conduct drone surveys and by implication, where they located risk. Due to battery limitations, drones have limited flight times. While these vary according to the model, Andy's research using a standard DGI Phantom Drone was able to image a 600 × 600 m area, flying for 13 minutes on a single battery. For fieldworkers, this was a significant amount of spatial information, but it paled in comparison to the global scope of the coarser satellite data that researchers were familiar working with. This punctual character of the drone gaze compelled researchers to target their studies in specific areas because as Andy pointed out 'we can't fly drones everywhere'. In this sense, while drones are closely associated with military usage and logics of surveillance (Wall and Monahan 2011) the visibilities they produce are not systematic or all-encompassing, but rather result in 'highly variable spatial logics and articulations' (Pauschinger and Klauser 2010, 443). To conclude his webinar on precision larvidicing in Zanzibar, Andy suggested 'broad scale mapping' as a method for planning future drone surveys. He explained that he had been involved in the development of a tropical wetland mapping tool 'TropWet' which used LANDSAT data to characterise the landscape according to percentage coverage of water and vegetation (Hardy, Oakes and Ettritch 2020). Because this data stretches back to the 1980's, Andy explained that TropWet allowed for the mapping of seasonal inundation patterns and the 'targeting of public health resources to tackle water-borne disease' (ibid., 18). This use of historical data to predict malaria hotspots was only one of the methods used to decide where to fly the drone. As Marta pointed out to me, the choice as to where to conduct a drone survey 'depend[ed] on what you want to know' and MACONDO members all had variable interests. While some were interested in mapping the impacts of land use change on human and host movement patterns, others were focused on mapping water bodies or understanding the behaviour of mosquito vectors. In other words, there is nothing given or definitive about the decision over where and what to map with the drone. The drone gaze was not so much panoptic as 'patchy' in character and, as Brighenti (2010, 187) points out, 'the decision as to who, where, when, and what is made visible [was] never of a neutral nature'. These choices were the first of many in a series of manoeuvres by researchers that gave rise to a patchy account of malaria risk.

4.2 *Compartmentalisation of landscape and risk variables*

The analysis of drone imagery involved a process of categorization and compartmentalisation that sought to locate and isolate 'risky' malaria places. According to Leach and Scoones (2013) the development of new technologies, such as drones, tends to favour the gaze from space or databases rather than the ground. This 'view from above' is associated with the 'ascendancy of quantitative modelling' (ibid, 15) that invokes the authority of 'evidence-based decision making' (Nutley *et al.* 2007, 23). In this discourse, 'sound scientific' risk assessment methods reduce the complex dimensions of the problem at hand to quantitative parameters of 'outcomes' and 'probabilities' that yield 'a single ostensibly definitive picture of risk' (Stirling and Scoones 2009, 1). In the context of malaria transmission, this segmentation of risk into scientific variables 'relies on the compartmentalism of human, parasite, insect and environmental realms' (Chandler and Beisel 2017, 415). Although my interviewees all expressed a desire to explore interactions between these categories, their analyses tended to achieve complexity by fragmenting components down further in each of their own niches rather than exploring *relations* between them. As a result, malaria risk was broken down into interrelated, but separate components and located in specific places of interaction.

For example, many MACONDO projects segmented the landscape in an effort to locate malaria risk, but these were not 'natural' categories found 'out there'. As Haraway (1988, 595) points out, 'boundaries are drawn by mapping practices; 'objects' do not pre-exist as such'. In another project, Fedra and Gabriel J's trained machine learning algorithms to classify drone images according to land cover classes. Fedra (an electronic engineer) explained that by working with training images which had been manually pre-labelled according to the land classes they wanted to use, the neural network could 'learn those patterns and recognise further images in order to classify them'. Importantly, these 'risky' land types were not self-evident but defined after careful discussion. Gabriel J (an electronic engineer) explained that when he first joined the MACONDO network, he had to meet weekly with the entomologists conducting the drone surveys and larval sampling to decide what categories they wanted to use to classify the landscape. In these meetings, there was a slight disconnect between the categories the engineers could train the network to recognise and the 'categories most critical for [the entomologists'] analysis'. For example, Gabriel J explained that while researchers wanted to know about mosquito presence in vegetated vs non-vegetated water bodies, he was unable to teach the algorithm to recognise this difference. Eventually, they shifted from 6–7 'very detailed land classes' down to a smaller number of simpler categories including rice, bare soil, households and forested areas. As such, classificatory systems 'are imagined holisms through which structures fit together' (Ton and Bubandt 2010, 17). The land classes used by Gabriel J and Fedra were not 'natural' but emerged from a series of deliberate manoeuvres shaped by a combination of research aims and objectives and technical limitations.

In compartmentalising the landscape into areas of supposed 'risk', researchers drew straight lines along blurred edges. Key to larval source management campaigns which target malaria breeding sites is the question 'What constitutes a water body?'. The answer to this is far from straightforward. When describing their efforts to classify water, researchers spoke of its slippery character, noting that water bodies can be natural or artificial, temporary or permanent, static or flowing and positive or negative for mosquito larvae. They also pointed to their varying scale (small containers, puddles, lakes, rivers) and biochemical composition (pH, level of vegetation, temperature, salinity, level of shade). During Andy's webinar on his work in Zanzibar, he showed an image from the field that illustrated the challenges of capturing this dynamic character of water. In the picture, which showed a 600 × 600 m area in rural Zanzibar, a range of land classes were visible including tilled soil, canopy cover and emergent vegetation. When this photo was digitally stitched together with other images to form a larger 'orthomosaic', yet more land cover categories were made visible, such as buildings, tracks, roads, open water and dense canopy cover. The water bodies visible in these images were heavy with sediment and similar in colour to surrounding soil. Furthermore, they had overflown into areas of vegetation at variable depths that were impossible to gauge accurately from the image. To the human eye, this liquid landscape was clearly difficult to arrange into distinct categories and, as Andy explained, it was even more difficult to train the computer to do this. The algorithm struggled to distinguish silted water from crops, shadows and inundated vegetation, and accuracy (compared to the manual classification) was only 57.9% due to the large number of false positives. Crucially, however, this blurriness between land categories was more than an obstacle to identifying water bodies and pinpointing malaria risk. Landscape 'blurriness' matters because it is often in the 'ecotones' (Lambin *et al.* 2010, 6) or transitional spaces between households and forests, water bodies and plantations where malaria transmission occurs. While MACONDO members compartmentalised the heterogenous landscape in an effort to locate malaria risk and target interventions, these land types did not exist 'out there'. Instead, researchers 'reify[ed] categories for the sake of the analysis' (Tsing *et al.* 2019, 190), often at their blurry edges where malaria risk is arguably highest.

4.3 *Indeterminate relationships between components of risk*

When MACONDO members broke risk down into component parts, there was often a lack of clarity about how these elements were connected, perpetuating overly simplistic or vague notions of dynamics. Stirling and Scoones (2009, 4) argue that conventional 'reductional-aggregative techniques' of risk assessment often fail to acknowledge the uncertainty entailed in establishing relationships between different indicators or components of risk. They define uncertainty as the state in which 'the available empirical information or analytical models simply do not present a definitive basis for assigning probabilities [to specific outcomes]' (ibid., 10). This was evident in Marta's comment that when you conduct larval surveys to assess where mosquitoes are breeding 'You kind of measure all these things, but there is not really a correlation or association with a specific measure or factor'. She continued, 'For example, it's not that if the pH is above or below seven, the mosquitoes are not going to be there. It is really variable and it depends on the species, it depends on the season, it depends on many other things.' This complexity was important to Marta's study because it prevented her from establishing a causal relationship between certain environmental variables and mosquito presence. Interestingly, however, Marta's awareness that mosquito behaviour could not be comprehensively captured as a sum of environmental variables did not deter her from attempting to locate areas of malaria risk. In fact, her study sought to identify a distinctive spectral signature for water bodies that were positive for mosquito larvae. While the correlation established between the mosquito habitats and a specific wavelength did not explain *why* the mosquitoes selected that aquatic habitat to breed in, Marta said this information was nonetheless useful for targeting the efforts of fieldworkers. MACONDO members understood that the connections between different environmental variables and risk factors were 'patchy' and riddled with uncertainty. Despite this, they made strategic choices to move forward with malaria control interventions. As Leach and Scoones (2013, 10) point out, disease models do not 'inform policy in a linear manner' but instead have 'social and political lives' that shape their development and application in public health projects. Although scientific methods make claims to 'rigour' and 'robustness' (Stirling and Scoones 2009, 13), what emerges from this study of mosquito behaviour was not a definitive picture of malaria risk, but rather an incomplete patchwork of component parts that did not fit together neatly.

4.4 *Uncertainty and ignorance*

Another important point to note about the mosaic of malaria risk articulated by MACONDO members is that while it included patches of 'precise' findings, these did not necessarily form a comprehensive account of malaria risk. This was reflected in the practice of ground-truthing which was shared across the network. Marta explained to me that ground-truthing is 'basically trying to match the satellite (or drone) image with what you're seeing on the ground'. For many of the researchers, this involved visiting areas that the drone had imaged to confirm the presence of a specific land type or water body. In Marta's study it also included larval sampling to establish a correlation between the spectral signature of the drone and the presence of anopheline larvae. This process of comparing the drone image with the 'reality' on the ground produced a narrow mathematical definition of accuracy. Marta's research, for example, concluded that 'high-resolution multispectral imagery can discriminate a profile of water bodies where *Ny. darlingi* is most likely to breed ... with an overall accuracy of 86.73%–96.98%' (Carrasco-Escobar *et al.* 2019, 1). While there was nothing factually incorrect about these findings, it is important to acknowledge that they were very narrow and assessed according to metrics that the researchers selected. Stirling and Scoones (2009, 15) argue that such quantitative analyses of risk often lead the policy makers who favour them to a fallacious conflation of 'accuracy and precision'. In the context of MACONDO's work, this means that although their findings were 'precise', they did not necessarily capture an 'accurate' picture of the full phenomenon of malaria transmission.

Another form of incertitude that pockmarked the character of malaria risk assessment in the MACONDO network was 'ignorance' (Stirling and Scoones 2009, 1). Simply put, this term encapsulates the 'unknown unknowns' of risk assessment or 'things we don't know we don't know' (ibid, 6). By definition, analyses based on probability 'cannot address possibilities that have not been defined or even anticipated' (Smithson 1989, 54). This is particularly relevant to complex phenomena such as malaria transmission where researchers cannot be confident that they are aware of all causal factors contributing to disease spread. For example, Kim noted in her webinar that *Plasmodium knowlesi* was only diagnosed in 2004, revealing the previously 'unknown' role of macaques in malaria transmission. It is also worth noting that for over 2,500 years, the idea persisted that malaria arose from miasmas rising from swamps (Cox 2010) and the origins of the word 'mal-aria' ('bad air') (Kelly and Beisel 2012, 74) suggests an association with those who worked in marshes, fought in the trenches of slept without a roof over their heads. It was not until the late 19th century that the role of parasites and mosquito vectors in malaria transmission was discovered (Cox 2010). More recently, the pace at which parasites and vector species are evolving has confounded efforts at disease prevention and control (Kelly and Beisel 2012). Many MACONDO members were racing to learn more about the behaviour of mosquitoes that have developed resistance to insecticides and are exhibiting new biting behaviours which evaded current control methods such as mosquito nets and indoor residual spraying. Going forward it was anticipated that processes of climate change, deforestation and biodiversity loss will have indeterminate impacts on malaria transmission both locally and globally (Fornace *et al.* 2021, Lambin *et al.* 2010). These 'unknown unknowns' (Stirling and Scoones 2009, 6) are an inevitable feature of malaria risk assessment. Consequently, the accounts of malaria risk offered by MACONDO members are understandably incomplete, with patches of 'precise' findings bordered by spaces of ignorance lurking somewhere in the shadows of the scientific gaze. Drawing attention to the 'multiple dimensions of incertitude' (ibid, 8) which checker scientific or evidence-based risk assessment methods is important because it questions the extent to which they can capture the indeterminate landscape interactions which shape malaria transmission and thus 'determine which interventions cause particular outcomes' (Adams Sandbrook 2013, 331).

4.5 *Multidisciplinarity and malaria multiple*

Finally, it is important to note that the accounts of malaria risk sketched by MACONDO members were stitched together using a range of disciplinary practices. The MACONDO network was deliberately composed of researchers from varying academic backgrounds including entomology, epidemiology, remote sensing and anthropology. One important driver behind this interdisciplinary collaboration was that many MACONDO researchers worked in residual transmission settings, where malaria elimination could not be achieved with conventional tools such as bednets and spraying. Edgar stressed to me that, in order to accomplish elimination, we need to 'broaden the tools that we have available.' He continued, 'it's not only, let's say epidemiology or entomology that are going to solve the problem, you have to have a multidisciplinary team'. Kim expressed a similar sentiment and stressed the value of 'people coming from different perspectives and backgrounds and looking at the same problem in different ways'.

This description of malaria as a stable problem that could be approached from different perspectives was certainly shared by other members of the network. However, recent relational theories in anthropology have argued that knowledge production is 'not only and epistemological act, but also a *doing* – a practice that involves creating worlds and that shapes ontologies' (Chandler and Beisel 2007, 415). In this sense, disease-making can be construed as a 'material-semiotic process' (Law 2004, 3) which conjures different articulations of malaria and enables certain practices of treatment and control (Langwick 2007). For example, when I asked Kallista to talk about how drone imagery was analysed, she said 'honestly I'm more of a mosquito person … I am more familiar with catching mosquitoes than using drones to take images of the environment'. As discussed in the introduction, this unitary focus on the vector has historically facilitated a focus on insecticides which has reshaped the biology of mosquitoes and parasites. On the other hand, Fedra (an electronic engineer) told me 'I am familiar with the images, but not with the process of being in the field, or taking images with drones. I mainly work with the images they acquire'. As mentioned above, this view of malaria as a visual and spatial phenomenon is linked to a shift towards environmental management strategies. The point to be drawn from this comparison is that different framings of malaria enable different intervention strategies which in turn shape the biology of the vector, the composition of the landscape, the behaviour of local populations and the focus of future studies. In other words, 'the fight against malaria can be understood as an ontological project' (Kelly and Beisel 2012, 72) which is constantly remaking the disease through its attempts to study and control it. The patchwork of malaria risk assessment is not simply comprised of different disciplinary viewpoints on a singular problem but rather constructs malaria as multiple and emergent from different disciplinary practices and geographical contexts.

4.6 *Summary*

In this section, we argued that just as the landscape imaged by drones was 'patchy', so too were the assessments of risk made by members of the MACONDO network. Pushing back against the idea that the scientific 'view from above' offers a comprehensive overview of malaria risk, we have argued instead that the picture of risk that emerged from drone use was distinctively incomplete. Due to their limited flying times, drones were only able to map small 'patches'of the landscape, requiring researchers to make deliberate choices about where to conduct their surveys. In the process of analysing their images, the landscape was separated into component parts which blurred together. Rather than offering an 'accurate' rendering of the 'full' picture of malaria risk, MACONDO researchers created small pockets of 'precise' findings which were bordered by spaces of uncertainty and ignorance, lurking somewhere in the shadows of the scientific gaze. This patchiness was also reflected in the multidisciplinary character of the network which entailed multiple malaria ontologies 'rubbing up against each other' (Tsing *et al.* 2019, 187) as researchers strove to generate knowledge that was useful for malaria control programmes.

5 Discussion – why patchiness matters?

In this chapter, we have argued that the MACONDO network's engagement with landscapes and risk was distinctively 'patchy'. Section 1 explored how drones facilitated a shift to thinking about malaria as emergent within heterogenous landscapes and constructed these as variably dynamic and static across macro and micro scales. In the process, specific landscape features were animated and flattened to produce an incomplete, but intelligible picture of multispecies processes relevant to malaria transmission. Section 2 explored how this 'patchy' character of the landscape was also reflected in MACONDO's engagement with risk. Contesting the notion that scientific methods of risk assessment are definitive and comprehensive, we pointed instead to their incomplete character. Due to their limited flying times, drones produced a punctual rather than panoptic view of malaria risk. Attempts to isolate 'risky' malaria places by compartmentalising the landscape were limited by the blurry and indeterminate relationships between environmental and spatial variables. MACONDO's quantitative and cartographic models did not capture the 'full' phenomenon of malaria risk, but instead offered patches of 'precise' findings, blemished by pockets of uncertainty and ignorance.

Why does patchiness matter? In short, because it leads us to question many of the received certainties upon which global health is predicated. Highlighting how malaria is emergent from 'patchy' landscapes, as MACONDO researchers inexplicitly do, questions the logic of biotechnical interventions that reify malaria as a stable natural entity that can be tackled with the same tools regardless of context (Iskander 2015). By pointing to the complex visual practice entailed in directing the drones punctual gaze on the landscape we additionally show that visualising technologies are never neutral or apolitical. Instead, we open the way for further discussion about how power is implicated in choices about what aspects of landscape, disease and community should be rendered visible.

Acknowledging the 'patchy' character of drone technology will be essential if drones are to become a more widespread and effective tool for malaria control intervention going forwards. This chapter has argued that making more effective use of drones is not simply a question of technical progress. While there will no doubt be improvements to flight times, photo quality and image processing as more training data is gathered and new drone hardware is released, we have cautioned against the pursuit of a 'perfect picture'. No matter how high resolution the image, researchers will continue to make choices about where to fly, what land type categories to use and how to present their findings. The 'patchy' character of drone imagery and its analysis will endure. If researchers want to improve and enrich their future studies, they need to be cognisant of the patchiness of their own work and be more deliberate in the way they engage with it. One way of doing this would be intertwining their scientific analyses of drone imagery with other ways of knowing. While many researchers acknowledge the importance of local communities to their work, there was little mention of these people's lived experiences of malaria. If researchers are to take seriously the idea that their imagery and analysis is 'patchy' then they should engage with these stories, not as lesser or more 'subjective' forms of knowledge, but rather as equally patchy, situated and powerful perspectives on malaria landscapes.

Patchiness also offers new incitements to anthropological theory and possibilities for multidisciplinary dialogue. Both anthropology and natural science have an interest in how disease emerges from multispecies landscapes, but this tends to be discussed in different registers. Science privileges scalable knowledge about the 'natural world' that can be applied across contexts, such as entomological data about the biting behaviours of specific vectors, or drone imagery that can be used to train classification algorithms. Anthropology, on the other hand, foregrounds the 'social' and presents lived experiences of space, place and disease which do not nest or translate easily. In the era of the Anthropocene, in which imbricated social and environmental processes are shaping new patterns of disease transmission, there is a growing need to bridge this divide between 'social' and 'natural' science. For anthropology, this means expanding the notion of the social to encompass more-than-human relationships (Tsing 2013). For science, this requires attention to the messy ways in which the social is enmeshed in 'natural' phenomena such as malaria and acknowledging how power is implicated in their models. This study has made small steps towards bridging this disciplinary divide by investigating how malaria emerges within 'patchy' multispecies landscapes. We have shown that disease and landscape are not exclusively 'natural' or 'social' concepts. Instead, they are co-constructed by researchers writing classification algorithms, mosquitoes searching rubber plantations for bloodmeals, parasites developing resistance against insecticides, timber-workers travelling along the riverbank, and macaques migrating into new habitats. Patchiness was a valuable analytical tool in this process because it encouraged attention to the uneven interactions of the 'natural' and the 'social' which public health discourse tends to flatten, but the intimate gaze of the drone on malaria landscapes cannot deny.

Acknowledgements

Funding for this project 'International collaborative network for the integration, standardization and assessment of the use of drones in malaria vector control strategies' was provided to DI by the Global Challenges Research Fund (GCRF) Networking Grants (GCRFNGR4\1140).

References

Adams W and Sandbrook C (2013) Conservation, evidence and policy. Oryx 47 (3): 329–335. https://doi.org/10.1017/s0030605312001470.

Brighenti A (2010) Visibility in social theory and social research. Palgrave Macmillan, London, UK.

Brown, H and Kelly AH (2014). Material proximities and hotspots: toward an anthropology of viral hemorrhagic fevers. Medical Anthropology Quarterly 28(2): 280–303.

Carrasco-Escobar G, Gamboa D, Castro MC, Bangdiwala SI, Rodriguez H, Contreras-Mancilla J and Alava F *et al.* (2017) Micro-epidemiology and spatial heterogeneity of *P. Vivax* parasitaemia in riverine communities of the Peruvian Amazon: a multilevel analysis. Scientific Reports 7(1): 8082. https://doi.org/10.1038/s41598-017-07818-0.

Carrasco-Escobar G, Manrique E, Ruiz-Cabrejos J, Saavedra M, Alava F, Bickersmith S and Prussing C *et al.* (2019) High-accuracy detection of malaria vector larval habitats using

drone-based multispectral imagery. PLOS Neglected Tropical Diseases 13(1): e0007105. https://doi.org/10.1371/journal.pntd.0007105.
Carrasco-Escobar G, Moreno M, Fornace K, Herrera-Varela M, Manrique E and Conn JE (2022) The use of drones for mosquito surveillance and control. Parasites, Vectors 15: 473. https://doi.org/10.1186/s13071-022-05580-5.
Chandler CIR and Beisel U (2017) The anthropology of Malaria: locating the social. Medical Anthropology 36(5): 411–421. https://doi.org/10.1080/01459740.2017.1306858.
Cox FEG (2010) History of the discovery of the malaria parasites and their vectors. Parasites & Vectors 3(1): 5. https://doi.org/10.1186/1756-3305-3-5.
Eckl J (2017) The social lives of global policies against malaria: conceptual considerations, past experiences, and current issues. Medical Anthropology 36(5): 422–435. https://doi.org/10.1080/01459740.2017.1315667.
Edwards P (2010) A vast machine: computer models, climate data, and the politics of global warming. MIT Press, Cambridge, MA, USA.
Fornace K, Diaz AV, Lines J and Drakeley CJ (2021) Achieving global malaria eradication in changing landscapes. Malaria Journal 20(1): 69. https://doi.org/10.1186/s12936-021-03599-0.
Fornace K, Drakeley CJ, William T, Espino F and Cox J (2014) Mapping infectious disease landscapes: unmanned aerial vehicles and epidemiology. Trends In Parasitology 30(11): 514–519. https://doi.org/10.1016/j.pt.2014.09.001.
Haraway D (1988) Situated knowledges: the science question in feminism and the privilege of partial perspective. Feminist Studies 14(3): 575. https://doi.org/10.2307/3178066.
Hardy A, Oakes G and Ettritch G (2020) Tropical wetland (Tropwet) Mapping tool: the automatic detection of open and vegetated waterbodies in Google Earth engine for tropical wetlands. Remote Sensing 12(7): 1182. https://doi.org/10.3390/rs12071182.
Hardy A, Makame M, Cross D, Majambere S and Msellem M (2017) Using low-cost drones to map malaria vector habitats. Parasites & Vectors 10(1): 29. https://doi.org/10.1186/s13071-017-1973-3.
Hausmann-Muela S and Eckl J (2015) Re-imagining malaria – a platform for reflections to widen horizons in malaria control. Malaria Journal 14(1): 180. https://doi.org/10.1186/s12936-015-0703-6.
Ingold T and Lee J (2021) Fieldwork on foot: perceiving, routing, socializing. In: Coleman S and Collinns P (eds) Locating the field: space, place and context in anthropology, 67–86. Routledge, Oxford, UK.
Iskander, D (2016) Parasites, power, and photography. Trends In Parasitology 32(1): 2–3. https://doi.org/10.1016/j.pt.2015.11.002.
Jumail A, Thor-Seng L, Salgado-Lynn M, Fornace KM and Stark DJ (2020) A comparative evaluation of thermal camera and visual counting methods for primate census in a Riparian forest at The Lower Kinabatangan Wildlife Sanctuary (LKWS), Malaysian Borneo. Primates 62(1): 143–151. https://doi.org/10.1007/s10329-020-00837-y.

Lambin EF, Tran A, Vanwambeke SO, Linard C and Soti V (2010) Pathogenic landscapes: interactions between land, people, disease vectors, and their animal hosts. International Journal of Health Geographics 9(1): 54. https://doi.org/10.1186/1476-072x-9-54.

Langwick SA (2007) Devils, parasites, and fierce needles: healing and the politics of translation in southern Tanzania. Science, Technology, & Human Values 32(1): 88–117. https://doi.org/10.1177/0162243906293887.

Latour, B (1988). The pasteurization of France / Bruno Latour translated by Alan Sheridan and John Law. Harvard University Press, Cambridge, MA, USA.

Latour B (2005) Reassembling the social: an introduction to actor-network-theory. Oxford University Press, Oxford, UK.

Law J (2004) After method: mess in social science research. Routledge, London, UK.

Law, J (2008). Actor network theory and material semiotics. In: Turner BS (ed.) The new Blackwell companion to social theory. Wiley-Blackwell, Oxford, UK, pp. 141–158.

Leach M and Scoones I (2013) The social and political lives of zoonotic disease models: narratives, science and policy. Social Science & Medicine 88: 10–17. https://doi.org/10.1016/j.socscimed.2013.03.017.

Lindsay S, Kirby M, Baris E and Bos R (2004) Environmental management for malaria control in the East Asia and Pacific (EAP) Region. World Bank, Washington D.C., USA.

MACONDO (2021) MACONDO × Network for the use of drones for malaria vector control. Available at: https://www.lshtm.ac.uk/research/centres-projects-groups/macondo#about.

Mitchell T (2012) Rule of experts. University of California Press, Berkeley, CA, USA.

Mol A (2002) The body multiple: ontology in medical practice. Duke University Press, London, UK.

Nájera JA, González-Silva M and Alonso PL (2011) Some lessons for the future from the global malaria eradication programme (1955–1969). Plos Medicine 8(1): e1000412. https://doi.org/10.1371/journal.pmed.1000412.

Nustad K and Swanson H (2021) Political ecology and the Foucault effect: a need to diversify disciplinary approaches to ecological management? Environment and Planning: Nature and Space 5(2) 1–23. https://doi.org/10.1177/25148486211015044.

Nutley S, Walter I and Davies H (2007) Using evidence: how research can inform public services. 1st ed. Bristol University Press, Bristol, UK.

Okumu F (2020) The fabric of life: what if mosquito nets were durable and widely available but insecticide-free? Malaria Journal 19(1): 260. https://doi.org/10.1186/s12936-020-03321-6.

Parker M and Allen T (2014) De-politicizing parasites: reflections on attempts to control the control of neglected tropical diseases. Medical Anthropology 33(3): 223–239. https://doi.org/10.1080/01459740.2013.831414.

Pauschinger D and Klauser F (2020) Aerial politics of visibility: actors, spaces, and drivers of professional drone usage in Switzerland. Surveillance & Society 18(4): 443–466. https://doi.org/10.24908/ss.v18i4.13434.

Randell HF, Dickinson KL, Shayo EH, Mboera LEG and Kramer RA (2010) Environmental management for malaria control: knowledge and practices in Mvomero, Tanzania. Ecohealth 7(4): 507–516. https://doi.org/10.1007/s10393-010-0343-9.

Ruckstuhl L, Lengeler C, Moyen JM, Garro H and Allan R (2017) Malaria case management by community health workers in the Central African Republic from 2009–2014: overcoming challenges of access and instability due to conflict. Malaria Journal 16(1): 388. https://doi.org/10.1186/s12936-017-2005-7.

Sandbrook C (2015) The social implications of using drones for biodiversity conservation. Ambio 44(S4): 636–647. https://doi.org/10.1007/s13280-015-0714-0.

Schiffman R (2014) Drones flying high as new tool for field biologists. Science 344(6183): 459. https://doi.org/10.1126/science.344.6183.459.

Scott J (1998) Seeing like a state: how certain schemes to improve the human condition have failed. Yale University Press, New Haven, CT, USA.

Smithson, M (1989) Ignorance and uncertainty: emerging paradigms. Springer, New York, NY, USA.

Stark DJ, Fornace K, Brock PM, Abidin TR, Gilhooly L, Jalius C, Goossens B, Drakeley CJ and Salgado-Lynn M (2019) Long-tailed macaque response to deforestation in a *Plasmodium knowlesi*-endemic area. Ecohealth 16(4): 638–646. https://doi.org/10.1007/s10393-019-01403-9.

Stirling AC and Scoones I (2009) From risk assessment to knowledge mapping: science, precaution, and participation in disease ecology. Ecology and Society 14(2): 14. https://doi.org/10.5751/es-02980-140214.

Ton O and Bubandt N (2010) Experiments in holism: theory and practice in contemporary anthropology. Wiley-Blackwell, Oxford, UK.

Tsing AL, Mathews AS and Bubandt N (2019) Patchy anthropocene: landscape structure, multispecies history, and the retooling of anthropology. Current Anthropology 60(S20): S186–S197. https://doi.org/10.1086/703391.

Tsing AL (2013) More-than-human sociality: a call for critical description. In: Hastrump K (ed.) Anthropology and nature. 1st ed. Routledge, New York, NY, USA, pp. 27–42.

Tusting LS, Thwing J, Sinclair D, Fillinger U, Gimnig J, Bonner KE, Bottomley C and Lindsay SW (2013) Mosquito larval source management for controlling malaria. Cochrane Database Of Systematic Reviews, no. 8: CD008923. https://doi.org/10.1002/14651858.cd008923.pub2.

Wall T and Monahan T (2011) Surveillance and violence from afar: the politics of drones and liminal security-scapes. Theoretical Criminology 15(3): 239–254. https://doi.org/10.1177/1362480610396650.

William T, Rahman HA, Jelip J, Ibrahim MY, Menon J, Grigg MJ, Yeo TW, Anstey NM and Barber BE (2013) Increasing incidence of *Plasmodium knowlesi* malaria following control of *P. falciparum* and *P. vivax* malaria in Sabah, Malaysia. Plos Neglected Tropical Diseases 7(1): e2026. https://doi.org/10.1371/journal.pntd.0002026.

World Health Organisation (2021) World Malaria Report 2020: 20 years of global progress and challenges. WHO, Geneva, Switzerland.

World Health Organization (2013) Larval source management – a supplementary measure for malaria vector control – an operational manual. WHO Global Malaria Programme, Geneva, Switzerland.

CHAPTER 8

Vector control and surveillance under lockdown: COVID-19 and future pandemics

Jose del Rosario Loaiza Rodríguez[1,2*], *Gillian Eastwood*[3] *and Luis F. Chaves Sanabria*[4]

[1]Instituto de Investigaciones Científicas y Servicios de Alta Tecnología (INDICASAT AIP), P.O. Box 0843–01103, 0843–01103, Panama 5, República de Panamá; [2]Programa Centroamericano de Maestría en Entomología, Universidad de Panamá, Bella Vista, Manuel E. Batista y Avenida Jose De Fábrega. Estafeta Universitaria. Apartado 3366, Panamá 4, República de Panamá; [3]Virginia Polytechnic Institute & State University, Department of Entomology, Center of Emerging Zoonotic & Arthropod-borne Pathogens (CeZAP), 309 Latham Hall, Blacksburg, VA 24061, USA; [4]Department of Environmental and Occupational Health, School of Public Health, Indiana University, 1025 E. 7th Street, Suite 111, Bloomington, IN 47405, USA; jloaiza@indicasat.org.pa

Abstract

Vector-borne diseases (VBDs) are widespread throughout the Americas, a region severely affected by the novel coronavirus disease 2019 (COVID-19). In order to curb the spread of the severe acute respiratory syndrome coronavirus 2 (SARS-CoV-2), health officials across the world established harsh constraints for people`s movement, including curfews and various levels of community lockdown. Although highly effective in dealing with the COVID-19 crisis initially, these containment tactics appear to have increased transmission likelihood for multiple vector-borne pathogens co-occurring with SARS-CoV-2. This could be due in part to logistical and safety challenges that prevent effective surveillance and control of arthropods that transmit pathogens affecting humans. This scenario is concerning since the Americas and other regions could be undergoing massive VBD outbreaks that might go unnoticed as a result of the COVID-19 pandemic. To reduce the risk of VBD exacerbation during a pandemic like COVID-19, i.e. the occurrence of a coronavirus-VBD syndemic, health personnel must be trained to adjust surveillance and control activities around households while respecting non-pharmaceutical disease prevention measures like social distancing. In this chapter, we examine the options to ensure effective vector monitoring and management in the face of large epidemics or pandemics of contagious diseases that consume public health resources and restrict individual human movement. We make recommendations for future investigation on vector surveillance and control strategies under various

 | DOI:10.3920/9789004688650_010

epidemiological scenarios and levels of community lockdown, as well as research methods for monitoring vector-borne pathogens during and after a pandemic.

Keywords

vector – surveillance – arthropod – vector-borne disease – control – pandemics – restrictions – Covid-19

1 Introduction

The coronavirus disease 2019 (COVID-19) pandemic caused by severe acute respiratory syndrome coronavirus 2 (SARS-CoV-2) has been so far the most significant public health emergency of the 21st century, with 308 million human cases and over 5.5 million deaths worldwide as of Jan 16, 2022 (WHO 2022). Developing countries in tropical regions are particularly vulnerable to infectious agents like SARS-CoV-2 due to the lack of potable water and sanitation, poor medical infrastructure, and limited access to health services (Miller *et al.* 2020). The exacerbated co-occurrence of COVID-19 and arthropod-borne viruses (i.e. arboviruses) or coronavirus-arbovirus syndemic, threatened to worsen the overall disease burden in the Americas (PAHO/WHO 2020). Health care systems in the Americas struggled to maintain sufficient human resources and medical supplies to tackle COVID-19 while being hit simultaneously by epidemics caused by dengue (DENV), yellow fever (YFV), chikungunya (CHIKV) and Zika viruses (ZIKV) (Magalhaes *et al.* 2020). This syndemic also extends to other vector-borne diseases (VBDs) including malaria, Chagas disease, leishmaniasis, tick-borne viruses and Lyme Disease. For example, ongoing efforts to eliminate malaria from countries in Central and South America were suspended due to the COVID-19 crisis, which will increase the likelihood of new epidemics and delay overall advances in regional malaria elimination programs (Siqueira *et al.* 2017, OPS/OMS 2020).

The overall number of cases and deaths due to arboviral diseases, including DENV, CHIKV and ZIKV, had decreased in the Americas during the first quarter of 2020 as compared to the previous year (Figure 1), as well as reported incidence of tick-borne Lyme Disease in the USA. Outpatient consultation and medical attention across the region also dropped due to strict lockdown regulations imposed by local governments, thus making diagnostic testing less available and case reporting unreliable. This scenario is worrisome because the region might be experiencing large VBD epidemics that are not being recognized due to a pandemic crisis such as COVID-19 (Wenman *et al.* 2020). Moreover, while developing countries had prioritized economic resources and human personnel to deal with the overwhelming

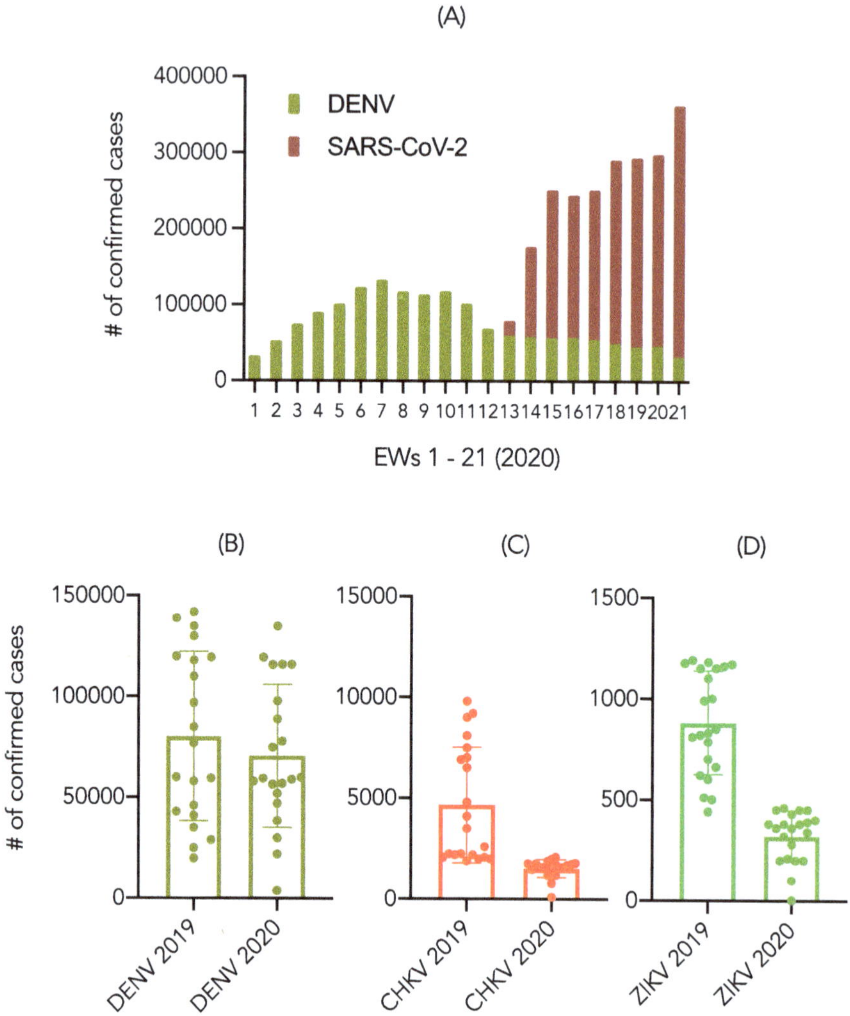

FIGURE 1 (A) Chronological relationship between laboratory confirmed cases of DENV and SARS-CoV-2 in the Americas by epidemiological weeks (EWS 1 to 21, 2020). We compared case data of DENV, CHIKV and ZIKV classified as '2019 EWS 1 to 21 and 2020 EWS 1 to 21' for countries and territories in the Americas. (B) DENV: (Wilcoxon ranked t test; Median of differences = 1,000.1; $P<0.5392$). (C) CHIKV: (Wilcoxon ranked t test; Median of differences = -2,300.2; $P<0.0001$). (D) ZIKV: (Wilcoxon ranked t test; Median of differences = -430.0; $P<0.0001$). Case data for COVID was obtained from the World Health Organization Coronavirus Disease (COVID-19) dashboard, accessed 12 July 2020. Available at https://covid19.who.int. Case data for DENV, CHIKV and ZIKV was extracted from the Health Information Platform for the Americas (PLISA, PAHO / WHO). Available at https://www.paho.org/data/index.php/es/

COVID-19 crisis, other public health actions such as vector surveillance and control were reduced drastically (Wilder-Smith *et al.* 2020, Grenadier 2020, Gomez-Dantés *et al.* 2020). Lack of logistical resources and insufficient personnel to survey vectors is a serious problem across both tropical and temperate regions where vector populations rapidly increase during summer (e.g. temperate areas) or the rainy season (e.g. tropical areas). Many locations remained under strictly enforced lockdowns triggering considerable restrictions in human mobility, which might have increased transmission by enhancing human-vector contact around households and residential areas (Cavany *et al.* 2021). An example is found in the poor communities of Panama City, where large families overcrowd housing units severely infested by abundant mosquito vectors that are only suppressed by actions from Panama`s national vector control programme (Whiteman *et al.* 2018, 2019a,b).

2 Human lifestyle changes during a pandemic

During the COVID-19 pandemic, the world observed a revolution in the way we live our daily lives and perform work activities. International travel almost stopped, and billions of people across the globe did not commute to their workplace and were working from home instead. While lockdowns and travel bans may minimize person-to-person contact for contagious agents such as coronaviruses, and reduce the likelihood of vector-borne infections contracted overseas, vector-borne pathogens continue to circulate locally in arthropods such as ticks, mosquitoes, and sandflies, and people may encounter them around their homes, yards and local community. In the United States, participation in outdoor activities soared during COVID-19, the sale of bicycles increased dramatically, visits to state parks boomed, and the number of people hiking, gardening, or spending time outdoors was at an all-time high due to indoor restrictions and social distancing under a pandemic setting (BBC 2020, Miller 2020, Ranzani *et al.* 2020). People who previously participated in outdoor activities during weekends were spending time outdoors almost daily.

Whilst generating many health benefits, outdoor activities without proper attention and precautions could lead to bites from hematophagous arthropods and exposure to vector-borne infections. A higher frequency of ticks found on people or pets was reported in some parts of the world following COVID-19 pandemic restrictions to indoor activities (Borsan *et al.* 2021). This was reflected also across the USA by increased submissions to passive vector surveillance programs, for example, in Connecticut and Maine (Spiegel 2020, UMaine 2020). However, the COVID-19 pandemic also altered how humans interacted with their healthcare systems, with reporting of some VBDs, e.g. Lyme disease in the USA, suggested to be artificially low due to healthcare-seeking behavior and avoidance of visits to medical facilities (McCormick *et al.* 2020). Similar perceived changes seen for VBD reporting during a pandemic might arise from the decrease in active tick and mosquito surveillance across the USA. Conducted by state, public health institutions, or county-level mosquito control districts, surveillance or pest control operations were variably impacted during the COVID-19 pandemic, for example, staff or funding being redirected, with many programs being reduced or even stopped completely (Jansen *et al.* 2021, NACCHO 2022).

3 Challenges of vector management during a pandemic

Vector surveillance monitors changes in the distribution and abundance of disease-transmitting arthropods such as ticks and mosquitoes. Vector surveillance also monitors the presence and prevalence of disease-causing pathogens transmitted by these arthropods to provide actionable, evidence-based information on infection risk to clinicians, the public, and policy makers (CDC 2020a). Failed implementation of vector control methods during COVID-19 has been observed in several regions of the world (Nurlaela and Mardliyah 2021, Seelig *et al.* 2020). In the USA, cutbacks that hindered staffing or redirected resources in efforts to tackle COVID-19 often took a toll on vector control, pathogen testing, and surveillance efforts; pandemic responses have the parallel potential to strain healthcare systems if management of arboviruses, including outreach and community education, is insufficient (NACCHO 2020, Santoro 2020). In order to decrease the likelihood of VBD exacerbation during a pandemic such as COVID-19, it is essential that vector surveillance and control continue in tropical and temperate settings (CDC 2020b, PAHO/WHO 2020). However, conventional methods to survey and control vectors require health personnel to work effectively around and inside houses, which may be inappropriate and ineffective by restrictions imposed during a pandemic (Wilder-Smith *et al.* 2020).

Due to a shortage of hospital beds and medical supplies, COVID-19 patients with mild symptoms (e.g. asymptomatic), representing roughly 70% of cases, often have been sent home to recover for a period of 10 to 14 days (WHO 2020). Nonetheless, in the case of COVID-19, asymptomatic people can remain infectious to relatives and visitors even under strict quarantine rules. Consequently, vector surveillance and control actions around households may expose health workers to asymptomatic pandemic-infected patients or vice-versa. In addition, indoor insecticide spraying, one of the most common methods to reduce vector populations, may incur negative effects on home-quarantined pandemic patients due to toxic chemicals worsening their respiratory manifestations of the infection (Sarwar 2016). Therefore, we posed the question – *Can health personnel in the Americas attain effective vector control and surveillance under the lockdown imposed during COVID-19 and future pandemics?*

4 Vector surveillance and control under community lockdown

Vector surveillance and control approaches during a pandemic can be adjusted to the various categories or epidemiological scenarios of transmission of the emergent pathogen. Supplementary Table S8.1 provides an outline of recommendations using SARS-CoV-2. Vector control personnel should receive specific and focused training about the use of any personal protective equipment (PPE) required by a pandemic situation and take extra precautions whenever they are working in neighborhoods with confirmed pandemic cases (Table 1).

TABLE 1 Summary of recommendations that people including vector control personnel need to follow to protect themselves from the COVID-19 disease under different categories or epidemiological scenarios of SARS-CoV-2 transmission in the Americas[a]

Categories 1 & 2	Category 3	Category 4
Containment and delay of spread	Delay of spread and mitigation	Full mitigation
No cases detected in the area or sporadic cases ('patient zero')	Cluster cases or limited community transmission	Wide community transmission
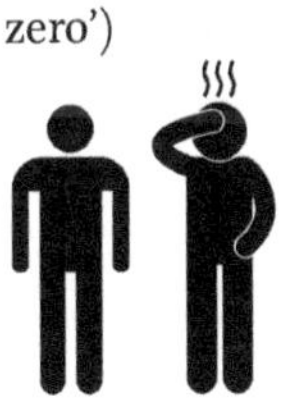	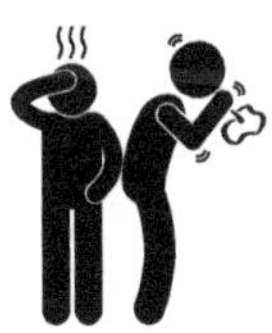	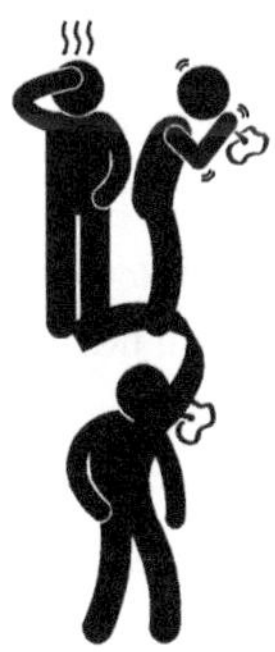
Wash hands with soap and water thoroughly and frequently. Hand sanitizers, well used, can also help. Always cough into elbow; no hand shaking, hugs or kisses.	Stay home if feeling unwell and practice even stricter social distancing, including from family members.	Face masks are protective against infection. Always wear a mask if going outside or if taking care of someone with symptoms.

TABLE 1 Summary of recommendations that people including vector control personnel (*cont.*)

Categories 1 & 2	Category 3	Category 4
Maintain social distancing (at least 2 meters distance) from anyone coughing or sneezing) and avoid large crowds.	Seek medical care early if experiencing a fever, cough and difficulty breathing. Call in advance to the health authority hotline. Do not go to the emergency room unless given the go-ahead by medical personnel.	Work from home. Take temperature daily. Upon development of high fever (>38 °C), dry cough and shortness of breath, seek medical care immediately.
The virus survives from 2 hours to 3 days in high traffic surfaces. Avoid touching eyes, nose, and mouth with unwashed hands. Disinfect frequently touched surfaces such as doorknobs.	Keep informed about the situation of COVID-19 in local district and home country. Follow instructions for school and work suspension in case of domicile close to the epidemic cluster.	Prepare for a possible regional or national 'lock-down' indicated by the local health authorities (probably 14 to 20 days). Try to have food, water and other basic essential supplies in sufficient inventory at home. Obey the regulations from the government closely and stay at home for as long as it is required.
Self-quarantine and call the health authority hotline in case of possible contact with the sporadic cases. Monitor and follow the directions of the local health authority.	Monitor and follow the directions of the local health authority.	Monitor and follow the directions of the local health authority.

a Information was partially obtained from published guidelines and management plans generated during the current COVID-19 pandemic (https://experience.arcgis.com/experience/685d0ace521648f8a5beeeee1b9125cd / https://www.who.int/emergencies/diseases/novel-coronavirus-2019/technical-guidance-publications).

Under the Categories 1 and 2 (Containment and delay of spread) with sporadic or no cases of disease detected in a particular region, countries can still employ conventional strategies of vector surveillance and control (Supplementary Table S8.1). In Panama, for example, large scale surveillance and control of urban *Aedes aegypti* and *Aedes albopictus* mosquitoes is accomplished by indoor pyrethroid thermal fogging to exterminate females when resting or seeking a blood meal and by searching for and eliminating natural and artificial water containers harboring immature stages (e.g. larvae and pupae) or treating them with organophosphates (Roiz *et al.* 2018). In Costa Rica, insecticide-based mosquito control is employed exclusively to combat focal VBD epidemics such as dengue, chikungunya, and Zika (Zardkoohi *et al.* 2020). Insecticide residual spraying and thermal fogging are also used following mass drug administration interventions in the context of malaria elimination in Costa Rica (Chaves *et al.* 2020a). The national program for integrated management of *Ae. aegypti* relies heavily on larval habitat mapping and elimination to assess the entomological risk of transmission prior to the rainy season, with efforts shifting to larval habitat treatment and insecticide fogging after the rainy season's increased transmission thresholds (Marín Rodríguez *et al.* 2012). Another strategy for guiding vector management in areas of Costa Rica prone to dengue epidemics since 2017 is the deployment of egg traps or oviposition traps (e.g. ovitraps are plastic cups partly filled with tap water and set with an egg-laying fiberboard paddle). High effectiveness in sites with notable changes in the abundance of *Ae. aegypti*, low cost, and ease of field deployment, with the potential involvement of local inhabitants in vector monitoring efforts, are some of the advantages of ovitrap-sampling (Chaves *et al.* 2021).

While many tick surveillance sites can be visited without the need for in-person contact (Whitlow *et al.* 2021), thus abiding by social distancing regulations in place during the COVID-19 pandemic, reduced staffing, lab access or capacity at tick-borne pathogen screening centers may necessitate prioritization among sites or diagnostic testing, pooling of samples (rather than testing specimens individually), or a community approach. Barriers to tick surveillance during a pandemic are already reduced by citizen science identifications, passive surveillance submissions, and co-ordination among stakeholders in a One Health approach to tick-borne disease prevention (Charles *et al.* 2021), and such tactics can be leveraged during a pandemic (Supplementary Table S8.1).

Under Category 3 (Delay of spread and mitigation) with clusters of cases and limited community transmission of the pandemic pathogen, countries can employ alternative approaches of vector control. Citizen science programs, in their most narrow definition, where data collection is outsourced to communities (Callaghan *et al.* 2019), can be implemented to gather large datasets from the community on mosquito occurrence, as is currently ongoing for kissing bugs (triatomines) in Texas, or ticks in parts of the UK and USA (Curtis-Robles *et al.* 2015, Cull 2021). Tick drags can easily be constructed from a 1 m^2 sheet of white cloth moved over vegetation following a standardized procedure (Salomon *et al.* 2020), enabling volunteers to participate in collections of ticks, the wooded or park locations of which allow for social distancing, and specimens can be mailed to a specific organization.

Citizen science involvement, for example *TickBlitz* that took place in New York state during the COVID-19 pandemic, can derive critical information on the presence of tick species and transmission risk, media attention, as well as tick biology training opportunities for participants (TickBlitz 2021).

Volunteers can take cellphone photos of mosquitoes (i.e. larvae and adult) or of other vector taxa, record the geographic locations using built-in mobile global positioning system (GPS) sensors, and send the data remotely to the vector control department for species identification (Mukundarajan *et al.* 2017, Tarter *et al.* 2019). Crowdsourced data and online platforms such as iNaturalist can complement vector surveillance efforts in determining seasonal occurrence and distribution patterns of medically important vector species, as well as monitoring range expansion (Cull 2021). Educational resources can be used as online guides to aid people in the recognition of anthropogenic and natural breeding sites (Smithsonian Science Education Center 2020).

Similar to remote-sensing satellite data, on a finer scale, drone technology can be applied to search for cryptic mosquito larval habitats on rooftops, tree holes or trash piles (Shragai *et al.* 2020); technologies that can be extended to other vectors, such as kissing bugs, phlebotomine sand flies and *Anopheles* spp. mosquitoes (Carrasco-Escobar *et al.* 2019). Such data can be mapped using geographic information system (GIS) with landscape spatial analysis to allow for more focused control tactics by pinpointing areas of high vector abundance (Whiteman *et al.* 2019b), while ensuring preventive practices in neighborhoods where small community transmission of the pandemic pathogen might be ongoing. In the USA, several programs by the National Association of County and City Health Officials (NACCHO) developed solutions to adapt and fulfill their critical role of vector control amid the COVID-19 pandemic. For example, some programs shifted to rely more heavily on GIS mapping tools to prioritize vector control in areas with a history of disease transmission. Similarly, partnerships with quantitative experts in academia could facilitate the use of predictive models to judge risk of transmission and action thresholds, even in the absence of present-day surveillance data (Karki *et al.* 2017).

Countries can employ a combination of surveillance with control approaches that respect social distancing and yet can target vectors, helping to achieve effective mitigation of VBD epidemics throughout the pandemic, while minimizing contact between health workers and the public (Roiz *et al.* 2018, Wilder-Smith *et al.* 2020). Mapping cases of VBDs and a pandemic disease such as COVID-19 can help to determine whether conventional (e.g. Categories 1 and 2 – Containment and delay of spread) or alternative vector management approaches such as citizen science or community enrolment (e.g. Categories 3 – Delay of spread and mitigation, and 4 – Full mitigation) can be applied, lessening the risk for both home-quarantined patients and vector control personnel while attaining successful mitigation of VBD outbreaks. Methods of high-resolution geospatial mapping can be run using disease occurrence points to develop a risk probability and to guide the distribution of insecticide treated bed nets (ITNs) in houses with cases of COVID-19 and substantial VBD-risk. This will aid in diminishing the possibility of a syndemic (i.e. *when nonlinear synergies among multiple diseases, social, and environmental factors at individual or societal scales can lead to higher burdens of disease or worse health outcomes*) (Singer *et al.* 2020), by reducing human-vector contact and vector longevity. This approach can be expanded to tackle various VBD systems collectively (e.g. malaria, leishmaniasis, Chagas Disease, tick-borne viruses and Lyme Disease), particularly in endemic areas where co-existing indoor biting and/or peridomestic vectors are not uncommon (Malone *et al.* 2019).

During the Category 4 (Full mitigation) phase of a pandemic, with widespread community transmission of COVID-19, vector surveillance and control measures will need to be set up outside houses and on domestic premises to prevent people (e.g. occupants and guests, or susceptible and infected) from coming into close contact. For diseases transmitted by *Aedes* (*Stegomyia*) spp., it is well-defined that effective biological larval control in small water containers can be achieved using long-lasting treatment with *Bacillus thuringiensis var. israelensis* (Bti) (Ritchie *et al.* 2010). Also, autocidal gravid oviposition traps (e.g. ovitraps with insecticide, oil, or adhesive glue), BG-Sentinel 2 traps (Biogents), and standard Gravid *Aedes* Traps (GAT), alone or in combination, can be set up outside homes to replace indoor pyrethroid spraying and ITNs, minimizing the risk of aggravated respiratory disease in home-quarantined pandemic patients, while disrupting the next generation of vectors by reducing egg-laying females (Barrera *et al.* 2014, Ramírez *et al.* 2018, Wipf *et al.* 2019). Backpack aspirators can be used to evaluate outdoor vector biting, and to remove both *Ae. aegypti* and *Ae. albopictus*, as well as other mosquito species, resting in backyards, gardens and surrounding vegetation (Roiz *et al.* 2018).

Community involvement and environmental methods targeting productive breeding sites, such as emptying of water containers and proper trash management, are even more crucial if municipal vector control services are halted (Espinal *et al.* 2019). The job may frequently be left up to each community, which under lockdown scenarios as experienced during COVID-19, could aid in mitigating mosquito populations through enhanced entomological surveillance and by promoting social awareness and education about VBDs (Predescu *et al.* 2006). For example, in Costa Rica, a campaign for community participation and social responsibility has been implemented to empower disadvantaged communities through encouragement to eliminate larval habitats in common community areas, but also in households, cleaning rain gutters and promoting the elimination of common larval habitats within the households. Similarly, there is an ongoing program aimed at the recycling of abandoned tires, which may serve as artificial breeding sites and facilitate the long-distance dispersal of *Aedes* mosquitoes, through rewards with virtual coins or 'Ecolones'.

Community re-emphasis on reduction of tick-habitats around yards (e.g. keeping grass short), wearing suitable clothing and checking for ticks after time spent outdoors, for instance, can stand in for conventional outreach by public health authorities. Public use of online platforms such as TickApp in the USA, where ticks and their geographical locations can be recorded, and tick prevention information gleaned, to encourage safer neighborhoods, maintain tick monitoring, and advance tick-borne disease research efforts even during a pandemic situation (Tickapp.us 2021).

Contemporary mechanisms of public participation in vector control or reduction of vector-borne pathogen risk involve large sections of the community, which open up new communication and data-sharing conduits, vital for achieving sustainable mitigation of VBDs, including those that have received less attention due to their encroachment mainly in socio-economically disadvantaged communities (Bartumeus *et al.* 2019). Procedures for vector surveillance and control must continue to follow the schedule of activities for a non-pandemic year. This will guarantee the effective mitigation of arthropod vectors while allowing adequate personnel and economic resources to tackle the pandemic crisis (Connelly *et al.* 2020). Although community surveillance and control efforts can reveal substantial evidence of vector distribution and seasonality, merely documenting the presence of tick, mosquito, sandfly or other vector species may be a poor indicator of human disease risk, thus pathogen testing should also be a necessary component of entomological risk assessments (CDC 2020a).

5 Assessing vector-borne pathogen infection during (and after) a pandemic

Arthropod vectors collected through the different categories of pandemic transmission should be tested for pathogen infection using integrative approaches to enable improved surveillance of both endemic and emerging VBDs. However, this is difficult to achieve in areas where diverse vector assemblages are pooled and screened through laborious taxonomic procedures involving hundreds of individuals and a cold chain to preserve pathogen nucleic acids (e.g. DNA / RNA) (Wipf *et al.* 2019). Pathogen infection rates in arthropod vectors are generally low in both tropical and temperate settings, owing to their large population sizes and the stochasticity of the infection process in animal host communities, making entomological risk assessment challenging (Ramírez *et al.* 2018).

Research methodologies to detect and isolate arboviral pathogen genetic material from vectors during and after a pandemic must avoid subjective sampling procedures that emphasize opportunistic rather than systematic surveillance schemes, as done in some of the best vector surveillance and control programs (Poh *et al.* 2019). The use of novel approaches that account for the heterogeneity of the urban or rural landscapes, a concept that previous studies frequently overlooked, can spur the design of even more effective and innovative methods for broad pathogen surveillance across various vector groupings (Heym *et al.* 2019). For example, Matrix-assisted laser desorption ionization (MALDI) methods can be used to identify field-collected vectors and the pathogens they harbor, with a minimal amount of tissue, in a short period of time, and without the need of expert taxonomists (Murugaiyan and Roesler 2017). Likewise, high-throughput metagenomic barcoding approaches not only can identify disease-causing agents across different vector groupings, but also microorganism taxa that could alter life history characteristics and viral replication in arthropod vectors (Bennett *et al.* 2019). Jointly or separately, MALDI mass spectra of highly abundant proteins from arthropod tissues and large-scale amplicon metagenomic sequencing of disease agents can be used to investigate the presence of endemic or emerging disease-causing pathogens across entire vector communities, while considering problematic vector taxonomy, low pathogen infection rates, and differences in habitat features (Murugaiyan and Roesler 2017, Bennett *et al.* 2019).

Recent advances in the identification of unknown pathogens with deep sequencing have enabled the rapid identification of novel or introduced VBDs. Whole genome analysis and landscape genomics of vector-associated pathogens through Nanopore MinION or Illumina next generation sequencing platforms can be conducted to examine vector-borne pathogen evolution (e.g. genomic recombination, selective sweep), demographic phenomena (e.g. introduction of multiple pathogen strains, bottlenecks) and molecular epidemiology (e.g. coinfection, virulence and pathogenicity) (Schwabl *et al.* 2017). The possibility of co-infection of arboviral disease and the pandemic pathogen in human communities exists. Mild cases of COVID-19 have been confused with dengue, resulting in delayed diagnosis and serious medical implications for patients (Yan *et al.* 2020). Therefore, pathogen surveillance from vector samples might be useful during and after the pandemic crisis to anticipate the potential co-circulation of DENV, CHIKV and ZIKV with the etiological agent of the pandemic, some of which could be difficult to disentangle using human samples due to various levels of cross-reactivity (Sharp *et al.* 2019). Moreover, genomic approaches for VBDs can aid scientists in detecting novel serotype/genotype combinations across areas where pandemic cases are being recorded, without the risk of obtaining human samples from potentially infected subjects. These approaches can also aid in alleviating the drawbacks of passive human case detection seen in the majority of arboviral diseases, which remain largely asymptomatic and unreported (Sharp *et al.* 2019). A recent study using mosquito saliva demonstrated the value of viral genomic sequencing to investigate the evolutionary forces shaping the genetic diversity of DENV within *Ae. aegypti* (Lequime *et al.* 2017), which is essential information to anticipate medical and epidemiological outcomes resulting from the spatiotemporal co-occurrence of particular serotype/genotype combinations of DENV and SARS-CoV-2. Gravid traps along with honey-baited nucleic acid preserving cards (FTA cards) have been recently proposed as an effective arbovirus detection method using female mosquitoes in areas of low disease prevalence. This approach can be complemented with additional pathogen mosquito screening methods for accurate arbovirus identification in sites where FTA cards are positive (Wipf *et al.* 2019).

Molecular blood meal analysis can be conducted throughout a pandemic such as COVID-19 to identify temporal shifts in vector feeding patterns, which could enable seasonal pathogen spillover events into humans and worsen overall disease burden. Blood meal sources from engorged arthropod vectors are routinely identified through conventional PCR protocols targeting various mitochondrial or nuclear gene fragments to incriminate reservoir hosts of endemic and emerging VBDs, including West Nile virus (WNV), visceral leishmaniasis, and Chagas Disease (Gonzalez *et al.* 2017, Goodman *et al.* 2018, Orantes *et al.* 2018). Molecular blood meal identification may be especially useful in areas that are currently undergoing significant ecological changes due to deforestation, agricultural development, and urbanization. For example, the intensive introduction of certain livestock animals could either dilute or amplify the spillover opportunities for some endemic and emerging VBPs by impacting vector feeding behavior (Navia-Gine *et al.* 2013). Therefore, not accounting for potentially changing vector-host interactions, and for the diversity of zoonotic VBPs that can co-circulate with pandemic pathogens like SARS-CoV-2 spatially and seasonally, will reduce our ability to forecast and prevent future syndemic events.

DNA aliquots can also be processed from vector samples to acquire baseline data about insecticide resistance, particularly for the most prevalent and competent vector species, including data on the presence of *kdr* mutations in populations of *Aedes* and *Anopheles* mosquitoes, but also in other vector species (Chaves *et al.* 2015, Zardkoohi *et al.* 2020). This will guarantee the effectiveness of conventional insecticide vector control approaches through reducing human-vector contact while considering mutations that may confer resistance against different insecticide classes (Roiz *et al.* 2018). This strategy can be practical during pre-epidemic periods to ensure that vector populations are effectively reduced before thresholds of increased human transmission occur during the rainy or summer seasons. Complementary research methods for monitoring VBPs during a pandemic could help to protect the overall health care system capacity by anticipating scenarios where the pandemic could potentially exacerbate the already complicated scenario of VBDs or vice-versa. This may be even more relevant during the post-pandemic era of COVID-19, which may well become the next neglected infection in poor communities around the world.

6 Conclusions

Vector surveillance and control approaches, in general, though especially as they pertain to pathogen transmission during pandemics, are inherently coupled natural-human systems where both the vector ecology and human behavior occur across diverse physical characteristics of the landscape, in addition to cultural, political, demographic, and socioeconomic contexts. Accordingly, in order to reduce the risk of coronavirus increasing transmission risk for VBDs in the Americas or vice-versa, it is imperative that vector surveillance efforts and pathogen transmission prevention campaigns examine multidisciplinary determinants of disease risk across different spatial and temporal scales.

In the case of COVID-19, while some countries have been able to reduce pandemic infection rates by applying stringent actions, like lockdowns, lately they have seen a significant increase in new cases as normal economic activities resume. This scenario is recurrently being reported in several countries, including South Korea, Germany, and Singapore, pushing their health authorities to enforce lockdowns once again, or in the USA, where some states that have limited their lockdowns have paid a high price in terms of exacerbated COVID-19 case and death burdens. Other countries like Costa Rica and Uruguay, have been able to rely on their socialized health systems to avoid major economic shutdowns while doing their best to prevent or at least maintain low SARS-CoV-2 transmission (Chaves *et al.* 2020b). Disruptions in control associated with reduced vector surveillance and monitoring activities are therefore expected to change transmission dynamics, likely exacerbating the transmission of endemic and emerging VBDs.

Despite the logistical and resource constraints posed by the COVID-19 epidemic, vector control programs across the Americas have adjusted to serve their critical public health role while restricting human mobility and maintaining social distance. Some of these adjustments are: (1) increasing the distribution of educational materials to local communities through various media outlets; (2) using mapping tools to search for vector habitat (Rhodes *et al.* 2022) and prioritizing efforts in areas where the most good can be done for the greatest number of residents; (3) focusing pathogen surveillance efforts on areas where infected arthropod specimens have previously been found; (4) forming a statewide group of vector control professionals to discuss methods for keeping the program running; and (5) enabling vector program staff to set and collect surveillance traps from their homes. Surveillance and vector control must continue under the enforcement of strict mitigation scenarios to reduce the severity of the COVID-19 pandemic. These restrictions are fertile territory for scientific research aimed at understanding how different vector mitigation strategies, implemented across the epidemiological, socioeconomic and cultural spectrum, can aid to maximize safety and effectiveness, while reducing the risk of a coronavirus-VBD syndemics.

Supplementary material

Supplementary material can be found online at https://doi.org/10.3920/978-90-8686-942-8_8.

Table S8.1. Summary of recommendations for vector surveillance and control approaches for different vector-borne disease systems under different categories or epidemiological scenarios of SARS-CoV-2 transmission in the Americas.

Acknowledgements

JL was funded by a grant from SENACYT 01 MOV 2018 (Panama); GE was supported by the USDA National Institute of Food and Agriculture, Hatch Project VA-160131; LFC was supported by the US National Science Foundation grant CNH2–1924200.

References

Barrera R, Amador M, Acevedo V, Caban B, Felix G and Mackay AJ (2014) Use of the CDC autocidal gravid ovitrap to control and prevent outbreaks of *Aedes aegypti* (Diptera: Culicidae). Journal of Medical Entomology 51(1): 145–154. https://doi.org/10.1603/ME13096.

Bartumeus F, Costa GB, Eritja R, Kelly AH, Finda M, Lezaun J, Okumu FM, Quinlan M, Thizy DC, Paré Toé L and Vaughan M (2019) Sustainable innovation in vector control requires strong partnerships with communities. PLOS Neglected Tropical Diseases 13(4): e0007204. https://doi.org/10.1371/journal.pntd.0007204.

BBC, 2020. The great bicycle boom of 2020. Available at: https://www.bbc.com/future/bespoke/made-on-earth/the-great-bicycle-boom-of-2020.html.

Bennett KL, Almanza A, McMillan WO, Saltonstall K, López Vdovenko E, Vinda JS, Mejia L, Driesse K, De León LF and Loaiza JR (2019) Habitat disturbance and the organization of bacterial communities in Neotropical hematophagous arthropods. PLoS ONE 14(9): e0222145. https://doi/10.1371/journal.pone.0222145.

Callaghan CT, Rowley JJL, Cornwell WK, Poore AGB and Major RE (2019) Improving big citizen science data: moving beyond haphazard sampling. PLoS Biology 17(6): e3000357. https://doi.org/10.1371/journal.pbio.3000357.

Carrasco-Escobar G, Manrique E, Ruiz-Cabrejos J, Saavedra M, Alava F, Bickersmith S, Prussing C, Vinetz JM, Conn JE, Moreno M and Gamboa D (2019) High-accuracy detection of malaria vector larval habitats using drone-based multispectral imagery. PLOS Neglected Tropical Diseases 13(1): e0007105. https://doi.org/10.1371/journal.pntd.0007105.

Cavany SM, España G, Vazquez-Prokopec GM, Scott TW and Perkins TA (2021) Pandemic-associated mobility restrictions could cause increases in dengue virus transmission. PLOS Neglected Tropical Diseases 15: e0009603. https://doi.org/10.1371/journal.pntd.0009603.

Centers for Disease Control and Prevention. (2020a) Guide to the Surveillance of Metastriate Ticks (Acari: Ixodidae) and their pathogens in the United States. Division of Vector-Borne Diseases, CDC. Atlanta & Ft. Collins. Available at: www.cdc.gov/ticks/surveillance.

Centers for Disease Control and Prevention. (2020b) CDC, National Center for Emerging and Zoonotic Infectious Diseases (NCEZID), Division of Vector-Borne Diseases (DVBD) Available at: https://www.cdc.gov/westnile/statsmaps/preliminarymapsdata2020/activitybystate2020.html.

Charles RA, Bermúdez S, Banović P, Alvarez DO, Díaz-Sánchez AA, Corona-González B, Etter EMC, Rodríguez González I, Ghafar A, Jabbar A, Moutailler S and Cabezas-Cruz A (2021) Ticks and tick-borne diseases in Central America and the Caribbean: A One Health perspective. Pathogens 10(10): 1273. https://doi.org/10.3390/pathogens10101273.

Chaves LF, Cordero V, Angel Delgado J, Aguilar-Avendaño G, Maynes C, Gutiérrez Alvarado E, Gutiérrez Alvarado JM, Ramírez Rojas M, Romero LM and Marín Rodríguez R (2021) Modeling the association between *Aedes aegypti* ovitrap egg counts, multi-scale remotely sensed environmental data and arboviral cases at Puntarenas, Costa Rica (2017–2018). Current Research in Parasitology and Vector-Borne Diseases, 1, 100014. https://doi.org/10.1016/j.crpvbd.2021.100014.

Chaves LF, Huber JH, Rojas Salas O, Ramírez Rojas M, Friberg MD, Marín Rodríguez R and Avila-Agüero ML (2020b) Coronavirus: Scientific insights and societal aspects. (2020). Mathematical Modelling of Natural Phenomena 15(32). https://doi.org/10.1051/mmnp/2020019.

Chaves LF, Huber JH, Rojas Salas O, Ramírez Rojas M, Romero LM, Gutiérrez Alvarado JM, Perkins TA, Prado M and Marín Rodríguez R (2020a) Malaria elimination in Costa Rica: changes in treatment and mass drug administration. Microorganisms 8(7): 984. https://doi.org/10.3390/microorganisms8070984.

Chaves LF, Kawashima E, Futami K, Minakawa N and Marin Rodriguez R (2015) Lack of KDR mutations in Asian tiger mosquitoes from Costa Rica. Bulletin of Insectology 68(1): 61–63.

Connelly CR, Gerding JA, Jennings SM, Ruiz A, Barrera R, Partridge S and Beard CB (2020) Morbidity and mortality weekly report continuation of mosquito surveillance and control during public health emergencies and natural disasters. Morb Mortal Wkly Rep 69: 938–940. https://doi.org/10.15585/mmwr.mm6928a6external icon.

Cull B (2021) Potential for online crowdsourced biological recording data to complement surveillance for arthropod vectors. PLoS ONE 16(4): e0250382. https://doi.org/10.1371/journal.pone.0250382.

Curtis-Robles R, Wozniak EJ, Auckland LD, Hamer GL, and Hamer SA (2015) Combining public health education and disease ecology research: using citizen science to assess Chagas disease entomological risk in Texas. PLOS Neglected Tropical Diseases 9(12): e0004235. https://doi.org/10.1371/journal.pntd.0004235.

Espinal MA, Andrus JK, Jauregui B, Waterman SH, Morens DM, Santos JI, Horstick O, Francis LA and Olson D (2019) Emerging and reemerging *Aedes*-transmitted arbovirus infections in the region of the Americas: implications for health policy. American Journal of Public Health 109(3) 387–392. https://doi.org/10.2105/AJPH.2018.304849.

Gómez Dantés H, Manrique-Saide P, Vazquez-Prokopec G, Correa Morales F, Siqueira Junior JB, Pimenta F, Coelho G and Bezerra H (2020) Prevention and control of *Aedes* transmitted infections in the post-pandemic scenario of COVID-19: challenges and opportunities for the region of the Americas. Memórias do Instituto Oswaldo Cruz 115: e200284. https://doi.org/10.1590/0074-02760200284

Goodman H, Egizi A, Fonseca D, Leisnham PT and LaDeau SL (2018) Primary blood-hosts of mosquitoes are influenced by social and ecological conditions in a complex urban landscape. Parasites and Vectors 11: 218. https://doi.org/10.1186/s13071-018-2779-7.

Grenadier A (2020) The impact of COVID-19 on local vector control response. NACCHO, May 04, 2020. Available at: https://www.naccho.org/blog/articles/the-impact-of-covid-19-on-local-vector-control-response.

Heym EC, Kampen H, Krone O, Schäfer M and Werner D (2019) Molecular detection of vector-borne pathogens from mosquitoes collected in two zoological gardens in Germany. Parasitology Research, 118: 2097–2105. https://doi.org/10.1007/s00436-019-06327-5.

Jansen CC, Darbro JM, Birrell FA, Shivas MA and Van den Hurk AF (2021) Impact of COVID-19 mitigation measures on mosquito-borne diseases in 2020 in Queensland, Australia. Viruses 16:13(6): 1150. https://doi.org/10.3390/v13061150.

Karki S, Westcott NE, Muturi EJ, Brown WM and Ruiz MO (2017) Assessing human risk of illness with West Nile virus mosquito surveillance data to improve public health Preparedness. Zoonoses Public Health 65: 177–184. https://doi.org/10.1111/zph.12386.

Lequime S, Richard V, Cao-Lormeau V and Lambrechts L (2017) Full-genome dengue virus sequencing in mosquito saliva shows lack of convergent positive selection during transmission by *Aedes aegypti*. Virus Evolution 3: vex031. https://doi.org/10.1093/ve/vex031.

Malone JB, Bergquist R, Martins M and Luvall JC (2019) Use of geospatial surveillance and response systems for vector-borne diseases in the elimination phase. Tropical Medicine and Infectious Disease 4(1): 15. https://doi.org/10.3390/tropicalmed4010015.

Marín Rodríguez R and Díaz Ríos M (2012) Sitios de Cría del *Aedes Aegypti* en la Región Pacífico Central de Costa Rica. Revista Costarricense de Salud Pública 21: 81–86.

McCormick DW, Kugeler KJ, Marx GE, Jayanthi P, Dietz S, Mead P and Hinckley AF (2021) Effects of COVID-19 Pandemic on reported lyme disease, United States, 2020. Emerging infectious diseases 27(10): 2715–2717. https://doi.org/10.3201/eid2710.210903.

Miller H (2020) Spending more time outside during the pandemic? Scientists say beware of ticks. Huffington Post 04/09/2020 updated 04/10/2020. Available at: https://www.huffpost.com/entry/coronavirus-tick-season-lyme_l_5e8f0a98c5b6b371812caabd.

Mukundarajan H, Hol FJH, Castillo EA, Newby C and Prakash M (2017) Using mobile phones as acoustic sensors for high-throughput mosquito surveillance. eLife 6: e27854. https://doi.org/10.7554/eLife.27854.

Murugaiyan J and Roesler U (2017) MALDI-TOF MS profiling-advances in species identification of pests, parasites, and vectors. Front. Cell. Infect. Microbiol. 7: 184. https://doi.org/10.3389/fcimb.2017.00184.

Navia-Gine WG, Loaiza JR and Miller MJ (2013) Mosquito-host interactions during and after an outbreak of equine viral encephalitis in eastern Panama. PLoS ONE 8(12): e81788. https://doi.org/10.1371/journal.pone.0081788.

Nurlaela L and Mardliyah E (2021) Integrated vector management on mosquito control during the COVID-19 pandemic. In: Proceedings of the International Symposium on Emergency Preparedness and Disaster Response during COVID 19 Pandemic. https://doi.org/10.2991/ahsr.k.210723.035.

Orantes LC, Monroy C, Dorn PL, Stevens L, Rizzo DM, Morrissey L, Hanley JP, Guadalupe Rodas A, Richards B, Wallin KF and Cahan SH (2018) Uncovering vector, parasite, blood meal and microbiome patterns from mixed-DNA specimens of the Chagas disease vector *Triatoma dimidiata*. PLOS Neglected Tropical Diseases 12(10): e0006730. https://doi.org/10.1371/journal.pntd.0006730.

PAHO/WHO (2019) Dengue. WHO, Washington DC, USA. Available at: https://www.paho.org/data/index.php/es/temas/indicadores-dengue.html.

Poh KC, Chaves LF, Reyna-Nava M, Roberts CM, Fredregill C, Bueno R, Debboun M and Hamer GL (2019) The influence of weather and weather variability on mosquito abundance and infection with West Nile virus in Harris County, Texas, USA. Science of The Total Environment 675: 260–272. https://doi.org/10.1016/j.scitotenv.2019.04.109.

Predescu M, Levins R and Awerbuch-Friedlander T (2006) Analysis of a nonlinear system for community intervention in mosquito control. Discrete and Continuous Dynamical Systems-Series B 6(3): 605–622. https://doi.org/10.3934/dcdsb.2006.6.605.

Ramírez AL, Van den Hurk AF, Meyer DB and Ritchie SA (2018) Searching for the proverbial needle in a haystack: advances in mosquito-borne arbovirus surveillance. Parasites and Vectors 11: 320. https://doi.org/10.1186/s13071-018.

Razani N, Radhakrishna R and Chan C (2020) Public lands are essential to public health during a pandemic. Pediatrics 146(2): e20201271. https://doi.org/10.1542/peds.2020-1271.

Ritchie SA, Rapley LP and Benjamin S (2010) *Bacillus thuringiensis* var. *israelensis* (BTI) provides residual control of *Aedes aegypti* in small containers. The American Journal of Tropical Medicine and Hygiene 82(6): 1053–1059. https://doi.org/10.4269/ajtmh.2010.09-0603.

Roiz D, Wilson AL, Scott TW, Fonseca DM, Jourdain F, Muller P, Velayudhan R and Corbel V (2018) Integrated *Aedes* management for the control of *Aedes*-borne diseases. PLOS Neglected Tropical Diseases 12(12): e0006845. https://doi.org/10.1371/journal.pntd.0006845.

Salomon J, Hamer SA and Swei A (2020) A beginner's guide to collecting questing hard ticks (Acari: Ixodidae): a standardized tick dragging protocol. Journal of Insect Science 20(6): 11. https://doi.org/10.1093/jisesa/ieaa073.

Santoro H (2020) COVID-19 is stripping resources from mosquito control programs. Future tense. Available at: https://www.newamerica.org/weekly/covid-19-stripping-resources-mosquito-control-programs/.

Sarwar M (2016) Indoor risks of pesticide uses are significantly linked to hazards of the family members. Cogent Medicine 3(1): 1155373. https://doi.org/10.1080/2331205X.2016.1155373.

Schwabl P, Llewellyn MS, Landguth EL, Andersson B, Kitron U, Costales JA, Ocaña S and Grijalva MJ (2017) Prediction and prevention of parasitic diseases using a landscape genomics framework. Trends parasitology 33(4): 264–275. https://doi.org/10.1016/j.pt.2016.10.008.

Sharp TM, Fischer M, Muñoz-Jordán JL, Paz-Bailey G, Staples JE, Gregory CJ and Waterman SH (2019) Dengue and Zika virus diagnostic testing for patients with a clinically compatible illness and risk for infection with both viruses. Morbidity and Mortality Weekly Report. Recommendations and Reports 68(1): 1–10. https://doi.org/10.15585/mmwr.rr6801a1.

Shragai E, Case T, Harrington L, Ren Y, Morreale S and Erickson D (2020) Evaluation of unmanned aerial vehicles and neural networks for integrated mosquito management of *Aedes albopictus* (Diptera: Culicidae). Journal of Medical Entomology 57(5): 1588–1595. https://doi.org/10.1093/jme/tjaa078.

Smithsonian Science Education Center (2020) Mosquito! community research guide: how can we ensure health for all from mosquito-borne diseases? Available at: https://ssec.si.edu/stemvisions-blog/introducing-mosquito-community-research-guide-how-can-we-ensure-health-all-mosquito.

Tarter KD, Levy GE, Yaglom HD, Adams LE, Plante L, Casal MG, Gouge DH, Rathman R, Stokka D, Weiss J, Venkat H and Walker KW (2019) Using citizen science to enhance surveillance of *Aedes aegypti* in Arizona. Journal of the American Mosquito Control Association 35(1): 11–18. https://doi.org/10.2987/18-6789.1.

TickBlitz (2021) New York State Tick Blitz. Available at: https://www.neregionalvectorcenter.com/new-york-state-tick-blitz.

UMaine (2020) UMaine tick surveillance program annual report – 2020. University of Maine Cooperative Extension, Diagnostic & Research Laboratory, Orono, ME, USA, 18 pp. Available at: https://tinyurl.com/2p9x6py7.

Wenham C, Lotta G and Pimenta D (2020) Mosquitoes and Covid-19 are a ticking time bomb for Latin America. Available at: https://blogs.lse.ac.uk/latamcaribbean/2020/03/31/mosquitoes-and-covid-19-are-a-ticking-time-bomb-for-latin-america/.

Whiteman A, Desjardins MR, Eskildsen GA and Loaiza JR (2019b) Detecting space-time clusters of dengue fever in Panama after adjusting for vector surveillance data. Plos Neglected Tropical Diseases 13(9): e0007266. https://doi.org/10.1371/journal.pntd.0007266.

Whiteman A, Gomez C, Rovira J, Loaiza JR and Chen G (2019a) *Aedes* mosquito infestation in socioeconomically contrasting neighborhoods of Panama City. EcoHealth 16(2): 210–221. https://doi.org/10.1007/s10393-019-014173.

Whiteman A, Mejia A, Hernandez I and Loaiza JR (2018) Socioeconomic and demographic predictors of resident knowledge, attitude, and practice regarding arthropod-borne viruses in Panama. BMC Public Health 18(1): 1261. https://doi.org/10.1186/s12889-018-6172-4.

Whitlow AM, Schürch R, Mullins D and Eastwood G (2021) The influence of southwestern Virginia environmental conditions on the potential ability of *Haemaphysalis longicornis*, *Amblyomma americanum*, and *Amblyomma maculatum* to overwinter in the region. Insects 12(11): 1000. https://doi.org/10.3390/insects12111000.

WHO (2020) Novel coronavirus (COVID-19) situation. Available at: https://experience.arcgis.com/experience/685d0ace521648f8a5beeeee1b9125cd.

WHO (2022) Coronavirus (COVID-19) dashboard. Available at: https://covid19.who.int/.

Wilder-Smith A, Tissera H, Eong Ooi E, Coloma J, Scott TW and Gubler DJ (2020) Preventing dengue epidemics during the COVID-19 pandemic. The American Journal of Tropical Medicine and Hygiene 103(2): 570–571. https://doi.org/10.4269/ajtmh.20-0480.

Wipf NC, Guidi V, Tonolla M, Ruinelli M, Müller P and Engler O (2019) Evaluation of honey-baited FTA cards in combination with different mosquito traps in an area of low arbovirus prevalence. Parasites and Vectors 12: 554 https://doi.org/10.1186/s13071-019-3798-8.

Zardkoohi A, Castañeda D, Lol JC, Castillo C, Lopez F, Marín Rodriguez R and Padilla N (2020) Co-occurrence of KDR mutations V1016I and F1534C and its association with phenotypic resistance to pyrethroids in *Aedes aegypti* (Diptera: Culicidae) populations from Costa Rica. Journal of Medical Entomology 57(3): 830–836. https://doi.org/10.1093/jme/tjz241.

CHAPTER 9

Agriculture and health: mitigating risks and optimising benefits

Isabel Byrne and Kallista Chan**

London School of Hygiene and Tropical Medicine, Keppel Street,
London WC1E 7HT, UK; *isabel.byrne@lshtm.ac.uk; *kallista.chan@lshtm.ac.uk;
the authors contributed equally

Abstract

Agriculture is a crucial component of our food system, providing nutrition, building materials, and economic stability around the world. These positive benefits of agriculture are those which tend to be highlighted by the agricultural sector. Agriculture and agricultural development can, however, also have negative outcomes on elements such as the environment and importantly on human health. Increases in infectious disease (especially vector-borne disease) risk and transmission are often linked to agriculture. These links can be driven by changes to the environment impacting disease vectors' ecologies, or socio-economic changes brought about by agricultural development impacting people's access to protection and healthcare. Although these negative consequences of agriculture on human health are unintended, they have wide-reaching impacts on the health of large, often poor, populations, with vector-borne disease burdens disproportionately higher in low-and-middle income countries. The world's growing population means that demand for agriculture is only going to increase to ensure food security. If left unmanaged, the vector-borne disease risks linked to agriculture and agricultural development are likely to intensify with this increase. We highlight the connections between agriculture and vector-borne disease, and the barriers which both the agricultural and health sector face in the challenge to tackle this issue. We introduce the co-benefits approach of finding 'win-win' solutions which optimize agricultural outputs while minimizing the negative impacts on human health. We provide examples of co-benefit approaches with a focus on agricultural irrigation projects which have reduced vector-borne disease risks and improved agricultural outputs. Finally, we suggest priority actions for both the agriculture and health sectors to overcome the challenges which impede the resolution of this problem.

 | DOI:10.3920/9789004688650_011

Keywords

co-benefits – agricultural development – intersectoral – deforestation – irrigation – intensification – rice

1 The health impact of agricultural development

Modern human populations are dependent on agriculture. It is a crucial part of our food systems, playing a key role in providing food security for our growing population. Industrial agricultural systems, despite generating negative impacts on some fronts, still supply global markets with large volumes of food and have boasted breakthroughs in crop productivity, food processing, distribution and improvements in food safety (Frison 2016). On the other hand, in low-and-middle-income countries, small-scale agriculture in rural communities provides sustenance, shelter, medicine, and income, thereby reducing hunger and poverty and improving livelihoods. Through these means, agriculture can create a pathway to improve the health and livelihoods of the poor. The positive impacts of agriculture on human health are far-reaching; from nutrition to economic development leading to improved access to healthcare (Hawkes and Ruel 2006a). These processes by which agriculture can improve human health tend to be those which are highlighted and focused on by the agricultural sector. There are, however, negative impacts on health created by agriculture and agricultural development, whereby agriculture also puts human health at risk (Hawkes and Ruel 2006a; Lines *et al.* 2020).

Unintended side effects of agriculture can impact negatively on human health, through processes such as disease transmission, occupational health hazards, and malnutrition (Hawkes and Ruel 2006b). In many cases, agriculture is associated with increased risk of infectious disease transmission, where agricultural drivers of transmission have been attributed to >25% of all infectious diseases which have emerged in humans (Alexandratos and Bruinsma 2012). These links between agriculture and poor health can reduce the productivity of farming communities where agricultural workers in ill health are less able to work. This in turn can jeopardize food security, income and economic development (Hawkes and Ruel 2006b), creating a barrier to the pathway out of poverty and undermining the benefits which agriculture provides to poor communities (Lines *et al.* 2020). There is a tendency in the agricultural sector to focus on the positive impacts which it has on health, with the processes producing negative health impacts being accepted as a 'necessary evil', or an inevitable by-product or trade-off of useful agricultural activities (Lines *et al.* 2020).

One such unintended negative consequence is increased vector-borne disease (VBD) risks due to agricultural practices. Tropical and low-and-middle-income countries bear a disproportionately high burden of VBDs, and also house an estimated three-quarters of global agricultural land cover (World Bank 2022; Wilson *et al.* 2020). The mechanisms through which agriculture can drive changes in VBDs are complex and often poorly understood, making them difficult to control for and manage when planning agricultural projects (WHO *et al.* 1996). Agricultural development can disrupt ecological and social systems through many mechanisms, leading to changes in VBD transmission. Land-use and land-cover changes for agriculture alter environmental conditions and subsequently can impact vector ecologies (Ferguson *et al.* 2010; Foley *et al.* 2005; Fornace *et al.* 2021; Jones *et al.* 2013). A common example of this is the creation of suitable breeding conditions for disease vectors by irrigation schemes for agricultural projects (Norris 2004; Patz *et al.* 2000). Changes in the local economy and human demographics driven by agricultural development can also impact population exposures and vulnerabilities to VBDs. Examples of this include the monetary gains of agricultural production leading to agricultural communities having improved access to healthcare, and better infrastructure and protections against vectors (WHO *et al.* 1996). Agricultural intensity generally rises with population density (Boserup 1965). The global population is projected to increase by around one-third by 2050, requiring a 70% increase in food production (FAO 2002). Agricultural intensification and expansion to support this growth will be fundamental for sustenance (Rohr *et al.* 2019). Current trends suggest that this expansion will likely lead to changes in VBD transmission. In the agricultural sector, plans for 'Sustainable Intensification' are at the forefront of agricultural development. Sustainable Intensification aims to create agricultural systems and methods which will increase agricultural yields to feed growing populations, while mitigating adverse impacts on the environment (Wezel *et al.* 2015). So far, however, these plans do no take mitigation of negative health impacts from agriculture into account.

As the agricultural sector develops to cope with changes in human populations, the environment, and the climate through Sustainable Intensification, it is imperative that VBDs are also considered. We must find effective ways to achieve high agricultural productivity without the unintended negative health costs from VBDs, and incorporate these methods into plans going forward (Lines *et al.* 2020). One of the major barriers to this goal currently is a lack of ownership of the problem. As the responsibility for disease surveillance, control and mitigation traditionally falls on the health sector, the agriculture sector tends not to be involved in these processes, despite the often deadly impacts of agriculture on disease ecology (Chan *et al.* 2022a). In some instances, in order to improve economic efficiency, agricultural development projects do include health components to mitigate sick labour (e.g. providing bed-nets, rapid diagnosis and treatment to agricultural workers in malarious settings (Packard 1986)). However, these 'downstream' solutions are not adequate. Instead, the agricultural sector needs to take accountability and take part in 'upstream' prevention. To do this, alliances between health and agriculture sectors are required to share the burden of mitigating and building out VBD risks created by agriculture through new methods which optimize the benefits of agriculture, while minimizing the risks on health (WHO *et al.* 1996; Lines *et al.* 2020). 'Adaptation co-benefits' have been described as a crucial step to break down such sectoral silos to allow for climate-resilient agricultural development. These are adaptations or developments to agricultural methods or policies which have a socially, economically or environmentally desirable outcome (Crumpler and Meybeck 2020). We believe that the definition of co-benefits can be expanded to include health outcomes, especially those linked to vector-borne disease transmission.

In this chapter, we aim to highlight the connections between agriculture and VBD, and to encourage collaborative disease and agriculture related research, planning and policy which can improve agricultural production while reducing risks to human health from VBD. We will provide an overview and examples of the common mechanisms by which agriculture impacts VBD transmission, then introduce the co-benefits approach and how it could be used to find 'win-win' solutions to the challenge of agriculture and VBD. The current barriers to overcoming this challenge will be outlined, with suggestions for both the agriculture and health sectors for how to overcome them in the future.

2 Drivers of agriculture-vector-borne disease associations

There are many driving forces which can increase or decrease VBD risks associated with agriculture and agricultural development. These drivers can be placed in three broad categories: socio-economic, demographic and environmental.

2.1 *Socio-economic drivers*

2.1.1 Economic

The economic drivers of agricultural impact on VBD are broadly linked to the improvements in conditions and quality of life which agriculture can offer through providing economic benefits. Poverty can enhance vulnerability to VBDs, primarily by limiting people's ability to manage and address health risks (Bardosh *et al.* 2017; Blas and Kurup 2010). It is the general consensus that socio-economic impacts in the wake of agricultural development follow a positive trend, where VBD risk and incidence is 'built-out' through local improvements to infrastructure, better access to health services and increased protection against vectors (WHO *et al.* 1996). Such positive impacts will in turn influence the health and well-being of the agricultural community, generating a positive feedback loop resulting in further improvements to the agricultural and economic productivity of the workforce (WHO *et al.* 1996).

Although there are many instances of agricultural development increasing wealth and hence improving health, they are rarely documented due to its indirect nature. Nonetheless, one example is the 'paddies paradox' hypothesis, which was used to partly explain why, until the early 2000s, there was often less malaria in African rice-growing villages despite higher numbers of mosquitoes in these areas (as rice paddies provide an ideal breeding environment for malaria vectors). Ijumba *et al.* (2001) argued that residents of rice-irrigation schemes became wealthier from their agricultural productivity, and part of this wealth trickles down into their health, by providing access to bed-nets and antimalarials to counter the higher vector abundances. However, this paradox may no longer be valid these days because malaria interventions have become more equitably distributed across Africa (Taylor *et al.* 2017). Upon a re-assessment of the paradox, Chan *et al.* (2022b) found that, compared to non-rice-farming communities, irrigated rice communities are now more exposed to greater malaria risk. This should be of concern to the agricultural sector as it plans to scale-up rice production across the continent.

2.1.2 Demographic

Agricultural development can often drive demographic changes which put populations at increased risk of ill health due to VBD. Large agricultural projects can create a demand for labor, resulting in the movement of populations of human workers. The migration of large groups of people with differing levels of immunity into new areas can pose VBD risks through two broad mechanisms. Firstly, an influx of previously unexposed people to an area with high or endemic disease transmission leaves them exposed to infections which have potential to be severe or fatal due to their naïve immunity (Prothero 2001; WHO *et al.* 1996). Ethiopia saw mass forced-resettlement schemes during the mid-80s. People without malaria immunity were moved from the northern plateau to lower lands where malaria is endemic, and were subsequently exposed to risks of high mortality and morbidity, further enhanced by exposure to higher vector abundances for those resettled to irrigation schemes (Kloos 1990; Prothero 2001). Secondly, human migration can introduce or reintroduce pathogens from other settings. Once a capable vector can transmit the introduced pathogen, this can lead to outbreaks in the workforce and in non-immune local communities. An example of this is the reintroduction of malaria to Eswatini in the 1960s and 1970s. Successful control measures (DDT spraying) had effectively eradicated malaria from the area by 1959, but a resurgence of malaria was driven by re-introduction of *Plasmodium* parasites to the area by migrant workers from malaria-endemic areas of Mozambique to work on sugarcane estates (Packard 1986; Martens and Hall 2000). As a more recent example, it has been shown that cross-border migrant workers play a role in spreading multidrug resistant malaria at the Thailand-Cambodia and Thailand-Myanmar borders (Bhumiratana *et al.* 2013; Tangena *et al.* 2016; Wangroongsarb *et al.* 2012).

These issues of VBD transmission and illness are often exacerbated by environmental and socio-economic drivers of disease which impact migrant workforces. Many crops which are cultivated in large agricultural schemes create a seasonal demand for temporary agricultural workers. This often occurs during or soon after the rainy season when VBD transmission is at its most intense (Wangroongsarb *et al.* 2012). These populations are often poor and marginalized groups who are subject to poor health infrastructure, inadequate basic services and vector control in housing (Prothero 2001).

2.2 *Environmental drivers*

Agriculture and agricultural development induce environmental and ecological changes which can often impact one of the variables which determine vectorial capacity. Examples of such environmental and ecological changes brought about by agricultural development include the creation of new breeding sites for vectors; changes in species dynamics; changes in microclimatic conditions which may favor vector longevity; and increases human-vector contact (Wangroongsarb *et al.* 2012). For brevity, we will focus on two major environmental drivers, irrigation and deforestation, though many others exist.

2.2.1 Irrigation

One of the most important ways in which environmental changes caused by agricultural development impact VBD is through water redistribution. Irrigation networks, dams and reservoirs increase with agricultural development and these changes in water distribution are widely associated with increases in disease vectors and hosts of human pathogens (Hawkes and Ruel 2006b). There exists a wealth of scientific literature highlighting how irrigation projects for agricultural development can induce changes in vector bionomics, species diversity, and disease transmission.

Through providing ideal habitats for the freshwater snail vectors, dam building has led to the introduction of schistosomiasis to previously unexposed populations (Mutero *et al.* 2006). Snail vectors had never been reported in the Hola settlement scheme in Kenya prior to an irrigation scheme in the 1950s. The following decade, a 70% prevalence of schistosomiasis was reported within the population, which rose to 90% by 1982 (Mutero 2002). In central Tunisia, the construction of irrigation facilities alongside unusually high temperatures created ideal conditions for an increase in leishmaniasis vector *Phlebotomine* sandflies. These changes have been linked to increases in human visceral and cutaneous leishmaniasis (Salah *et al.* 2000). Irrigated rice agriculture has been notoriously linked to malaria vector production, with rice fields acting as a major source of the primary malaria vector species in central China, sub-Saharan Africa, parts of central Asia, Indonesia, and Peru (Lacey and Lacey 1990). Ultimately, rice-growing areas in sub-Saharan Africa often harbour high malaria transmission capacity (Haileselassie *et al.* 2021; Chan *et al.* 2022b). In Sri Lanka and the Thar Desert in India irrigation development has been linked to both increases in malaria vectors and changes in malaria transmission from mild to frequent epidemics (Amerasinghe and Ariyasena 1991; Tyagi and Chaudhary 1997).

2.2.2 Deforestation and plantations

The clearing of land for agricultural activities is the largest single cause of deforestation (FAO 2022). Deforestation alters the ecology of a landscape, impacting temperature, humidity, vegetation, water retention, and soil composition. Disease vectors are sensitive to such changes, and thus, deforestation and the knock-on effects it has on a landscape's ecology influence the transmission of VBDs through changes in vector ecology, alongside human behavior patterns (Yasuoka and Levins 2007).

Deforestation has been shown to increase the risk of scrub-typhus in Korea, and agriculture-related work activities have been shown as risk factors transmission (Kim *et al.* 2018; Ma *et al.* 2017; Min *et al.* 2019). This is driven by the secondary growth of scrub vegetation after deforestation which provides an ideal habitat for the mite vectors, resulting in higher vector densities (Min *et al.* 2019). The distribution of lymphatic filariasis is impacted by deforestation and agriculture, and may be linked to the generation of suitable vector habitats (Duker and Kwarteng 2021), with many of the important mosquito vectors of lymphatic filariasis shown to be positively associated with deforestation (Burkett-Cadena and Vittor 2018). In south-west Nigeria, lymphatic filariasis was found to be higher in communities with lower canopy height and tree coverage (Brant *et al.* 2018). In south-east Cote d'Ivoire, the abundance and distribution of *Aedes* vectors of lymphatic filariasis were found to be impacted by landcover and landuse change from rainforest to oil palm plantations (Zahouli *et al.* 2017). In the Democratic Republic of Congo, deforestation and agricultural expansion were associated with increased indoor biting rates of malaria vectors, causing an increase in malaria prevalence in children (Janko *et al.* 2018). Increases in the human incidence of the simian malaria *Plasmodium knowlesi* has been shown to be strongly associated with deforestation in Sabah, Malaysia (Fornace *et al.* 2016, 2019b). Deforestation and land-use change for agriculture have been linked to changes in the reservoir macaque behavior and increased contact between people and mosquito vectors and forest edges, and the creation of favorable vector breeding habitats (Byrne *et al.* 2021; Fornace *et al.* 2019a; Stark *et al.* 2019).

Deforestation activities are often the first steps in the creation of plantation farms. In recent decades monoculture-based agriculture for crops such as oil palm and rubber have expanded extensively, especially in South East Asia (Ahrends *et al.* 2015; Bartholomé and Belward 2005; Shah *et al.* 2019; Tangena *et al.* 2016). Here, multiple studies have shown increases in these two agriculture types to be associated with outbreaks and increases in prevalence of VBDs such as dengue, malaria and chikungunya (Morand and Lajaunie 2021; Shah *et al.* 2019). Monocultures tend to have lower species richness compared to primary and secondary forests and altered ecology in terms of canopy, undergrowth, humidity, greater human disturbance (Shah *et al.* 2019). Rubber plantations provide suitable environments for long-lived forest vectors such as *Anopheles dirus sensu lato* malaria vector and *Aedes albopictus* dengue and chikungunya vectors (Jomon and Valamparampil 2014; Sulaiman and Jeffery 1986), and create a wide range of man-made and natural larval habitats (Tangena *et al.* 2016). Multiple epidemics of dengue and chikungunya have been reported from plantations in Malaysia and India in the past two decades, each occurrence infecting thousands of people in plantation working communities (Kumar *et al.* 2011; Nakhapakorn and Tripathi 2005; Tangena *et al.* 2016). Regular malaria outbreaks have been reported across Southeast Asia in rubber plantations and other monocrop plantations. Yasuoka and Levins (2007) describe changes in vector composition increasing malaria transmission among cassava and sugarcane plantation workers in Thailand. The initial development of the plantations led to decreases in the shade-loving vector *Anopheles dirus*, however the species was replaced by the sun-loving vector *Anopheles minimus*.

It is important to note that the impact of deforestation on VBD transmission is complex and not uniform in every setting, as it depends on many factors involved in different vector ecologies and disease transmission cycles (Kalbus *et al.* 2021). In some African settings deforestation can actually lead to reductions in malaria transmission by reducing suitable habitats of forest dwelling vectors (Guerra *et al.* 2006). Additionally, to our knowledge no positive association has yet been shown dengue and deforestation, although studies are sparse (Husnina *et al.* 2019). Broadly speaking however, a systematic review by Burkett-Cadena and Vittor (2018) has shown that the net effect of deforestation favors human disease vectors, and that non-deforested forest habitats favor non-vectors.

2.3 *The complexity of drivers*

We have highlighted that the impact of agriculture and agricultural development on VBD transmission can be driven by multiple drivers and varying mechanisms working within them. These drivers do not work in isolation and are often working in conjunction with each other. In Lowland Eswatini, malaria had been successfully controlled, prompting the expansion of sugarcane agriculture. This required the construction of irrigation schemes, providing a niche for *Anopheles* vectors to breed in, resulting in resurgences in malaria (Packard 1986). These resurgences were intensified by poor infrastructure and frequent importation of migrant labourers from endemic-Mozambique (Tejedor-Garavito *et al.* 2017). This example highlights how the environmental, socio-economic and demographic drivers can overlap to exacerbate the negative impacts of agricultural development on VBD transmission. Another example is the Mahaweli rice development project in Sri Lanka, where irrigation created breeding sites for Japanese encephalitis virus (JEV) vector *Culex tritaeniorhyncus*, resulting in increases in human-vector contacts (Amerasinghe and Indrajith 1994). A separate agricultural development project nearby encouraged pig production, which are the reservoir host for JEV. Subsequent JEV epidemics severely impacted the newly settled and non-immune communities of agricultural workers (Mutero *et al.* 2006).

When there are multiple drivers of transmission working at varying scales, untangling the cause-effect relationship of agriculture on VBD transmission becomes a hugely complex task. Showing that there is a relationship between an agricultural activity and disease transmission is the first step, but understanding the mechanisms underlying this relationship would require multiple robust field studies and analyses. In order to translate this knowledge into policy change or change which will be accepted within the agricultural sector, further studies and trials to develop 'win-win' solutions, or co-benefits, for agriculture and health need to be found.

3 Co-benefits: the concept

By definition, a co-benefit is an additional benefit from an action or intervention that is undertaken to achieve a particular purpose. It implies a 'win-win' strategy to address multiple goals with a single policy, and can be implemented across different scales and sectors (Crumpler and Meybeck 2020). The term emerged in the 1990s and is popular amongst the climate change community (Mayrhofer and Gupta 2016). A classic example of a climate co-benefit is reducing fossil fuel combustion, which not only helps tackle climate change but also improves air quality and thus has significant health and environmental benefits. In contrast to co-benefits, an intervention can sometimes create conflicts or trade-offs, which need to be taken account of and minimised.

Whilst co-benefits can arise from climate change adaptation in agriculture, this term can be extended to not only cover climate actions but also agricultural interventions. Health co-benefits which are generated by agricultural development strategies exist, but these are often unintended positive side effects, similar to the aforementioned unintended negative side effects. More effort needs to be placed in recognising, developing, and adopting co-benefits with intended positive side effects. This is especially important as discussions at the agriculture-health interface currently place a lot of emphasis on trade-offs, rather than co-benefit solutions.

4 Agriculture-vector-borne disease co-benefits: case studies

Co-benefits, a new term at the interface between agriculture and VBDs, aims to optimise health and productivity benefits of agriculture, whilst minimising the health risks to the agricultural community. To provide better understanding of this new term, we will highlight a number of case studies, largely in the context of irrigation, rice and mosquito-borne diseases.

4.1 *Irrigated rice: water management techniques*

Irrigated rice is typically grown in fields which are continuously flooded from transplanting to around one week before harvest. Providing a constant flow of water can increase rice productivity, not only because rice is a water-loving plant but also because water helps control competition from weeds. Unfortunately, this stable body of water, continuously present for at least 3–4 months (depending on variety), permits many cycles of mosquito vector breeding. Consequently, irrigated rice cultivation in many parts of the world (sub-Saharan Africa, Asia and South America) are associated with increased transmission of mosquito-borne diseases such as malaria, Japanese encephalitis, lymphatic filariasis and zoonotic arboviruses (Lacey and Lacey 1990). Whilst medical entomologists have been advocating alternative water management techniques such as intermittent irrigation to control vector proliferation, these techniques are often not taken up by farmers as they do not necessarily produce greater yields (Van der Hoek *et al.* 2001; Keiser *et al.* 2002). There are several exceptions, which include intermittent irrigation in Peru and China, both of which are model examples of co-benefits.

In north-western Peru, intermittent irrigation was applied to rice crops in four regions by the National Institute of Agrarian Innovation, under an agreement with the Ministry of Health (FAO). Although farmers were hesitant to change their practices at first, they were incentivised by the reflected 20–25% increase in crop yields and 26–57% water-saving capabilities (RTI International 2012). In terms of its health co-benefits, intermittent irrigation in rice was not only able to reduce malaria vector production by 70–93% but also reduced malaria transmission and the number of outbreaks (Chang 2007).

Irrespective of mosquito production, agronomists in conjunction with climate change scientists have also been developing water-saving technologies as water for agriculture is becoming increasingly scarce. Alternate wetting and drying irrigation (AWD) is another variation of intermittent irrigation which was implemented in numerous Asian countries including Vietnam, Bangladesh and Thailand. Its benefits are diverse: reduced greenhouse gas emissions, improved soil structure, greater yields, reduced environmental impact and increased farm efficiency (Allen and Sander 2019). Whilst their effects on mosquito production and VBD (namely Japanese encephalitis) transmission have not been explored, it is suspected that AWD can disrupt mosquito life cycles and hence reduce vector abundance in rice areas (Allen and Sander 2019).

System of rice intensification (SRI) is a package of management methods concerning soil, water and nutrients to increase the productivity of rice whilst saving water and seed requirements. As intermittent irrigation (or AWD, used interchangeably) is part of this package, SRI also has the potential to reduce vector densities in rice fields (Mati *et al.* 2021). Only one study has been conducted so far, in an irrigation scheme in Kenya, and observed that larvae were completely eliminated following two days of drying (Omwenga *et al.* 2014).

Another water management technique in rice cultivation which can potentially bring co-benefits is drip irrigation. By precisely watering plants or small planted areas directly, drip irrigation is highly effective in water productivity whilst reducing greenhouse gas emissions and other negative environmental effects such as groundwater pollution (Tas 2021). Without any standing water, mosquito vectors would not be able to develop.

By limiting mosquito development, these water management techniques (AWD, intermittent irrigation, SRI and drip irrigation) do not only mitigate problems in water scarcity but also malaria risk.

4.2 *Irrigated rice: nutrient management techniques*

Various studies have shown that the application of synthetic nitrogenous fertilisers in rice fields is associated with increased mosquito populations, possibly through increased nutrients for larval development or reducing water turbidity and hence increasing attractiveness for oviposition (Mutero *et al.* 2000, 2004; Victor and Reuben 2000). However, with very few exceptions, fertiliser application cannot be avoided; it is necessary to increase rice productivity. Whilst synthetic chemicals are primarily used, organic materials such as neem, *Azolla*, manure and biochar are viable options that may also provide climate co-benefits by reducing the amount of greenhouse gas emissions.

Recognising the necessity of fertilisers and their frequency and timing of application, Tanzanian malariologists tested combining fertiliser application with biolarvicides (*Bti*). This was highly effective in reducing mosquito larval densities (*An. gambiae* s.l. and *Cx. quinquefasciatus*), reaching up to 78.9% reduction (Mazigo *et al.* 2019b). This agricultural-VBD intervention provides co-benefits by improving rice grain output whilst reducing malaria transmission. Moreover, social science studies have revealed that willingness to contribute to and adopt this fertiliser-biolarvicide within their practices were high amongst farmers (Mazigo *et al.* 2019a).

Neem (or *Azadirachta indica*) is a natural extract that has many uses in a farming system: pest and insect control, animal feed, and fertilisers. Its insecticidal properties work indirectly, where it acts as an anti-feedant, repellent and egg-laying deterrent and eventually causes insects to starve to death (Benelli *et al.* 2015; Nicoletti *et al.* 2016). Neem cake is often used as an organic fertiliser by providing nitrogen and phosphorus. Given these co-beneficial properties, neem has been tested in rice fields for its efficacy against mosquito vectors and in enhancing grain yield. Laboratory trials have demonstrated that neem, including leaf extracts, are effective against malaria vectors, through repellence, oviposition deterrence, preventing adult emergence and reducing *Anopheles* survival (Vatandoost and Vaziri 2004; Nathan *et al.* 2005; Elsiddig 2007). In rice fields, neem cake powder enhanced grain yield, resulting in a greater number of productive tillers, plant height and grains per panicle, all whilst significantly reducing culicine mosquito vectors (Rao *et al.* 1995).

Like neem, mosquito fern (or *Azolla*) can have diverse benefits in a farming system too: as a biofertiliser, livestock feed and, sometimes, mosquito control. They occur naturally and in large quantities in rice fields. As an agricultural input, it is a source of green manure due to its symbiotic relationship with nitrogen-fixing cyanobacteria, and hence enhances the fertility of rice paddy soil. It has also been proposed as a way to promote carbon sequestration (Kollah *et al.* 2016). When grown into a thick carpet on the surface, *Azolla* can act as mosquito control by making it difficult for larvae to breathe and interfering with oviposition (IRRI 1988). In India, when *Azolla* covered more than 80% of the water surface, it was found to significantly reduce immature mosquito populations. Unfortunately, since such coverage can only be achieved two weeks after transplanting, its usefulness to control the early peak in vector production (in the 5–6 weeks following transplanting) is limited (Rajendran and Reuben 1991). However, because vector production is not restricted to the initial post-transplanting period, it can be useful during other rice-growing phases. At the farmer level, *Azolla* is beneficial as it keeps soil moist, reducing the labour and cost necessary for weeding and increasing grain yield by 9–14% at virtually no cost (Lines *et al.* 1992). However, *Azolla* can be labour intensive, where farmers may not have any economic advantage in choosing it over chemical fertilisers.

4.3 *Rice-fish/duck co-culture systems*

Fish provide a multitude of co-benefits when introduced to a rice system. They generate higher economic return by providing an additional source of income and minimising use of additional fertilisers, in turn increasing rice growth and yield. In some settings, they also generate fewer mosquito vectors. In a meta-analysis on malaria vector control in experimental rice fields, rice-fish co-culture reduced anopheline immatures by 82–87% (Chan *et al.* 2022a). Rice systems are not only limited to one species of fish; herbivorous fish have been released in combination with larvivorous fish to complement them by consuming aquatic weeds which would otherwise obstruct larvivorous fish movement. In one such study, this combination allowed 75–82% suppression of larvae, including the first 3–5 weeks after transplanting when peak mosquito production occurs. Nonetheless, more research is required to optimise using fish as vector control, as more than 100 fish species eat mosquito larvae, so species must be carefully selected for rice fields to ensure these co-benefits (Lacey and Lacey 1990).

Popular in China, rice-fish cultivation had increased from 11 provinces in the 1980s to 25 provinces by the 2000s. This expansion in rice-fish system use was not only correlated with a significant decrease in malaria vector abundance, but also in malaria incidence[1] (Zhao and Xue 2022). To our knowledge, rice-fish systems have only been trialled once in sub-Saharan Africa, in a study which found that *Tilapia* was effective not only as a food and protein source but also in suppressing *An. gambiae* s.l. by 88% (Bolay *et al.* 1990). Mosquito control using rice-fish co-culture in Californian rice fields were less evident, possibly due to the fish species and their feeding preferences (omnivorous or preference for predators)(Blaustein 1992; Kramer *et al.* 1987). Nonetheless, many studies saw a net profit in rice-fish systems over rice-only systems, up to 2.5 times (Victor *et al.* 1994).

Integrated rice-duck farming (IRDF) has been extensively explored in East Asian countries. Various studies have reported higher rice yields of 10–20% compared to traditional rice systems. Ducks did not only control weeds and insect pests very effectively, they also provided an additional source of income for farmers (Hossain *et al.* 2005; Pernollet *et al.* 2015). Moreover, climate change researchers had found that by significantly reducing methane emissions, IRDF can mitigate global warming potential (Xu *et al.* 2017). In China, ducks were also seen to forage on mosquito larvae, achieving 92–99% mosquito control (Zhao and Xue 2022). With this multitude of transectoral benefits (increased food security, climate change mitigation, income generation), the potential of IRDF as malaria vector control is worth further exploration, especially in African rice fields.

Nowadays, in China, other rice co-culture systems are being explored, such as combinations of rice with crab, crayfish, turtle, frog and/or shrimp.

4.4 *Wet-crop dry-crop rotation*

Practising crop rotation provides many benefits to a farmer, both economically and socially. It diversifies the array of crops or products, avoids build-up of resistance of insects, pathogens and weeds, and spreads labour demand, which allows equipment costs to reduce. Studies on the rotation of rice fields and dry-crop fields by alternating seasons and its effect on anopheline larvae have only been documented in China. The review by Zhao and Xue (2022) provide a summary of wet-crop dry-crop rotation, demonstrating its ability to increase crop productivity, whilst reducing vector breeding and hence malaria incidence. For example, Gao *et al.* found that biannual rotation of rice fields with dry fields (wheat or rapeseed) changed vector breeding sites significantly, reducing *An. lesteri* and *An. sinensis* densities around

1 Note that only associations were observed in these Chinese field trials, and confounding variables (such as other malaria interventions) were not necessarily accounted for.

93–100% (Zhao and Xue 2022). Another study found that vector breeding was also reduced when rice fields were left fallow throughout winter (Qunhua *et al.* 2004).

4.5 *Aquaculture in dams*

Whilst dams are crucial for agricultural and economic development, they can also increase the transmission of VBDs such as schistosomiasis. To promote co-benefits in equity, health, sustainable development and climate resilience, Lund *et al.* proposed several agricultural innovations based in sub-Saharan African dams (Lund *et al.* 2021). The first is the introduction of the African river prawn to target schistosomiasis-infected snails and thus reduce human disease prevalence. Despite requiring some adjustments such as infrastructure modification to accommodate prawn migration, this investment in aquaculture also leads to an additional source of income and protein for farmers. The authors also proposed transforming removed vegetation in dams and nearby canals into compost for crop production, livestock feed or biofuel. They emphasise that through sound ecological design and management, dams can play an important role not only in alleviating poverty and food insecurity but also VBD transmission (Hopkins *et al.* 2021).

5 Barriers to overcome

It is clear from the examples of the consequences of agriculture on VBD ecology that although they are always unintended, these consequences have important and often negative impacts on human health, especially for poor and marginalised groups. With the necessity for a global agricultural scale-up to feed our ever-growing population, there is strong potential for these unintended side-effects of VBD transmission to increase alongside it (Rohr *et al.* 2019). The main barriers to solving this issue is a lack of problem ownership and a lack of intersectoral collaboration which leaves the agricultural and health sectors disjointed (Hawkes and Ruel 2006a).

The issue of problem ownership persists and is a barrier to efforts to tackle this issue. Traditionally, the health sector bears the burden of tackling problems relating to infectious disease transmission. On the other hand, development within the agricultural sector tends to focus on economic benefits to production and, more recently with Sustainable Intensification, on mitigating negative impacts on the environment. However, as we have highlighted, agriculture plays a role in VBD transmission, and it is crucial for the agricultural sector to take its fair share of responsibility for the health problems it creates (Lines *et al.* 2020).

There have been numerous calls over the past three decades (Hawkes and Ruel 2006b; Lines *et al.* 2020; WHO *et al.* 1996) for these sectors to align and begin to work together to overcome this 'unavoidable' and 'unintentional' issue, by acknowledging its existence and developing methods to avoid it. This, however, remains a daunting task (Hawkes and Ruel 2006b) which will require concerted collaborative efforts and resources from both sides. Researchers are often taught to work within their research silos and to disseminate their findings to like-minded researchers who have been trained in the same methods. As a result, it can be difficult to bridge disciplines and to find a common language between sectors. To tackle this issue of VBD transmission being driven by aspects of agricultural development we need innovation and strong will to facilitate interdisciplinary discussion, research and planning between the agriculture and health sectors, and indeed the water sector too. Such intersectoral collaboration can, however, often be held up by financial constraints. Generally, health sectors do not generate their own revenue, whereas agricultural sectors do.

One way in which the agricultural sector can be held accountable for their role in creating health risks is to share revenue with Ministries of Health and institutions focused on researching the links and possible solutions to this agriculture and VBD issue. An example of intersectoral research with resources provided by the agricultural sector is the CGIAR (agricultural organisation) funded Agriculture and Infectious Disease Group at the London School of Hygiene and Tropical Medicine (https://www.lshtm.ac.uk/research/centres-projects-groups/agriculture-infectious-disease-group). This is a multidisciplinary group involving infectious disease researchers collaborating with CGIAR centres such as International Livestock Research Institute (ILRI), the International Food Policy Research Institute (IFPRI), the International Institute for Tropical Agriculture (IITA), and Africa Rice Center. Their research is focused on the side-effects of agriculture on infectious disease with projects running on VBD, neglected zoonotic diseases and antimicrobial resistance.

Such collaborations create an ideal environment for the development of innovative co-benefits which include human health or vector-borne disease transmission as an outcome. It is important for experts from each sector to engage in dialogue on the issue and develop solutions which benefit them both. This will require robust research firstly into the cause-effect nature of agricultural impacts on VBD transmission and secondly into field-trials for innovative agricultural methods which can minimise this 'cause' from practices in the future. It is important for organisations within the agricultural sector to foot the bill of such research. Whilst they are conducting regular research on and developing agricultural practices that improve crop yield, it is important for them to consider the impact that these new practices may have on VBDs. Similarly, it is important for researchers within the health sector to be flexible and adapt their methods to fit within the framework of agricultural research, to ensure the smooth integration and bridging of agricultural and public health disciplines. This bridging of disciplines is not only required at the level of research communities, but also when it comes to funding: donor communities need to create more opportunities and prioritise these intersectoral issues.

Box 1: Priority actions for the health sector to overcome barriers and develop co-benefit solutions to agriculture-VBD issue

- Develop capacity for dialogue and common research language with agricultural sector
- Lead robust studies into the cause-effect of impacts of agriculture on VBD transmission
- Adapt research methods to integrate within agricultural field trials

Box 2: Priority actions for the agricultural sector to overcome barriers and develop co-benefit solutions to agriculture-VBD issue

- Develop capacity for dialogue and common research language with health sector
- Provide expertise on agricultural research methodologies to facilitate integration of health research into trials
- Fund agricultural research projects which prioritise health outcomes linked to vector-borne disease

6 Conclusions

In order to feed the world's growing population, an increase in food production alongside policies to enhance food access are necessary. With expansion in agricultural development therefore an inevitable part of this strategy, it is imperative that the linked issue of agriculture increasing VBD transmission is acknowledged and tackled. It is clear that we need intersectoral work which bridges the two most involved disciplines of health and agriculture to begin to tackle this issue. This will involve disentangling the cause-effect relationships between the environmental drivers and VBD transmission, and facing issues such as the movement of vulnerable or infected populations. We need a co-benefits approach to find solutions which provide attractive outcomes for both sectors in order for them to be taken up and utilised as agriculture continues to develop. This will require concerted efforts by both sides to enable dialogue, sharing of resources and knowledge to develop innovative solutions, and to lead strong and robust research and field trials. We have seen that this is possible with the development and widespread uptake of Sustainable Intensification to mitigate agricultural impacts on the climate and the environment. This is promising and encourages the belief that agriculture can too be adapted to mitigate negative impacts on human health.

Acknowledgements

This work was partially funded by, and is a contribution to, the CGIAR Research Program on Agriculture for Nutrition and Health (A4NH). The opinions expressed here belong to the authors, and do not necessarily reflect those of A4NH or CGIAR. KC was supported by the Wellcome Trust's Our Planet Our Health programme (grant number 216098/Z/19/Z), and IB was funded by the Bill and Melinda Gates Foundation (OPP# 1177272). We would like to thank the editors and reviewers for their feedback.

References

Ahrends A, Hollingsworth PM, Ziegler AD, Fox JM, Chen H, Su Y and Xu J (2015) Current trends of rubber plantation expansion may threaten biodiversity and livelihoods. Global Environmental Change 34: 48–58. https://doi.org/10.1016/j.gloenvcha.2015.06.002.

Alexandratos N and Bruinsma J (2012) World agriculture towards 2030/2050: the 2012 revision. FAO, Rome, Italy, 147 pp. https://doi.org/10.22004/ag.econ.288998.

Allen J and Sander BO (2019). The diverse benefits of alternate wetting and drying (AWD). International Rice Research Institute (IRRI), Los Baños, Philippines. Available at: https://hdl.handle.net/10568/101399.

Amerasinghe F and Indrajith N (1994) Postirrigation breeding patterns of surface water mosquitoes in the Mahaweli Project, Sri Lanka, and comparisons with preceding developmental phases. Journal of Medical Entomology 31: 516–523.

Amerasinghe FP and Ariyasena TG (1991) Survey of adult mosquitoes (Diptera: Culicidae) during irrigation development in the Mahaweli project, Sri Lanka. Journal of Medical Entomology 28: 387–393. 10.1093/jmedent/28.3.387.

Bardosh KL, Ryan SJ, Ebi K, Welburn S and Singer B (2017) Addressing vulnerability, building resilience: community-based adaptation to vector-borne diseases in the context of global change. Infectious Diseases of Poverty 6: 1–21.

Bartholomé E and Belward AS (2005) GLC2000: a new approach to global land cover mapping from Earth observation data. International Journal of Remote Sensing 26: 1959–1977. https://doi.org/10.1080/01431160412331291297.

Benelli G, Murugan K, Panneerselvam C, Madhiyazhagan P, Conti B and Nicoletti M (2015) Old ingredients for a new recipe? Neem cake, a low-cost botanical by-product in the fight against mosquito-borne diseases. Parasitology Research 114: 391–397.

Bhumiratana A, Intarapuk A, Sorosjinda-Nunthawarasilp P, Maneekan P and Koyadun S (2013) Border malaria associated with multidrug resistance on Thailand-Myanmar and Thailand-Cambodia borders: transmission dynamic, vulnerability, and surveillance. Biomed Research International 2013: 363417. https://doi.org/10.1155/2013/363417.

Blas E and Kurup AS (2010) Equity, social determinants and public health programmes. World Health Organization.

Blaustein L (1992) Larvivorous fishes fail to control mosquitoes in experimental rice plots. Hydrobiologia 232: 219–232.

Bolay FK, Trpis M, Davidson E, Faust R, Margalit J and Tahori A (1990) Control of mosquitoes with *Bacillus thuringiensis* var. *israelensis* and larvivorous fish, *Tilapia nilotica*, in rice fields in Liberia, West Africa. Israel J Entomol 23: 77–82.

Boserup E (1965) The conditions of agricultural growth: the economics of agrarin change under population pressure. Allen & Unwin, London, UK.

Brant TA, Okorie PN, Ogunmola O, Ojeyode NB, Fatunade S, Davies E, Saka Y, Stanton MC, Molyneux DH and Stothard JR (2018) Integrated risk mapping and landscape characterisation of lymphatic filariasis and loiasis in South West Nigeria. Parasite Epidemiology and Control 3: 21–35.

Burkett-Cadena ND and Vittor AY (2018) Deforestation and vector-borne disease: forest conversion favors important mosquito vectors of human pathogens. Basic and applied ecology 26: 101–110.

Byrne I, Aure W, Manin BO, Vythilingam I, Ferguson HM, Drakeley CJ, Chua TH and Fornace KM (2021) Environmental and spatial risk factors for the larval habitats of *Plasmodium knowlesi* vectors in Sabah, Malaysian Borneo. Scientific Reports 11: 11. https://doi.org/10.1038/s41598-021-90893-1.

Chan K, Bottomley C, Saito K, Lines J and Tusting LS (2022a) The control of malaria vectors in rice fields: a systematic review and meta-analysis. Scientific Reports 12: 17. https://doi.org/10.1038/s41598-022-24055-2.

Chan K, Tusting LS, Bottomley C, Saito K, Djouaka R and Lines J (2022b) Malaria transmission and prevalence in rice-growing versus non-rice-growing villages in Africa: a systematic review and meta-analysis. Lancet Planetary Health 6: E257–E269.

Chang J (2007). Intermittent rice irrigation (IRI) for malaria control in Peru: a win-win intervention based on a multi-sector and trans-disciplinary approach. Available at: https://www.linksglobal.org/AMI/extras/Manuscript3.IntermittentRiceIrrigation.FINAL.100511.pdf.

Crumpler K and Meybeck A (2020) Adaptation in the agriculture sectors: leveraging co-benefits for mitigation and sustainable development. FAO, Rome, Italy. https://doi.org/10.13140/RG.2.2.35243.87842.

Duker AA and Kwarteng EVS (2021) Lymphatic filariasis: a snap shot of a neglected tropical disease. International Journal of Community Medicine and Public Health 8: 3611–3617. https://doi.org/10.18203/2394-6040.ijcmph20212625.

Elsiddig F (2007) Effect of neem, cafure and rehan organic extracts compared to other chemical and biological standard insecticides on *Anopheles arabiensis* patton mosquito, Sudan University of Science & Technology.

Ferguson HM, Dornhaus A, Beeche A, Borgemeister C, Gottlieb M, Mulla MS, Gimnig JE, Fish D and Killeen GF (2010) Ecology: a prerequisite for malaria elimination and eradication. PLoS Medicine 7: e1000303.

Foley JA, DeFries R, Asner GP, Barford C, Bonan G, Carpenter SR, Chapin FS, Coe MT, Daily GC and Gibbs HK (2005) Global consequences of land use. Science 309: 570–574.

Food and Agriculture Organization (FAO) (2002). How to feed the world in 2050. Food and Agriculture Organization, Rome, Italy.

Food and Agriculture Organisation (FAO) (2022) FRA 2020 remote sensing survey. FAO Forestry Paper:186. FAO, Rome, Italy. https://doi.org/10.4060/cb9970en.

Fornace KM, Abidin TR, Alexander N, Brock P, Grigg MJ, Murphy A, William T, Menon J, Drakeley CJ and Cox J (2016) Association between landscape factors and spatial patterns of *Plasmodium knowlesi* infections in Sabah, Malaysia. Emerging Infectious Diseases 22: 201–208. https://doi.org/10.3201/eid2202.150656.

Fornace KM, Alexander N, Abidin TR, Brock PM, Chua TH, Vythilingam I, Ferguson HM, Manin BO, Wong ML, Ng SH, Cox J and Drakeley C (2019a) Local human movement patterns and land use impact exposure to zoonotic malaria in Malaysian Borneo. Elife 8: 17. https://doi.org/10.7554/eLife.47602.

Fornace KM, Brock PM, Abidin TR, Grignard L, Herman LS, Chua TH, Daim S, William T, Patterson C, Hall T, Grigg MJ, Anstey NM, Tetteh KKA, Cox J and Drakeley CJ (2019b) Environmental risk factors and exposure to the zoonotic malaria parasite *Plasmodium knowlesi* across northern Sabah, Malaysia: a population-based cross-sectional survey. Lancet Planetary Health 3: E179–E186. https://doi.org/10.1016/s2542-5196(19)30045-2.

Fornace KM, Diaz AV, Lines J and Drakeley CJ (2021) Achieving global malaria eradication in changing landscapes. Malaria Journal 20: 14. https://doi.org/10.1186/s12936-021-03599-0.

Frison EA (2016). From uniformity to diversity: a paradigm shift from industrial agriculture to diversified agroecological systems. Available at: https://www.ipes-food.org/_img/upload/files/UniformityToDiversity_FULL.pdf.

Guerra C, Snow R and Hay S (2006) A global assessment of closed forests, deforestation and malaria risk. Annals of Tropical Medicine and Parasitology 100: 189.

Haileselassie W, Zemene E, Lee MC, Zhong D, Zhou G, Taye B, Dagne A, Deressa W, Kazura JW and Yan G (2021) The effect of irrigation on malaria vector bionomics and transmission intensity in western Ethiopia. Parasites & Vectors 14: 1–11.

Hawkes C and Ruel M (2006a) The links between agriculture and health: an intersectoral opportunity to improve the health and livelihoods of the poor. Bulletin of the World Health Organization 84: 984–990.

Hawkes C and Ruel MT (2006b) Understanding the links between agriculture and health. International Food Policy Research Institute Washington, DC, USA.

Hopkins SR, Sokolow SH, Buck JC, De Leo GA, Jones IJ, Kwong LH, LeBoa C, Lund AJ, MacDonald AJ and Nova N (2021) How to identify win-win interventions that benefit human health and conservation. Nature sustainability 4: 298–304.

Hossain ST, Sugimoto H, Ahmed GJU and Islam M (2005). Effect of integrated rice-duck farming on rice yield, farm productivity, and rice-provisioning ability of farmers. Asian Journal of Agriculture and Development 2: 79–86.

Husnina Z, Clements AC and Wangdi K (2019). Forest cover and climate as potential drivers for dengue fever in Sumatra and Kalimantan 2006–2016: a spatiotemporal analysis. Tropical Medicine & International Health 24: 888–898.

Ijumba J and Lindsay S (2001) Impact of irrigation on malaria in Africa: paddies paradox. Medical and Veterinary Entomology 15: 1–11.

International Rice Research Institute (IRRI) (1988) Vector-borne disease control in humans through rice agroecosystem management: Proceedings of the Workshop on Research and Training Needs in the Field of integrated vector-borne disease control in riceland agroecosystems of developing countries. 9–14 March 1987, Manila, Philippines.

Janko MM, Irish SR, Reich BJ, Peterson M, Doctor SM, Mwandagalirwa MK, Likwela JL, Tshefu AK, Meshnick SR and Emch ME (2018) The links between agriculture, *Anopheles* mosquitoes, and malaria risk in children younger than 5 years in the Democratic Republic of the Congo: a population-based, cross-sectional, spatial study. The Lancet Planetary Health 2: e74–e82.

Jomon K and Valamparampil T (2014) Medically important mosquitoes in the rubber plantation belt of central Kerala, India. Southeast Asian Journal of Tropical Medicine and Public Health 45: 796.

Jones BA, Grace D, Kock R, Alonso S, Rushton J, Said MY, McKeever D, Mutua F, Young J and McDermott J (2013) Zoonosis emergence linked to agricultural intensification and environmental change. Proceedings of the national academy of sciences 110: 8399–8404.

Kalbus A, de Souza Sampaio V, Boenecke J and Reintjes R (2021). Exploring the influence of deforestation on dengue fever incidence in the Brazilian Amazonas state. Plos One 16: e0242685.

Keiser J, Utzinger J and Singer BH (2002). The potential of intermittent irrigation for increasing rice yields, lowering water consumption, reducing methane emissions, and controlling malaria in African rice fields. Journal of the American Mosquito Control Association 18: 329–340.

Kim DS, Acharya D, Lee K, Yoo SJ, Park JH and Lim HS (2018) Awareness and work-related factors associated with scrub typhus: a case-control study from South Korea. International Journal of Environmental Research and Public Health 15: 1143.

Kloos H (1990) Health aspects of resettlement in Ethiopia. Social Science & Medicine 30: 643–656.

Kollah B, Patra AK and Mohanty SR (2016) Aquatic microphylla *Azolla*: a perspective paradigm for sustainable agriculture, environment and global climate change. Environmental Science and Pollution Research 23: 4358–4369.

Kramer VL, Garcia R and Colwell A (1987) An evaluation of the mosquitofish, *Gambusia affinis*, and the inland silverside, *Menida beryllina*, as mosquito control agents in California wild rice fields. Journal of the American Mosquito Control Association 3(4): 626–632.

Kumar NP, Suresh A, Vanamail P, Sabesan S, Krishnamoorthy KG, Mathew J, Jose VT and Jambulingam P (2011) Chikungunya virus outbreak in Kerala, India, 2007: a seroprevalence study. Memorias Do Instituto Oswaldo Cruz 106: 912–916.

Lacey LA and Lacey CM (1990) The medical importance of riceland mosquitoes and their control using alternatives to chemical insecticides. Journal of the American Mosquito Control Association. Supplement 2: 1–93.

Lines J, Bett B, Fèvre E, Moodley A and Waage J (2020) Mitigating health risks in sustainable agricultural intensification. International Food Policy Research Institute, Washington, DC, USA.

Lines J, Nicholson E, Haji H, Yusuf S, Juma M, Dunn D and Msimbe M (1992) The effects of *Azolla* on *Anopheles gambiae s.l.* in ricefields in Zanzibar. Parasit Vectors 4: 110. https://doi.org/10.1186/1756-3305-4-110.

Lund AJ, Lopez-Carr D, Sokolow SH, Rohr JR and De Leo GA (2021) Agricultural innovations to reduce the health impacts of dams. Sustainability 13: 1869.

Ma CJ, Oh GJ, Kang GU, Lee JM, Lee DU, Nam HS, Ryu SY and Lee YH, 2017. Differences in agricultural activities related to incidence of scrub typhus between Korea and Japan. Epidemiology and Health 39: e2017051. https://doi.org/10.4178/epih.e2017051.

Martens P and Hall L (2000). Malaria on the move: human population movement and malaria transmission. Emerging Infectious Diseases 6: 103.

Mati B, Nyangau W, Ndiiri J and Wanjogu R (2021) Enhancing production while saving water through the system of rice intensification (sri) in Kenya's irrigation schemes. Journal of Agriculture, Science and Technology 20: 24–40.

Mayrhofer JP and Gupta J (2016) The science and politics of co-benefits in climate policy. Environmental Science & Policy 57: 22–30.

Mazigo HD, Massawe IS, Rumisha SF, Kweka EJ and Mboera LE (2019a) Rice farmers' perceptions and acceptability in the use of a combination of biolarvicide (*Bacillus thuringiensis* var. *israeliensis*) and fertilizers application for malaria control and increase rice productivity in a rural district of central Tanzania. Malaria Journal 18: 1–11.

Mazigo HD, Mboera LE, Rumisha SF and Kweka EJ (2019b) Malaria mosquito control in rice paddy farms using biolarvicide mixed with fertilizer in Tanzania: semi-field experiments. Malaria Journal 18: 1–10.

Min KD, Lee JY, So Y and Cho SI (2019) Deforestation increases the risk of scrub typhus in Korea. International Journal of Environmental Research and Public Health 16: 1518.

Morand S and Lajaunie C (2021) Outbreaks of vector-borne and zoonotic diseases are associated with changes in forest cover and oil palm expansion at global scale. Frontiers in veterinary science: 230.

Mutero CM (2002). Health impact assessment of increased irrigation in the Tana River Basin, Kenya. The changing face of irrigation in Kenya: opportunities for anticipating change in eastern and southern Africa: 211–229.

Mutero CM, Blank H, Konradsen F and Van Der Hoek W (2000) Water management for controlling the breeding of *Anopheles* mosquitoes in rice irrigation schemes in Kenya. Acta Tropica 76: 253–263.

Mutero CM, McCartney M and Boelee E (2006). Agriculture, malaria, and water-associated diseases: understanding the links between agriculture and health, International Food Policy Research Institute (IFPRI), Washington, DC, USA.

Mutero CM, Wekoyela P, Githure J and Konradsen F (2004) Ammonium sulphate fertiliser increases larval populations of *Anopheles arabiensis* and culicine mosquitoes in rice fields. Acta Tropica 89: 187–192.

Nakhapakorn K and Tripathi NK (2005) An information value based analysis of physical and climatic factors affecting dengue fever and dengue haemorrhagic fever incidence. International Journal of Health Geographics 4: 1–13.

Nathan SS, Kalaivani K and Murugan K (2005). Effects of neem limonoids on the malaria vector *Anopheles stephensi* Liston (Diptera: Culicidae). Acta Tropica 96: 47–55.

Nicoletti M, Murugan K, Canale A and Benelli G 2016. Neem-borne molecules as eco-friendly control tools against mosquito vectors of economic importance. Current Organic Chemistry 20: 2681–2689.

Norris DE (2004) Mosquito-borne diseases as a consequence of land use change. Ecohealth 1: 19–24.

Omwenga KG, Mati BM and Home PG (2014). Determination of the effect of the system of rice intensification (SRI) on rice yields and water saving in Mwea irrigation scheme, Kenya. Journal of Water Resource and protection 2014.

Packard RM (1986) Agricultural development, migrant labor and the resurgence of malaria in Swaziland. Social Science & Medicine 22: 861–867.

Patz JA, Graczyk TK, Geller N and Vittor AY (2000). Effects of environmental change on emerging parasitic diseases. International Journal for Parasitology 30: 1395–1405.

Pernollet CA, Simpson D, Gauthier-Clerc M and Guillemain M (2015). Rice and duck, a good combination? Identifying the incentives and triggers for joint rice farming and wild duck conservation. Agriculture, Ecosystems & Environment 214: 118–132.

Prothero RM (2001). Migration and malaria risk. Health, Risk & Society 3: 19–38.

Qunhua L, Xin K, Changzhi C, Shengzheng F, Yan L, Rongzhi H, Zhihua Z, Gibson G and Wenmin K (2004) New irrigation methods sustain malaria control in Sichuan Province, China. Acta Tropica 89: 241–247.

Rajendran R and Reuben R (1991). Evaluation of the water fern *Azolla microphylla* for mosquito population management in the rice-land agro-ecosystem of south India. Medical and Veterinary Entomology 5: 299–310.

Rao D, Reuben R and Nagasampagi B (1995) Development of combined use of neem (*Azadirachta indica*) and water management for the control of culicine mosquitoes in rice fields. Medical and Veterinary Entomology 9: 25–33.

Rohr JR, Barrett CB, Civitello DJ, Craft ME, Delius B, DeLeo GA, Hudson PJ, Jouanard N, Nguyen KH and Ostfeld RS (2019) Emerging human infectious diseases and the links to global food production. Nature sustainability 2: 445–456.

RTI International (2012). Peru vector control needs assessment report – integrated vector management (IVM) Task Order 2 USAID PMI.

Salah AB, Ismail RB, Amri F, Chlif S, Rzig FB, Kharrat H, Hadhri H, Hassouna M and Dellagi K (2000) Investigation of the spread of human visceral leishmaniasis in central Tunisia. Transactions of the Royal Society of Tropical Medicine and Hygiene 94: 382–386.

Shah HA, Huxley P, Elmes J and Murray KA (2019) Agricultural land-uses consistently exacerbate infectious disease risks in Southeast Asia. Nature Communications 10: 4299.

Stark DJ, Fornace KM, Brock PM, Abidin TR, Gilhooly L, Jalius C, Goossens B, Drakeley CJ and Salgado-Lynn M (2019) Long-tailed macaque response to deforestation in a *Plasmodium knowlesi*-endemic area. Ecohealth 16: 638–646.

Sulaiman S and Jeffery J (1986) The ecology of *Aedes albopictus* (Skuse)(Diptera: Culicidae) in a rubber estate in Malaysia. Bulletin of Entomological Research 76: 553–557.

Tangena JAA, Thammavong P, Wilson AL, Brey PT and Lindsay SW (2016). Risk and control of mosquito-borne diseases in Southeast Asian rubber plantations. Trends in parasitology 32: 402–415.

Tas I (2021). Production cost and water savings of paddy produced by drip irrigation. Current Trends in Natural Sciences 10: 151–165.

Taylor C, Florey L and Ye Y (2017) Equity trends in ownership of insecticide-treated nets in 19 sub-Saharan African countries. Bulletin of the World Health Organization 95: 322.

Tejedor-Garavito N, Dlamini N, Pindolia D, Soble A, Ruktanonchai NW, Alegana V, Le Menach A, Ntshalintshali N, Dlamini B and Smith DL (2017) Travel patterns and demographic characteristics of malaria cases in Swaziland, 2010–2014. Malaria Journal 16: 1–18.

Tyagi B and Chaudhary R (1997) Outbreak of *falciparum* malaria in the Thar Desert (India), with particular emphasis on physiographic changes brought about by extensive canalization and their impact on vector density and dissemination. Journal of Arid Environments 36: 541–555.

Van Der Hoek W, Sakthivadivel R, Renshaw M, Silver JB, Birley MH and Konradsen F (2001) Alternate wet/dry irrigation in rice cultivation: a practical way to save water and control malaria and Japanese encephalitis? International Water Management Institute (IWMI), Colombo, Sri Lanka, 30 pp. https://doi.org/10.3910/2009.053.

Vatandoost H and Vaziri V (2004). Larvicidal activity of a neem tree extract [Neemarin] against mosquito larvae in the Islamic Republic of Iran. EMHJ-Eastern Mediterranean Health Journal 10(4–5): 573–581.

Victor T, Chandrasekaran B and Reuben R (1994) Composite fish culture for mosquito control in rice fields in southern India. The Southeast Asian Journal of Tropical Medicine and Public Health 25: 522–527.

Victor T and Reuben R (2000) Effects of organic and inorganic fertilisers on mosquito populations in rice fields of southern India. Medical and Veterinary Entomology 14: 361–368.

Wangroongsarb P, Sudathip P and Satimai W (2012) Characteristics and malaria prevalence of migrant populations in malaria-endemic areas along the Thai-Cambodian border. Southeast Asian J Trop Med Public Health 43: 261–269.

Wezel A, Soboksa G, McClelland S, Delespesse F and Boissau A (2015) The blurred boundaries of ecological, sustainable, and agroecological intensification: a review. Agronomy for Sustainable Development 35: 1283–1295.

WHO/FAO/UNEP/UNCHS Panel of Experts on Environmental Management for Vector Control & World Health Organization (1996) Agricultural development and vector-borne diseases: training and information materials on vector biology and control in the VBC slide set series. World Health Organization, Geneva, Switzerland.

Wilson AL, Courtenay O, Kelly-Hope LA, Scott TW, Takken W, Torr SJ and Lindsay SW (2020) The importance of vector control for the control and elimination of vector-borne diseases. Plos Neglected Tropical Diseases 14: e0007831.

World Bank (2022) The World Bank open data catalog – agricultural land (% of land area). Available at: https://data.worldbank.org/indicator/AG.LND.AGRI.ZS.

Xu G, Liu X, Wang Q, Yu X and Hang Y (2017). Integrated rice-duck farming mitigates the global warming potential in rice season. Science of the Total Environment 575: 58–66.

Yasuoka J and Levins R (2007) Impact of deforestation and agricultural development on anopheline ecology and malaria epidemiology. The American Journal of Tropical Medicine and Hygiene 76: 450–460.

Zahouli JB, Koudou BG, Müller P, Malone D, Tano Y and Utzinger J (2017) Effect of land-use changes on the abundance, distribution, and host-seeking behavior of *Aedes* arbovirus vectors in oil palm-dominated landscapes, southeastern Côte d'Ivoire. Plos One 12: e0189082.

Zhao, T.-Y. and Xue, R.-D., 2022. Integrated mosquito management in rice field in China. Wetlands Ecology and Management 30: 963–973. https://doi.org/10.1007/s11273-021-09840-6.

PART 3

VBD surveillance and control in changing environments

CHAPTER 10

Modelling the effects of climate and climate change on transmission of vector-borne disease

Marta S. Shocket[1*], *Jamie M. Caldwell*[2], *Paul J. Huxley*[3], *Catherine A. Lippi*[1,4], *Francis A. Windram*[5] and *Alexander C. Keyel*[6,7]

[1]Department of Geography, University of Florida, 3141 Turlington Hall, 330 Newell Dr, Gainesville, FL 32611, USA; [2]High Meadows Environmental Institute, Princeton University, Guyot Hall, Princeton, NJ 08540, USA; [3]Department of Statistics, Virginia Polytechnic and State University, 250 Drillfield Drive, Blacksburg, VA 24061, USA; [4]Emerging Pathogens Institute, University of Florida, P.O. Box 100009, 2055 Mowry Road, Gainesville, FL 32610, USA; [5]Department of Life Sciences, Imperial College London, Silwood Park, Buckhurst Road, Ascot, Berkshire, SL5 7PY, UK; [6]Department Division of Infectious Diseases, Wadsworth Center, New York State Department of Health, 120 New Scotland Road, Albany, NY 12208, USA; [7]Department of Atmospheric and Environmental Sciences, University at Albany, 1400 Washington Ave, Albany, NY 12222, USA; *marta.shocket@gmail.com

Abstract

Mathematical and statistical models are critical tools for both understanding how climate can influence patterns of vector-borne disease transmission, and predicting how climate change might affect these patterns in the future. This chapter focuses primarily on quantitative approaches for modelling the effects of climate on mosquito-borne disease (MBD), although we also briefly consider tick-borne disease. We initially describe how the biological mechanisms that contribute to transmission of vector-borne disease can respond to changes in climate and other environmental factors. Importantly, transmission of MBD responds nonlinearly over gradients of both temperature and rainfall. When building or interpreting models for the effects of climate on MBD dynamics, it is important to consider that the effects of temperature and rainfall on disease may be positive, negative, or both depending on circumstance. This context-dependence can limit the transferability of models beyond the setting in which they were fit. Next, we provide an overview of important concepts and approaches for modelling vector-borne diseases using mechanistic and statistical models. This includes the most commonly used modelling methods, techniques for model evaluation and validation, and climate re-analysis products used as model predictors.

 | DOI:10.3920/9789004688650_012

The best choices of methods for model construction and evaluation depend on the goals of the model and the structure of the underlying data, including their spatial and temporal scales. Then, we explore three case studies of MBD in more detail and use them to illustrate representative modelling approaches across a gradient of spatiotemporal scales: (1) local time series models of dengue fever in San Juan, Puerto Rico; (2) regional models of West Nile virus in the United States; and (3) continental and global models for how climate change may impact future transmission risk for malaria and dengue fever. Finally, we note some key challenges, knowledge gaps, and research frontiers for modelling climate and MBD.

Keywords

dengue – malaria – mosquito-borne disease – rainfall – temperature – tick-borne disease – West Nile virus

1 Introduction

Mathematical and statistical models are critical tools for understanding how climate can influence patterns of vector-borne disease transmission, and predicting how climate change might affect these patterns in the future. This chapter focuses primarily on quantitative approaches for modelling the effects of climate on mosquito-borne disease (MBD). We start by describing how biological mechanisms that contribute to transmission of vector-borne disease can respond to changes in climate and other environmental factors. Next, we provide an overview of important concepts and approaches for modelling vector-borne diseases. Then, we explore three case studies of MBD in more detail and use them to illustrate representative modelling approaches across a gradient of spatiotemporal scales: (1) local time series models of dengue fever in San Juan, Puerto Rico; (2) regional models of West Nile virus in the United States; and (3) continental and global models for how climate change may impact future transmission risk for malaria and dengue fever. Finally, we note some key challenges, knowledge gaps, and research frontiers for modelling climate and MBD.

Additionally, we briefly discuss tick-borne disease (TBD) at several points in the chapter. In the section on biological mechanisms for transmission, we summarise key differences between mosquitoes and ticks as disease vectors. In the modelling overview section, we describe how these biological features influence the mechanistic modelling approaches used for tick-borne disease. After the case studies, we summarise major conclusions from models investigating the impacts of climate change on tick-borne disease.

2 Biological mechanisms for climate drivers of vector-borne disease

Temperature, rainfall, humidity, and other environmental factors can strongly affect the physiology and life history traits (e.g. development, survival, and reproduction) of small ectothermic animals like mosquitoes and other arthropod disease vectors. These individual-level effects can propagate through the system to dramatically affect the extent to which vector populations transmit pathogens to their vertebrate hosts. In this section, we describe some key biological mechanisms that determine how climatic factors can impact transmission of vector-borne disease. We also describe how interactions between climatic and non-climatic factors (e.g. human behaviour, host immunity and resource competition) can affect risk of vector-borne disease transmission.

2.1 *Pathogen transmission*

Vector-borne pathogens are usually transmitted when: (1) an uninfected vector bites an infected host to acquire the pathogen; (2) the vector survives long enough for the pathogen to complete the relevant portion of its life cycle and migrate to the salivary glands (making the vector infectious); and (3) the vector bites a new uninfected, susceptible host to pass on the pathogen. Infected hosts typically remain infectious to vectors for a limited amount of time before they recover from their infection. Recovered hosts often gain short-term or long-term immunity to future infections. Some pathogens are maintained primarily by transmission cycles between vectors and humans (e.g. dengue virus, *Plasmodium falciparum* malaria), while others are maintained primarily within vertebrate reservoir host populations and only occasionally spillover to infect humans (e.g. West Nile virus). Some pathogens are associated with multiple types of transmission cycles. For example, yellow fever virus can have sylvatic (i.e. based in forest-dwelling wildlife), urban (human-based), or intermediate patterns of transmission.

Some vector-borne diseases can be transmitted in other ways besides a bite from an infectious vector. For example, Zika virus can also be transmitted sexually between humans (Gao *et al.* 2016), and the transmission of mosquito and tick-borne pathogens via blood transfusion is an important health concern on every inhabited continent (Owusu-Ofori *et al.* 2010; Pantanowitz *et al.* 2002; Petersen and Busch 2010; Pisani *et al.* 2016; Tambyah *et al.* 2008). West Nile virus can be transmitted directly between bird reservoir hosts (Komar *et al.* 2003), which may be particularly important for pathogen maintenance over the winter when mosquitoes are not active (Montecino-Latorre and Barker 2018). Rift Valley fever virus is most often transmitted to humans by direct contact with livestock that were infected by bites from infectious mosquitoes (Sang *et al.* 2017). Additionally, many vector-borne pathogens can be transmitted vertically between arthropod adults and their offspring

(Adams and Boots 2010; Ciota *et al.* 2017). Although such different modes of transmission can be important, in this chapter we focus on the horizontal transmission that comprises the vast majority of mosquito-borne infections in humans and is the foundation of most models for MBD.

2.2 *Temperature*

Arthropod vectors and their pathogens are ectothermic organisms whose body temperature depends on the surrounding environment. Accordingly, they are extremely sensitive to the environmental temperature, which is a strong driver of nearly all of the organism-level traits that are relevant to vector population abundance and pathogen transmission: the vector population growth rate, death rate, and biting rate; and the pathogen development rate (which determines the extrinsic incubation period) and probability of successfully making the vector infectious (Eikenberry and Gumel 2018; Mordecai *et al.* 2019). More specifically, these traits typically respond to temperature in a nonlinear, unimodal way: first they increase with temperature up to a peak value, and then decrease if temperature rises further (Dell *et al.* 2011; Mordecai *et al.* 2019). This general pattern for the thermal responses of traits is predicted to scale up and also describe the thermal response for mosquito population abundance and the transmission of MBD (Figure 1A) (Mordecai *et al.* 2019; Shocket *et al.* 2018). The increasing portion of the thermal response for transmission (left side of Figure 1A) is largely driven by enhanced mosquito survival at all life stages and faster development of juvenile mosquitoes and pathogens, while the decreasing portion (right side of Figure 1A) is largely driven by declining adult survival (Mordecai *et al.* 2019). The specific temperature that maximises transmission varies across different mosquito-pathogen systems, but generally falls between 22–30 °C (Mordecai *et al.* 2019). These intermediate optima for transmission – a 'Goldilocks' thermal zone that, like the classic fairy tale, is not too cold or too hot, but just right – suggest that ongoing warming from climate change will lead to shifts in transmission patterns of MBD. Locations and times of year that are currently optimal for transmission could become too warm and see declining disease, while locations and times of year that are currently too cool will likely move closer to the optimum and see increasing disease.

The basic thermal response framework described above (and illustrated in Figure 1A) assumes that the vector and pathogen traits that contribute to transmission (e.g. birth, death, development, biting, and transmission rates) depend on mean temperatures over relatively short time scales. However, aspects of temperature beyond the mean can also affect transmission of MBD. Fluctuating temperatures can yield outcomes that differ substantially from constant temperatures with the same mean (Bernhardt *et al.* 2018; Ruel and Ayres 1999). For MBD transmission, daily temperature variation can be particularly important (Boser *et al.* 2021; Lambrechts *et al.* 2011). In general, fluctuations increase performance

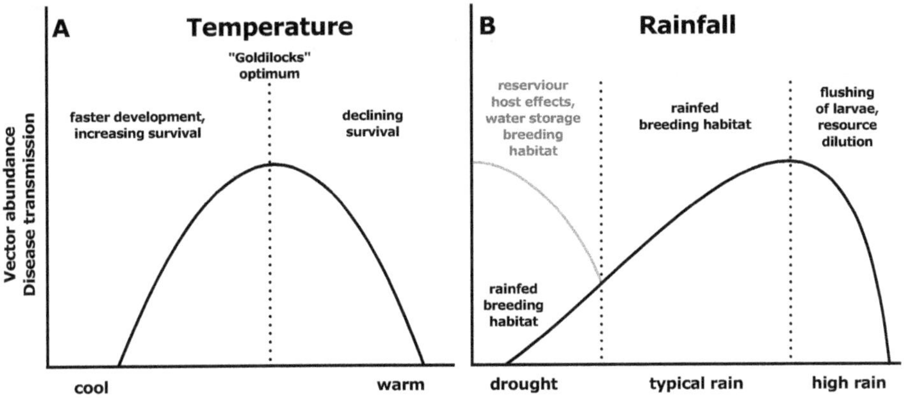

FIGURE 1 Vector abundance and transmission of mosquito-borne disease respond nonlinearly to both temperature and rainfall. (A) The thermal responses for vector abundance and disease transmission increase at first (left of dotted line), largely driven by enhanced mosquito survival and faster development of mosquito larvae and pathogens. After reaching the optimal 'Goldilocks' value at an intermediate temperature, they decrease (right of dotted line), largely driven by declining mosquito survival. The general shape of the thermal response for mosquito-borne disease is consistent, but the specific temperatures of the optimum and thermal limits vary between vector-pathogen systems. (B) Vector abundance and disease transmission often respond positively to rainfall, which increases the availability of rainfed breeding habitat (black line, left and middle section). However, high levels of rain can sometimes flush larvae out or dilute food resources, lowering vector abundance and transmission (right section). Additionally, some vector-pathogen systems show increases in transmission in drought conditions (grey line), either due to increased breeding habitat in water storage containers (dengue virus and other *Aedes aegypti*-transmitted arboviruses) or changes in reservoir hosts (West Nile virus). Thus, the response of mosquito-borne disease to rainfall is less consistent than its response the temperature, both between vector-pathogen systems and in different locations.

when mean temperatures are cooler and decrease performance when mean temperatures are near the optimum or warmer (Beck-Johnson *et al.* 2017; Lambrechts *et al.* 2011; Liu-Helmersson *et al.* 2014; Paaijmans *et al.* 2010, 2013). In temperate areas, winter temperatures outside the main transmission seasons can also impact patterns of disease. Milder winter temperatures can increase survival of mosquito adults (Reisen *et al.* 2008; Vinogradova 2000) and eggs (Fischer *et al.* 2011; Thomas *et al.* 2012), making the seasonal bottleneck in vector abundance less severe and allowing populations to increase more quickly during the following year. Surviving adults may also help maintain pathogens in vector and host populations, by either remaining infected or acquiring new infections through low levels of biting activity (Poh *et al.* 2019). Conversely, severe freezes lead to outbreaks of St. Louis encephalitis, likely by killing understory vegetation, which then increases the foraging and reproductive success of bird reservoir hosts (Day and Shaman 2009). Additionally, mosquito tolerance to thermal extremes may change seasonally based on thermal acclimation (Oliveira *et al.* 2021). Thus, while thermal response frameworks based on mean temperatures provide key insights and explanatory power, it can also be important to consider more nuanced aspects of temporal variation in temperature when modelling MBD.

Thermal heterogeneity at fine spatial scales can also have important impacts on MBD transmission. There can be substantial variation in temperature across land use gradients or large differences between indoor and outdoor settings that impact mosquito physiology and capacity for transmission (Afrane *et al.* 2005; Boser *et al.* 2021; Cator *et al.* 2013; Erraguntla *et al.* 2021; Murdock *et al.* 2017; Ngowo *et al.* 2017; Paaijmans and Thomas 2011). Additionally, in extreme hot and cold environments, mosquitoes and other vectors may be able to select favourable microclimates to provide a buffer and protect themselves from the negative impacts of adverse temperatures (Blanford *et al.* 2009; Danforth *et al.* 2016; Kirby and Lindsay 2004; Ngowo *et al.* 2017; Pincebourde and Woods 2020; Sauer *et al.* 2021; Woods *et al.* 2015). Modellers may want to consider temperature variation at multiple spatial scales, or think carefully about whether coarse-scale temperature data will match the microclimate that a target mosquito population experiences in the field.

2.3 *Rainfall*

Mosquitoes lay their eggs and complete the juvenile portion of their life cycle in aquatic habitats, including ponds, puddles, and human-created environments like discarded waste, water storage containers, and drainage ditches. The availability and quality of these breeding habitats often depends on the amount of rainfall and its interaction with the physical environment (e.g. topography, soil type, land cover, and hydrological features), other aquatic species present (competitors and food resources), and human behaviour. The complexity of these interactions can lead to nonlinear responses of mosquito populations and pathogen transmission to variation in rainfall (Figure 1B). Substantial variation in the breeding ecology of different vector species means that responses to rainfall are less consistent than responses to temperature across vector-pathogen systems (Shocket *et al.* 2020a).

The nonlinear responses of mosquito populations and pathogen transmission to rainfall result from the combination of multiple mechanisms that act over different parts of the rainfall gradient (Figure 1B). Most simply, more rainfall can lead to increased rainfed breeding habitat, more abundant mosquito populations, and higher risk of MBD transmission (Shocket *et al.* 2020a). However, in some cases very low rainfall can also increase breeding habitat or MBD transmission. For instance, *Aedes aegypti*, an urban specialist, often breeds in water storage containers, so low rainfall during the dry season or drought can increase human water storage behaviours and lead to higher mosquito abundance and outbreaks of dengue fever and chikungunya fever (Anyamba *et al.* 2012; Chandran and Azeez 2015; Livdahl 1982; Padmanabha *et al.* 2010; Pontes *et al.* 2000; Trewin *et al.* 2013). Drought can also increase transmission of West Nile virus and St. Louis Encephalitis virus without affecting mosquito abundance, due to increased contact between birds and vectors congregating at the few remaining water sources (Paull *et al.* 2017; Shaman *et al.* 2002, 2005), and possibly also due to physiological stress on bird reservoir hosts (Gervasi *et al.* 2016). Conversely, too much rainfall can be detrimental, diluting food resources (Livdahl 1982) but see (Kaufman *et al.* 1999; Walker *et al.* 1991) or flushing larvae from their habitats before they can complete development to emerge as adults and thus lowering disease transmission (Barros *et al.* 2011; Benedum *et al.* 2018; Koenraadt and Harrington 2008; Olson *et al.* 2009; Paaijmans *et al.* 2007).

2.4 *Humidity, wind, and tides*

Some models for climate and MBD investigate or incorporate less commonly utilised aspects of climate and related environmental factors, including humidity, wind, and tides. In general, higher humidity increases vector survival and reproduction (Bayoh 2001; Costa *et al.* 2010; Gaaboub *et al.* 1971), increasing transmission (Santos-Vega *et al.* 2022). Wind can be important at multiple spatial scales. Wind-assisted, long-distance dispersal of mosquitoes has been observed for *Anopheles* malaria vectors (Huestis *et al.* 2019) and linked to outbreaks of Japanese Encephalitis (Ritchie and Rochester 2001) and Rift Valley fever (Mapaco *et al.* 2012). Local wind patterns can structure spatial patterns of malaria risk within a community by increasing vector abundance in specific areas (Midega *et al.* 2012). Finally, some mosquitoes breed in brackish estuaries rather than freshwater habitats, and tidal height can drive the abundance of these species and the pathogens they transmit, such as Ross River virus (Jacups *et al.* 2008; Kokkinn *et al.* 2009). Accordingly, sea level rise due to climate change may directly impact transmission of disease by saltmarsh mosquitoes.

2.5 *Non-climatic factors*

Mosquito abundance and transmission of MBD is also strongly affected by a variety of non-climatic factors, including land cover and land use; the immunity, behaviour, population density, and vector control activities of humans; the immunity, behaviour, abundance, and species composition of non-human reservoir hosts; and the interactions of vectors with competitors, predators, and food resources (Edman and Scott 1987; Shocket *et al.* 2020a). Immunity can be a particularly important factor: cycles of infectious disease outbreaks are often caused by the acquisition of immunity from infection and then the subsequent waning of protection or demographic replacement of immune hosts with susceptible hosts (Grenfell *et al.* 2001; Keyel *et al.* 2021b; Paull *et al.* 2017). Land use is another critical factor, because different habitats types support different species and yield vastly different arthropod community compositions and abundances of important vectors (Diuk-Wasser *et al.* 2021; Shocket *et al.* 2020a). Human-modified environments like agricultural or newly deforested areas often provide ideal habitats for highly competent vector species and are places where humans spend substantial time outdoors at work, resulting in high levels of transmission (Calderón-Arguedas *et al.* 2015; Chaves *et al.* 2018; MacDonald and Mordecai 2019; Santos and Almeida 2018; Shah *et al.* 2019a, 2022; Tucker Lima *et al.* 2017). More generally, human behaviour is a major determinant of exposure to infectious mosquitoes that bite outdoors, and is often dictated by the economic need to earn a living, particularly in the Global South (Gryseels *et al.* 2015; Tangena *et al.* 2017). Models investigating the effect of climate on MBD may need to incorporate or control for the impact of these factors in order to detect and accurately characterise the impact of climate on transmission.

Non-climatic factors can interact with climate to impact MBD transmission in a variety of ways. For instance, intraspecific competition and the availability of food resources in the larval stages can modify the effect of temperature, changing the optimal temperatures for important vector and pathogen traits and thus for overall transmission (Huxley *et al.* 2021, 2022; Shapiro *et al.* 2016). These shifts may lead to differences between the thermal responses experienced by field populations of vectors (that are often food limited) and the thermal responses predicted by mathematical models that are parameterised using data from optimally-fed lab populations. Climate, immunity, and land use together can create complicated, multi-year cycles of malaria infections in the East African highlands (spanning Ethiopia, Kenya, and Uganda) (Pascual *et al.* 2008; Zhou *et al.* 2004). Climate and socio-ecological factors like population density, quantity of travellers, and land use interact to determine the dynamics of dengue fever in southern China (Li *et al.* 2021b). Climate can also complicate vector-control activities: regions prone to high winds or rain may have fewer opportunities for spraying aerial insecticides.

Non-climatic factors can also provide a means by which climate indirectly impacts transmission. Three such examples have already been described above: drought increasing household water storage (Chandran and Azeez 2015; Padmanabha *et al.* 2010; Trewin *et al.* 2013), winter freezes increasing bird reservoir host reproduction and abundance (Day and Shaman 2009), and drought influencing bird reservoir host behaviour and physiology (Gervasi *et al.* 2016; Paull *et al.* 2017; Shaman *et al.* 2002, 2005). For Ross River virus, specific sequences of seasonal rainfall affect the abundance and immune status of kangaroo reservoirs that drive transmission. High rainfall in summer typically leads to high transmission; however, if rainfall was sparse the previous winter, low recruitment of juvenile kangaroos can inhibit epidemics (Mackenzie *et al.* 2000). Conversely, low rainfall the previous summer can enhance transmission and lead to explosive epidemics because more of the kangaroo population is unexposed and susceptible to infection (Woodruff *et al.* 2002). Climate can also indirectly impact human contact with mosquitoes that bite outdoors by influencing the amount of time that people spend outside and the amount of skin left exposed by clothing.

2.6 *Ticks as disease vectors*

The lifecycle and physiology of ticks differ from those of mosquitoes in ways that fundamentally alter how climate impacts vector populations and pathogen transmission (Ogden and Lindsay 2016). Ticks have a fixed life cycle that spans over multiple years. Thus, unlike mosquitoes and other continually reproducing vectors (including sand flies, blackflies, and tsetse flies, as well plant disease vectors like aphids, whiteflies, and leafhoppers), tick populations cannot increase rapidly in response to short-term changes in temperature or rainfall (Ogden and Lindsay 2016; Shocket *et al.* 2020a). Instead, tick abundance is primarily affected by extreme temperatures and levels of humidity that create population bottlenecks (Brunner *et al.* 2012; Ogden *et al.* 2014; Ogden and Lindsay 2016; Ostfeld and Brunner 2015; Padgett and Lane 2001). Ticks also take very infrequent blood meals – only one per life stage. Accordingly, the pathogen development rate that is so important for MBD becomes basically irrelevant (Ogden and Lindsay 2016). Instead, the probability that a tick becomes infectious is determined by the effects of climate on their phenology (seasonal timing) of blood meals (Gatewood *et al.* 2009; Ostfeld and Brunner 2015; Randolph *et al.* 2000) and behaviour while they 'quest' for hosts (Arsnoe *et al.* 2015; Ginsberg *et al.* 2017; Vail and Smith 2002).

Reservoir host transmission competence and population abundance are critically important for determining the dynamics of tick-borne diseases (TBDs) (Tsao *et al.* 2021). No tick-borne diseases are maintained solely by transmission cycles in humans, nor are any tick populations sustained solely by feeding on humans, so both processes depend on reservoir hosts. Ticks also depend on reservoir hosts for dispersal over any distance farther than a few meters, so host movement drives many landscape-scale patterns of TBD (Madhav *et al.* 2004; Tsao *et al.* 2021). Nonetheless, the reservoir hosts for many medically important tick-borne pathogens are currently unknown (Eremeeva and Dasch 2015; Michelitsch *et al.* 2019; Tsao *et al.* 2021). Each species of mosquito generally transmits a small group of diseases (e.g. *Anopheles spp.* and malaria parasites, or *Ae. aegypti* and a handful of arboviruses). In contrast, medically important ticks can be competent vectors for an array of taxonomically diverse pathogens, meaning that interactions between pathogens during co-infection may be more important for transmission dynamics (Cutler *et al.* 2021; Moutailler *et al.* 2016). Some TBDs are caused by currently unknown agents (Kannangara and Patel 2018), which may be problematic for modelling efforts. Even when etiologic agents are known, diagnostic limitations have led to reporting groups comprised of several diseases (e.g. spotted fever group rickettsioses; SFGR) (Tijsse-Klasen *et al.* 2014) that may have different transmission dynamics. There are many knowledge gaps about the basic biology and ecology of TBDs.

2.7 *Section summary*

Temperature and rainfall have nonlinear impacts on vector abundance and transmission of vector-borne disease due to biological mechanisms that drive these effects (Figure 1). Additionally, climate can interact with non-climatic factors like human behaviour, and the abundance and immunity of reservoir hosts in complex and unexpected ways. When building or interpreting models for the effects of climate on MBD, it is important to keep in mind that the effects of temperature and rainfall on disease may be positive, negative, both, or neither depending on circumstance, including the spatial and temporal scale of the data (Cohen *et al.* 2016; Uelmen *et al.* 2021a). This context-dependence can limit the transferability of models beyond the setting in which they were fit.

3 Overview of concepts and approaches for modelling vector-borne disease

Models for transmission of MBD may be used to predict a variety of outcome variables, including mosquito abundance, mosquito infection prevalence, human infection prevalence, total quantity of human cases over an epidemic period, peak prevalence during an epidemic period, or timing of peak prevalence. MBD models are often divided into two broad categories: mechanistic (or process-based/trait-based) models and statistical (or phenomenological/correlative) models. Mechanistic models use equations to explicitly represent the biological processes or traits that contribute to mosquito population growth and disease transmission. Conversely, statistical models make inferences purely based on the relationships between observed data: they use equations to predict an observed outcome variable based on hypothesised driver variables without explicitly describing the underlying biology. The distinction between the two classes of models is not always clear-cut: hybrid models exist that combine both types (Stensgaard *et al.* 2016), many mechanistic models use the output from statistical models as inputs (or vice versa), and statistical models often work best when their construction and interpretation is informed by mechanistic insights (e.g. the nonlinear responses to climate described in the previous section). Both types of models have advantages and disadvantages and together they provide complimentary forms of evidence. In general, mechanistic models may be better for understanding biological processes, while statistical models often make better predictions.

3.1 *Mechanistic models of MBD*

Mechanistic models for transmission of MBD are typically based on a Susceptible-Infected-Recovered (SIR) or similar structure that tracks the numbers of hosts and/or mosquito vectors moving through infection categories or 'compartments'

(Anderson and May 1979; Cator *et al.* 2020; Reiner *et al.* 2013) (Figure 2A). Some of these SIR-type compartment models also explicitly track the numbers of vectors as they move through stages of the mosquito lifecycle (Ermert *et al.* 2011; Morin *et al.* 2015) (Figure 2B), and even the hydrology of water accumulating in breeding sites (Tompkins and Ermert 2013). Alternatively, SIR-type models can assume that mosquito abundance is constant (DeFelice *et al.* 2018), that it depends on a function for carrying capacity (Caldwell *et al.* 2021; Romeo-Aznar *et al.* 2018), or they can represent vectors implicitly by adding a delay to the force of infection between infected and susceptible hosts (Santos-Vega *et al.* 2022). Individual-based or agent-based models track each host and their infection status rather than tracking the total number of hosts in each category (Smith *et al.* 2018) (Figure 2C). Some models also track individual vectors (Bershteyn *et al.* 2018; Bomblies *et al.* 2008), whereas others count them like a compartment model (Mahmood *et al.* 2020). Another common approach is to condense the SIR system into a single expression – typically a form of the Ross-Macdonald equation (Simoy and Aparicio 2020; Smith *et al.* 2012) – that represents the force of transmission as a function of mosquito and human traits (Lambrechts *et al.* 2011; Mordecai *et al.* 2019) (Figure 2D). This approach is powerful in its simplicity: it predicts threshold conditions for a pathogen to invade and establish in a host population that are relatively easy to analyse and translate into potential targets for intervention (Smith *et al.* 2012). For this reason, models based on the Ross-MacDonald framework are commonly used and have been extended and applied in numerous different contexts (Simoy and Aparicio 2020; Smith *et al.* 2012). Mechanistic model frameworks are generally quite flexible, and all of approaches described here can be adapted to operate at a variety of spatial and temporal scales.

Mechanistic models are especially useful for predicting transmission under novel environments that we can simulate but cannot currently observe, for example, warming beyond current temperatures (Mordecai *et al.* 2019; Ryan *et al.* 2015) or responses to potential public health or vector control interventions (Artzy-Randrup *et al.* 2015; ten Bosch *et al.* 2020). Another strength of mechanistic models is providing insight into the specific biological processes or traits that drive transmission (e.g. the importance of adult vs juvenile mosquito mortality for limiting abundance) and therefore identifying specific targets for intervention. Mechanistic models may also generate general predictions that can be tested in specific locations or disease systems (Romeo-Aznar *et al.* 2018). However, mechanistic models are data hungry: they require substantial data from previous experimental and/or observational studies to provide numerical values for all of the specified biological processes. They can also be computationally intensive compared to statistical models. Additionally, because of their reliance on experimental data, mechanistic models typically focus on a small number of causative factors while holding 'all else equal', which can limit their relevance to transmission in natural settings. For this

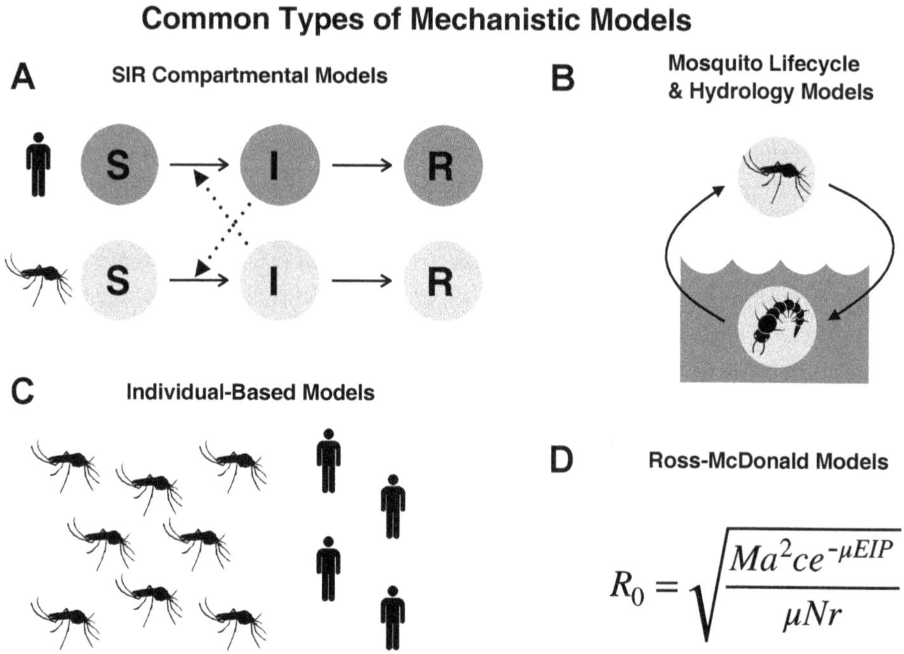

FIGURE 2 Common types of mechanistic models of mosquito-borne disease. (A) Susceptible-Infected-Recovered (SIR) models track the numbers of human hosts (top row) and mosquito vectors (bottom row) moving through the different infection categories (solid lines). New human infections are driven by currently-infected mosquitoes and vice versa (dotted lines). (B) Many models track the numbers of vectors as they move through stages of the mosquito lifecycle. Some models also track the hydrology of breeding sites. (C) Individual- or agent-based models track each host and their infection status; some models also track individual vectors while others count them as in an SIR model. (D) Many models condense the SIR system into a single expression – the Ross-McDonald equation – representing the force of transmission as a function of mosquito and human traits. In this equation, the basic reproduction number (R_0, the average number of new infections caused by a single infection in a fully susceptible population) is a function of adult mosquito density (M), mosquito biting rate (a), vector competence (c), adult mosquito mortality (μ), the extrinsic incubation period (EIP, the time required for the pathogen to complete development inside the mosquito), the density of human hosts (N), and the rate of recovery from infection (r).

reason, ideally the results from mechanistic models should be validated with results from a statistical model of field observations, but finding appropriate data to do so can be challenging.

3.2 *Statistical models of MBD*

Statistical models for MBD incorporate the extremely broad array of statistical models used for ecological and epidemiological data more generally. These methods include regression models, wavelet analysis, and machine learning techniques (including decision-tree-based and network-based approaches) (Table 1), some of which are highlighted in our case studies below. Regression models are an extremely broad category of models that can be generalised to accommodate many different types of response variables and data structures (Table 1) and can be fit using either frequentist or Bayesian methods. Time series data are often analysed using classical techniques such as cross-correlations and ARIMA or SARIMA models ([seasonal] autoregressive integrated moving average). Regression models of MBD often must be extended to account for multilevel or hierarchical data structures, where observations are clustered within groups and therefore are not independent. One option is to fit a mixed model where, in addition to the fixed effects of climate (and other variables of interest), random effects account for repeated observations from the same location or year that may vary together randomly as a group (Karki *et al.* 2020; Little *et al.* 2016). Multilevel or hierarchical data structures are also frequently modelled with Bayesian methods (Lowe *et al.* 2017). Multiple methods for statistical modelling can be combined into hybrid approaches. For zero-inflated (excess data points with zero values) or unbalanced data, hurdle models combine a logistic model for the presence or absence of disease with a second model that predicts the quantity of disease for only the observations with disease present (Mordecai *et al.* 2017). Another hybrid method takes the residuals (unexplained variation or error) from one model and passes to another model as the variable to be fitted (Chakraborty *et al.* 2019, but see McElreath 2020 for why this may not be ideal). The most appropriate and commonly-used methods vary based on the research goals and the data structure, including the spatial and temporal scales of the data.

TABLE 1 Statistical approaches that are commonly used to model mosquito abundance or incidence of mosquito-borne disease, their response variable data type/structure and spatiotemporal scale, and examples from the literature.

Statistical model	**Response variable data type/structure and spatio-temporal scale**	**Examples from MBD literature**
Simple linear regression	Normally-distributed continuous data; flexible spatiotemporal scale	Caldwell *et al.* 2021; Landesman *et al.* 2007
Logistic regression	Binary data; flexible spatio-temporal scale	Benedum *et al.* 2020; Davis *et al.* 2018; Karki *et al.* 2020; Méndez-Lázaro *et al.* 2014; Uelmen *et al.* 2021b
Poisson or negative binomial generalised linear model (GLM) regression	Count (integer) data; flexible spatiotemporal scale	Benedum *et al.* 2020; Bi *et al.* 2009; Little *et al.* 2016; Lowe *et al.* 2017

TABLE 1 Statistical approaches that are commonly used to model mosquito abundance (*cont.*)

Statistical model	Response variable data type/structure and spatiotemporal scale	Examples from MBD literature
Gamma GLM regression	Over-dispersed or skewed continuous data >0; flexible spatiotemporal scale	Mordecai *et al.* 2017; Ripoche *et al.* 2019
Generalised additive model (GAM)	Flexible	Colón-González *et al.* 2018; Li *et al.* 2019; Smith *et al.* 2020
Correlation analysis (cross-correlations, Spearman correlation)	Times series data; flexible spatiotemporal scale, often used for weekly data	Bi *et al.* 2004, 2009; Karki *et al.* 2020; Méndez-Lázaro *et al.* 2014
(Seasonal) autoregressive integrated moving average (ARIMA, SARIMA)	Times series data; flexible spatiotemporal scale, often used for weekly data	Bi *et al.* 2004; Chakraborty *et al.* 2019; Johansson *et al.* 2016; Keyel and Kilpatrick 2021; Poh *et al.* 2019
Wavelet analysis	Times series data; flexible spatial scale, fine temporal scale	Cazelles *et al.* 2005, 2007; Pascual *et al.* 2008; Poh *et al.* 2019; Santos-Vega *et al.* 2022
Markov chain model	Flexible	Damos *et al.* 2021; Santos-Vega *et al.* 2016
Decision tree machine learning methods (e.g. random forest)	Flexible	Benedum *et al.* 2020; Hess *et al.* 2018; Keyel *et al.* 2019, 2021b
Neural network and support vector machine (SVM) learning methods	Flexible	Akhtar *et al.* 2019; Chakraborty *et al.* 2019; Laureano-Rosario *et al.* 2018; McGough *et al.* 2021
Environmental niche model (ENM), species distribution model (SDM)	Spatially explicit presence or presence/absence data, usually at large spatial scales	Kraemer *et al.* 2019; Messina *et al.* 2019; Tjaden *et al.* 2018

Statistical models are often better than mechanistic models at reproducing patterns found in field observations (Johansson *et al.* 2016) because they can capture phenomena without specifying the cause *a priori* in the model structure. As a simple example, sampling from a historical distribution of cases may have high predictive skill and provide insights into how many cases a region may expect in a typical year, but does not provide any insights into why those cases will occur. Statistical models that lack mechanistic insight can be difficult to generalise to other contexts even if they perform well in their original setting. However, statistical models can also include variables with known biological relevance, and the resulting model fits may provide insight into causal relationships or even allow for formal causal inference (MacDonald and Mordecai 2019; Nova *et al.* 2021). Statistical models can also screen larger numbers of environmental driver variables for relevance (see paragraph on feature selection below). However, statistical models can also be overfit, and models that perform well on the data used to develop the model do not necessarily perform well on new independent data sets (see *Model validation, evaluation, and selection* below). Statistical models trained on an insufficient data range may also produce incorrect predictions. For example, MBD models trained with data that does not capture the upper end of the unimodal temperature relationship (Figure 1A) may yield predictions that MBD will only increase with climate change.

Choosing which variables to include as predictors (sometimes called 'feature selection') is an important part of building statistical models with climate data (Pol *et al.* 2016), yet is rarely straightforward for several reasons. Firstly, there are multiple ways to quantify variation in both temperature and rainfall and in how the two interact, particularly over larger timescales (e.g. mean temperature of wettest quarter, precipitation of warmest quarter, maximum temperature of warmest period, etc.) (Harris *et al.* 2013). Second, due to the time lags inherent in mosquito population growth and disease transmission, climatic variables can impact these processes over a range of potential time delays. Finally, many predictors can be highly collinear, or nonlinearly correlated (e.g. daily mean temperature and daily minimum/maximum temperature typically covary strongly with each other, as do instances of the same climate variable lagged at different time steps). One approach to dealing with multiple time lags and covariation among predictors is to select specific climate variables *a priori* based on knowledge about the relevant ecology or research questions (but see Pol *et al.* 2016). Alternatively, there are several empirical options: (1) fitting a model to all variables and then reducing the number of variables based on their predictive power (Benedum *et al.* 2018; Poh *et al.* 2019); (2) fitting a model to each climate variable individually and then either (a) selecting the best-performing model (Bi *et al.* 2004, 2009) or (b) using the variable from the best-performing model to include in further analyses (Stewart Ibarra *et al.* 2013; Uelmen *et al.* 2021b). Methods for species distribution models (SDMs) are relatively robust to collinearity in predictors, but it can also be a major source of uncertainty and reduce model transferability (Braunisch *et al.* 2013; De Marco and Nóbrega 2018; Feng *et al.* 2019). Ordination methods (e.g. non-metric multidimensional scaling; NMDS, principle components analysis; PCA, etc.) can reduce the number of variables and eliminate covariation between predictors, but can make interpreting and transferring the model results more challenging. The best strategy for variable selection will depend on the research goals, the modelling approach, and the specific climate-disease relationships embedded within the dataset.

3.3 *Models of tick-borne disease*

The same statistical modelling methods used for MBD (Table 1) are also applied to tick-borne disease (TBD). However, the unique biological features of ticks require mechanistic models for TBD that use different structures than those for MBD. While these models are fundamentally still SIR-type compartment models, the specific compartments differ. The models typically track multiple behavioural statuses (questing, feeding, and engorged) for each life stage (larvae, nymphs, adults) (Dobson *et al.* 2011; Ogden *et al.* 2005, 2007; Ostfeld and Brunner 2015). They may also track multiple host species that play specific ecological roles (Ogden *et al.* 2005, 2007). For example, deer are critical for the feeding and reproduction of blacklegged tick adults (*Ixodes scapularis*) but they do not transmit the Lyme disease pathogen (*Borrelia burgdorferi*), whereas rodents are common hosts for larvae and nymphs and are excellent reservoirs for transmitting infection (Ostfeld *et al.* 2006). (Models of MBD may also track multiple hosts, but it is less common.)

3.4 *Climate reanalysis products and future climate models*

One of the first steps for fitting a model investigating the effect of climate on MBD transmission is acquiring appropriate climate data to use as predictor variables. For models that incorporate climate at smaller spatial scales, researchers often collect weather data from their own field-deployed sensors or use data produced by local weather stations. However, models at larger spatial scales typically need input from continental or global-scale climate products. These large-scale climate products process and synthesise climate data from multiple sources to provide output in a standardised, spatially continuous gridded format. This process often involves 'reanalysis,' which compensates for known biases produced by different instruments over time and is an important step for generating high-quality, continuous long-term datasets. Reanalysed climate products are available across a range of spatial and temporal scales, ranging from ~1 km to several hundred km and produced at hourly, daily, monthly, or annual time scales. Examples of organizations that create and provide climate products used for modelling MBD include WorldClim (www.worldclim.org), the U.S. National Oceanic and Atmospheric Administration's (NOAA) National Centers for Environmental Information (NCEI; https://www.ncei.noaa.gov/products/weather-climate-models), NASA's Land Data Assimilation System (LDAS; https://ldas.gsfc.nasa.gov/data), the European Centre for Medium-Range Weather Forecasts (ECMWF; https://www.ecmwf.int/en/research/climate-reanalysis), Oregon State's PRISM Climate Group (https://prism.oregonstate.edu/), and University of East Anglia's Climatic Research Unit (https://www.uea

.ac.uk/web/groups-and-centres/climatic-research-unit/data). Google Earth Engine also provides access to a variety of climate data (https://developers.google.com/earth-engine/datasets/).

Models investigating the impacts of future climate change on MBD also need output from a general circulation model (GCM) predicting future climatic conditions based on the physical processes of the earth's atmosphere and oceans. The availability of models varies across data products, and a number of different GCMs are routinely used in MBD modelling efforts. For example, WorldClim (www.worldclim.org) provides output from 23 different GCMs across a range of spatiotemporal scales. Different GCMs can vary widely in their predictions for temperature and rainfall at specific locations for the same level of radiative forcing (net energy input or warming to the earth-atmosphere system) at the global scale (Kamruzzaman *et al.* 2021; Raju and Kumar 2020). Accordingly, many analyses use an ensemble approach that averages or compares the results based on output from multiple GCMs (but see Ribes *et al.* 2021 and the 'hot models' discussion in the paragraph below). Fortunately, tools have been developed to help researchers select a GCM or set of GCMs that are best-suited for their climate variables and region of interest (Parding *et al.* 2020).

Climate change modelling is organised by the Coupled Model Intercomparison Project (CMIP; https://www.wcrp-climate.org/wgcm-cmip). At the time of writing this chapter, recent models of MBD typically use GCM output from the previous phase (CMIP5) based on representative concentration pathways (RCPs) for different future scenarios of greenhouse gas concentrations. The four CMIP5 scenarios (RCP2.6, RCP4.5, RCP6.0, and RCP8.5) are based on the maximum level of global warming (radiative forcing in W/m^2) predicted by the year 2100 (van Vuuren *et al.* 2011). The current phase (CMIP6) uses a framework that couples levels of radiative forcing with five shared socioeconomic pathways (SSP 1 – SSP 5) representing different scenarios of demographic, social, economic, political, and technological development (O'Neill *et al.* 2016). Three of the four primary scenarios in CMIP6 match the previous RCPs: SSP1–2.6 (sustainability), SSP2–4.5 (middle of the road), and SSP5–8.5 (fossil-fuelled development), while the fourth main scenario has a slight increase in warming over the previous RCP (SSP3–7.0, regional rivalry), and radiative forcing of 6.0 W/m^2 has been downgraded to one of several secondary scenarios (SSP4–6.0, inequality) (O'Neill *et al.* 2016). CMIP6 also includes new GCMs, some of which have increased sensitivity and predict higher levels of warming compared to the GCMs from CMIP5; accordingly, some researchers have advocated for using ensembles that exclude these so-called 'hot models' (Hausfather *et al.* 2022; Ribes *et al.* 2021). The best practices for choosing the most appropriate GCMs and RCPs/SSPs are an active area of research and debate and will continue to evolve over time.

3.5 *Model evaluation, validation, and selection*

The steps taken to evaluate or validate a model will depend on its purpose (see review by Rykiel 1996), and several validation frameworks have been developed (Augusiak *et al.* 2014; Grimm *et al.* 2014). If more than one model has been developed, selecting a subset of one or more models may be desirable. Alternatively, models may be combined into a model ensemble and used in combination. Model ensembles often perform better than individual models for predicting spatial distributions (McIntyre *et al.* 2017) and forecasting dynamics (Johansson *et al.* 2019; Oidtman *et al.* 2021). Moreover, ensembles can balance the advantages and disadvantages of different modelling approaches, even in cases where their predicative skill is not significantly better than the best-performing individual model (Beeman *et al.* 2021).

There are many metrics available for assessing the fit of models. One of the most common is a model R^2, or similar derived metrics, which represent the variation in the dependent variable explained by a model. For some applications, Root Mean Squared Error (RMSE) may be useful, while presence/absence models are often evaluated with AUC (Area Under the Receiver Operating Curve) (but see Beale *et al.* 2008 as a caution against overly relying on high AUC scores). Probabilistic models, or models where the prediction takes the form of a probability distribution rather than a single point estimate, can be evaluated using the logarithmic score or the continuous ranked probability score (Wilks 2011), and software implementations are freely available (e.g. *scoringRules* package in R: Jordan *et al.* 2019). While p-values are not without their criticisms (Greenland *et al.* 2016), they can be a useful to assess the confidence in a model's outcome. The significance of specific variables is often evaluated using the p-value of the corresponding coefficient in a statistical model. It is important, however, to also consider the model's statistical power to detect a meaningful effect size, as large datasets can detect effects that are statistically significant but not biologically meaningful (Cohen 2013).

Two other important evaluation accuracy metrics for outbreak presence/absence models are sensitivity (the proportion of correctly predicted presences) and specificity (the proportion of correctly predicted absences). These two quantities necessarily trade off with each other, a fact that is illustrated by the trivial models of predicting that disease is always present (sensitivity = 1, specificity = 0) or always absent (sensitivity = 0, specificity = 1). An ideal model will balance and maximise both, and the Receiver Operating Curve can help visualise the trade-offs. Balanced accuracy (the mean of specificity and sensitivity) is often used to evaluate model performance when the outcomes are unbalanced (i.e. more observations with outbreaks than without, or vice versa). Additionally, presences or absences can be weighted in the optimization process, as sometimes it is worse to miss the presence of a disease than to predict the disease is present when it is actually absent.

For models where prediction skill is important, it is important to examine a model's performance using a data set that was not used to build the model, i.e. conduct cross-validation (Roberts *et al.* 2017). The simplest method is to split the available data into two sections: a training set used to build the model and a testing set used to evaluate the model performance. However, this approach potentially yields underpowered models, because model skill generally increases with the size of the training set. Leave-one-out cross-validation and k-fold cross-validation are two other related options. In leave-one-out cross-validation each individual data point is removed from the dataset sequentially, the model is refit, and the model's ability to predict the missing data point is evaluated. K-fold cross-validation works similarly: the data are randomly divided into *k* number of groups and the model is re-fit *k* times with each group of data withheld for testing one time. While these methods give a less biased estimate of the model skill than splitting the data into training and testing sets, it is not possible in all cases, such as with time series. Blocked cross-validation, where data are split strategically by leaving an entire year or spatial unit out (Roberts *et al.* 2017), is commonly used for infectious disease data sets. Using an independent data set collected after a model was finalised is an ideal test, particularly for testing its transferability, but such data may be difficult to come by.

Current practices for model selection use information theoretic approaches like AIC (Akaike information criterion) or BIC (Bayesian information criterion (Burnham *et al.* 2011; Burnham and Anderson 2010; Neath and Cavanaugh 2012). These metrics aim to avoid overfitting a model by balancing model predictive skill and simplicity: a predictor variable must improve model fit sufficiently to justify its inclusion. The likelihood ratio test is also frequently used to compare two nested models (i.e. when a smaller model contains a subset of variables from a larger model) and, like other frequentist statistical methods, generates a *p*-value.

Model evaluation and selection often include comparison against a null model, i.e. a model where the response variable is predicted in the absence of hypothesised mechanisms (Gotelli and Graves 1996), in this case disease incidence predicted in the absence of climate drivers as model input. While standard null models assume that every observation is the same value (the mean of the dataset), there has been a recent call for inclusion of more sophisticated and individually-tailored null models (Table 2) that give better insight into model prediction skill (Keyel and Kilpatrick 2021) or the relevant scales of different climate impacts (Nova *et al.* 2021). This practice can help avoid situations where models appear to have high predictive skill (i.e. high accuracy scores), but provide no information on the process being studied (Olden *et al.* 2002). For instance, an 'always absent' null model may perform extremely well for low-incidence diseases (Keyel and Kilpatrick 2021).

TABLE 2 A selection of null models (i.e. models without climate predictors) that can be used to evaluate climate-driven models of mosquito-borne disease. Comparing a climate-driven model to appropriate null models can avoid situations where a model appears to have high predictive skill (i.e. high accuracy scores), but provides no useful information on how climate affects transmission of mosquito-borne disease. Adapted from prior studies (Johansson *et al.* 2019; Keyel and Kilpatrick 2021; Nova *et al.* 2021).

Null model	Model description	Comments
Always absent null (non-probabilistic)	Disease is always absent.	This model can perform very well for low-incidence diseases. If a model cannot outperform this null model, it provides no useful information, even if it has high accuracy scores.
Mean value null (non-probabilistic)	All observations are the mean value of disease cases.	This model is equivalent to the standard null hypothesis and rarely performs well.
Seasonal mean value null (non-probabilistic)	All observations are the mean value of disease cases during that week or month of year.	This model can perform well for diseases with strong seasonality. If a model cannot outperform this null model, climate may still be important, but primarily for determining seasonality.
Auto-regressive null (non-probabilistic or probabilistic)	ARIMA (for annual time series) or SARIMA (for weekly time series) fit based on relationships within the time series at various time lags.	ARIMA models can perform well for diseases with strong biennial immunity-driven cycles. SARIMA models can perform well for diseases with strong seasonality. If a model cannot outperform a SARIMA null model, climate may still be important, but primarily for determining seasonality.
Historical null (probabilistic)	Samples are taken from a pool of all observations.	This model performs better with more observations to sample from. It performs worse at higher spatial and temporal resolutions because cases become rarer (and it approaches the always absent null model).

TABLE 2 A selection of null models (*cont.*)

Null model	Model description	Comments
Negative binomial null (probabilistic)	Samples are taken from a negative binomial distribution fit to all observations.	This model is similar to historical null, but often performs better at small sample sizes because it estimates the full distribution of cases.
Uniform null (probabilistic)	Samples are taken from a uniform distribution set between 0 and the maximum number of observed cases, i.e. equal probability for all theoretically possible outcomes.	This model provides a very general baseline, but is limited to the range of historical observations and likely will not perform as well as a null model that better reflects the structure of the underlying data.

In conclusion, a variety of techniques exist for model evaluation and validation. The choice of methods will depend on the goals of the model and the structure of the underlying data. Cross-validation, sensitivity, specificity, accuracy, and AUC scores are often used to evaluate individual models, while AIC, BIC, and null models are often used to compare between models.

4 Case study #1: local time series models of dengue fever in San Juan, Puerto Rico

4.1 *Background*

Dengue fever is globally distributed across tropical areas, particularly in low-income urban areas where it is transmitted by its primary vector *Aedes aegypti* (Bhatt *et al.* 2013; Lowe *et al.* 2020). The estimated 390 million annual infections result in ~96 million symptomatic cases that cause substantial morbidity and mortality (Bhatt *et al.* 2013). Dengue virus is primarily maintained by infection cycles in humans (Vasilakis *et al.* 2011). Cases in San Juan, Puerto Rico exhibit a strong, consistent seasonal pattern; however, there are also high levels of interannual variation, with large epidemics occurring every 3–5 years (Johansson *et al.* 2019; Méndez-Lázaro *et al.* 2014). Multiple serotypes of dengue virus (DENV1 – DENV4) circulate and interact via host immunity, producing a complex range of phenomena including long-term protection (lifelong immunity to a specific strain after infection), short-term protection (temporary cross-protection against the other three serotypes lasting several months), antibody-dependent enhancement (exposure to

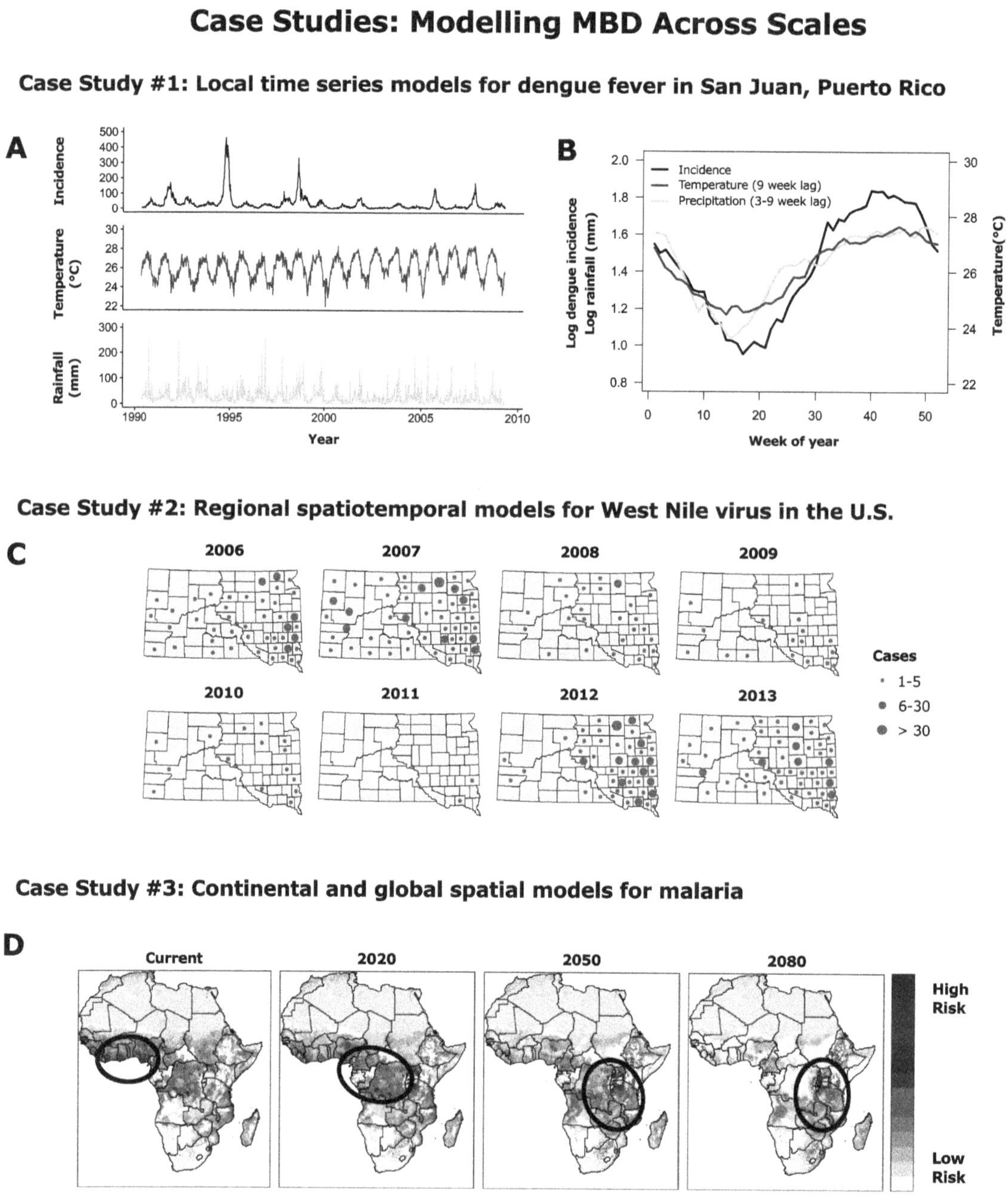

FIGURE 3 Examples of output from three case studies of modelling mosquito-borne disease. (A) Case study #1: Time series for 23 years of dengue incidence, temperature, and precipitation in San Juan, Puerto Rico used in the dengue forecasting challenge (Johansson *et al.* 2019). (B) The average seasonal patterns for the variables in A with time lags identified by pairwise cross-correlations, adapted from (Nova *et al.* 2021). (C) Case study #2: Output from the spatiotemporal South Dakota model for West Nile virus, adapted from (Davis *et al.* 2018). (D) Case study #3: Output from a mechanistic Ross-McDonald model predicting future patterns for people at risk of malaria infection with climate change (RCP8.5), adapted from a figure originally in colour from (Ryan *et al.* 2015)

a second strain yields higher risk of severe disease), and partial cross-protection (reduction in risk of severe disease from new strains after exposure to two or more different strains) (Dejnirattisai *et al.* 2016; Gibbons *et al.* 2007).

The time series of weekly dengue cases in San Juan (Figure 3A) is one of the most well-documented and thoroughly analysed MBD datasets due to being included in a forecasting challenge launched by multiple U.S. government agencies in 2015 (Johansson *et al.* 2019). It is also one of the longest, spanning 23 years at the time of the contest. The goal of the forecasting challenge was to improve prediction of when the periodic large epidemics are likely to occur in order to better prevent them and mitigate their negative impacts on human health and the economy (Johansson *et al.* 2019). Modelling teams were provided with total incidence data, partial serotype data, and climate data and asked to make probabilistic predictions for three targets: maximum incidence, the timing of the peak, and the total number of cases over the entire epidemic season. Model predictions were submitted as probabilities assigned to bins of possible outcomes. Retrospective forecasts were submitted for four-week intervals in the dataset to determine how forecast skill changed over the course of the epidemic season (Johansson *et al.* 2019). Prior studies using the San Juan time series indicated that climate data could explain substantial variation in dengue infections dynamics (Laureano-Rosario *et al.* 2018; Méndez-Lázaro *et al.* 2014; Morin *et al.* 2015).

4.2 *Modelling approaches and results*

Sixteen teams created models and submitted predictions for the forecasting challenge, covering a wide range of modelling methods. Mechanistic approaches included SIR-type compartment models, both with and without a vector population component. Statistical approaches included logistic regression, negative binomial generalised linear regression, SARIMA, approximating the seasonal pattern with a sine or cosine function, a neural network, and a Gaussian process model (Johansson *et al.* 2019). Ten teams (63%) used climate data as predictors, two teams (13%) used serotype data in their models, and seven teams (44%) used multi-model ensembles that combined predictions from multiple models (Johansson *et al.* 2019). Many teams used lagged versions of the climate variables (e.g. Figure 3B), as it takes several weeks for changes in climate to impact vector populations and 8–10 weeks to impact human cases (Hu *et al.* 2006; Jacups *et al.* 2008; Mordecai *et al.* 2017; Shocket *et al.* 2018; Stewart Ibarra *et al.* 2013). Predictions from the submitted models were compared to an ensemble combining all of the submissions and null models, and two null models without any climate predictors: a uniform model that gave equal probabilities to each possible outcome and a SARIMA model that captured the average seasonal response in incidence.

In addition to the standard climate variables (temperature, rainfall, and humidity), one team used two climate-related indices as input for their model: the normalized difference vegetation index (NDVI) and an El Niño-Southern Oscillation (ENSO) index. Vegetation indices use remotely-sensed observations of specific wavelengths of light to assess the 'greenness' of an area (Pettorelli *et al.* 2011), which can be used as a proxy for water availability and rainfall integrated over the recent past. Vegetation indices have been used to model vector abundance and/or disease cases for Rift Valley fever (Linthicum *et al.* 1999), West Nile virus (Brown *et al.* 2008; Ward 2009; Ward *et al.* 2005), and malaria (Dantur Juri *et al.* 2015; Fastring and Griffith 2009; Haque *et al.* 2010; Lourenço *et al.* 2011). ENSO is a multi-year climate oscillation impacting global temperature, rainfall, and wind patterns. ENSO has been used to successfully forecast outbreaks of dengue (Adde *et al.* 2016; Cazelles *et al.* 2005; Colón-González *et al.* 2011; van Panhuis *et al.* 2015), Rift Valley fever (Anyamba *et al.* 2009; Linthicum *et al.* 1999), and malaria (Bouma *et al.* 2016), and can increase model accuracy beyond including temperature and rainfall alone (Earnest *et al.* 2012). ENSO metrics are especially attractive for use in forecasting MBD because the changes in sea surface temperature and air pressure that indicate a forthcoming change in climate drivers provide several months of lead time for potential interventions.

There was substantial variation in forecast skill among the submitted models. In general, purely statistical models scored better than models with mechanistic components, and models without climate data as input scored better than those using climate variables as predictors (Johansson *et al.* 2019). Additionally, predictions from ensembles scored better than those from individual models. In fact, the ensemble of all models performed better than almost all of the individual submitted models (Johansson *et al.* 2019). Early season forecasts were generally poor, with many submitted models scoring worse than the uniform null model. Unsurprisingly, most models increased in accuracy as the season progressed and they acquired more information about the infection dynamics (Johansson *et al.* 2019). Different submitted models provided the best early season forecast for each target, making it difficult to identify a single best forecast model. The best model for week of peak incidence was a Gaussian process model using cases at the end of the previous season, a seasonal sine wave, and an estimate of the severity of the current season. The best model for peak incidence was an ensemble of two models: an SIR-type model parameterised using the case data and an extremely random trees machine learning model using case data and climate variables. The best model for total incidence was an ensemble of three statistical models, two of which used only case data and one of which used case data and climate variables (Johansson *et al.* 2019).

4.3 *Synthesis and discussion*

Results from the dengue forecasting challenge highlight both a key strength and key weakness of statistical models. First, they often perform better than mechanistic models when the primary goal is prediction. Complex mechanistic models may perform poorly due to the inherent difficulty in characterising the uncertainty and variability across the large number of parameters. However, successfully replicating a pattern does not necessarily yield insight into the biological mechanisms generating that pattern. Three different models with very divergent approaches performed best at predicting each target, and it is unclear exactly why those specific combinations of modelling methods and predictors worked best for the different aspects of dengue dynamics. This case study also demonstrates that model ensembles are a powerful tool for predicting disease dynamics, and often perform better than the individual component models (Buczak *et al.* 2018; Johansson *et al.* 2019; Oidtman *et al.* 2021; Wimberly *et al.* 2022; Yamana *et al.* 2016b). In this example, the ensemble constructed from all the submitted and null models scored well because it averaged out uncertainty where different models disagreed while reinforcing certainty where all the models agreed (Johansson *et al.* 2019).

The results also pose an interesting question: if temperature and rainfall are so important for the mechanisms of transmission (Figure 1), why did models with climate input perform worse? One potential answer is that forecasts of climate itself are uncertain, so any predictions based on them will incorporate this error (Johansson *et al.* 2019; Lowe *et al.* 2017). Another likely answer is that information about climate can be encoded indirectly. For instance, if climate primarily determines the seasonality of transmission while interannual variation is primarily driven by other factors (like serotype dynamics and host immunity), then the effects of climate at a single location may be adequately captured phenomenologically via a sine function or SARIMA model. A subsequent analysis of the time series partially supports this interpretation and outperformed all models from the challenge when forecasting the three targets (Nova *et al.* 2021). It used a causal inference method called empirical dynamic modelling (Sugihara *et al.* 2012) to argue that (for dengue in San Juan) temperature only influences the seasonality of transmission, while population susceptibility and rainfall contribute to both seasonality and interannual variation (Nova *et al.* 2021).

Models investigating the relationship between climate and dengue may benefit from considering or incorporating other factors that are important for dengue transmission. Host immunity from prior exposure is critical for the probability of both acquiring the infection and development of symptomatic disease, and the serotype and strain replacement dynamics for dengue make that process particularly complex, as shown by studies from Malaysia, Thailand, and Vietnam (Adams *et al.* 2006; Aguas *et al.* 2019; Tan *et al.* 2017; Zhang *et al.* 2005). *Ae. aegypti*'s preference for breeding in human containers means that dengue transmission can be particularly dependent on human behaviour and larger structural forces like poverty and access to piped water that drive water storage activity, as shown in Ecuador (Stewart Ibarra *et al.* 2013; Stewart Ibarra and Lowe 2013). Finally, human mobility can have important impacts on dengue dynamics, with connectivity between different regions influencing local dynamics in Thailand (Kiang *et al.* 2021), as well as travel within cities affecting district-level transmission in Pakistan (Kraemer *et al.* 2018; Wesolowski *et al.* 2015).

5 Case study #2: regional models of West Nile virus in the United States

5.1 *Background*

West Nile virus (WNV) is globally distributed and the most common mosquito-borne pathogen across temperate North America and Europe. The virus is transmitted by a diverse set of mosquito species, primarily in the genus *Culex*, and maintained in a similarly diverse set of wildlife species that act as reservoir hosts. While birds are considered the primary reservoirs, mammals may also play a role (Root and Bosco-Lauth 2019). Each year during the late summer and fall, WNV spills over into humans, dead-end hosts that are unlikely to infect new vectors. The vast majority of human and equine reported cases in the U.S. (90%) occur between July and September (Petersen 2019). Between 20 and 30% of infections cause clinical symptoms and <1% of infections become neuroinvasive and cause encephalitis, which can lead to permanent cognitive impairment or death (Petersen 2019). As with dengue in San Juan, there is strong seasonality and high levels of interannual variation. However, the incidence of severe West Nile disease is much lower than severe dengue: annual incidence for neuroinvasive WNV in the U.S. is 0.4 per 100,000 individuals (McDonald *et al.* 2021) compared to an annual reported incidence for dengue hospitalizations in Puerto Rico of 10 per 100,000 individuals (Shankar *et al.* 2018). Additionally, there is substantial spatial variation in WNV infections. Incidence is generally highest in the central and western U.S. (Petersen 2019), and although the number of annual neuroinvasive cases in the U.S. is relatively constant, cases peak in different areas of the country in different years (McDonald *et al.* 2021).

Modelling efforts for WNV in the U.S. often focus on regional scale models investigating spatial variation at the county or sub-county level. Many of these models also incorporate temporal variation at weekly or annual time scales. In this case study, we examine four such models for different regions – the Chicago metropolitan area (Karki *et al.* 2020), New York/Connecticut (Keyel *et al.* 2019), and two for South Dakota (Davis *et al.* 2018; Hess *et al.* 2018) (Table 3) – that were among those recently compared by (Keyel *et al.* 2021a). Unlike in the dengue forecasting challenge, three of the models were able to access mosquito infection rate (IR) data collected by vector control districts in addition to human case data and environmental predictors. These mosquito infection data are versatile and incredibly useful: they can be modelled as outcomes that depend on environmental factors or as input variables for predicting human cases (Table 3). Infection rates can be calculated in several ways. Typically, multiple mosquitoes are pooled together and tested at the same time (often ~50 per pool). Maximum likelihood methods are recommended for calculating infection rates, as they can provide more refined estimates with associated confidence intervals (Chiang and Reeves 1962), and can easily be calculated in Excel (Centers for Disease Control and Prevention 2022) or R (Williams and Moffitt 2005). Minimum infection rates, calculated by assuming only a single mosquito per pool was infected are also frequently used in the historical literature but do not provide as much information as maximum likelihood approaches.

TABLE 3 Regional models found that climate variables explained spatial and temporal variation in West Nile Virus (WNV) risk. IR = infection rate in mosquitoes; Q1 = 1st quarter (January–March); and Q3 = 3rd quarter (July–September)

Location (reference)	**Model type**	**Spatial and temporal resolution of model output (years of data)**	**Main results**
Chicago area (Karki *et al.* 2020)	Mixed effects logistic regression	Weekly presence/ absence of human cases in 1 km hexagons (2005–2016)	Higher mosquito infection rate (IR), warmer temperatures 2–4 weeks prior, and warmer temperatures in January increased risk of WNV.
New York + Connecticut (Keyel *et al.* 2019)	Random forest	Annual human cases and mosquito IR by county (2000–2015)	Warmer mean minimum temperature in Q1 and Q3, and drought in Q3 increased human WNV cases. Warmer mean minimum temperature in Q3 increased IR; soil moisture had complex, nonlinear effects on IR (drought always increased IR, high moisture only did so sometimes).
South Dakota (Davis *et al.* 2018)	Logistic regression	Weekly presence/ absence of human cases by county (2002–2017)	Warmer temperature and more humid air increased risk of WNV, but only when IR began increasing early in the season.
South Dakota (Hess *et al.* 2018)	Boosted regression tree	Human incidence in 300 m grid (pooled from 2004–2017)	Early season soil moisture and late-season relative humidity predicted spatial distribution.

5.2 *Modelling approaches and results*

One challenge for modelling variation in West Nile virus activity over time *and* space is that the number of observed cases is often very low and zero-inflated, likely due to genuinely low prevalence (which can be evaluated using sentinel chicken data: Dunphy *et al.* 2019; Snyder *et al.* 2020) that is exacerbated by difficulties detecting and reporting cases that are either asymptomatic or mildly symptomatic. These low-prevalence data often violate the distributional assumptions of most traditional modelling techniques and make the data harder to fit. For instance, in the spatiotemporal dataset for South Dakota, only 4.1% of county-weeks contained any observations of WNV, and of those, 82% had just one case (Davis *et al.* 2018). Two of the models compensated for this issue by using logistic regression to model the presence/absence of disease in each analytical unit rather than the number of cases (Davis *et al.* 2018; Karki *et al.* 2020). Other methods used in the examples here include aggregating cases into annual totals (Keyel *et al.* 2019) or removing the temporal component entirely to model only spatial variation (Hess *et al.* 2018). While all of these approaches make the modelling process more robust, they also limit the utility of the resulting models to make quantitative predictions for outbreak severity (for the former two models) or to inform public health responses at finer temporal scales (for the latter two models).

All four models were able to reproduce regional variation in WNV activity and found that climate variables were important for explaining the spatial and temporal patterns of human cases or mosquito infection rate (Table 3, Figure 3C) (Davis *et al.* 2018; Hess *et al.* 2018; Karki *et al.* 2020; Keyel *et al.* 2019). The New York/Connecticut model explicitly estimated how much climate information improved model skill, increasing the explained variance by 17–19% for mosquito infection rate, and 7–12% for human cases (Keyel *et al.* 2019). These estimates are consistent with another analysis using a mechanistic model to forecast WNV time series in 12 counties spread across the U.S. (DeFelice *et al.* 2018). Warmer temperatures during the transmission season increased WNV risk in all three models that included temporal variation, indicating that temperature is important for both seasonal and interannual variation in transmission (Davis *et al.* 2018; Karki *et al.* 2020; Keyel *et al.* 2019). Additionally, in New York/Connecticut and Chicago, warmer winter temperatures also increased WNV risk, indicating that overwintering temperature is likely important for the mosquito population dynamics or viral maintenance in both locations (Karki *et al.* 2020; Keyel *et al.* 2019). Measures of precipitation, soil moisture, or humidity were also important in all models except the Chicago model (Davis *et al.* 2018; Hess *et al.* 2018; Karki *et al.* 2020; Keyel *et al.* 2019).

Mosquito infection rate (IR) was also important for the performance of models that included it as a predictor (Davis *et al.* 2018; Karki *et al.* 2020). In metropolitan Chicago, fine-scale spatial variation in IR significantly predicted WNV risk for humans (Karki *et al.* 2020). Additionally, a simple regression model pooling the IR data over space up to week 33 (mid-way through August) was able to predict 93% of the interannual variation in human cases for the whole region (Karki *et al.* 2020). In the spatiotemporal South Dakota model, increases in IR early in the season were required for climate variables to translate into human cases, making climate suitability necessary but not sufficient for predicting WNV risk (Davis *et al.* 2018). In the New York/Connecticut model, IR was a significant predictor, but explained a small proportion of the total variation (2–5%) (Keyel *et al.* 2019). In both studies the IR data came from a limited subset of counties (for the New York study: 8/62 = 13%), which greatly reduced the sample size of the models and may have influenced the performance of the New York model.

As with dengue in San Juan, more accurate forecasting methods for WNV are needed to better direct vector control activities and other public health interventions, although substantial progress is being made. In 2016, an earlier version of the spatiotemporal South Dakota model (Davis *et al.* 2018) was used to make prospective forecasts for WNV at two points early in the transmission season (early and late July). In early July, the model successfully predicted that the WNV season would be larger and start earlier than normal based solely on record-high temperatures (relevant IR data were not yet available), although it underestimated the eventual case total (Davis *et al.* 2017). By late July, including IR data drove the model prediction even higher, making the predicted case total more accurate (Davis *et al.* 2017). The model (updated slightly each year) was used to make real-time, prospective weekly forecasts every year for the next three years (through 2019). At that point, the current model was systematically evaluated for its forecasting accuracy over the four year period, and demonstrated a clear ability to distinguish between years with high (2016 and 2018) and low (2017 and 2019) numbers of human cases using the data available by early July (Wimberly *et al.* 2022). Fortunately, this time frame is sufficient to increase vector control efforts and implement public outreach programs, as human cases typically peak in August (Wimberly *et al.* 2022).

Longer-term predictions for WNV under climate change are also critical. A model based on the New York/Connecticut approach predicted cases of WNV in the region under future climate change (using an ensemble of GCMs for RCP8.5 from Liu *et al.* 2017) and estimated that average cases of neuroinvasive WNV would increase by 28% (from 68 to 87 annually) (Keyel *et al.* 2021b). As expected based on the unimodal thermal response for transmission of West Nile virus (Figure 1) (Shocket *et al.* 2020b), this outcome is the net effect of shifts in disease, with increases in some places and decreases in others. The model also predicts that transmission will become more geographically homogenous, with more counties experiencing at least one case but fewer counties experiencing more than 5 cases in a single year (Keyel *et al.* 2021b).

5.3 *Synthesis and discussion*

Regional models of WNV in the U.S. support the idea that climate shapes spatial and temporal variation in transmission and improves model performance. While there were some consistent patterns for the effect of temperature (warmer temperatures during the transmission season and winter months generally increased transmission), the effect of moisture was more complex. The specific moisture-related variables that were most important for predicting WNV differed between the regions. This context-dependence may stem from differences in the ecology of the local vector species, geographical features that interact with moisture (e.g. land cover, topography, soil type, etc.), or the numerical range of each variable experienced in a given region.

Metrics of mosquito infection rate (IR) also helped predict WNV risk. For South Dakota, IR growth rate early in the transmission season was critical for determining human cases (Davis *et al.* 2018), timing that is ideal for forecasting because it provides early warning. In Chicago, mid-summer IR predicted final human case load with extremely high accuracy (Karki *et al.* 2020). While this timing (halfway through the transmission season) is less optimal, it could still provide some lead time for increased public health messaging. IR data are particularly useful for modelling pathogens like WNV that persist in non-human reservoir hosts and exhibit low-incidence in humans. Surveillance programs can pool mosquitoes and test thousands of individual vectors per week in order to detect prevalence increasing in reservoir and vector populations before spillover to humans occurs. Unfortunately, IR data is expensive and labour-intensive to collect, which helps explain why it was only available for a subset (13%) of counties in New York (those with most consistent burdens of WNV). Additionally, incorporating IR data in models can be challenging, due to difficulties standardizing regional-scale mosquito data that are collected by multiple vector control districts, which often use different mosquito trap types and trapping protocols. Novel tools such as VectorSurv (https://maps.vectorsurv.org/arbo), an online, multi-state vector surveillance and data management platform, may help to overcome these difficulties and leverage IR data to improve modelling efforts and better inform public policy, which in turn, may incentivise the collection of additional IR data.

Models investigating the effect of climate on transmission of WNV may benefit from considering other factors, particularly patterns arising from the complex community of vectors and reservoir hosts and their interactions with each other. For instance, in late summer vector species may shift their blood meal sources from birds to humans (Kilpatrick *et al.* 2006) or from more competent bird species to less competent ones as seasonal bird migrations affect the relative abundance of these hosts (Hamer *et al.* 2009). The composition of bird communities also strongly influences variation in transmission at regional spatial scales. Highly abundant species that dominate low-diversity bird communities tend to be highly competent reservoirs, creating a biodiversity-disease 'dilution effect' where transmission of WNV is lower in areas of high bird diversity and higher in areas of low bird diversity (Kain and Bolker 2019; Keesing and Ostfeld 2021). The abundance of American robins can be particularly helpful for predicting WNV infection rates (Kilpatrick *et al.* 2006). Additionally, human behaviour may reinforce the effects of climate on transmission of WNV, for example, if people spend less time outside and wear more protective clothing as temperatures become less suitable and school terms begin simultaneously.

6 Case study #3: continental and global models for the impact of climate change on malaria and dengue fever

6.1 *Background*

Malaria remains the deadliest mosquito-borne disease, causing over 200 million cases and killing over half a million people each year (World Health Organization 2021). The vast majority of cases (95%) occur in Africa (World Health Organization 2021) where malaria and other vector-borne diseases interact with the ongoing legacy of colonialism, underdevelopment, and economic exploitation in complex ways (Acemoglu *et al.* 2001; Alsan 2015; Athni *et al.* 2021; Tilley 2016). Since 2019, disruptions in public health interventions and medical treatments due to the COVID-19 pandemic have led to substantial increases in malaria burden, partially reversing two decades of progress (World Health Organization 2021). Malaria is caused by parasites in the genus *Plasmodium* and transmitted by a broad array of mosquitoes in the genus *Anopheles* (Kiszewski *et al.* 2004). The main African parasite (*Plasmodium falciparum*) is primarily maintained in cycles between humans (Sundararaman *et al.* 2013), although spillover and spillback with primates is more important for transmission of other malaria species (*P. knowlesi* and *P. vivax*) in southeast Asia and Latin America (Antinori *et al.* 2021; Chaves *et al.* 2022; Lempang *et al.* 2022; Ribeiro de Castro Duarte *et al.* 2021). Within Africa, malaria transmission occurs along a temporal spectrum from marginal (1–3 months a year) to endemic (10–12 months a year), with differences largely determined by climatic suitability (Ryan *et al.* 2020).

The question of how malaria transmission will respond to climate change motivated some of the earliest research investigating climate change impacts on infectious disease and has inspired the development of a large body of modelling efforts (Eikenberry and Gumel 2018). These models often focus on predicting responses over large spatial and temporal scales, producing continental or global maps of disease risk over decadal time scales (Figure 3D). Longer term analyses are important for motivating current investments in reducing greenhouse gas emissions and planning future investments in public health infrastructure.

6.2 *Modelling approaches and results*

The first model for the impacts of climate change on malaria used a temperature-dependent adaptation of the Ross-Macdonald equation (Figure 2D) to predict large, ubiquitous increases in transmission across most of the world as global temperatures warmed (Martens *et al.* 1995). A central assumption in this prediction is that malaria transmission is optimised at 31 °C. An updated Ross-Macdonald equation model incorporating more realistic thermal biology argued that the optimum for malaria transmission is much cooler (around 25 °C) and predicts that warming from climate change will cause shifts in disease rather than universal increases (Mordecai *et al.* 2013). Specifically, the current hotspot for transmission in West Africa (where mean temperatures are currently optimal and will become too warm) will shift eastward into higher elevation areas in East Africa (where mean temperatures are currently too cool and will move closer to the optimum) (Figure 3D) (Ryan *et al.* 2015). While the total land area that permits any malaria transmission in Africa is expected to increase, the land area that is highly suitable for transmission and the total number of people at risk for malaria will decrease (Ryan *et al.* 2015, 2020).

Other methods concur that climate change will shift current patterns of malaria burden. A study comparing five models using a mix of mechanistic and statistical approaches found agreement that malaria transmission will decrease in West Africa but increase in East Africa (Caminade *et al.* 2014). These models also predicted reduced transmission in other warm, tropical areas (coastal India, Australia, Southeast Asia, and South America) (Caminade *et al.* 2014). More detailed predictions for West Africa are revealed by two mechanistic models that incorporate the effects of temperature and rainfall on transmission. HYDREMATS combines breeding habitat hydrology and individual-based simulations of vectors and hosts (Figure 2B and 2C) (Yamana *et al.* 2016a), and the Liverpool Malaria Model simulates vector and host populations using SIR-type compartments (Figure 2A) (Diouf *et al.* 2022). Most general circulation models predict that under future climate change the western sub-region of West Africa will get warmer and drier while the eastern sub-region will get warmer and wetter (Yamana *et al.* 2016a). Thus, HYDREMATS predicts that transmission will decrease in the western sub-region with little change to the eastern sub-region (Yamana *et al.* 2016a). The Liverpool Malaria Model study considered two different climate change scenarios, and found that more intense warming (RCP8.5) will cause larger reductions in transmission than the milder scenario (RCP4.5) (Diouf *et al.* 2022).

Species distribution models (SDMs), also commonly referred to as ecological niche models (ENMs), are statistical approaches for modelling how the environment shapes where species can persist, typically over large spatial scales (Stevens and Pfeiffer 2011; Tjaden *et al.* 2018). These methods take spatial presence or presence/absence data and use gridded environmental data to build a multivariate regression model (or sometimes another type of correlative model) of environmental suitability. SDMs made for a given location are sometimes projected to different geographic areas or time horizons to predict new species ranges, for example, to predict potential shifts in future distributions in response to future climate projected by a GCM. SDMs are more commonly generated for vectors than for pathogens themselves (but see Stevens and Pfeiffer 2011); however, predicted suitability for vectors alone can be a reasonable proxy for diseases where pathogen transmission is limited by the range limits of specific, highly competent vectors (Laporta *et al.* 2015; Tjaden *et al.* 2018).

SDMs are commonly used to predict how *Anopheles* vectors will respond to climate change. In general, SDMs predict that *Anopheles* vectors will expand their range into more temperate areas like Europe (Hertig 2019) and China (Ren *et al.* 2016) and increase malaria risk as the climate warms, although there is some variation among different species (Ren *et al.* 2016). In tropical South America, SDMs also predict the range expansion of many *Anopheles* vectors, although there is disagreement about the range of one of the most important vectors (*An. darlingi*), which may contract due to the climate becoming drier (Alimi *et al.* 2015; Laporta *et al.* 2015). Although there are currently no SDMs predicting the impact of climate change on Africa's most important vector (*An. gambiae*) within the continent, the total suitable area worldwide is expected to decrease (Li *et al.* 2021a). Additionally, the range of another vector (*An. arabiensis*) will likely contract within Africa (Drake and Beier 2014). This effect of climate could counteract the hypothesis that *An. arabiensis* will become more important as a malaria vector in the future with continued public health investments because it primarily feeds outdoors and is therefore unaffected by insecticide-treated bed nets and indoor spraying (Drake and Beier 2014).

Similar modelling approaches have also been used to predict future global distributions of dengue fever, including mechanistic models for transmission (Mordecai *et al.* 2017), statistical models for incidence (Colón-González *et al.* 2018; Messina *et al.* 2019), and SDMs of vector species *Ae. aegypti* and *Ae. albopictus* (Kraemer *et al.* 2015, 2019). As for *Anopheles* vectors, at decadal time scales climate change will likely cause *Aedes* vectors to expand poleward (Kraemer *et al.* 2019) and higher in elevation (Lippi *et al.* 2019). Additionally, the optimal temperature for transmission of dengue by *Ae. aegypti* is substantially warmer than for transmission of malaria by *Anopheles spp.* (29 vs 25 °C) (Mordecai *et al.* 2013, 2017, 2019). Thus, warming from climate change is predicted to cause widespread increases in transmission of dengue (Colón-González *et al.* 2018; Messina *et al.* 2019). Moreover, the current distribution of cases in Kenya demonstrates that dengue transmission is favoured relative to malaria in warmer conditions (Shah *et al.* 2019b). Together, these findings suggest that climate change may lead the disease burden in Africa to shift from malaria to dengue (Mordecai *et al.* 2020). This change will require a simultaneous shift in public health strategies, as malaria interventions (anti-parasitic therapies, insecticide-treated bed nets, and indoor spraying) are ineffective against the dengue virus and its vectors (*Ae. aegypti* and *Ae. albopictus*, which feed outdoors during the day) (Ferguson *et al.* 2016; Mordecai *et al.* 2020). These vectors also breed in different types of habitats (human containers vs natural water bodies), and so will require different approaches for larval source reduction and control.

6.3 *Synthesis and discussion*

Climate change is shifting patterns of MBD at large spatial scales. In the current hot spots for malaria, transmission will likely decrease as temperatures become too warm. These parts of Africa may see a shift from malaria to dengue, which is favoured at higher temperatures. However, malaria and dengue will both increase in other places, especially at higher latitudes and elevations, as temperatures in these relatively cool locations become more conducive for transmission. Part of this shift will be driven by the expanding geographic ranges of vector species into new areas as they warm and become suitable habitat. Changes in rainfall will also be important for determining regional patterns of transmission, as some places are getting wetter and others are getting drier. The net effect of all of these changes on the total global burden of a MBDs like malaria and dengue will depend on the distribution of human population density across all of these locations, as well as investments in public health interventions and medical treatment.

Climate is predicted to be particularly important for shaping patterns of disease transmission at larger spatial scales (Cohen *et al.* 2016), but including other factors can still inform and improve these modelling efforts. While climate determines the potential for expansions of vectors' geographic ranges in the long-term, human movement drives the short-term spread of *Aedes* vectors of dengue, with long-distance importations being particularly important for *Ae. aegypti* (Kraemer *et al.* 2019). The Asian malaria vector *An. stephensi* was recently introduced into Africa and has been slowly expanding over the past decade (Sinka *et al.* 2020). This urban specialist may shift future malaria burden from rural areas to cities, and has already shown signs of successfully adapting from seasonal to year-round transmission activity (Sinka *et al.* 2020). At regional scales, human mobility can be important for spreading malaria just as with dengue (Buckee *et al.* 2013; Wesolowski *et al.* 2012). Additionally, malaria exhibits unique patterns of immunity stemming from the parasite's complex life cycle and its interaction with the immune system. These within-host dynamics combined with partial or waning immunity can be important for modelling dynamics at regional and local scales (Alonso *et al.* 2019).

7 Results from models of tick-borne disease

General predictions for the impact of climate change on TBD are similar to those for MBD in cooler, temperate areas. Based on statistical relationships between climate and incidence of Lyme disease, warming temperatures from climate change are predicted to increase transmission across the U.S. (Dumic and Severnini 2018; Robinson *et al.* 2015), particularly in the northeast region (Couper *et al.* 2021b). Simulations with mechanistic models indicate that warmer temperatures contributed to the emergence of Lyme disease in Canada over the past 50 years, and predict that transmission will continue to increase with climate change (Ogden *et al.* 2014). Across Europe, warmer temperatures are correlated with tick populations expanding both farther north and higher in elevation (Ostfeld and Brunner 2015). Species distribution models (SDM) using projections of future climate conditions predict that European ticks will continue to expand their geographic ranges into higher latitudes as these areas warm and experience milder winters (Porretta *et al.* 2013). Thus, the warming climate has generally increased the ranges of tick species and enhanced transmission of TBD, and is likely to continue doing so in the future.

8 Challenges, knowledge gaps, and research frontiers

Major challenges for modelling MBD fall into three categories: data generation and availability, model construction, and translating model output into action. In this section, we describe some of these challenges, list knowledge gaps in MBD research that would improve modelling efforts, and identify active research frontiers where the field is advancing.

8.1 *Challenges: data generation and availability*

Many data availability challenges relate to basic surveillance of mosquitoes and human cases. Mosquito populations are extremely patchy and heterogenous over space and time (Jian *et al.* 2016; Vazquez-Prokopec *et al.* 2016). Sampling this variation can be challenging, as intensive trapping effort is needed to overcome stochastic noise and species identification may be difficult and time consuming. Multiple species with different vectoral capabilities or different life histories may be grouped in surveillance data. Data sets on mosquito surveillance are typically not shared publicly, which limits nationwide syntheses. Even within a state or province, mosquito control districts may function independently, data sharing between agencies may be limited or non-existent, and resources or technological infrastructure needed to support widespread data sharing are not available. Many MBDs are rare, especially during the early season, which makes early detection difficult. Asymptomatic cases in humans are difficult to identify, and even symptomatic cases of rare diseases may be missed by clinicians. This can make estimating human case numbers challenging because only a fraction of total cases is reported to relevant health authorities through passive surveillance. In MBD where humans are not dead-end hosts, asymptomatic individuals may allow the disease to persist, as asymptomatic individuals are unlikely to seek medical care and may contribute to ongoing transmission (Coura *et al.* 2006). Detecting asymptomatic infections can be challenging, even in wealthy nations with more developed health infrastructure. This can make it difficult to tease out disease-climate relationships, as model predictions of climatic suitability accompanied by an absence of reported cases may not represent an actual absence of disease. Consistent monitoring, infrastructure, and data reporting protocols, as well as open data and/or data sharing agreements among agencies could facilitate more widely available and user-friendly data. One recent paper has suggested minimum data standards for vector competence experiments (Wu *et al.* 2022), a strategy that could be utilized for other types of vector data.

One key subset of this mosquito surveillance data challenge is obtaining vector control data and integrating it into models (Caputo and Manica 2020). While there are many mechanistic models designed specifically to study the theoretical impact of various types of vector control (Cailly *et al.* 2012; Wijaya *et al.* 2014; Zhu *et al.* 2019), data for the actual impact of these measures in the field is rare (Reiner *et al.* 2016) (but see Ng'habi *et al.* 2018; Senapati *et al.* 2019). Furthermore, even basic data such as the extent and timing of vector control activities are generally not available in a form that can be used in models. Accordingly, most statistical models of MBD do not incorporate the effects vector of control. Assuming that vector control methods are effective, this decision means that most models are omitting a major factor, which may impact model accuracy. For example, we may be underestimating the impact of climate on transmission or mosquito population abundance if there is widespread aerial spraying or larviciding occurring that the models do not account for. One relatively simple way to address this issue is to simulate counterfactual scenarios to assess likely differences between actual and potential vector abundances.

Other data availability challenges relate to climate predictors. While high-quality data on regional climate and landcover exist, data can be lacking at fine spatial scales. Diurnal air temperatures at coarse scales may not be representative of the microclimate in mosquito resting sites due to spatial heterogeneity (Afrane *et al.* 2005; Boser *et al.* 2021; Cator *et al.* 2013; Murdock *et al.* 2017; Ngowo *et al.* 2017; Paaijmans and Thomas 2011) and mosquito thermoregulation (Blanford *et al.* 2009; Danforth *et al.* 2016; Kirby and Lindsay 2004; Ngowo *et al.* 2017; Pincebourde and Woods 2020; Sauer *et al.* 2021; Woods *et al.* 2015). For instance, mosquitoes breeding in catch basins experience very different temperatures and relative humidity levels than the conditions recorded by weather stations in open fields, and may serve as refugia that function to buffer mosquitoes against otherwise prohibitive environmental extremes (Erraguntla *et al.* 2021). Additionally, key data on host infection rates are not collected at the same scale as mosquito infection rates (or made less precise intentionally to protect patient identities), and host immunity is important for determining outbreaks of zoonotic MBDs (Mackenzie *et al.* 2000; Paull *et al.* 2017; Woodruff *et al.* 2002). Researchers could partially address these issues by determining whether there are consistent relationships between local scale climate variability and regional scale climate data, which could allow for better downscaling of available climate data.

8.2 *Challenges: model construction*

Relationships between MBD and climate predictor variables are non-linear and complex (see section on *Biological mechanisms for climate drivers of MBD*). Accordingly, models must be constructed and analysed carefully to accurately detect and characterise these relationships. Identifying the critical factors among several colinear predictor variables may be a challenge. Temperature can be measured in a multitude of ways (mean, minimum, maximum, daily temperature range), across multiple scales (daily, weekly, monthly, quarterly, annually), at a variety of time lags, and many of these metrics will be highly correlated with each other. There is little consensus for which measures are most predictive or how to select among them, and including too many predictors risks overfitting or finding false relationships by chance. Additionally, even when qualitative patterns are identified, translating them into quantitative predictive models may be difficult.

Models may be limited by the inherent stochasticity of the MBD systems, especially when disease incidence is low. At low infection rates, very different outcomes could occur based on random chance: whether an infected mosquito happened to feed, or if it fed, and how susceptible the host was. This stochasticity in biotic interactions could be the difference between kick-starting the amplification process or an outbreak fizzling out, making it inherently difficult to generate accurate predictions even if climatic conditions are suitable. At higher infection rates, these types of chance events should be less influential. In low incidence settings, machine learning may be particularly useful, as these techniques are generally more robust to data inadequacies.

For predictive models to be useful in a policy-making context, models must be able to provide actionable information. A useful thought experiment is to ask how a model might change a public health or vector control decision, and what accuracy level would be needed to change the decision. If the decision would not change, or would require an accuracy beyond the model's capabilities, time and effort could be better spent on other decisions or activities.

8.3 *Challenges: translating model output into action*

Once a model generates a forecast or set of results, there are social, political, and economic barriers to effective implementation as policy (Dickinson and Paskewitz 2012; Dickinson *et al.* 2016; Keyel *et al.* 2021a; Moise *et al.* 2019; Tedesco *et al.* 2010). For instance, in the Midwestern U.S., interest and attention from local news organizations in producing stories about WNV peaks around Memorial Day when people begin spending more time outside for the summer, but by the time human risk peaks around Labor Day their focus has already shifted to 'back to school' stories (R. Smith, personal communication). Additionally, in many cases, decisions must be made before forecasts are available. Some local governments and vector control agencies must allocate their budgets during the prior fiscal year, and by the time WNV forecasts have been generated, most vector control districts have already made their seasonal hiring decisions (Keyel *et al.* 2021a). Vector control activities may not be a budget priority (Dickinson and Paskewitz 2012; Dickinson *et al.* 2016), or there may not be funds available in resource poor communities regardless of desire. Successful model implementation should also take local characteristics and culture into account. Studies on Knowledge, Attitudes, and Perceptions/Practices (KAP) can be extremely useful at generating qualitative and quantitative data to inform public health interventions (Jones *et al.* 2014; Potter *et al.* 2016; Vijayakumar *et al.* 2009).

Real time data processing and logistics are also a key challenge for using forecasts to make operational decisions. The dengue 'forecasting' challenge was actually hindcasting past data that were not publicly available yet. Accordingly, the data were already collected, processed, and prepared for release. However, during a live epidemic season, the logistics of data reporting and processing will delay data availability and reduce the accuracy of forecasts (DeFelice *et al.* 2019; Johansson *et al.* 2019). Even short delays on the order of 1–2 weeks could lower the efficacy of vector control and public health interventions. Many solutions to these types of data-related challenges rely heavily on investment in infrastructure and technology and thus are exacerbated in low- and middle-income countries with fewer resources (Lowe *et al.* 2020). However, the COVID-19 pandemic highlighted the need for fast and accurate public health data, and many governments and institutions have invested time and money to streamline this process in ways that will improve ongoing real-time collection of data for other diseases.

8.4 *Knowledge gaps*

There are several knowledge gaps where additional research would improve modelling efforts. Current models for the impacts of climate change on vectors or MBD do not consider the possibility that mosquitoes may evolve in response to warmer temperatures. There are theoretical reasons to suggest that mosquito species have high potential to thermally adapt: short generation times, high population growth rates, and strong selection on mortality rates due to hot temperatures (Couper *et al.* 2021a). However, we currently lack sufficient data characterizing the standing genetic variation for thermal responses or local thermal adaptation in existing populations (Couper *et al.* 2021a), which would provide better evidence that adaptation to climate change is a likely outcome and guidance for how to include such evolution in models. Passage studies suggest viruses have the capacity to adapt to changing temperatures (Fay *et al.* 2021). Additionally, for pathogens that circulate and are maintained in reservoir hosts (such as WNV and Ross River virus, the most common vector-borne disease in Australia), major questions remain about how much different hosts contribute to transmission cycles. Increased surveillance of these pathogens in non-human animals could increase our understanding of current patterns and improve predictions for the future since these vertebrate hosts are also affected by climate change. Finally, more clarity is needed on how climatic factors impact transmission of MBD at different spatial and temporal scales. There is broad consensus that climate is key for determining seasonality and patterns at large spatial scales, but debate over its importance at finer scales. One study of WNV and the tick-borne Lyme disease pathogen across the U.S. found that climate was important for determining patterns at larger spatial scales, whereas biotic interactions were more important at local scales (Cohen *et al.* 2016). However, other studies of WNV have detected the effects of climate at much finer scales (Keyel *et al.* 2019; Uelmen *et al.* 2021b, a).

8.5 *Research frontiers*

Advances in data generation, processing, and availability may improve future modelling efforts. Incorporating data from internet searches and social media improved models of Zika cases during the rapidly unfolding outbreak in five Latin American countries (McGough *et al.* 2017). New smart traps, drone technology, and machine learning approaches for mosquito identification aim to make processing mosquito surveillance data more efficient (Fouet and Kamdem 2019; Goodwin *et al.* 2021; Joshi and Miller 2021; Microsoft 2019). More generally, machine learning techniques are an area of rapid growth across a wide variety of tasks used for mosquito control and modelling (Joshi and Miller 2021). Additionally, there is a growing movement to standardise data collection and increase the availability of data on vector populations and vector-borne diseases through public databases like VectorBASE (https://www.vectorbase.org/), Vector Byte (https://vectorbyte.org), the datasets for the dengue forecasting challenge (https://predict.cdc.gov), and the CDC Zika data repository (https://github.com/cdcepi/zika).

9 Conclusions

Models are a critical tool for understanding how climate shapes patterns of vector-borne disease and predicting how these patterns might change in response to future climate change. The relationships between transmission and climate predictor variables like temperature and rainfall are non-linear and complex. There is a wide array of methods available for modelling, including mechanistic, statistical, and hybrid approaches. The most appropriate method will depend on the research questions and the spatial and temporal scale of the data. Comparing results from different approaches can often yield insight or combine to provide complimentary evidence. Ensembles of models may be useful – both for global circulation models (GCMs) predicting future conditions (to account for uncertainty in the changing climate), and for models forecasting outbreaks of mosquito-borne disease (because ensembles often perform better than individual models). Generating accurate short-term local and regional forecasts is challenging, but can provide critical information for preventing and mitigating outbreaks. At larger scales, we expect climate change to lead to shifts in spatial and temporal patterns of vector-borne disease transmission.

Acknowledgements

JMC was supported by the High Meadows Environmental Institute (HMEI) Grand Challenges, HMEI Studies Strategic Fund, and the Gatto Fund; PH was funded through US National Science Foundation CAREER award NSF DMS/DEB #1750113 and VectorBiTE Research Coordination Network; ACK acknowledges funding from US National Institutes of Health grant R01AI168097.

References

Acemoglu D, Johnson S and Robinson JA (2001) The Colonial origins of comparative development: an empirical investigation. American Economic Review, 91: 1369–1401. https://doi.org/10.1257/aer.91.5.1369.

Adams B and Boots M (2010) How important is vertical transmission in mosquitoes for the persistence of dengue? Insights from a mathematical model. Epidemics, 2: 1–10. https://doi.org/10.1016/j.epidem.2010.01.001.

Adams B, Holmes EC, Zhang C, Mammen MP, Nimmannitya S, Kalayanarooj S and Boots M (2006) Cross-protective immunity can account for the alternating epidemic pattern of dengue virus serotypes circulating in Bangkok. Proceedings of the National Academy of Sciences, 103: 14234–14239. https://doi.org/10.1073/pnas.0602768103.

Adde A, Roucou P, Mangeas M, Ardillon V, Desenclos J-C, Rousset D, Girod R, Briolant S, Quenel P and Flamand C (2016) Predicting Dengue Fever Outbreaks in French Guiana Using Climate Indicators. PLoS neglected tropical diseases, 10: e0004681. https://doi.org/10.1371/journal.pntd.0004681.

Afrane YA, Lawson BW, Githeko AK and Yan G (2005) Effects of microclimatic changes caused by land use and land cover on duration of gonotrophic cycles of *Anopheles gambiae* (Diptera: Culicidae) in western Kenya highlands. Journal of Medical Entomology, 42: 974–980. https://doi.org/10.1093/jmedent/42.6.974.

Aguas R, Dorigatti I, Coudeville L, Luxemburger C and Ferguson NM (2019) Cross-serotype interactions and disease outcome prediction of dengue infections in Vietnam. Scientific Reports, 9: 9395. https://doi.org/10.1038/s41598-019-45816-6.

Akhtar M, Kraemer MUG and Gardner LM (2019) A dynamic neural network model for predicting risk of Zika in real time. BMC Medicine, 17: 171. https://doi.org/10.1186/s12916-019-1389-3.

Alimi TO, Fuller DO, Qualls WA, Herrera SV, Arevalo-Herrera M, Quinones ML, Lacerda MVG and Beier JC (2015) Predicting potential ranges of primary malaria vectors and malaria in northern South America based on projected changes in climate, land cover and human population. Parasites & Vectors, 8: 431. https://doi.org/10.1186/s13071-015-1033-9.

Alonso D, Dobson A and Pascual M (2019) Critical transitions in malaria transmission models are consistently generated by superinfection. Philosophical Transactions of the Royal Society B: Biological Sciences, 374: 20180275. https://doi.org/10.1098/rstb.2018.0275.

Alsan M (2015) The Effect of the TseTse Fly on African Development. American Economic Review, 105: 382–410. https://doi.org/10.1257/aer.20130604.

Anderson RM and May RM (1979) Population biology of infectious diseases: Part I. Nature, 280: 361–367. https://doi.org/10.1038/280361a0.

Antinori S, Bonazzetti C, Giacomelli A, Corbellino M, Galli M, Parravicini C and Ridolfo AL (2021) Non-human primate and human malaria: past, present and future. Journal of Travel Medicine, 28: taab036. https://doi.org/10.1093/jtm/taab036.

Anyamba A, Chretien J-P, Small J, Tucker CJ, Formenty PB, Richardson JH, Britch SC, Schnabel DC, Erickson RL and Linthicum KJ (2009) Prediction of a Rift Valley fever outbreak. Proceedings of the National Academy of Sciences, 106: 955–959. https://doi.org/10.1073/pnas.0806490106.

Anyamba A, Linthicum KJ, Small JL, Collins KM, Tucker CJ, Pak EW, Britch SC, Eastman JR, Pinzon JE and Russell KL (2012) Climate teleconnections and recent patterns of human and animal disease outbreaks. PLoS Neglected Tropical Diseases, 6: e1465. https://doi.org/10.1371/journal.pntd.0001465.

Arsnoe IM, Hickling GJ, Ginsberg HS, McElreath R and Tsao JI (2015) Different populations of blacklegged tick nymphs exhibit differences in questing behavior that have implications for human lyme disease risk. PLoS ONE, 10: e0127450. https://doi.org/10.1371/journal.pone.0127450.

Artzy-Randrup Y, Dobson AP and Pascual M (2015) Synergistic and antagonistic interactions between bednets and vaccines in the control of malaria. Proceedings of the National Academy of Sciences, 112: 3014–3019. https://doi.org/10.1073/pnas.1409467112.

Athni TS, Shocket MS, Couper LI, Nova N, Caldwell IR, Caldwell JM, Childress JN, Childs ML, De Leo GA, Kirk DG, MacDonald AJ, Olivarius K, Pickel DG, Roberts SO, Winokur OC, Young HS, Cheng J, Grant EA, Kurzner PM, Kyaw S, Lin BJ, Lopez RC, Massihpour DS, Olsen EC, Roache M, Ruiz A, Schultz EA, Shafat M, Spencer RL, Bharti N and Mordecai

EA (2021) The influence of vector-borne disease on human history: socio-ecological mechanisms. Ecology Letters, 24: 829–846. https://doi.org/10.1111/ele.13675.

Augusiak J, Van den Brink PJ and Grimm V (2014) Merging validation and evaluation of ecological models to 'evaludation': A review of terminology and a practical approach. Ecological Modelling, 280: 117–128. https://doi.org/10.1016/j.ecolmodel.2013.11.009.

Barros FSM, Arruda ME, Gurgel HC and Honório NA (2011) Spatial clustering and longitudinal variation of *Anopheles darlingi* (Diptera: Culicidae) larvae in a river of the Amazon: the importance of the forest fringe and of obstructions to flow in frontier malaria. Bulletin of Entomological Research, 101: 643–658. https://doi.org/10.1017/S0007485311000265.

Bayoh MN (2001) Studies on the development and survival of *Anopheles gambiae* sensu stricto at various temperatures and relative humidities. Doctoral thesis. Durham University.

Beale CM, Lennon JJ and Gimona A (2008) Opening the climate envelope reveals no macroscale associations with climate in European birds. Proceedings of the National Academy of Sciences, 105: 14908–14912. https://doi.org/10.1073/pnas.0803506105.

Beck-Johnson LM, Nelson WA, Paaijmans KP, Read AF, Thomas MB and Bjørnstad ON (2017) The importance of temperature fluctuations in understanding mosquito population dynamics and malaria risk. Royal Society Open Science, 4: 160969. https://doi.org/10.1098/rsos.160969.

Beeman SP, Morrison AM, Unnasch TR and Unnasch RS (2021) Ensemble ecological niche modeling of West Nile virus probability in Florida. PLOS ONE, 16: e0256868. https://doi.org/10.1371/journal.pone.0256868.

Benedum CM, Seidahmed OME, Eltahir EAB and Markuzon N (2018) Statistical modeling of the effect of rainfall flushing on dengue transmission in Singapore. PLoS Neglected Tropical Diseases, 12: e0006935. https://doi.org/10.1371/journal.pntd.0006935.

Benedum CM, Shea KM, Jenkins HE, Kim LY and Markuzon N (2020) Weekly dengue forecasts in Iquitos, Peru; San Juan, Puerto Rico; and Singapore. PLOS Neglected Tropical Diseases, 14: e0008710. https://doi.org/10.1371/journal.pntd.0008710.

Bernhardt JR, Sunday JM, Thompson PL and O'Connor MI (2018) Nonlinear averaging of thermal experience predicts population growth rates in a thermally variable environment. Proceedings of the Royal Society B: Biological Sciences, 285: 20181076. https://doi.org/10.1098/rspb.2018.1076.

Bershteyn A, Gerardin J, Bridenbecker D, Lorton CW, Bloedow J, Baker RS, Chabot-Couture G, Chen Y, Fischle T, Frey K, Gauld JS, Hu H, Izzo AS, Klein DJ, Lukacevic D, McCarthy KA, Miller JC, Ouedraogo AL, Perkins TA, Steinkraus J, ten Bosch QA, Ting H-F, Titova S, Wagner BG, Welkhoff PA, Wenger EA, Wiswell CN, and for the Institute for Disease Modeling (2018) Implementation and applications of EMOD, an individual-based multi-disease modeling platform. Pathogens and Disease, 76. https://doi.org/10.1093/femspd/fty059.

Bhatt S, Gething PW, Brady OJ, Messina JP, Farlow AW, Moyes CL, Drake JM, Brownstein JS, Hoen AG, Sankoh O, Myers MF, George DB, Jaenisch T, Wint GRW, Simmons CP, Scott TW, Farrar JJ and Hay SI (2013) The global distribution and burden of dengue. Nature, 496: 504–507. https://doi.org/10.1038/nature12060.

Bi P, Hiller JE, Cameron AS, Zhang Y and Givney R (2009) Climate variability and Ross River virus infections in Riverland, South Australia, 1992–2004. Epidemiology and infection, 137: 1486–93. https://doi.org/10.1017/S0950268809002441.

Bi P, Parton. K.A. and Donald K (2004) Climate variability and the transmission of Ross River virus infection in coastal regions of Queensland, Australia., 4 (2), 90–96. Environmental Health, 4: 90–96.

Blanford S, Read AF and Thomas MB (2009) Thermal behaviour of *Anopheles stephensi* in response to infection with malaria and fungal entomopathogens. Malaria Journal, 8: 72. https://doi.org/10.1186/1475-2875-8-72.

Bomblies A, Duchemin J-B and Eltahir EAB (2008) Hydrology of malaria: Model development and application to a Sahelian village: hydrology of malaria. Water Resources Research, 44. https://doi.org/10.1029/2008WR006917.

ten Bosch QA, Wagman JM, Castro-Llanos F, Achee NL, Grieco JP and Perkins TA (2020) Community-level impacts of spatial repellents for control of diseases vectored by *Aedes aegypti* mosquitoes. PLOS Computational Biology, 16: e1008190. https://doi.org/10.1371/journal.pcbi.1008190.

Boser A, Sousa D, Larsen A and MacDonald A (2021) Micro-climate to macro-risk: mapping fine scale differences in mosquito-borne disease risk using remote sensing. Environmental Research Letters, 16: 124014. https://doi.org/10.1088/1748-9326/ac3589.

Bouma MJ, Siraj AS, Rodo X and Pascual M (2016) El Niño-based malaria epidemic warning for Oromia, Ethiopia, from August 2016 to July 2017. Tropical Medicine & International Health, 21: 1481–1488. https://doi.org/10.1111/tmi.12776.

Braunisch V, Coppes J, Arlettaz R, Suchant R, Schmid H and Bollmann K (2013) Selecting from correlated climate variables: a major source of uncertainty for predicting species distributions under climate change. Ecography, 36: 971–983. https://doi.org/10.1111/j.1600-0587.2013.00138.x.

Brown H, Diuk-Wasser M, Andreadis T and Fish D (2008) Remotely-Sensed Vegetation Indices Identify Mosquito Clusters of West Nile Virus Vectors in an Urban Landscape in the Northeastern United States. Vector-Borne and Zoonotic Diseases, 8: 197–206. https://doi.org/10.1089/vbz.2007.0154.

Brunner JL, Killilea M and Ostfeld RS (2012) Overwintering survival of nymphal *Ixodes scapularis* (Acari: Ixodidae) under natural conditions. Journal of Medical Entomology, 49: 981–987. https://doi.org/10.1603/ME12060.

Buckee CO, Wesolowski A, Eagle NN, Hansen E and Snow RW (2013) Mobile phones and malaria: Modeling human and parasite travel. Travel Medicine and Infectious Disease, 11: 15–22. https://doi.org/10.1016/j.tmaid.2012.12.003.

Buczak AL, Baugher B, Moniz LJ, Bagley T, Babin SM and Guven E (2018) Ensemble method for dengue prediction. PLOS ONE, 13: e0189988. https://doi.org/10.1371/journal.pone.0189988.

Burnham KP and Anderson DR (2010) *Model selection and multimodel inference: a practical information-theoretic approach.* 2. ed. Springer, New York, NY.

Burnham KP, Anderson DR and Huyvaert KP (2011) AIC model selection and multimodel inference in behavioral ecology: some background, observations, and comparisons. Behavioral Ecology and Sociobiology, 65: 23–35. https://doi.org/10.1007/s00265-010-1029-6.

Cailly P, Tran A, Balenghien T, L'Ambert G, Toty C and Ezanno P (2012) A climate-driven abundance model to assess mosquito control strategies. Ecological Modelling, 227: 7–17. https://doi.org/10.1016/j.ecolmodel.2011.10.027.

Calderón-Arguedas O, Troyo A, Moreira-Soto RD, Marín R and Taylor L (2015) Dengue viruses in *Aedes albopictus* Skuse from a pineapple plantation in Costa Rica. Journal of Vector Ecology, 40: 184–186. https://doi.org/10.1111/jvec.12149.

Caldwell JM, LaBeaud AD, Lambin EF, Stewart-Ibarra AM, Ndenga BA, Mutuku FM, Krystosik AR, Ayala EB, Anyamba A, Borbor-Cordova MJ, Damoah R, Grossi-Soyster EN, Heras FH, Ngugi HN, Ryan SJ, Shah MM, Sippy R and Mordecai EA (2021) Climate predicts geographic and temporal variation in mosquito-borne disease dynamics on two continents. Nature Communications, 12: 1233. https://doi.org/10.1038/s41467-021-21496-7.

Caminade C, Kovats S, Rocklov J, Tompkins AM, Morse AP, Colón-González FJ, Stenlund H, Martens P and Lloyd SJ (2014) Impact of climate change on global malaria distribution. Proceedings of the National Academy of Sciences, 111: 3286–3291. https://doi.org/10.1073/pnas.1302089111.

Caputo B and Manica M (2020) Mosquito surveillance and disease outbreak risk models to inform mosquito-control operations in Europe. Current Opinion in Insect Science, 39: 101–108. https://doi.org/10.1016/j.cois.2020.03.009.

Cator LJ, Johnson LR, Mordecai EA, El Moustaid F, Smallwood TRC, LaDeau SL, Johansson MA, Hudson PJ, Boots M, Thomas MB, Power AG and Pawar S (2020) The Role of Vector Trait Variation in Vector-Borne Disease Dynamics. Frontiers in Ecology and Evolution, 8: 189. https://doi.org/10.3389/fevo.2020.00189.

Cator LJ, Thomas S, Paaijmans KP, Ravishankaran S, Justin JA, Mathai MT, Read AF, Thomas MB and Eapen A (2013) Characterizing microclimate in urban malaria transmission settings: a case study from Chennai, India. Malaria Journal, 12: 84. https://doi.org/10.1186/1475-2875-12-84.

Cazelles B, Chavez M, Magny GC de, Guégan J-F and Hales S (2007) Time-dependent spectral analysis of epidemiological time-series with wavelets. Journal of The Royal Society Interface, 4: 625–636. https://doi.org/10.1098/rsif.2007.0212.

Cazelles B, Chavez M, McMichael AJ and Hales S (2005) Nonstationary Influence of El Niño on the Synchronous Dengue Epidemics in Thailand. PLoS Medicine, 2: e106. https://doi.org/10.1371/journal.pmed.0020106.

Centers for Disease Control and Prevention (2022) *Mosquito Surveillance Software*. Available at: https://www.cdc.gov/westnile/resourcepages/mosqSurvSoft.html.

Chakraborty T, Chattopadhyay S and Ghosh I (2019) Forecasting dengue epidemics using a hybrid methodology. Physica A: Statistical Mechanics and its Applications, 527: 121266. https://doi.org/10.1016/j.physa.2019.121266.

Chandran R and Azeez PA (2015) Outbreak of dengue in Tamil Nadu, India. Current Science, 109: 171–176.

Chaves A, Dolz G, Ibarra-Cerdeña CN, Núñez G, Ortiz-Malavasi E E, Bernal-Valle S and Gutiérrez-Espeleta GA (2022) Presence and potential distribution of malaria-infected New World primates of Costa Rica. Malaria Journal, 21: 17. https://doi.org/10.1186/s12936-021-04036-y.

Chaves LSM, Conn JE, López RVM and Sallum MAM (2018) Abundance of impacted forest patches less than 5 km2 is a key driver of the incidence of malaria in Amazonian Brazil. Scientific Reports, 8: 1–11. https://doi.org/10.1038/s41598-018-25344-5.

Chiang CL and Reeves WC (1962) STATISTICAL ESTIMATION OF VIRUS INFECTION RATES IN MOSQUITO VECTOR POPULATIONS1. American Journal of Epidemiology, 75: 377–391. https://doi.org/10.1093/oxfordjournals.aje.a120259.

Ciota AT, Bialosuknia SM, Ehrbar DJ and Kramer LD (2017) Vertical Transmission of Zika Virus by *Aedes aegypti* and *Ae. albopictus* Mosquitoes. Emerging Infectious Diseases, 23: 880–882. https://doi.org/10.3201/eid2305.162041.

Cohen J (2013) *Statistical Power Analysis for the Behavioral Sciences*. 0 edn. Routledge. https://doi.org/10.4324/9780203771587.

Cohen JM, Civitello DJ, Brace AJ, Feichtinger EM, Ortega CN, Richardson JC, Sauer EL, Liu X and Rohr JR (2016) Spatial scale modulates the strength of ecological processes driving disease distributions. Proceedings of the National Academy of Sciences, 113: E3359–E3364. https://doi.org/10.1073/pnas.1521657113.

Colón-González FJ, Bentham G and Lake IR (2011) Climate Variability and Dengue Fever in Warm and Humid Mexico. The American Journal of Tropical Medicine and Hygiene, 84: 757–763. https://doi.org/10.4269/ajtmh.2011.10-0609.

Colón-González FJ, Harris I, Osborn TJ, Steiner São Bernardo C, Peres CA, Hunter PR, Warren R, van Vuurene D and Lake IR (2018) Limiting global-mean temperature increase to 1.5–2 °C could reduce the incidence and spatial spread of dengue fever in Latin America. Proceedings of the National Academy of Sciences, 115: 6243–6248. https://doi.org/10.1073/pnas.1718945115.

Costa EAP de A, Santos EM de M, Correia JC and Albuquerque CMR de (2010) Impact of small variations in temperature and humidity on the reproductive activity and survival of *Aedes aegypti* (Diptera, Culicidae). Revista Brasileira de Entomologia, 54: 488–493. https://doi.org/10.1590/S0085-56262010000300021.

Couper LI, Farner JE, Caldwell JM, Childs ML, Harris MJ, Kirk DG, Nova N, Shocket M, Skinner EB, Uricchio LH, Exposito-Alonso M and Mordecai EA (2021a) How will mosquitoes adapt to climate warming? eLife, 10: e69630. https://doi.org/10.7554/eLife.69630.

Couper LI, MacDonald AJ and Mordecai EA (2021b) Impact of prior and projected climate change on US Lyme disease incidence. Global Change Biology, 27: 738–754. https://doi.org/10.1111/gcb.15435.

Coura JR, Suárez-Mutis M and Ladeia-Andrade S (2006) A new challenge for malaria control in Brazil: asymptomatic *Plasmodium* infection – a review. Memórias do Instituto Oswaldo Cruz, 101: 229–237. https://doi.org/10.1590/S0074-02762006000300001.

Cutler SJ, Vayssier-Taussat M, Estrada-Peña A, Potkonjak A, Mihalca AD and Zeller H (2021) Tick-borne diseases and co-infection: Current considerations. Ticks and Tick-borne Diseases, 12: 101607. https://doi.org/10.1016/j.ttbdis.2020.101607.

Damos PT, Dorrestijn J, Thomidis T, Tuells J and Caballero P (2021) A Temperature Conditioned Markov Chain Model for Predicting the Dynamics of Mosquito Vectors of Disease. Insects, 12: 725. https://doi.org/10.3390/insects12080725.

Danforth ME, Reisen WK and Barker CM (2016) The Impact of Cycling Temperature on the Transmission of West Nile Virus. Journal of Medical Entomology, 53: 681–686. https://doi.org/10.1093/jme/tjw013.

Dantur Juri MJ, Estallo E, Almirón W, Santana M, Sartor P, Lamfri M and Zaidenberg M (2015) Satellite-derived NDVI, LST, and climatic factors driving the distribution and abundance of *Anopheles* mosquitoes in a former malarious area in northwest Argentina. Journal of Vector Ecology, 40: 36–45. https://doi.org/10.1111/jvec.12130.

Davis JK, Vincent G, Hildreth MB, Kightlinger L, Carlson C and Wimberly MC (2017) Integrating environmental monitoring and mosquito surveillance to predict vector-borne disease: prospective forecasts of a West Nile Virus outbreak. PLoS Currents. https://doi.org/10.1371/currents.outbreaks.90e80717c4e67e1a830f17feeaaf85de.

Davis JK, Vincent GP, Hildreth MB, Kightlinger L, Carlson C and Wimberly MC (2018) Improving the prediction of arbovirus outbreaks: a comparison of climate-driven models for West Nile virus in an endemic region of the United States. Acta Tropica, 185: 242–250. https://doi.org/10.1016/j.actatropica.2018.04.028.

Day JF and Shaman J (2009) Severe winter freezes enhance St. Louis Encephalitis Virus amplification and epidemic transmission in Peninsular Florida. Journal of Medical Entomology, 46: 1498–1506. https://doi.org/10.1603/033.046.0638.

De Marco P and Nóbrega CC (2018) Evaluating collinearity effects on species distribution models: An approach based on virtual species simulation. PLOS ONE, 13: e0202403. https://doi.org/10.1371/journal.pone.0202403.

DeFelice NB, Birger R, DeFelice N, Gagner A, Campbell SR, Romano C, Santoriello M, Henke J, Wittie J, Cole B, Kaiser C and Shaman J (2019) Modeling and surveillance of reporting delays of mosquitoes and humans infected with West Nile Virus and associations with accuracy of West Nile Virus forecasts. JAMA Network Open, 2: e193175. https://doi.org/10.1001/jamanetworkopen.2019.3175.

DeFelice NB, Schneider ZD, Little E, Barker C, Caillouet KA, Campbell SR, Damian D, Irwin P, Jones HMP, Townsend J and Shaman J (2018) Use of temperature to improve West Nile virus forecasts. PLOS Computational Biology, 14: e1006047. https://doi.org/10.1371/journal.pcbi.1006047.

Dejnirattisai W, Supasa P, Wongwiwat W, Rouvinski A, Barba-Spaeth G, Duangchinda T, Sakuntabhai A, Cao-Lormeau V-M, Malasit P, Rey FA, Mongkolsapaya J and Screaton

GR (2016) Dengue virus sero-cross-reactivity drives antibody-dependent enhancement of infection with zika virus. Nature Immunology, 17: 1102–1108. https://doi.org/10.1038/ni.3515.

Dell AI, Pawar S and Savage VM (2011) Systematic variation in the temperature dependence of physiological and ecological traits. Proceedings of the National Academy of Sciences, 108: 10591–10596. https://doi.org/10.1073/pnas.1015178108.

Dickinson K and Paskewitz S (2012) Willingness to pay for mosquito control: how important is West Nile Virus risk compared to the nuisance of mosquitoes? Vector-Borne and Zoonotic Diseases, 12: 886–892. https://doi.org/10.1089/vbz.2011.0810.

Dickinson KL, Hayden MH, Haenchen S, Monaghan AJ, Walker KR and Ernst KC (2016) Willingness to Pay for Mosquito Control in Key West, Florida and Tucson, Arizona. The American Journal of Tropical Medicine and Hygiene, 94: 775–779. https://doi.org/10.4269/ajtmh.15-0666.

Diouf I, Adeola AM, Abiodun GJ, Lennard C, Shirinde JM, Yaka P, Ndione J-A and Gbobaniyi EO (2022) Impact of future climate change on malaria in West Africa. Theoretical and Applied Climatology, 147: 853–865. https://doi.org/10.1007/s00704-021-03807-6.

Diuk-Wasser MA, VanAcker MC and Fernandez MP (2021) Impact of Land Use Changes and Habitat Fragmentation on the Eco-epidemiology of Tick-Borne Diseases. Journal of Medical Entomology, 58: 1546–1564. https://doi.org/10.1093/jme/tjaa209.

Dobson ADM, Finnie TJR and Randolph SE (2011) A modified matrix model to describe the seasonal population ecology of the European tick *Ixodes ricinus*: *Ixodes ricinus* population model. Journal of Applied Ecology, 48: 1017–1028. https://doi.org/10.1111/j.1365-2664.2011.02003.x.

Drake JM and Beier JC (2014) Ecological niche and potential distribution of *Anopheles arabiensis* in Africa in 2050. Malaria Journal, 13: 213. https://doi.org/10.1186/1475-2875-13-213.

Dumic I and Severnini E (2018) 'Ticking Bomb': the impact of climate change on the incidence of lyme disease. Canadian Journal of Infectious Diseases and Medical Microbiology, 2018: 1–10. https://doi.org/10.1155/2018/5719081.

Dunphy BM, Kovach KB, Gehrke EJ, Field EN, Rowley WA, Bartholomay LC and Smith RC (2019) Long-term surveillance defines spatial and temporal patterns implicating *Culex tarsalis* as the primary vector of West Nile virus. Scientific Reports, 9: 6637. https://doi.org/10.1038/s41598-019-43246-y.

Earnest A, Tan SB and Wilder-Smith A (2012) Meteorological factors and El Niño Southern Oscillation are independently associated with dengue infections. Epidemiology and Infection, 140: 1244–1251. https://doi.org/10.1017/S095026881100183X.

Edman JD and Scott TW (1987) Host defensive behaviour and the feeding success of mosquitoes. International Journal of Tropical Insect Science, 8: 617–622. https://doi.org/10.1017/S1742758400022694.

Eikenberry SE and Gumel AB (2018) Mathematical modeling of climate change and malaria transmission dynamics: a historical review. Journal of Mathematical Biology, 77: 857–933. https://doi.org/10.1007/s00285-018-1229-7.

Eremeeva ME and Dasch GA (2015) Challenges posed by tick-borne rickettsiae: eco-epidemiology and public health implications. Frontiers in Public Health, 3. https://doi.org/10.3389/fpubh.2015.00055.

Ermert V, Fink AH, Jones AE and Morse AP (2011) Development of a new version of the Liverpool Malaria Model. I. Refining the parameter settings and mathematical formulation of basic processes based on a literature review. Malaria Journal, 10: 35. https://doi.org/10.1186/1475-2875-10-35.

Erraguntla M, Dave D, Zapletal J, Myles K, Adelman ZN, Pohlenz TD and Lawley M (2021) Predictive model for microclimatic temperature and its use in mosquito population modeling. Scientific Reports, 11: 18909. https://doi.org/10.1038/s41598-021-98316-x.

Fastring DR and Griffith JA (2009) Malaria incidence in Nairobi, Kenya and dekadal trends in NDVI and climatic variables. Geocarto International, 24: 207–221. https://doi.org/10.1080/10106040802491835.

Fay RL, Ngo KA, Kuo L, Willsey GG, Kramer LD and Ciota AT (2021) Experimental evolution of West Nile Virus at higher temperatures facilitates broad adaptation and increased genetic diversity. Viruses, 13: 1889. https://doi.org/10.3390/v13101889.

Feng X, Park DS, Liang Y, Pandey R and Papeş M (2019) Collinearity in ecological niche modeling: Confusions and challenges. Ecology and Evolution, 9: 10365–10376. https://doi.org/10.1002/ece3.5555.

Ferguson NM, Rodríguez-Barraquer I, Dorigatti I, Mier-y-Teran-Romero L, Laydon DJ and Cummings DAT (2016) Benefits and risks of the Sanofi-Pasteur dengue vaccine: modeling optimal deployment. Science, 353: 1033–1036. https://doi.org/10.1126/science.aaf9590.

Fischer S, Alem IS, De Majo MS, Campos RE and Schweigmann N (2011) Cold season mortality and hatching behavior of *Aedes aegypti* L. (Diptera: Culicidae) eggs in Buenos Aires City, Argentina. Journal of Vector Ecology, 36: 94–99. https://doi.org/10.1111/j.1948–7134.2011.00145.x.

Fouet C and Kamdem C (2019) Integrated mosquito management: is precision control a luxury or necessity? Trends in Parasitology, 35: 85–95. https://doi.org/10.1016/j.pt.2018.10.004.

Gaaboub IA, El-Sawaf SK and El-Latif MA (1971) Effect of different relative humidities and temperatures on egg-production and longevity of adults of *Anopheles* (Myzomyia) *pharoensis* Theob.1. Zeitschrift für Angewandte Entomologie, 67: 88–94. https://doi.org/10.1111/j.1439-0418.1971.tb02098.x.

Gao D, Lou Y, He D, Porco TC, Kuang Y, Chowell G and Ruan S (2016) Prevention and control of zika as a mosquito-borne and sexually transmitted disease: a mathematical modeling analysis. Scientific Reports, 6: 28070. https://doi.org/10.1038/srep28070.

Gatewood AG, Liebman KA, Vourc'h G, Bunikis J, Hamer SA, Cortinas R, Melton F, Cislo P, Kitron U, Tsao J, Barbour AG, Fish D and Diuk-Wasser MA (2009) Climate and tick seasonality are predictors of *Borrelia burgdorferi* genotype distribution. Applied and Environmental Microbiology, 75: 2476–2483. https://doi.org/10.1128/AEM.02633-08.

Gervasi SS, Burkett-Cadena N, Burgan SC, Schrey AW, Hassan HK, Unnasch TR and Martin LB (2016) Host stress hormones alter vector feeding preferences, success, and productivity. Proceedings of the Royal Society B: Biological Sciences, 283: 20161278. https://doi.org/10.1098/rspb.2016.1278.

Gibbons RV, Kalanarooj S, Jarman RG, Nisalak A, Vaughn DW, Endy TP, Mammen MP and Srikiatkhachorn A (2007) Analysis of repeat hospital admissions for dengue to estimate the frequency of third or fourth dengue infections resulting in admissions and dengue hemorrhagic fever, and serotype sequences. The American Journal of Tropical Medicine and Hygiene, 77: 910–913.

Ginsberg HS, Albert M, Acevedo L, Dyer MC, Arsnoe IM, Tsao JI, Mather TN and LeBrun RA (2017) Environmental factors affecting survival of immature *Ixodes scapularis* and implications for geographical distribution of lyme disease: the climate/behavior hypothesis. PLoS ONE, 12: e0168723. https://doi.org/10.1371/journal.pone.0168723.

Goodwin A, Padmanabhan S, Hira S, Glancey M, Slinowsky M, Immidisetti R, Scavo L, Brey J, Sai Sudhakar BMM, Ford T, Heier C, Linton Y-M, Pecor DB, Caicedo-Quiroga L and Acharya S (2021) Mosquito species identification using convolutional neural networks with a multitiered ensemble model for novel species detection. Scientific Reports, 11: 13656. https://doi.org/10.1038/s41598-021-92891-9.

Gotelli NJ and Graves GR (1996) Null models in ecology. Smithsonian Institution Press, Washington.

Greenland S, Senn SJ, Rothman KJ, Carlin JB, Poole C, Goodman SN and Altman DG (2016) Statistical tests, P values, confidence intervals, and power: a guide to misinterpretations. European Journal of Epidemiology, 31: 337–350. https://doi.org/10.1007/s10654-016-0149-3.

Grenfell BT, Bjørnstad ON and Kappey J (2001) Travelling waves and spatial hierarchies in measles epidemics. Nature, 414: 716–723. https://doi.org/10.1038/414716a.

Grimm V, Augusiak J, Focks A, Frank BM, Gabsi F, Johnston ASA, Liu C, Martin BT, Meli M, Radchuk V, Thorbek P and Railsback SF (2014) Towards better modelling and decision support: Documenting model development, testing, and analysis using TRACE. Ecological Modelling, 280: 129–139. https://doi.org/10.1016/j.ecolmodel.2014.01.018.

Gryseels C, Durnez L, Gerrets R, Uk S, Suon S, Set S, Phoeuk P, Sluydts V, Heng S, Sochantha T, Coosemans M and Peeters Grietens K (2015) Re-imagining malaria: heterogeneity of human and mosquito behaviour in relation to residual malaria transmission in Cambodia. Malaria Journal, 14: 165. https://doi.org/10.1186/s12936-015-0689-0.

Hamer GL, Kitron K Uriel D, Goldberg TL, Brawn JD, Loss SR, Ruiz MO, Hayes DB and Walker ED (2009) Host selection by *Culex pipiens* mosquitoes and West Nile Virus amplification. The American Journal of Tropical Medicine and Hygiene, 80: 268–278. https://doi.org/10.4269/ajtmh.2009.80.268.

Haque U, Hashizume M, Glass GE, Dewan AM, Overgaard HJ and Yamamoto T (2010) The role of climate variability in the spread of malaria in Bangladeshi Highlands. PLoS ONE, 5: e14341. https://doi.org/10.1371/journal.pone.0014341.

Harris RMB, Porfirio LL, Hugh S, Lee G, Bindoff NL, Mackey B and Beeton NJ (2013) To Be Or Not to Be? Variable selection can change the projected fate of a threatened species under future climate. Ecological Management & Restoration, n/a-n/a. https://doi.org/10.1111/emr.12055.

Hausfather Z, Marvel K, Schmidt GA, Nielsen-Gammon JW and Zelinka M (2022) Climate simulations: recognize the 'hot model' problem. Nature, 605: 26–29. https://doi.org/10.1038/d41586-022-01192-2.

Hertig E (2019) Distribution of *Anopheles* vectors and potential malaria transmission stability in Europe and the Mediterranean area under future climate change. Parasites & Vectors, 12: 18. https://doi.org/10.1186/s13071-018-3278-6.

Hess A, Davis JK and Wimberly MC (2018) Identifying environmental risk factors and mapping the distribution of West Nile Virus in an endemic region of North America. GeoHealth, 2: 395–409. https://doi.org/10.1029/2018GH000161.

Hu W, Tong S, Mengersen K, Oldenburg B and Dale P (2006) Mosquito species (Diptera: Culicidae) and the transmission of Ross River virus in Brisbane, Australia. Journal of Medical Entomology, 43: 375–381. https://doi.org/10.1603/0022-2585(2006)043[0375:MSDCAT]2.0.CO;2.

Huestis DL, Dao A, Diallo M, Sanogo ZL, Samake D, Yaro AS, Ousman Y, Linton Y-M, Krishna A, Veru L, Krajacich BJ, Faiman R, Florio J, Chapman JW, Reynolds DR, Weetman D, Mitchell R, Donnelly MJ, Talamas E, Chamorro L, Strobach E and Lehmann T (2019) Windborne long-distance migration of malaria mosquitoes in the Sahel. Nature, 574: 404–408. https://doi.org/10.1038/s41586-019-1622-4.

Huxley PJ, Murray KA, Pawar S and Cator LJ (2021) The effect of resource limitation on the temperature dependence of mosquito population fitness. Proceedings of the Royal Society B: Biological Sciences, 288: rspb.2020.3217, 20203217. https://doi.org/10.1098/rspb.2020.3217.

Huxley PJ, Murray KA, Pawar S and Cator LJ (2022) Competition and resource depletion shape the thermal response of population fitness in *Aedes aegypti*. Communications Biology, 5: 66. https://doi.org/10.1038/s42003-022-03030-7.

Jacups SP, Whelan PI, Markey PG, Cleland SJ, Williamson GJ and Currie BJ (2008) Predictive indicators for Ross River virus infection in the Darwin area of tropical northern Australia, using long-term mosquito trapping data. Tropical Medicine and International Health, 13: 943–952. https://doi.org/10.1111/j.1365-3156.2008.02095.x.

Jian Y, Silvestri S, Brown J, Hickman R and Marani M (2016) The predictability of mosquito abundance from daily to monthly timescales. Ecological Applications, 26: 2611–2622. https://doi.org/10.1002/eap.1405.

Johansson MA, Apfeldorf KM, Dobson S, Devita J, Buczak AL, Baugher B, Moniz LJ, Bagley T, Babin SM, Guven E, Yamana TK, Shaman J, Moschou T, Lothian N, Lane A, Osborne G, Jiang G, Brooks LC, Farrow DC, Hyun S, Tibshirani RJ, Rosenfeld R, Lessler J, Reich NG, Cummings DAT, Lauer SA, Moore SM, Clapham HE, Lowe R, Bailey TC, García-Díez M, Carvalho MS, Rodó X, Sardar T, Paul R, Ray EL, Sakrejda K, Brown AC, Meng X, Osoba O, Vardavas R, Manheim D, Moore M, Rao DM, Porco TC, Ackley S, Liu F, Worden L, Convertino M, Liu Y, Reddy A, Ortiz E, Rivero J, Brito H, Juarrero A, Johnson LR, Gramacy RB, Cohen JM, Mordecai EA, Murdock CC, Rohr JR, Ryan SJ, Stewart-Ibarra

AM, Weikel DP, Jutla A, Khan R, Poultney M, Colwell RR, Rivera-García B, Barker CM, Bell JE, Biggerstaff M, Swerdlow D, Mier-y-Teran-Romero L, Forshey BM, Trtanj J, Asher J, Clay M, Margolis HS, Hebbeler AM, George D and Chretien J-P (2019) An open challenge to advance probabilistic forecasting for dengue epidemics. Proceedings of the National Academy of Sciences, 116: 24268–24274. https://doi.org/10.1073/pnas.1909865116.

Johansson MA, Reich NG, Hota A, Brownstein JS and Santillana M (2016) Evaluating the performance of infectious disease forecasts: A comparison of climate-driven and seasonal dengue forecasts for Mexico. Scientific Reports, 6: 33707. https://doi.org/10.1038/srep33707.

Jones CH, Benítez-Valladares D, Guillermo-May G, Dzul-Manzanilla F, Che-Mendoza A, Barrera-Pérez M, Selem-Salas C, Chablé-Santos J, Sommerfeld J, Kroeger A, O'Dempsey T, Medina-Barreiro A and Manrique-Saide P (2014) Use and acceptance of long lasting insecticidal net screens for dengue prevention in Acapulco, Guerrero, Mexico. BMC Public Health, 14: 846. https://doi.org/10.1186/1471-2458-14–846.

Jordan A, Krüger F and Lerch S (2019) Evaluating Probabilistic Forecasts with **scoringRules**. Journal of Statistical Software, 90. https://doi.org/10.18637/jss.v090.i12.

Joshi A and Miller C (2021) Review of machine learning techniques for mosquito control in urban environments. Ecological Informatics, 61: 101241. https://doi.org/10.1016/j.ecoinf.2021.101241.

Kain MP and Bolker BM (2019) Predicting West Nile virus transmission in North American bird communities using phylogenetic mixed effects models and eBird citizen science data. Parasites & Vectors, 12: 395. https://doi.org/10.1186/s13071-019-3656-8.

Kamruzzaman M, Shahid S, Islam AT, Hwang S, Cho J, Zaman MdAU, Ahmed M, Rahman MdM and Hossain MdB (2021) Comparison of CMIP6 and CMIP5 model performance in simulating historical precipitation and temperature in Bangladesh: a preliminary study. Theoretical and Applied Climatology, 145: 1385–1406. https://doi.org/10.1007/s00704-021-03691-0.

Kannangara DW and Patel P (2018) Report of Non-Lyme, Erythema Migrans Rashes from New Jersey with a Review of Possible Role of Tick Salivary Toxins. Vector-Borne and Zoonotic Diseases, 18: 641–652. https://doi.org/10.1089/vbz.2018.2278.

Karki S, Brown WM, Uelmen J, Ruiz MO and Smith RL (2020) The drivers of West Nile virus human illness in the Chicago, Illinois, USA area: Fine scale dynamic effects of weather, mosquito infection, social, and biological conditions. PLOS ONE, 15: e0227160. https://doi.org/10.1371/journal.pone.0227160.

Kaufman MG, Walker ED, Smith TW, Merritt RW and Klug MJ (1999) Effects of Larval Mosquitoes (*Aedes triseriatus*) and Stemflow on Microbial Community Dynamics in Container Habitats. Applied and Environmental Microbiology, 65: 2661–2673. https://doi.org/10.1128/AEM.65.6.2661-2673.1999.

Keesing F and Ostfeld RS (2021) Dilution effects in disease ecology. Ecology Letters, 24: 2490–2505. https://doi.org/10.1111/ele.13875.

Keyel AC, Elison Timm O, Backenson PB, Prussing C, Quinones S, McDonough KA, Vuille M, Conn JE, Armstrong PM, Andreadis TG and Kramer LD (2019) Seasonal temperatures and hydrological conditions improve the prediction of West Nile virus infection rates in

Culex mosquitoes and human case counts in New York and Connecticut. PLOS ONE, 14: e0217854. https://doi.org/10.1371/journal.pone.0217854.

Keyel AC, Gorris ME, Rochlin I, Uelmen JA, Chaves LF, Hamer GL, Moise IK, Shocket M, Kilpatrick AM, DeFelice NB, Davis JK, Little E, Irwin P, Tyre AJ, Helm Smith K, Fredregill CL, Elison Timm O, Holcomb KM, Wimberly MC, Ward MJ, Barker CM, Rhodes CG and Smith RL (2021a) A proposed framework for the development and qualitative evaluation of West Nile virus models and their application to local public health decision-making. PLOS Neglected Tropical Diseases, 15: e0009653. https://doi.org/10.1371/journal.pntd.0009653.

Keyel AC and Kilpatrick AM (2021) Probabilistic Evaluation of Null Models for West Nile Virus in the United States. bioRxiv.

Keyel AC, Raghavendra A, Ciota AT and Elison Timm O (2021b) West Nile virus is predicted to be more geographically widespread in New York State and Connecticut under future climate change. Global Change Biology, 27: 5430–5445. https://doi.org/10.1111/gcb.15842.

Kiang MV, Santillana M, Chen JT, Onnela J-P, Krieger N, Engø-Monsen K, Ekapirat N, Areechokchai D, Prempree P, Maude RJ and Buckee CO (2021) Incorporating human mobility data improves forecasts of Dengue fever in Thailand. Scientific Reports, 11: 923. https://doi.org/10.1038/s41598-020-79438-0.

Kilpatrick AM, Kramer LD, Jones MJ, Marra PP and Daszak P (2006) West Nile Virus Epidemics in North America Are Driven by Shifts in Mosquito Feeding Behavior. PLoS Biology, 4: e82. https://doi.org/10.1371/journal.pbio.0040082.

Kirby MJ and Lindsay SW (2004) Responses of adult mosquitoes of two sibling species, *Anopheles arabiensis* and *A. gambiae* s.s. (Diptera: Culicidae), to high temperatures. Bulletin of Entomological Research, 94: 441–448. https://doi.org/10.1079/BER2004316.

Kiszewski A, Mellinger A, Spielman A, Malaney P, Sachs SE and Sachs J (2004) A global index representing the stability of malaria transmission. The American Journal of Tropical Medicine and Hygiene, 70: 486–498. https://doi.org/10.4269/ajtmh.2004.70.486.

Koenraadt CJM and Harrington LC (2008) Flushing Effect of Rain on Container-Inhabiting Mosquitoes *Aedes aegypti* and *Culex pipiens* (Diptera: Culicidae). Journal of Medical Entomology, 45: 28–35. https://doi.org/10.1603/0022-2585(2008)45[28:FEOROC]2.0.CO;2.

Kokkinn MJ, Duval DJ and Williams CR (2009) Modelling the ecology of the coastal mosquitoes *Aedes vigilax* and *Aedes camptorhynchus* at Port Pirie, South Australia. Medical and Veterinary Entomology, 23: 85–91. https://doi.org/10.1111/j.1365-2915.2008.00787.x.

Komar N, Langevin S, Hinten S, Nemeth N, Edwards E, Hettler D, Davis B, Bowen R and Bunning M (2003) Experimental infection of North American birds with the New York 1999 strain of West Nile Virus. Emerging Infectious Diseases, 9: 311–322. https://doi.org/10.3201/eid0903.020628.

Kraemer MU, Sinka ME, Duda KA, Mylne AQ, Shearer FM, Barker CM, Moore CG, Carvalho RG, Coelho GE, Van Bortel W, Hendrickx G, Schaffner F, Elyazar IR, Teng H-J, Brady OJ, Messina JP, Pigott DM, Scott TW, Smith DL, Wint GW, Golding N and Hay SI (2015) The global distribution of the arbovirus vectors *Aedes aegypti* and *Ae. albopictus*. eLife, 4: e08347. https://doi.org/10.7554/eLife.08347.

Kraemer MUG, Bisanzio D, Reiner RC, Zakar R, Hawkins JB, Freifeld CC, Smith DL, Hay SI, Brownstein JS and Perkins TA (2018) Inferences about spatiotemporal variation in dengue virus transmission are sensitive to assumptions about human mobility: a case study using geolocated tweets from Lahore, Pakistan. EPJ Data Science, 7: 16. https://doi.org/10.1140/epjds/s13688-018-0144-x.

Kraemer MUG, Reiner RC, Brady OJ, Messina JP, Gilbert M, Pigott DM, Yi D, Johnson K, Earl L, Marczak LB, Shirude S, Davis Weaver N, Bisanzio D, Perkins TA, Lai S, Lu X, Jones P, Coelho GE, Carvalho RG, Van Bortel W, Marsboom C, Hendrickx G, Schaffner F, Moore CG, Nax HH, Bengtsson L, Wetter E, Tatem AJ, Brownstein JS, Smith DL, Lambrechts L, Cauchemez S, Linard C, Faria NR, Pybus OG, Scott TW, Liu Q, Yu H, Wint GRW, Hay SI and Golding N (2019) Past and future spread of the arbovirus vectors *Aedes aegypti* and *Aedes albopictus*. Nature Microbiology, 4: 854–863. https://doi.org/10.1038/s41564-019-0376-y.

Lambrechts L, Paaijmans KP, Fansiri T, Carrington LB, Kramer LD, Thomas MB and Scott TW (2011) Impact of daily temperature fluctuations on dengue virus transmission by *Aedes aegypti*. Proceedings of the National Academy of Sciences, 108: 7460–7465. https://doi.org/10.1073/pnas.1101377108.

Landesman WJ, Allan BF, Langerhans RB, Knight TM and Chase JM (2007) Inter-Annual Associations Between Precipitation and Human Incidence of West Nile Virus in the United States. Vector-Borne and Zoonotic Diseases, 7: 337–343. https://doi.org/10.1089/vbz.2006.0590.

Laporta GZ, Linton Y-M, Wilkerson RC, Bergo ES, Nagaki SS, Sant'Ana DC and Sallum MAM (2015) Malaria vectors in South America: current and future scenarios. Parasites & Vectors, 8: 426. https://doi.org/10.1186/s13071-015-1038-4.

Laureano-Rosario A, Duncan A, Mendez-Lazaro P, Garcia-Rejon J, Gomez-Carro S, Farfan-Ale J, Savic D and Muller-Karger F (2018) Application of Artificial Neural Networks for Dengue Fever Outbreak Predictions in the Northwest Coast of Yucatan, Mexico and San Juan, Puerto Rico. Tropical Medicine and Infectious Disease, 3: 5. https://doi.org/10.3390/tropicalmed3010005.

Lempang MEP, Dewayanti FK, Syahrani L, Permana DH, Malaka R, Asih PBS and Syafruddin D (2022) Primate malaria: An emerging challenge of zoonotic malaria in Indonesia. One Health, 14: 100389. https://doi.org/10.1016/j.onehlt.2022.100389.

Li C, Gao Y, Zhao Z, Ma D, Zhou R, Wang J, Zhang Q and Liu Q (2021a) Potential geographical distribution of *Anopheles gambiae* worldwide under climate change. Journal of Biosafety and Biosecurity, 3: 125–130. https://doi.org/10.1016/j.jobb.2021.08.004.

Li C, Wu X, Sheridan S, Lee J, Wang X, Yin J and Han J (2021b) Interaction of climate and socio-ecological environment drives the dengue outbreak in epidemic region of China. PLOS Neglected Tropical Diseases, 15: e0009761. https://doi.org/10.1371/journal.pntd.0009761.

Li R, Xu L, Bjørnstad ON, Liu K, Song T, Chen A, Xu B, Liu Q and Stenseth NC (2019) Climate-driven variation in mosquito density predicts the spatiotemporal dynamics of dengue. Proceedings of the National Academy of Sciences, 116: 3624–3629. https://doi.org/10.1073/pnas.1806094116.

Linthicum KJ, Anyamba A, Tucker CJ, Kelley PW, Myers MF and Peters CJ (1999) Climate and satellite indicators to forecast Rift Valley fever epidemics in Kenya. Science (New York, N.Y.), 285: 397–400.

Lippi CA, Stewart-Ibarra AM, Loor MEFB, Zambrano JED, Lopez NAE, Blackburn JK and Ryan SJ (2019) Geographic shifts in *Aedes aegypti* habitat suitability in Ecuador using larval surveillance data and ecological niche modeling: Implications of climate change for public health vector control. PLOS Neglected Tropical Diseases, 13: e0007322. https://doi.org/10.1371/journal.pntd.0007322.

Little E, Campbell SR and Shaman J (2016) Development and validation of a climate-based ensemble prediction model for West Nile Virus infection rates in *Culex* mosquitoes, Suffolk County, New York. Parasites & Vectors, 9: 443. https://doi.org/10.1186/s13071-016-1720-1.

Liu C, Ikeda K, Rasmussen R, Barlage M, Newman AJ, Prein AF, Chen F, Chen L, Clark M, Dai A, Dudhia J, Eidhammer T, Gochis D, Gutmann E, Kurkute S, Li Y, Thompson G and Yates D (2017) Continental-scale convection-permitting modeling of the current and future climate of North America. Climate Dynamics, 49: 71–95. https://doi.org/10.1007/s00382-016-3327-9.

Liu-Helmersson J, Stenlund H, Wilder-Smith A and Rocklöv J (2014) Vectorial capacity of *Aedes aegypti*: Effects of temperature and implications for global dengue epidemic potential. PLoS ONE, 9. https://doi.org/10.1371/journal.pone.0089783.

Livdahl TP (1982) Competition within and between hatching chorots of a treehole mosquito. Ecology, 63: 1751. https://doi.org/10.2307/1940117.

Lourenço PM, Sousa CA, Seixas J, Lopes P, Novo MT and Almeida APG (2011) *Anopheles atroparvus* density modeling using MODIS NDVI in a former malarious area in Portugal. Journal of Vector Ecology, 36: 279–291. https://doi.org/10.1111/j.1948–7134.2011.00168.x.

Lowe R, Ryan SJ, Mahon R, Van Meerbeeck CJ, Trotman AR, Boodram L-LG, Borbor-Cordova MJ and Stewart-Ibarra AM (2020) Building resilience to mosquito-borne diseases in the Caribbean. PLOS Biology, 18: e3000791. https://doi.org/10.1371/journal.pbio.3000791.

Lowe R, Stewart-Ibarra AM, Petrova D, García-Díez M, Borbor-Cordova MJ, Mejía R, Regato M and Rodó X (2017) Climate services for health: predicting the evolution of the 2016 dengue season in Machala, Ecuador. The Lancet Planetary Health, 1: e142–e151. https://doi.org/10.1016/S2542-5196(17)30064-5.

MacDonald AJ and Mordecai EA (2019) Amazon deforestation drives malaria transmission, and malaria burden reduces forest clearing. Proceedings of the National Academy of Sciences, 116: 22212–22218. https://doi.org/10.1073/pnas.1905315116.

Mackenzie JS, Lindsay MD and Broom AK (2000) Effect of climate and weather on the transmission of Ross River and Murray Valley encephalitis viruses. Microbiology Australia, 21: 20–25.

Madhav NK, Brownstein JS, Tsao JI and Fish D (2004) A Dispersal Model for the Range Expansion of Blacklegged Tick (Acari: Ixodidae). Journal of Medical Entomology, 41: 842–852. https://doi.org/10.1603/0022-2585-41.5.842.

Mahmood I, Jahan M, Groen D, Javed A and Shafait F (2020) An Agent-Based Simulation of the Spread of Dengue Fever. In: Computational Science – ICCS 2020, Lecture Notes in

Computer Science (eds. Krzhizhanovskaya VV, Závodszky G, Lees MH, Dongarra JJ, Sloot PMA, Brissos S and Teixeira J). Springer International Publishing, Cham, pp. 103–117. https://doi.org/10.1007/978-3-030-50420-5_8.

Mapaco LP, Coetzer JAW, Paweska JT and Venter EH (2012) An investigation into an outbreak of Rift Valley fever on a cattle farm in Bela-Bela, South Africa, in 2008. Journal of the South African Veterinary Association, 83: 47–54. https://doi.org/10.4102/jsava.v83i1.132.

Martens WJ, Niessen LW, Rotmans J, Jetten TH and McMichael AJ (1995) Potential impact of global climate change on malaria risk. Environmental Health Perspectives, 103: 458–464. https://doi.org/10.1289/ehp.95103458.

McDonald E, Mathis S, Martin SW, Staples JE, Fischer M and Lindsey NP (2021) Surveillance for West Nile Virus Disease – United States, 2009–2018. MMWR. Surveillance Summaries, 70: 1–15. https://doi.org/10.15585/mmwr.ss7001a1.

McElreath R (2020) Statistical rethinking: a Bayesian course with examples in R and Stan. CRC texts in statistical science. 2nd edn. Taylor and Francis, CRC Press, Boca Raton.

McGough SF, Brownstein JS, Hawkins JB and Santillana M (2017) Forecasting Zika Incidence in the 2016 Latin America Outbreak Combining Traditional Disease Surveillance with Search, Social Media, and News Report Data. PLOS Neglected Tropical Diseases, 11: e0005295. https://doi.org/10.1371/journal.pntd.0005295.

McGough SF, Clemente L, Kutz JN and Santillana M (2021) A dynamic, ensemble learning approach to forecast dengue fever epidemic years in Brazil using weather and population susceptibility cycles. Journal of The Royal Society Interface, 18: 20201006. https://doi.org/10.1098/rsif.2020.1006.

McIntyre S, Rangel EF, Ready PD and Carvalho BM (2017) Species-specific ecological niche modelling predicts different range contractions for Lutzomyia intermedia and a related vector of Leishmania braziliensis following climate change in South America. Parasites & Vectors, 10: 157. https://doi.org/10.1186/s13071-017-2093-9.

Méndez-Lázaro P, Muller-Karger F, Otis D, McCarthy M and Peña-Orellana M (2014) Assessing Climate Variability Effects on Dengue Incidence in San Juan, Puerto Rico. International Journal of Environmental Research and Public Health, 11: 9409–9428. https://doi.org/10.3390/ijerph110909409.

Messina JP, Brady OJ, Golding N, Kraemer MUG, Wint GRW, Ray SE, Pigott DM, Shearer FM, Johnson K, Earl L, Marczak LB, Shirude S, Davis Weaver N, Gilbert M, Velayudhan R, Jones P, Jaenisch T, Scott TW, Reiner RC and Hay SI (2019) The current and future global distribution and population at risk of dengue. Nature Microbiology, 4: 1508–1515. https://doi.org/10.1038/s41564-019-0476-8.

Michelitsch A, Wernike K, Klaus C, Dobler G and Beer M (2019) Exploring the Reservoir Hosts of Tick-Borne Encephalitis Virus. Viruses, 11: 669. https://doi.org/10.3390/v11070669.

Microsoft (2019) Project Premonition. Microsoft.

Midega JT, Smith DL, Olotu A, Mwangangi JM, Nzovu JG, Wambua J, Nyangweso G, Mbogo CM, Christophides GK, Marsh K and Bejon P (2012) Wind direction and proximity to larval sites determines malaria risk in Kilifi District in Kenya. Nature Communications, 3. https://doi.org/10.1038/ncomms1672.

Moise IK, Zulu LC, Fuller DO and Beier JC (2019) Persistent barriers to implementing efficacious mosquito control activities in the continental United States: insights from vector control experts. In: Rodriguez-Morales, A.J. (ed.) Current topics in neglected tropical diseases. IntechOpen. https://doi.org/10.5772/intechopen.76774.

Montecino-Latorre D and Barker CM (2018) Overwintering of West Nile virus in a bird community with a communal crow roost. Scientific Reports, 8: 6088. https://doi.org/10.1038/s41598-018-24133-4.

Mordecai EA, Caldwell JM, Grossman MK, Lippi CA, Johnson LR, Neira M, Rohr JR, Ryan SJ, Savage V, Shocket MS, Sippy R, Stewart Ibarra AM, Thomas MB and Villena O (2019) Thermal biology of mosquito-borne disease. Ecology Letters, 22: 1690–1708. https://doi.org/10.1111/ele.13335.

Mordecai EA, Cohen JM, Evans MV, Gudapati P, Johnson LR, Lippi CA, Miazgowicz K, Murdock CC, Rohr JR, Ryan SJ, Savage V, Shocket MS, Stewart Ibarra A, Thomas MB and Weikel DP (2017) Detecting the impact of temperature on transmission of Zika, dengue, and chikungunya using mechanistic models. PLoS Neglected Tropical Diseases, 11: e0005568. https://doi.org/10.1371/journal.pntd.0005568.

Mordecai EA, Paaijmans KP, Johnson LR, Balzer C, Ben-Horin T, de Moor E, McNally A, Pawar S, Ryan SJ, Smith TC and Lafferty KD (2013) Optimal temperature for malaria transmission is dramatically lower than previously predicted. Ecology letters, 16: 22–30. https://doi.org/10.1111/ele.12015.

Mordecai EA, Ryan SJ, Caldwell JM, Shah MM and LaBeaud AD (2020) Climate change could shift disease burden from malaria to arboviruses in Africa. The Lancet Planetary Health, 4: e416–e423. https://doi.org/10.1016/S2542-5196(20)30178-9.

Morin CW, Monaghan AJ, Hayden MH, Barrera R and Ernst K (2015) Meteorologically Driven Simulations of Dengue Epidemics in San Juan, PR. PLoS Neglected Tropical Diseases, 9: e0004002. https://doi.org/10.1371/journal.pntd.0004002.

Moutailler S, Valiente Moro C, Vaumourin E, Michelet L, Tran FH, Devillers E, Cosson J-F, Gasqui P, Van VT, Mavingui P, Vourc'h G and Vayssier-Taussat M (2016) Co-infection of Ticks: The Rule Rather Than the Exception. PLOS Neglected Tropical Diseases, 10: e0004539. https://doi.org/10.1371/journal.pntd.0004539.

Murdock C, Evans M, McClanahan T, Miazgowicz K and Tesla B (2017) Fine-scale variation in microclimate across and urban landscape changes the capacity of *Aedes albopictus* to vector arboviruses. PLoS Neglected Tropical Diseases, 11: e0005640. https://doi.org/10.5061/dryad.s3953.

Neath AA and Cavanaugh JE (2012) The Bayesian information criterion: background, derivation, and applications. WIREs Computational Statistics, 4: 199–203. https://doi.org/10.1002/wics.199.

Ng'habi K, Viana M, Matthiopoulos J, Lyimo I, Killeen G and Ferguson HM (2018) Mesocosm experiments reveal the impact of mosquito control measures on malaria vector life history and population dynamics. Scientific Reports, 8: 13949. https://doi.org/10.1038/s41598-018-31805-8.

Ngowo HS, Kaindoa EW, Matthiopoulos J, Ferguson HM and Okumu FO (2017) Variations in household microclimate affect outdoor-biting behaviour of malaria vectors. Wellcome Open Research, 2: 102. https://doi.org/10.12688/wellcomeopenres.12928.1.

Nova N, Deyle ER, Shocket MS, MacDonald AJ, Childs ML, Rypdal M, Sugihara G and Mordecai EA (2021) Susceptible host availability modulates climate effects on dengue dynamics. Ecology Letters, 24: 415–425. https://doi.org/10.1111/ele.13652.

Ogden NH, Bigras-Poulin M, O'Callaghan CJ, Barker IK, Kurtenbach K, Lindsay LR and Charron DF (2007) Vector seasonality, host infection dynamics and fitness of pathogens transmitted by the tick *Ixodes scapularis*. Parasitology, 134: 209–227. https://doi.org/10.1017/S0031182006001417.

Ogden NH, Bigras-Poulin M, O'Callaghan CJ, Barker IK, Lindsay LR, Maarouf A, Smoyer-Tomic KE, Waltner-Toews D and Charron D (2005) A dynamic population model to investigate effects of climate on geographic range and seasonality of the tick *Ixodes scapularis*. International Journal for Parasitology, 35: 375–389. https://doi.org/10.1016/j.ijpara.2004.12.013.

Ogden NH and Lindsay LR (2016) Effects of Climate and Climate Change on Vectors and Vector-Borne Diseases: Ticks Are Different. Trends in Parasitology, 32: 646–656. https://doi.org/10.1016/j.pt.2016.04.015.

Ogden NH, Radojevic′ M, Wu X, Duvvuri VR, Leighton PA and Wu J (2014) Estimated effects of projected climate change on the basic reproductive number of the lyme disease vector *Ixodes scapularis*. Environmental Health Perspectives, 122: 631–638. https://doi.org/10.1289/ehp.1307799.

Oidtman RJ, Omodei E, Kraemer MUG, Castañeda-Orjuela CA, Cruz-Rivera E, Misnaza-Castrillón S, Cifuentes MP, Rincon LE, Cañon V, Alarcon P de, España G, Huber JH, Hill SC, Barker CM, Johansson MA, Manore CA, Reiner, RC, Rodriguez-Barraquer I, Siraj AS, Frias-Martinez E, García-Herranz M and Perkins TA (2021) Trade-offs between individual and ensemble forecasts of an emerging infectious disease. Nature Communications, 12: 5379. https://doi.org/10.1038/s41467-021-25695-0.

Olden JD, Jackson DA and Peres-Neto PR (2002) Predictive Models of Fish Species Distributions: A Note on Proper Validation and Chance Predictions. Transactions of the American Fisheries Society, 131: 329–336. https://doi.org/10.1577/1548-8659(2002)131<0329:PMOFSD>2.0.CO;2.

Oliveira BF, Yogo WIG, Hahn DA, Yongxing J and Scheffers BR (2021) Community-wide seasonal shifts in thermal tolerances of mosquitoes. Ecology, 102. https://doi.org/10.1002/ecy.3368.

Olson SH, Gangnon R, Elguero E, Durieux L, Guégan J-F, Foley JA and Patz JA (2009) Links between climate, malaria, and wetlands in the Amazon Basin. Emerging Infectious Diseases, 15: 659–662. https://doi.org/10.3201/eid1504.080822.

O'Neill BC, Tebaldi C, van Vuuren DP, Eyring V, Friedlingstein P, Hurtt G, Knutti R, Kriegler E, Lamarque J-F, Lowe J, Meehl GA, Moss R, Riahi K and Sanderson BM (2016) The Scenario

Model Intercomparison Project (ScenarioMIP) for CMIP6. Geoscientific Model Development, 9: 3461–3482. https://doi.org/10.5194/gmd-9-3461-2016.

Ostfeld RS and Brunner JL (2015) Climate change and *Ixodes* tick-borne diseases of humans. Philosophical Transactions of the Royal Society B: Biological Sciences, 370: 20140051. https://doi.org/10.1098/rstb.2014.0051.

Ostfeld RS, Canham CD, Oggenfuss K, Winchcombe RJ and Keesing F (2006) Climate, deer, rodents, and acorns as determinants of variation in lyme-disease risk. PLoS Biology, 4: e145. https://doi.org/10.1371/journal.pbio.0040145.

Owusu-Ofori AK, Parry C and Bates I (2010) Transfusion-transmitted malaria in countries where malaria is endemic: a review of the literature from Sub-Saharan Africa. Clinical Infectious Diseases, 51: 1192–1198. https://doi.org/10.1086/656806.

Paaijmans KP, Blanford S, Bell AS, Blanford JI, Read AF and Thomas MB (2010) Influence of climate on malaria transmission depends on daily temperature variation. Proceedings of the National Academy of Sciences of the United States of America, 107: 15135–9. https://doi.org/10.1073/pnas.1006422107.

Paaijmans KP, Heinig RL, Seliga RA, Blanford JI, Blanford S, Murdock CC and Thomas MB (2013) Temperature variation makes ectotherms more sensitive to climate change. Global Change Biology, 19: 2373–2380. https://doi.org/10.1111/gcb.12240.

Paaijmans KP and Thomas MB (2011) The influence of mosquito resting behaviour and associated microclimate for malaria risk. Malaria Journal, 10: 183. https://doi.org/10.1186/1475-2875-10-183.

Paaijmans KP, Wandago MO, Githeko AK and Takken W (2007) Unexpected High Losses of *Anopheles gambiae* Larvae Due to Rainfall. PLoS ONE, 2: e1146. https://doi.org/10.1371/journal.pone.0001146.

Padgett KA and Lane RS (2001) Life cycle of *Ixodes pacificus* (Acari: Ixodidae): timing of developmental processes under field and laboratory conditions. Journal of Medical Entomology, 38: 684–693. https://doi.org/10.1603/0022-2585-38.5.684.

Padmanabha H, Soto E, Mosquera M, Lord CC and Lounibos LP (2010) Ecological links between water storage behaviors and *Aedes aegypti* production: implications for dengue vector control in variable climates. EcoHealth, 7: 78–90. https://doi.org/10.1007/s10393-010-0301-6.

van Panhuis WG, Choisy M, Xiong X, Chok NS, Akarasewi P, Iamsirithaworn S, Lam SK, Chong CK, Lam FC, Phommasak B, Vongphrachanh P, Bouaphanh K, Rekol H, Hien NT, Thai PQ, Duong TN, Chuang J-H, Liu Y-L, Ng L-C, Shi Y, Tayag EA, Roque VG, Lee Suy LL, Jarman RG, Gibbons RV, Velasco JMS, Yoon I-K, Burke DS and Cummings DAT (2015) Region-wide synchrony and traveling waves of dengue across eight countries in Southeast Asia. Proceedings of the National Academy of Sciences of the United States of America, 112: 13069–13074. https://doi.org/10.1073/pnas.1501375112.

Pantanowitz L, Telford SR and Cannon ME (2002) Tick-borne diseases in transfusion medicine. Transfusion Medicine, 12: 85–106. https://doi.org/10.1046/j.1365–3148.2002.00358.x.

Parding KM, Dobler A, McSweeney CF, Landgren OA, Benestad R, Erlandsen HB, Mezghani A, Gregow H, Räty O, Viktor E, El Zohbi J, Christensen OB and Loukos H (2020)

GCMeval – An interactive tool for evaluation and selection of climate model ensembles. Climate Services, 18: 100167. https://doi.org/10.1016/j.cliser.2020.100167.

Pascual M, Cazelles B, Bouma MJ, Chaves LF and Koelle K (2008) Shifting patterns: malaria dynamics and rainfall variability in an African highland. Proceedings of the Royal Society B: Biological Sciences, 275: 123–132. https://doi.org/10.1098/rspb.2007.1068.

Paull SH, Horton DE, Ashfaq M, Rastogi D, Kramer LD, Diffenbaugh NS and Kilpatrick AM (2017) Drought and immunity determine the intensity of West Nile virus epidemics and climate change impacts. Proceedings of the Royal Society B: Biological Sciences, 284: 20162078. https://doi.org/10.1098/rspb.2016.2078.

Petersen LR (2019) Epidemiology of West Nile Virus in the United States: Implications for Arbovirology and Public Health. Journal of Medical Entomology, 56: 1456–1462. https://doi.org/10.1093/jme/tjz085.

Petersen LR and Busch MP (2010) Transfusion-transmitted arboviruses. Vox Sanguinis, 98: 495–503. https://doi.org/10.1111/j.1423-0410.2009.01286.x.

Pettorelli N, Ryan S, Mueller T, Bunnefeld N, Jedrzejewska B, Lima M and Kausrud K (2011) The Normalized Difference Vegetation Index (NDVI): unforeseen successes in animal ecology. Climate Research, 46: 15–27. https://doi.org/10.3354/cr00936.

Pincebourde S and Woods HA (2020) There is plenty of room at the bottom: microclimates drive insect vulnerability to climate change. Current Opinion in Insect Science, 41: 63–70. https://doi.org/10.1016/j.cois.2020.07.001.

Pisani G, Cristiano K, Pupella S and Liumbruno GM (2016) West Nile Virus in Europe and Safety of Blood Transfusion. Transfusion Medicine and Hemotherapy, 43: 158–167. https://doi.org/10.1159/000446219.

Poh KC, Chaves LF, Reyna-Nava M, Roberts CM, Fredregill C, Bueno R, Debboun M and Hamer GL (2019) The influence of weather and weather variability on mosquito abundance and infection with West Nile virus in Harris County, Texas, USA. Science of The Total Environment, 675: 260–272. https://doi.org/10.1016/j.scitotenv.2019.04.109.

Pol M, Bailey LD, McLean N, Rijsdijk L, Lawson CR and Brouwer L (2016) Identifying the best climatic predictors in ecology and evolution. Methods in Ecology and Evolution, 7: 1246–1257. https://doi.org/10.1111/2041-210X.12590.

Pontes RJ, Spielman A, Oliveira-Lima JW, Hodgson JC and Freeman J (2000) Vector densities that potentiate dengue outbreaks in a Brazilian city. The American Journal of Tropical Medicine and Hygiene, 62: 378–383. https://doi.org/10.4269/ajtmh.2000.62.378.

Porretta D, Mastrantonio V, Amendolia S, Gaiarsa S, Epis S, Genchi C, Bandi C, Otranto D and Urbanelli S (2013) Effects of global changes on the climatic niche of the tick *Ixodes ricinus* inferred by species distribution modelling. Parasites & Vectors, 6: 271. https://doi.org/10.1186/1756-3305-6-271.

Potter A, Jardine A and Neville PJ (2016) A Survey of Knowledge, Attitudes, and Practices in Relation to Mosquitoes and Mosquito-Borne Disease in Western Australia. Frontiers in Public Health, 4. https://doi.org/10.3389/fpubh.2016.00032.

Raju KS and Kumar DN (2020) Review of approaches for selection and ensembling of GCMs. Journal of Water and Climate Change, 11: 577–599. https://doi.org/10.2166/wcc.2020.128.

Randolph SE, Green RM, Peacey MF and Rogers DJ (2000) Seasonal synchrony: the key to tick-borne encephalitis foci identified by satellite data. Parasitology 121(1): 15–23.

Reiner RC, Achee N, Barrera R, Burkot TR, Chadee DD, Devine GJ, Endy T, Gubler D, Hombach J, Kleinschmidt I, Lenhart A, Lindsay SW, Longini I, Mondy M, Morrison AC, Perkins TA, Vazquez-Prokopec G, Reiter P, Ritchie SA, Smith DL, Strickman D and Scott TW (2016) Quantifying the Epidemiological Impact of Vector Control on Dengue. PLOS Neglected Tropical Diseases, 10: e0004588. https://doi.org/10.1371/journal.pntd.0004588.

Reiner RC, Perkins TA, Barker CM, Niu T, Chaves LF, Ellis AM, George DB, Le Menach A, Pulliam JRC, Bisanzio D, Buckee C, Chiyaka C, Cummings DAT, Garcia AJ, Gatton ML, Gething PW, Hartley DM, Johnston G, Klein EY, Michael E, Lindsay SW, Lloyd AL, Pigott DM, Reisen WK, Ruktanonchai N, Singh BK, Tatem AJ, Kitron U, Hay SI, Scott TW and Smith DL (2013) A systematic review of mathematical models of mosquito-borne pathogen transmission: 1970–2010. Journal of The Royal Society Interface, 10: 20120921. https://doi.org/10.1098/rsif.2012.0921.

Reisen WK, Cayan D, Tyree M, Barker CM, Eldridge B and Dettinger M (2008) Impact of climate variation on mosquito abundance in California. Journal of Vector Ecology, 33: 89–98. https://doi.org/10.3376/1081-1710(2008)33[89:IOCVOM]2.0.CO;2.

Ren Z, Wang D, Ma A, Hwang J, Bennett A, Sturrock HJW, Fan J, Zhang W, Yang D, Feng X, Xia Z, Zhou X-N and Wang J (2016) Predicting malaria vector distribution under climate change scenarios in China: Challenges for malaria elimination. Scientific Reports, 6: 20604. https://doi.org/10.1038/srep20604.

Ribeiro de Castro Duarte AM, Fernandes LN, Silva FS, Sicchi IL, Mucci LF, Curado I, Fernandes A, Medeiros-Sousa AR, Ceretti-Junior W, Marrelli MT, Evangelista E, Teixeira R, Summa JL, Nardi MS, Garnica MR, Loss AC, Buery JC, Cerutti Jr. C, Pacheco MA, Escalante AA, Mureb Sallum MA and Laporta GZ (2021) Complexity of malaria transmission dynamics in the Brazilian Atlantic Forest. Current Research in Parasitology & Vector-Borne Diseases, 1: 100032. https://doi.org/10.1016/j.crpvbd.2021.100032.

Ribes A, Qasmi S and Gillett NP (2021) Making climate projections conditional on historical observations. Science Advances, 7: eabc0671. https://doi.org/10.1126/sciadv.abc0671.

Ripoche M, Campagna C, Ludwig A, Ogden NH and Leighton PA (2019) Short-term Forecasting of Daily Abundance of West Nile Virus Vectors *Culex pipiens-restuans* (Diptera: Culicidae) and *Aedes vexans* Based on Weather Conditions in Southern Québec (Canada). Journal of Medical Entomology, 56: 859–872. https://doi.org/10.1093/jme/tjz002.

Ritchie SA and Rochester W (2001) Wind-Blown Mosquitoes and Introduction of Japanese Encephalitis into Australia. Emerging Infectious Diseases, 7: 900–908. https://doi.org/10.3201/eid0705.017524.

Roberts DR, Bahn V, Ciuti S, Boyce MS, Elith J, Guillera-Arroita G, Hauenstein S, Lahoz-Monfort JJ, Schröder B, Thuiller W, Warton DI, Wintle BA, Hartig F and Dormann CF (2017) Cross-validation strategies for data with temporal, spatial, hierarchical, or phylogenetic structure. Ecography, 40: 913–929. https://doi.org/10.1111/ecog.02881.

Robinson SJ, Neitzel DF, Moen RA, Craft ME, Hamilton KE, Johnson LB, Mulla DJ, Munderloh UG, Redig PT, Smith KE, Turner CL, Umber JK and Pelican KM (2015) Disease Risk in a Dynamic Environment: The Spread of Tick-Borne Pathogens in Minnesota, USA. EcoHealth, 12: 152–163. https://doi.org/10.1007/s10393-014-0979-y.

Romeo-Aznar V, Paul R, Telle O and Pascual M (2018) Mosquito-borne transmission in urban landscapes: the missing link between vector abundance and human density. Proceedings of the Royal Society B: Biological Sciences, 285: 20180826. https://doi.org/10.1098/rspb.2018.0826.

Root JJ and Bosco-Lauth AM (2019) West Nile Virus Associations in Wild Mammals: An Update. Viruses, 11: 459. https://doi.org/10.3390/v11050459.

Ruel JJ and Ayres MP (1999) Jensen's inequality predicts effects of environmental variation. Trends in Ecology & Evolution, 14: 361–366. https://doi.org/10.1016/S0169-5347(99)01664-X.

Ryan SJ, Lippi CA and Zermoglio F (2020) Shifting transmission risk for malaria in Africa with climate change: a framework for planning and intervention. Malaria Journal, 19: 170. https://doi.org/10.1186/s12936-020-03224-6.

Ryan SJ, McNally A, Johnson LR, Mordecai EA, Ben-Horin T, Paaijmans KP and Lafferty KD (2015) Mapping physiological suitability limits for malaria in Africa under climate change. Vector borne and zoonotic diseases, 15: 718–25. https://doi.org/10.1089/vbz.2015.1822.

Rykiel EJ (1996) Testing ecological models: the meaning of validation. Ecological Modelling, 90: 229–244. https://doi.org/10.1016/0304–3800(95)00152-2.

Sang R, Arum S, Chepkorir E, Mosomtai G, Tigoi C, Sigei F, Lwande OW, Landmann T, Affognon H, Ahlm C and Evander M (2017) Distribution and abundance of key vectors of Rift Valley fever and other arboviruses in two ecologically distinct counties in Kenya. PLoS Neglected Tropical Diseases, 11: e0005341. https://doi.org/10.1371/journal.pntd.0005341.

Santos AS and Almeida AN (2018) The Impact of Deforestation on Malaria Infections in the Brazilian Amazon. Ecological Economics, 154: 247–256. https://doi.org/10.1016/j.ecolecon.2018.08.005.

Santos-Vega M, Bouma MJ, Kohli V and Pascual M (2016) Population Density, Climate Variables and Poverty Synergistically Structure Spatial Risk in Urban Malaria in India. PLOS Neglected Tropical Diseases, 10: e0005155. https://doi.org/10.1371/journal.pntd.0005155.

Santos-Vega M, Martinez PP, Vaishnav KG, Kohli V, Desai V, Bouma MJ and Pascual M (2022) The neglected role of relative humidity in the interannual variability of urban malaria in Indian cities. Nature Communications, 13: 533. https://doi.org/10.1038/s41467-022-28145-7.

Sauer FG, Grave J, Lühken R and Kiel E (2021) Habitat and microclimate affect the resting site selection of mosquitoes. Medical and Veterinary Entomology, 35: 379–388. https://doi.org/10.1111/mve.12506.

Senapati A, Sardar T, Ganguly KS, Ganguly KS, Chattopadhyay AK and Chattopadhyay J (2019) Impact of adult mosquito control on dengue prevalence in a multi-patch setting: A case study in Kolkata (2014–2015). Journal of Theoretical Biology, 478: 139–152. https://doi.org/10.1016/j.jtbi.2019.06.021.

Shah HA, Carrasco LR, Hamlet A and Murray KA (2022) Exploring agricultural land-use and childhood malaria associations in sub-Saharan Africa. Scientific Reports, 12: 4124. https://doi.org/10.1038/s41598-022-07837-6.

Shah HA, Huxley P, Elmes J and Murray KA (2019a) Agricultural land-uses consistently exacerbate infectious disease risks in Southeast Asia. Nature Communications, 10: 4299. https://doi.org/10.1038/s41467-019-12333-z.

Shah MM, Krystosik AR, Ndenga BA, Mutuku FM, Caldwell JM, Otuka V, Chebii PK, Maina PW, Jembe Z, Ronga C, Bisanzio D, Anyamba A, Damoah R, Ripp K, Jagannathan P, Mordecai EA and LaBeaud AD (2019b) Malaria smear positivity among Kenyan children peaks at intermediate temperatures as predicted by ecological models. Parasites & Vectors, 12: 288. https://doi.org/10.1186/s13071-019-3547-z.

Shaman J, Day JF and Stieglitz M (2002) Drought-Induced Amplification of *Saint Louis encephalitis virus*, Florida. Emerging Infectious Diseases, 8: 575–580. https://doi.org/10.3201/eid0806.010417.

Shaman J, Day JF and Stieglitz M (2005) Drought-Induced Amplification and Epidemic Transmission of West Nile Virus in Southern Florida. Journal of Medical Entomology, 42: 134–141. https://doi.org/10.1093/jmedent/42.2.134.

Shankar MB, Rodríguez-Acosta RL, Sharp TM, Tomashek KM, Margolis HS and Meltzer MI (2018) Estimating dengue under-reporting in Puerto Rico using a multiplier model. PLOS Neglected Tropical Diseases, 12: e0006650. https://doi.org/10.1371/journal.pntd.0006650.

Shapiro LLM, Murdock CC, Jacobs GR, Thomas RJ and Thomas MB (2016) Larval food quantity affects the capacity of adult mosquitoes to transmit human malaria. Proceedings of the Royal Society B: Biological Sciences, 283: 20160298. https://doi.org/10.1098/rspb.2016.0298.

Shocket MS, Anderson CB, Caldwell JM, Childs ML, Couper LI, Han S, Harris MJ, Howard ME, Kain MP, MacDonald AJ, Nova N and Mordecai EA (2020a) Environmental Drivers of Vector-Borne Disease. In: Population Biology of Vector-Borne Diseases. Oxford University Press, Oxford, UK.

Shocket MS, Ryan SJ and Mordecai EA (2018) Temperature explains broad patterns of Ross River virus transmission. eLife, 7: e37762. https://doi.org/10.7554/eLife.37762.

Shocket MS, Verwillow AB, Numazu MG, Slamani H, Cohen JM, El Moustaid F, Rohr J, Johnson LR and Mordecai EA (2020b) Transmission of West Nile and five other temperate mosquito-borne viruses peaks at temperatures between 23 °C and 26 °C. eLife, 9: e58511. https://doi.org/10.7554/eLife.58511.

Simoy MI and Aparicio JP (2020) Ross-Macdonald models: Which one should we use? Acta Tropica, 207: 105452. https://doi.org/10.1016/j.actatropica.2020.105452.

Sinka ME, Pironon S, Massey NC, Longbottom J, Hemingway J, Moyes CL and Willis KJ (2020) A new malaria vector in Africa: Predicting the expansion range of *Anopheles stephensi* and identifying the urban populations at risk. Proceedings of the National Academy of Sciences, 202003976. https://doi.org/10.1073/pnas.2003976117.

Smith DL, Battle KE, Hay SI, Barker CM, Scott TW and McKenzie FE (2012) Ross, macdonald, and a theory for the dynamics and control of mosquito-transmitted pathogens. PLoS pathogens, 8: e1002588. https://doi.org/10.1371/journal.ppat.1002588.

Smith KH, Tyre AJ, Hamik J, Hayes MJ, Zhou Y and Dai L (2020) Using Climate to Explain and Predict West Nile Virus Risk in Nebraska. GeoHealth, 4. https://doi.org/10.1029/2020GH000244.

Smith NR, Trauer JM, Gambhir M, Richards JS, Maude RJ, Keith JM and Flegg JA (2018) Agent-based models of malaria transmission: a systematic review. Malaria Journal, 17: 299. https://doi.org/10.1186/s12936-018-2442-y.

Snyder RE, Feiszli T, Foss L, Messenger S, Fang Y, Barker CM, Reisen WK, Vugia DJ, Padgett KA and Kramer VL (2020) West Nile virus in California, 2003–2018: A persistent threat. PLOS Neglected Tropical Diseases, 14: e0008841. https://doi.org/10.1371/journal.pntd.0008841.

Stensgaard A-S, Booth M, Nikulin G and McCreesh N (2016) Combining process-based and correlative models improves predictions of climate change effects on Schistosoma mansoni transmission in eastern Africa. Geospatial Health, 11. https://doi.org/10.4081/gh.2016.406.

Stevens KB and Pfeiffer DU (2011) Spatial modelling of disease using data- and knowledge-driven approaches. Spatial and Spatio-temporal Epidemiology, 2: 125–133. https://doi.org/10.1016/j.sste.2011.07.007.

Stewart Ibarra AM and Lowe R (2013) Climate and Non-Climate Drivers of Dengue Epidemics in Southern Coastal Ecuador. The American Journal of Tropical Medicine and Hygiene, 88: 971–981. https://doi.org/10.4269/ajtmh.12-0478.

Stewart Ibarra AM, Ryan SJ, Beltrán E, Mejía R, Silva M and Muñoz Á (2013) Dengue Vector Dynamics (*Aedes aegypti*) Influenced by Climate and Social Factors in Ecuador: Implications for Targeted Control. PLoS ONE, 8: e78263. https://doi.org/10.1371/journal.pone.0078263.

Sugihara G, May R, Ye H, Hsieh C -h., Deyle E, Fogarty M and Munch S (2012) Detecting Causality in Complex Ecosystems. Science, 338: 496–500. https://doi.org/10.1126/science.1227079.

Sundararaman SA, Liu W, Keele BF, Learn GH, Bittinger K, Mouacha F, Ahuka-Mundeke S, Manske M, Sherrill-Mix S, Li Y, Malenke JA, Delaporte E, Laurent C, Mpoudi Ngole E, Kwiatkowski DP, Shaw GM, Rayner JC, Peeters M, Sharp PM, Bushman FD and Hahn BH (2013) *Plasmodium falciparum*-like parasites infecting wild apes in southern Cameroon do not represent a recurrent source of human malaria. Proceedings of the National Academy of Sciences, 110: 7020–7025. https://doi.org/10.1073/pnas.1305201110.

Tambyah PA, Koay ESC, Poon MLM, Lin RVTP and Ong BKC (2008) Dengue Hemorrhagic Fever Transmitted by Blood Transfusion. New England Journal of Medicine, 359: 1526–1527. https://doi.org/10.1056/NEJMc0708673.

Tan K-K, Zulkifle N-I, Abd-Jamil J, Sulaiman S, Yaacob CN, Azizan NS, Che Mat Seri NAA, Samsudin NI, Mahfodz NH and AbuBakar S (2017) Disruption of predicted dengue virus type 3 major outbreak cycle coincided with switching of the dominant circulating virus genotype. Infection, Genetics and Evolution, 54: 271–275. https://doi.org/10.1016/j.meegid.2017.07.008.

Tangena J-AA, Thammavong P, Lindsay SW and Brey PT (2017) Risk of exposure to potential vector mosquitoes for rural workers in Northern Lao PDR. PLOS Neglected Tropical Diseases, 11: e0005802. https://doi.org/10.1371/journal.pntd.0005802.

Tedesco C, Ruiz M and McLafferty S (2010) Mosquito politics: Local vector control policies and the spread of West Nile Virus in the Chicago region. Health & Place, 16: 1188–1195. https://doi.org/10.1016/j.healthplace.2010.08.003.

Thomas SM, Obermayr U, Fischer D, Kreyling J and Beierkuhnlein C (2012) Low-temperature threshold for egg survival of a post-diapause and non-diapause European aedine strain, *Aedes albopictus* (Diptera: Culicidae). Parasites & Vectors, 5: 100. https://doi.org/10.1186/1756-3305-5-100.

Tijsse-Klasen E, Koopmans MPG and Sprong H (2014) Tick-Borne Pathogen â€' Reversed and Conventional Discovery of Disease. Frontiers in Public Health, 2. https://doi.org/10.3389/fpubh.2014.00073.

Tilley H (2016) Medicine, Empires, and Ethics in Colonial Africa. AMA Journal of Ethics, 18: 743–753. https://doi.org/10.1001/journalofethics.2016.18.7.mhst1-1607.

Tjaden NB, Caminade C, Beierkuhnlein C and Thomas SM (2018) Mosquito-Borne Diseases: Advances in Modelling Climate-Change Impacts. Trends in Parasitology, 34: 227–245. https://doi.org/10.1016/j.pt.2017.11.006.

Tompkins AM and Ermert V (2013) A regional-scale, high resolution dynamical malaria model that accounts for population density, climate and surface hydrology. Malaria Journal, 12: 65. https://doi.org/10.1186/1475-2875-12-65.

Trewin BJ, Kay BH, Darbro JM and Hurst TP (2013) Increased container-breeding mosquito risk owing to drought-induced changes in water harvesting and storage in Brisbane, Australia. International Health, 5: 251–258. https://doi.org/10.1093/inthealth/iht023.

Tsao JI, Hamer SA, Han S, Sidge JL and Hickling GJ (2021) The contribution of wildlife hosts to the rise of ticks and tick-borne diseases in North America. Journal of Medical Entomology, 58: 1565–1587. https://doi.org/10.1093/jme/tjab047.

Tucker Lima JM, Vittor A, Rifai S and Valle D (2017) Does deforestation promote or inhibit malaria transmission in the Amazon? A systematic literature review and critical appraisal of current evidence. Philosophical Transactions of the Royal Society of London. Series B, Biological Sciences, 372: 20160125. https://doi.org/10.1098/rstb.2016.0125.

Uelmen JA, Irwin P, Bartlett D, Brown W, Karki S, Ruiz MO, Fraterrigo J, Li B and Smith RL (2021a) Effects of Scale on Modeling West Nile Virus Disease Risk. The American Journal of Tropical Medicine and Hygiene, 104: 151–165. https://doi.org/10.4269/ajtmh.20-0416.

Uelmen JA, Irwin P, Brown WM, Karki S, Ruiz MO, Li B and Smith RL (2021b) Dynamics of data availability in disease modeling: An example evaluating the trade-offs of ultra-fine-scale factors applied to human West Nile virus disease models in the Chicago area, USA. PLOS ONE, 16: e0251517. https://doi.org/10.1371/journal.pone.0251517.

Vail SG and Smith G (2002) Vertical Movement and Posture of Blacklegged Tick (Acari: Ixodidae) Nymphs as a Function of Temperature and Relative Humidity in Laboratory Experiments. Journal of Medical Entomology, 39: 842–846. https://doi.org/10.1603/0022-2585-39.6.842.

Vasilakis N, Cardosa J, Hanley KA, Holmes EC and Weaver SC (2011) Fever from the forest: prospects for the continued emergence of sylvatic dengue virus and its impact on public health. Nature Reviews Microbiology, 9: 532–541. https://doi.org/10.1038/nrmicro2595.

Vazquez-Prokopec GM, Perkins TA, Waller LA, Lloyd AL, Reiner RC, Scott TW and Kitron U (2016) Coupled Heterogeneities and Their Impact on Parasite Transmission and Control. Trends in Parasitology, 32: 356–367. https://doi.org/10.1016/j.pt.2016.01.001.

Vijayakumar KN, Gunasekaran K, Sahu SS and Jambulingam P (2009) Knowledge, attitude and practice on malaria: A study in a tribal belt of Orissa state, India with reference to use of long lasting treated mosquito nets. Acta Tropica, 112: 137–142. https://doi.org/10.1016/j.actatropica.2009.07.011.

Vinogradova EB (2000) *Culex pipiens pipiens* mosquitoes taxonomy, distribution, ecology, physiology, genetics, applied importance and control. Pensoft, Sofia.

van Vuuren DP, Edmonds J, Kainuma M, Riahi K, Thomson A, Hibbard K, Hurtt GC, Kram T, Krey V, Lamarque J-F, Masui T, Meinshausen M, Nakicenovic N, Smith SJ and Rose SK (2011) The representative concentration pathways: an overview. Climatic Change, 109: 5–31. https://doi.org/10.1007/s10584-011-0148-z.

Walker ED, Lawson DL, Merritt RW, Morgan WT and Klug MJ (1991) Nutrient Dynamics, Bacterial Populations, and Mosquito Productivity in Tree Hole Ecosystems and Microcosms. Ecology, 72: 1529–1546. https://doi.org/10.2307/1940953.

Ward MP (2009) Equine West Nile virus disease occurrence and the Normalized Difference Vegetation Index. Preventive Veterinary Medicine, 88: 205–212. https://doi.org/10.1016/j.prevetmed.2008.10.003.

Ward MP, Ramsay BH and Gallo K (2005) Rural Cases of Equine West Nile Virus Encephalomyelitis and the Normalized Difference Vegetation Index. Vector-Borne and Zoonotic Diseases, 5: 181–188. https://doi.org/10.1089/vbz.2005.5.181.

Wesolowski A, Eagle N, Tatem AJ, Smith DL, Noor AM, Snow RW and Buckee CO (2012) Quantifying the Impact of Human Mobility on Malaria. Science, 338: 267–270. https://doi.org/10.1126/science.1223467.

Wesolowski A, Qureshi T, Boni MF, Sundsøy PR, Johansson MA, Rasheed SB, Engø-Monsen K and Buckee CO (2015) Impact of human mobility on the emergence of dengue epidemics in Pakistan. Proceedings of the National Academy of Sciences, 112: 11887–11892. https://doi.org/10.1073/pnas.1504964112.

Wijaya KP, Götz T and Soewono E (2014) An optimal control model of mosquito reduction management in a dengue endemic region. International Journal of Biomathematics, 07: 1450056. https://doi.org/10.1142/S1793524514500569.

Wilks DS (2011) Statistical Methods in the Atmospheric Sciences. Elsevier/Academic Press, Amsterdam. Available at: http://site.ebrary.com/lib/alltitles/docDetail.action?docID=10468912.

Williams CJ and Moffitt CM (2005) Estimation of pathogen prevalence in pooled samples using maximum likelihood methods and open-source software. Journal of Aquatic Animal Health, 17: 386–391. https://doi.org/10.1577/H04-066.1.

Wimberly MC, Davis JK, Hildreth MB and Clayton JL (2022) Integrated forecasts based on public health surveillance and meteorological data predict West Nile Virus in a high-risk region of North America. Environmental Health Perspectives, 130: 087006. https://doi.org/10.1289/EHP10287.

Woodruff RE, Guest CS, Garner MG, Becker N, Lindesay J, Carvan T and Ebi K (2002) Predicting Ross River virus epidemics from regional weather data. Epidemiology, 13: 384–393. https://doi.org/10.1097/01.EDE.0000016601.23748.1D.

Woods HA, Dillon ME and Pincebourde S (2015) The roles of microclimatic diversity and of behavior in mediating the responses of ectotherms to climate change. Journal of Thermal Biology, 54: 86–97. https://doi.org/10.1016/j.jtherbio.2014.10.002.

World Health Organization (2021) World malaria report 2021. World Health Organization, Geneva. Available at: https://apps.who.int/iris/handle/10665/350147.

Wu VY, Chen B, Christofferson R, Ebel G, Fagre AC, Gallichotte EN, Sweeny AR, Carlson CJ and Ryan SJ (2022) A minimum data standard for vector competence experiments. Scientific Data, 9: 634. https://doi.org/10.1038/s41597-022-01741-4.

Yamana TK, Bomblies A and Eltahir EAB (2016a) Climate change unlikely to increase malaria burden in West Africa. Nature Climate Change, 6: 1009–1013. https://doi.org/10.1038/nclimate3085.

Yamana TK, Kandula S and Shaman J (2016b) Superensemble forecasts of dengue outbreaks. Journal of The Royal Society Interface, 13: 20160410. https://doi.org/10.1098/rsif.2016.0410.

Zhang C, Mammen MP, Chinnawirotpisan P, Klungthong C, Rodpradit P, Monkongdee P, Nimmannitya S, Kalayanarooj S and Holmes EC (2005) Clade Replacements in Dengue Virus Serotypes 1 and 3 Are Associated with Changing Serotype Prevalence. Journal of Virology, 79: 15123–15130. https://doi.org/10.1128/JVI.79.24.15123-15130.2005.

Zhou G, Minakawa N, Githeko AK and Yan G (2004) Association between climate variability and malaria epidemics in the East African highlands. Proceedings of the National Academy of Sciences, 101: 2375–2380. https://doi.org/10.1073/pnas.0308714100.

Zhu G, Liu T, Xiao J, Zhang B, Song T, Zhang Y, Lin L, Peng Z, Deng A, Ma W and Hao Y (2019) Effects of human mobility, temperature and mosquito control on the spatiotemporal transmission of dengue. Science of The Total Environment, 651: 969–978. https://doi.org/10.1016/j.scitotenv.2018.09.182.

CHAPTER 11

Leveraging Earth observation data for surveillance of vector-borne diseases in changing environments

Kimberly M. Fornace[1,2,3*], *Emilia Johnson*[1,2], *Marta Moreno*[2,4], *Andy Hardy*[5] *and Gabriel Carrasco-Escobar*[6,7]

[1]School of Biodiversity, One Health and Veterinary Medicine, University of Glasgow, Graham Kerr Building, College of Medical, Veterinary & Life Sciences, Glasgow G12 8QQ, UK; [2]Centre for Climate Change and Planetary Health, London School of Hygiene and Tropical Medicine, Keppel Street, London, WC1N 7HT, UK; [3]Saw Swee Hock School of Public Health, National University of Singapore, 12 Science Drive 2, 117549, Singapore; [4]Department of Infection Biology, London School of Hygiene and Tropical Medicine, Keppel Street, London, WC1N 7HT, UK; [5]Department of Geography and Earth Sciences, Aberystwyth University, Penglais, Aberystwth, SY23 3DB, UK; [6]Institute of Tropical Medicine 'Alexander von Humboldt', Universidad Peruana Cayetano Heredia, Av. Honorio Delgado 430, San Martin de Porres, Peru; [7]University of California, San Diego, 9500 Gilman Drive, La Jolla, CA 92093, USA; *kimberly.fornace@glasgow.ac.uk

Abstract

Vector-borne disease transmission is driven by environmental factors determining the distribution and spread of pathogens, vectors and human and animal populations. Earth observation (EO) data, such as satellite and drone imagery, can be used to characterise these factors and identify high risk geographical areas and populations. While the use of EO data to understand vector-borne disease epidemiology has a long history, the rapid expansion of satellite and aerial data, analysis methods and computing power offer new opportunities to integrate EO data into disease surveillance. We review sources and characteristics of EO data and analysis methods, identify commonly used EO-derived metrics for a range of diseases and present case studies on specific applications of EO data for disease surveillance. We additionally describe key considerations for disease control programmes considering the use of EO data, highlighting the applicability of different data types and analysis methods for different ecological contexts and use-cases.

 | DOI:10.3920/9789004688650_013

Keywords

Earth observation – geographical information systems – remote sensing – spatial epidemiology – surveillance

1 Background

Vector-borne diseases (VBDs), such as malaria and dengue, are well-established as highly sensitive to environmental conditions. Local land use practices and meteorological factors directly determine the spatial and temporal distributions of mosquito larval aquatic habitats (Fornace *et al.* 2021, Patz *et al.* 2004, Thomson *et al.* 2006, Vittor *et al.* 2009). Wider climatic changes and disruptions to existing ecosystems can alter the abundance and behaviour of mosquito species and lead to expansion of these vectors into new locations (Caminade *et al.* 2019, Iwamura *et al.* 2020, Jones *et al.* 2008, Metcalf *et al.* 2017). These ecological changes interact with socioeconomic systems in complex and context-specific ways to impact VBD transmission risks (Baeza *et al.* 2017, de Castro *et al.* 2006, Keiser *et al.* 2005).

With unprecedented levels of global environmental change, it is increasingly critical to monitor changing VBD dynamics. Increasing quality and availability of Earth observation (EO) data provides new opportunities to characterise the impacts of environmental change on VBD transmission and develop targeted surveillance methods. EO refers to the collection of physical and biological data on planetary surfaces obtained using remote sensing methods, typically sensors based on satellites or aircraft. These data can be used to monitor factors such as land cover, vegetation levels, water body distribution and extents of human settlements (Finer *et al.* 2018, Lloyd *et al.* 2017, Pekel *et al.* 2016, Wardrop *et al.* 2018, Wimberly *et al.* 2021). Since the launch of the satellite Landsat-1 in 1972, the quantity and quality of satellite-based EO data has grown exponentially (Finer *et al.* 2018). Simultaneously, aerial technologies, such as low-cost drones, are increasingly accessible and are now widely used to collect EO data at user-defined locations (Koh and Wich 2012). This expansion of EO data has been accompanied by technological developments in computing and imagery analysis methods enabling processing and interpretation of these data sources.

The potential utility of EO data for VBD epidemiological studies has been widely recognised since the 1970s (Cline 1970). Motivated by increasing mosquito resistance to insecticides and bans on the widespread use of chemicals such as DDT and outdoor disease transmission, early uses of EO data focused on characterising aquatic mosquito larval habitats to better target control measures. In 1971, the National Aeronautics and Space Administration (NASA) conducted targeted aerial surveys in New Orleans, demonstrating the capacity of multispectral imaging using the visible to near-infrared region of the electromagnetic spectrum to identify mosquito breeding sites (NASA 1973). These techniques were later deployed operationally within other areas of the United States to target the breeding sites of mosquito vectors during an outbreak of St. Louis encephalitis virus (Wagner *et al.* 1979). Subsequent studies illustrated how different types of aerial and space-borne EO data could be used to locate aquatic habitats of mosquito larvae and characterise wider types of land cover associated with abundance of adult mosquitoes and malaria transmission (Bergquist *et al.* 2021, Hay 2000, Hay *et al.* 1998).

Since these early uses of EO data to characterise vector habitats at local scales, there has been a rapid increase in the use of spatial and environmental data for VBD studies. Initiatives such as the Malaria Atlas Project use geo-referenced data and covariates (e.g. precipitation, temperature, vegetation) derived from planetary-level EO data to develop high resolution maps of global vector and VBD distributions (e.g. (Bhatt *et al.* 2013, Sinka *et al.* 2016, Weiss *et al.* 2019)). EO data is also increasingly incorporated into VBD early warning systems, with metrics derived from EO data used to inform predictions of disease outbreaks and trigger VBD control measures (e.g. (Lowe *et al.* 2013, Thomson *et al.* 2006)). These data are also used to plan and inform surveillance activities, such as mapping health facility catchment areas, defining survey populations or identifying high priority areas for vector monitoring (e.g. (Fornace *et al.* 2018, Franke *et al.* 2015, Noor *et al.* 2009, Stresman *et al.* 2014)). At much finer scales, very high resolution EO data has been used to monitor changes in land cover, mosquito breeding sites and human and wildlife disease reservoir distribution to understand the mechanisms driving infectious disease emergence (e.g. (Carrasco-Escobar *et al.* 2019, Fornace *et al.* 2014, Minakawa *et al.* 2005)).

However, despite these advances, only a relatively small proportion of available EO data is actively used for VBD surveillance. There remain significant barriers to integrating EO data into health surveillance systems in many high VBD burden countries; these challenges often include limited access to equipment, computing infrastructure or specialised technical remote sensing expertise within disease control departments. Additionally, with the wide range of types of EO data and analysis methods now available, it can be challenging to identify the best data for specific use cases. Within this chapter, we review available EO data sources, characteristics and analysis methods. We then examine existing applications of EO data to study VBD epidemiology, present examples of how EO data can be leveraged to improve VBD surveillance in changing environments and discuss considerations for the use of EO data, highlighting the need for knowledge of local vector ecology to inform EO data selection and applications.

2 Sources and characteristics of Earth observation data

EO involves the use of sensors to collect data used to measure characteristics of planetary surfaces from reflected or emitted radiation from a distance. Although EO can be conducted using aerial and ground-based platforms, spaceborne satellites

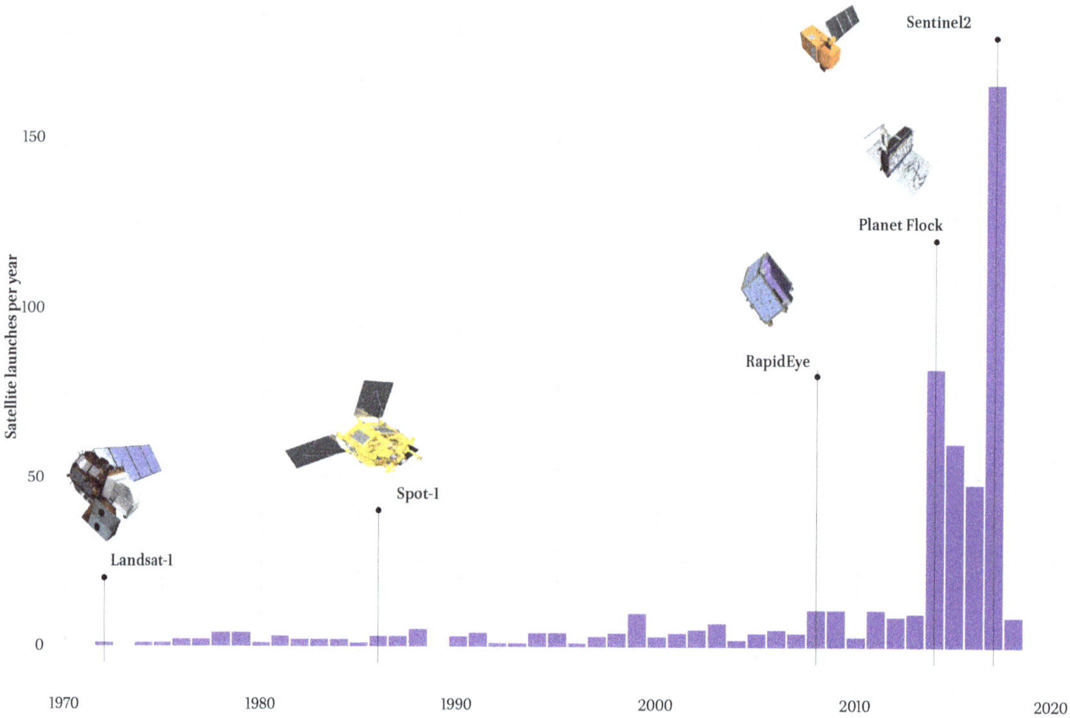

FIGURE 1 Earth Observation satellites launched by year (data obtained from Union of Concerned Scientists 2021)

are by far the largest source of EO data. Since the first launch of the EO satellite Sputnik 1 by the former Soviet Union in 1957, over a thousand EO satellites have been launched (Figure 1), (Tatem *et al.* 2008, Union of Concerned Scientists 2021). These data are available through a range of public and private sources, such as the European Space Agency, NASA and commercial companies such as Maxar Technologies (https://www.maxar.com/) and Planet (https://www.planet.com/). Costs for these data range from freely available to thousands of dollars for specifically tasking commercial satellites to cover target areas. While most free EO data is available through government or intergovernmental agencies, corporate partnerships and outreach programmes have vastly increased access to high resolution EO data. For example, a partnership between Planet and Norway's International Climate and Forests Initiative provides free access to high resolution satellite data for tropical areas for non-profit uses (https://www.planet.com/nicfi/). These data can be further supplemented by local EO data collection using aerial platforms such as drones and other aircraft (e.g. (Carrasco-Escobar *et al.* 2019, Fornace *et al.* 2014, Hardy *et al.* 2017, Wagner *et al.* 1979)).

The characteristics of the EO data collected are determined by the specific type of sensor used for data collection. Passive sensors measure light reflected by the sun while active sensors have their own source of electromagnetic energy and measure the backscatter reflected from this source. While passive sensors include instruments such as cameras, active systems use technologies such as radar and lidar. These systems are characterised by radiometric resolution based on the sensitivity of sensors to measure these differences in reflected or emitted energy. The region of the electromagnetic spectrum covered and the number of bands or channels used to sample this region of the spectrum determines the spectral resolution of a system. This spectral resolution represents the degree of precision to which reflected energy from the Earth's surface is being sampled. For example, low spectral resolution systems (e.g. many cameras carried by low-cost drones) sample the visible part of the spectrum in three bands: blue, green and red. In contrast, more sophisticated systems sample the spectrum from the visible to the near infrared and shortwave infrared over a number of bands (e.g. Landsat TM system with six bands, MODIS with 32 bands) which enables spectral detection of more complex features, such as different habitat types or calculation of vegetation indices (Wimberly *et al.* 2021).

All EO data is additionally characterised by temporal resolution, the frequency at which data are collected, and spatial resolution, the pixel size of data collected. With satellite-based EO data, the temporal resolution is determined by the satellite orbit or specific tasking requests determining the frequency at which a satellite passes over a specific location and collects data. Temporal resolution may be additionally determined by the availability of usable data; critically, for optical satellite-based systems, cloud cover is a major limitation for obtaining usable data over areas within the tropics (Burke *et al.* 2021). These limitations have led to a rapid expansion of other types of platforms used to collect EO data underneath the clouds, such as drones (also known as unmanned aerial vehicles or UAVs). These technologies allow targeted collection of EO data at user defined time intervals. Drones additionally allow collection of data with a much higher spatial resolution than most satellites (e.g. <10 cm/pixel for standard drone data vs >10 m/pixel for most freely available satellite data). These resolutions, as well as the cost and feasibility of using different platforms, impact the suitability of different types of EO data for VBD applications (Figure 2). Due to the difficulties in obtaining cloud-free satellite imagery, increasingly, studies look towards the use of radar imagery resulting from active satellite-based systems operate within the microwave part of the spectrum that is not inhibited by cloud cover. Radar imagery can provide valuable information for vector disease applications, such as wetland mapping, land cover mapping and forest cover. Some sources of radar imagery are free and are routinely collected (e.g. Sentinel-1 with a 12-day return period for the tropics) adding to its value within operational monitoring programs. But, like optical satellite imagery, its spatial resolution is currently limited to 10 m which may be inadequate for many vector disease applications.

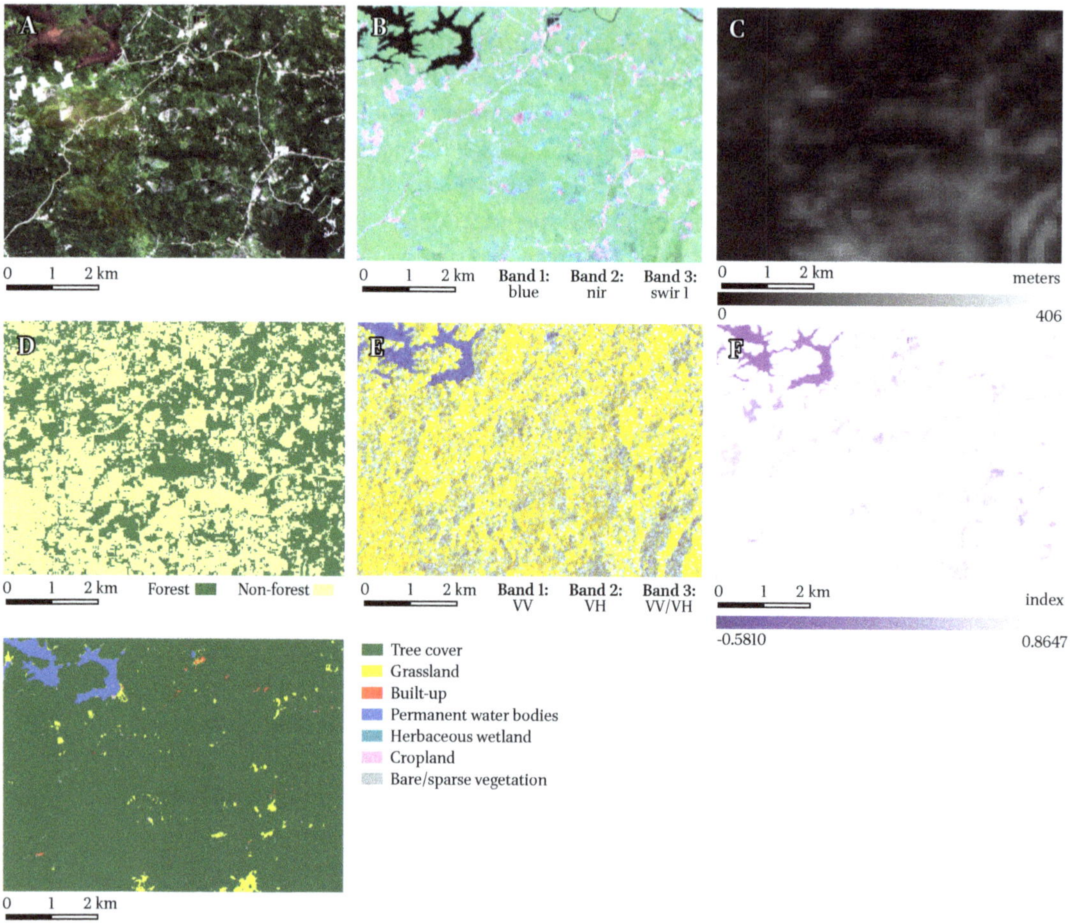

FIGURE 2 Example of sources, spatial resolutions and spectral capacity of Earth Observation data in April 2021 in Sabah, Malaysia (A) PlanetScope Tropical Visual Archive; (B) Landsat 8 (Band 1 = Blue, Band 2 = near infrared (NIR), Band 3 = short wave infrared (SWIR); (C) Elevation (SRTM 1 arc-second); (D) Classified forest cover (0, 1) (Hansen *et al.* 2013); (E) Sentinal-1 radar image (Band 1 = VV, Band 2 = VH, Band 3 = VV/VH composite); (F) Normalised Difference Vegetation Index (NVDI), derived from Landsat 8; (G) Land cover thematic map (WorldCover)

3 Analysing Earth observation data

After acquiring EO data, these data are typically analysed to identify features of interest. For example, these may include specific land classes associated with vector habitats, types of water bodies where vectors breed or locations of houses comprising the target population at risk. EO-derived metrics are often used as covariates in models to identify risk factors or predict risks of vector occurrence or disease risks (Weiss *et al.* 2015). On more operational levels, EO data may inform planning of

VBD surveillance and control measures through identification of high-risk areas or target populations.

The intended end use of the data, the feature(s) of interest and available resources determine the analysis approach used for EO data. Prior to analysis, a number of pre-processing steps are typically conducted to improve the data quality before analysis. This can include radiometric calibration to transform the radiance measured by the sensor to reflectance, the proportion of solar radiation reflected back to the sensor, to adjust for atmospheric effects. Additional pre-processing steps may include masking clouds or unreliable values (i.e. due to a fault in the sensor) and excluding these from further analysis. Orthorectification methods may also be used to adjust for distortions from the terrain and satellite or platform motion.

After pre-processing steps have been completed, the EO data can be analysed using a range of different methods. One of the most frequently used methods is the calculation of spectral indices as a ratio between two or more bands in optical data. Commonly used indices include the normalised vegetation index (NDVI), enhanced vegetation index (EVI) and soil adjusted vegetation index (SAVI), measures of greenness used to assess vegetation (Weiss *et al.* 2015, Wimberly *et al.* 2021). Different band combinations may also be used to create natural colour and false colour composites to visualise EO imagery and aid manual identification of key features of interest.

EO data are also frequently classified into thematic maps to identify key features of interest, such as water bodies or land cover types. These classification approaches can use a wide range of methods spanning simple visual identification to advanced machine learning and artificial intelligence methods. Visualising and manually digitising EO data remains one of the simplest, and often the most accurate and quickest, methods of identifying features in complex images. This requires informed users to detect and label features or classes of interest. Although this can be labour-intensive, increasingly citizen science approaches have been used to engage volunteers in labelling large numbers of images using online platforms such as Zooniverse (Simpson *et al.* 2014). Additionally, digitally assisted technological approaches, such as region growing, allow users to identify features and rapidly label similar surrounding pixels more efficiently (Hardy *et al.* 2022a).

Alternatively, model-based methods can be used to automatically identify features in EO data. These model-based methods can be split into two categories: supervised learning, in which labelled data are used to fit a model of predetermined features of interest, and unsupervised learning, which analyses unlabelled datasets to group features into different categories (Mather and Koch 2010). Supervised learning approaches require labelled training data of the specific classes to be identified; these can include ground-truthed data (such as from field surveys of vector breeding sites) or labelled examples of features of interest. While unsupervised approaches do not require training data, results may be more challenging to interpret and require an operator to match an unsupervised class to an information class of interest.

Traditionally, pixel-based classification is one of the most commonly utilised methods of image classification. This method assigns individual pixels into different class types, typically on the basis of spectral information available for individual pixels. In contrast, object-oriented classification methods classify groups of similar pixels using both pixel-level values and the spatial relationships of pixels to each other (Liu and Fan 2010). Images are typically segmented into groups of similar pixels which are subsequently assigned to specific objects or classes. More recently, deep learning approaches, such as convolutional neural networks (CNN), have revolutionised image analysis. These methods allow efficient analysis of image textures, patterns and spectral characteristics by using artificial intelligence approaches to identify features in complex environments (Cheng *et al.* 2020). Although computationally intensive, more efficient deep-learning architecture and cloud-based computing are increasingly accessible and applied for ecological analysis of EO data, e.g. (Bravo *et al.* 2021, Gray *et al.* 2019, Kattenborn *et al.* 2019). While these approaches can capture complex patterns in the data to improve classification output, these typically require very large training datasets.

4 Existing use of Earth observation-derived data for vector-borne disease surveillance: a scoping review

These different data sources and analysis methods can be used to generate a wide range of environmental covariates to integrate into VBD epidemiological studies. To evaluate the most commonly used EO-derived metrics and data sources, a brief scoping review was conducted using Medline (through PubMed) and Scopus since 2012. We sought studies which used satellite data to describe, analyse or forecast human vector-borne diseases. We restricted the search strategy on the last 10 years but did not restrict the studies to population ages or countries.

Based on identification of relevant VBD, the following search strategy was used: ('Chikungunya' OR 'Lyme Disease' OR 'Plague' OR 'Relapsing Fever' OR 'Rocky Mountain Spotted Fever' OR 'Tularemia' OR 'Typhus' OR 'West Nile Virus' OR 'Zika' OR 'trypanosomiasis' OR 'schistosomiasis' OR 'leishmaniasis' OR 'dengue' OR 'malaria' OR 'vector-borne disease' OR 'mosquito-borne disease' OR 'WNV' OR 'chikungunya' OR 'filariasis' OR 'yellow fever' OR 'Japanese encephalitis' OR 'onchocerciasis' OR 'tungiasis' OR 'crimean-congo haemorrhagic fever' OR 'lyme disease' OR 'spotted fever' OR 'Q fever' OR 'chagas') AND ('Earth observation' OR 'Remote sensing' OR 'Satellite data'). We used EndNote20 and Rayyan to remove duplicates from the search results. Data on the disease focus, EO data source and metrics used were extracted by four reviewers; discrepancies were solved by consensus. A qualitative synthesis was conducted whereby the characteristics of the variables which were used by the satellites.

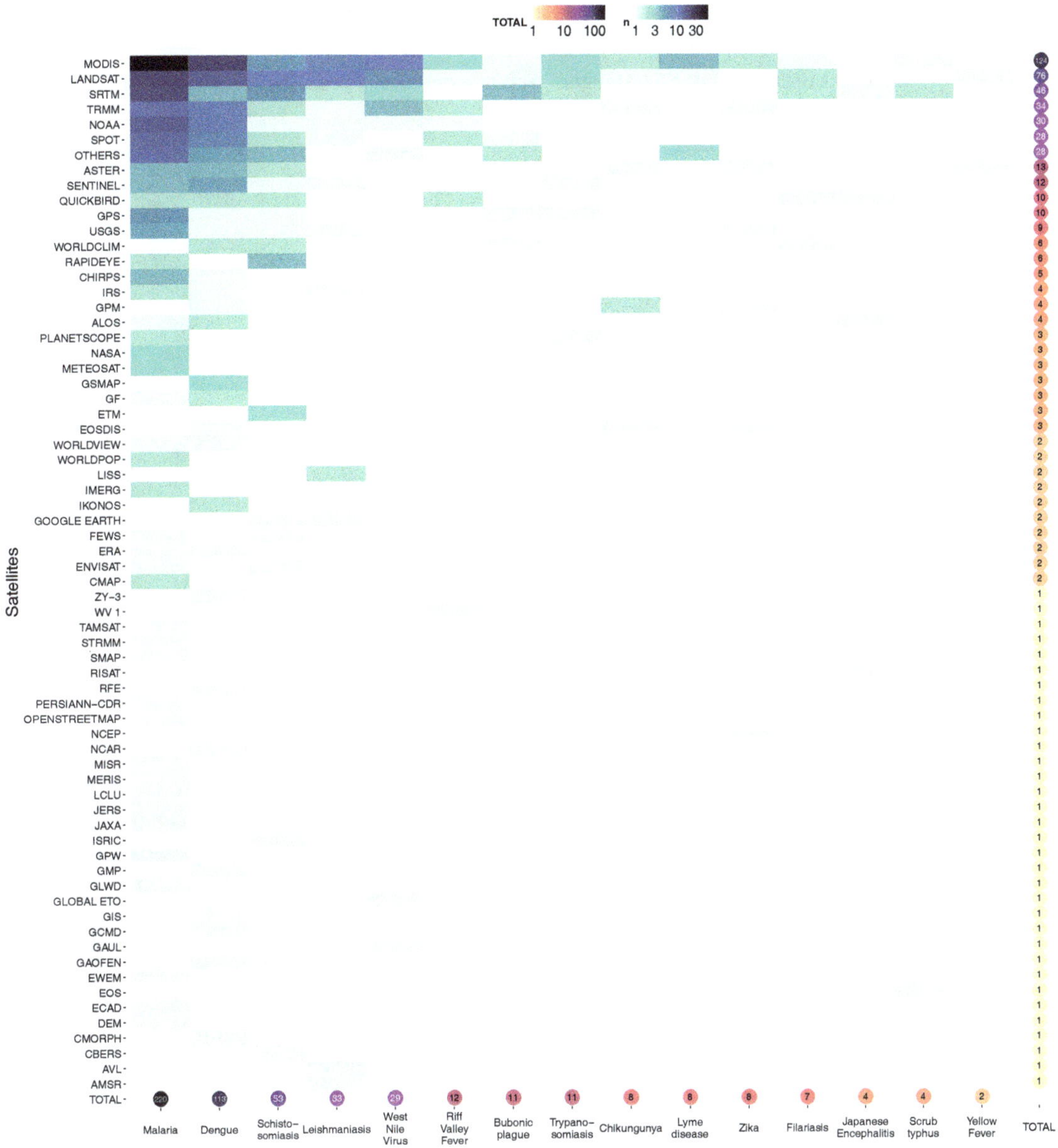

FIGURE 3 Use of sources of Earth observation data by VBD (results from scoping review)

Within this review, there was an initial total of 963 studies identified; out of these, 714 studies were excluded due to duplicates, out of scope or not specifying the vector-borne disease they were studying. From the 249 studies which were included, we extracted the name of the EO source data, type of data used, and the vector-borne disease which were studied. Figure 3 summarizes the number of EO data sources used for each vector-borne disease's studies. The most popular EO data

TABLE 1 Earth observation-derived variables used per vector-borne disease

Variables used	Malaria	Dengue	Schistosomiasis	Leishmaniasis	West Nile Virus	Chikunguny
Normalized difference vegetation index	61	28	23	17	10	6
Precipitation	54	35	7	7	9	6
Land surface temperature	53	26	13	7	9	4
Land cover	32	28	6	8	4	
Altitude	42	7	11	4	4	1
Temperature	22	21	5	4	4	3
Soil-related information	21	4	7	5	2	2
Water-related information	19	6	13	3	2	
Total	304	155	85	55	44	22

sources are the Moderate-Resolution Imaging Spectroradiometer (MODIS) and the Landsat satellite, possibly due to the open data repositories and long-term existence, respectively. In terms of mosquito-borne diseases, the use of these EO data sources is predominantly reported for malaria, dengue, leishmaniasis, and West Nile virus. However, a substantial number of studies using MODIS, Landsat, and the Shuttle Radar Topography Mission (SRTM) sources assessed infectious diseases transmitted by other arthropod and non-arthropod vectors such as freshwater snails (schistosomiasis), fleas (bubonic plague), triatomine bugs, and flies (trypanosomiasis).

The distribution and epidemiology of all vectors transmitting these diseases depend on their interactions with the environment, with varying characteristics important for the ecology of different vectors. Table 1 describes the most common EO-derived variables used for each vector-borne disease. Normalized Difference Vegetation Index (NDVI), precipitation and land surface temperature are the most common types of data used to study the distribution of these diseases, especially for mosquito-borne diseases. In contrast, other variables are more frequently used for non-mosquito-borne diseases; for example, hydrological variables are most frequently reported for studies on schistosomiasis due to the habitats of the snail vector. It is important to take into consideration that the use of a specific type of data will depend on the type of vector, reservoirs, transmission mechanism, and the distribution of each disease.

Rift Valley Fever	Zika	Bubonic plague	Lyme disease	Trypano-somiasis	Filariasis	Yellow Fever	Scrub typhus	Japanese Encephalitis	Total
5	4	2	2	3		1	1		163
3	6	2	1	1	1	1	0	0	133
	3		1	2					118
2			2	1	3	1	1		88
3	1	2	0	0	1	1	1	0	78
1	4	2	2	1	1	1			71
6	2	2	1			1		1	54
				1					44
[illegible]0	20	10	9	9	6	6	3	1	749

5 Applications of Earth observation-derived data for VBD surveillance and control

These studies use EO-derived data for a wide range of applications, from understanding the basic epidemiology and distributions of the vectors to designing early warning systems and surveillance approaches. EO data can be used to describe habitats of vectors or hosts, identify larval breeding sites or target control measures. Within this section, we describe case studies of specific applications of EO data and integration into VBD surveillance and control measures.

5.1 *Spatial distribution of vector species*

One of the primary uses of EO-derived data in VBD epidemiology is the development of maps of distribution of vector species. This spatial distribution of particular vector species has often been used as a proxy for risk of disease exposure (Kraemer *et al.* 2019, Messina *et al.* 2019, Ryan *et al.* 2019), contributing to strategic planning and informed management decisions. Ecological niche models (ENMs, also known as Species Distribution Models), which determine environmental conditions that meet a species' ecological requirements and predict the relative suitability of habitat have been employed in spatial epidemiology to determine environmental conditions associated with disease occurrence (Peterson 2014,

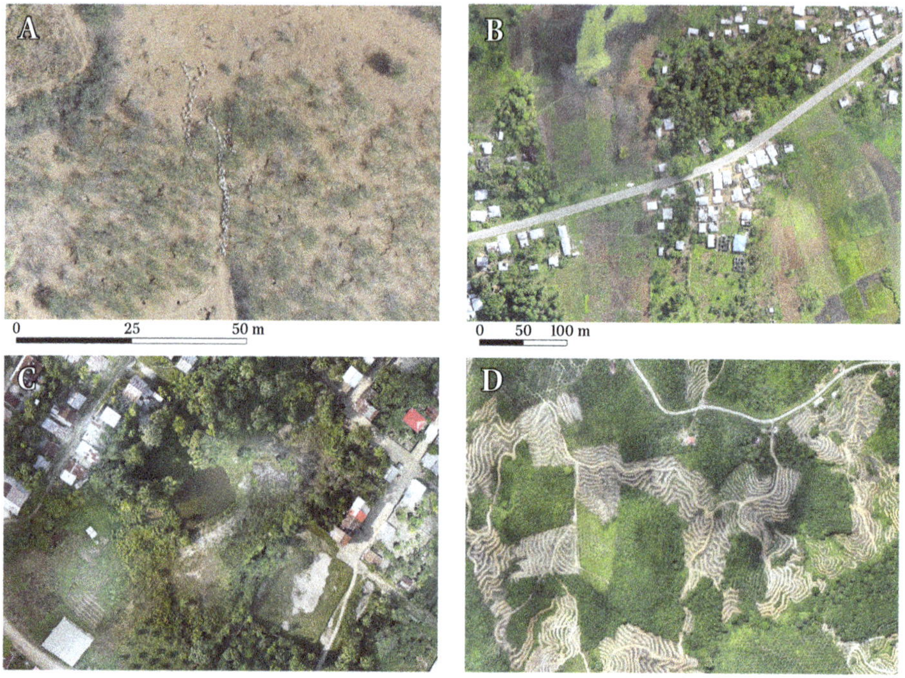

FIGURE 4 Example drone imagery in VBD surveillance, detecting (A) goats in Kenya; (B) human settlements in Zanzibar; (C) vector breeding sites in Peru; (D) landscape modification in Malaysia

Phillips *et al.* 2006). These models can be also used to predict the range of vectors, usually merging ground-based observations (e.g. from surveillance records) and potential environmental predictors. For example, in Ecuador, the distribution of *Ae. aegypti* was projected to the year 2050 under a variety of models of climate change, predicting shifts in the mosquito range and reinforcing surveillance on human populations that may be at risk of exposure to diseases vectored by *Aedes* (Lippi *et al.* 2019). Species distribution models have been also used to optimise a tsetse fly eradication campaign in Senegal, allowing more efficient control operations for the deployment of insecticide-treated targets and release of sterile males in the fight against human and animal trypanosomiasis (Dicko *et al.* 2014). Pareyn *et al.* (2021) identified that suitable habitats for *Phlebotomus pedifer*, vector of cutaneous leishmaniasis in Ethiopia, are more extensive than thought and that the main environmental drivers of their distribution were mean annual temperature, precipitation seasonality and Enhanced Vegetation Index, among others (Pareyn *et al.* 2020). In seven predominant *Culex* mosquito species in the Americas, temperature, humidity, urban/built-up land class, and cultivated and managed vegetation were important environmental drivers structuring the spatial distribution of these species (Gorris *et al.* 2021).

On finer spatial scales, monitoring changes in landscape can be used to identify changes to vector habitats and design targeted entomological surveillance. A study in Sabah, Malaysia and Palawan in the Philippines demonstrated the use of UAVs to map environmental risk factors for transmission of the zoonotic malaria *Plasmodium knowlesi* (Fornace *et al.* 2014). Due to the difficulty obtained cloud-free satellite data, a UAV was used to provide data with higher spatial and temporal resolution. Consolidated and adaptive mapping of an area over a set time period (December 2013 to May 2014) also allows for repeat sampling of areas seen to be undergoing rapid land use change, which generates datasets of land cover that are accurate for the desired timeframes. This ability to adapt and map study areas in real-time and produce maps with high temporal and spatial granularity is an essential tool for understanding the dynamic interactions between environmental factors, vector ecology and local transmission patterns (Figure 4). Resulting maps can then be used to systematically characterise land use types over the study area and create accurate spatial sampling frames for entomological surveys in areas undergoing rapid deforestation (Byrne *et al.* 2021a).

5.2 *Surveillance of invasive mosquito species*

The use of EO might be particularly useful to identify pathways for vector introduction from abroad and to support strong surveillance systems and effective interventions (Caminade *et al.* 2012). *Anopheles stephensi*, an endemic malaria vector in Asia, has been detected in Africa, particularly in the Horn of Africa – Djibouti (Faulde *et al.* 2014), Ethiopia (Carter *et al.* 2018), Somalia (World Health Organisation 2019) – and now spread to several regions in the continent (Ahmed *et al.* 2021), raising concerns about the impact on malaria transmission. This mosquito species thrives in clean water containers, abundant in urban landscapes. Because most malaria vector control strategies in Africa target rural environments, the prospect of this malaria vector in urban areas is of great concern for the malaria control and elimination programs (World Health Organisation 2019). Due to the confirmed vector competence in *An. stephensi* Ethiopian and Djibutian populations (Seyfarth *et al.* 2019), its association to malaria outbreaks and increased reported cases in Djibuti (Faulde *et al.* 2014), extended mosquito presence in the dry season (Seyfarth *et al.* 2019) and reduced susceptibility to multiple insecticides classes (Yared *et al.* 2020), WHO considers the spread of *An. stephensi* a major potential threat to malaria control and elimination in Africa and Southern Asia (World Health Organisation 2019). As a result, several measures have been recommended to tackle its invasion and spread. One of the core interventions is to conduct active surveillance for *An. stephensi* aquatic stages in urban and peri-urban areas – in addition to routine surveillance in rural environments. EO data could be extremely advantageous for mapping and monitoring typical breeding sites – water storage containers outside the home, rainwater collections, roof tops, wells or large human-made cisterns – to identify high risk urban areas in which *An. stephensi* will have the best conditions to establish.

The potential for *An. stephensi* invasion across sub-Saharan Africa has been predicted combining occurrence data from 1985–2016 with satellite imagery data sets (Sinka *et al.* 2020). The habitat suitability modelling study, which includes several environmental variables extracted from MODIS (annual mean temperature, Index and Tasselled Cap Wetness, Enhanced Vegetation and land cover classification) ((Deblauwe *et al.* 2016), CHIRPS (seasonal precipitation)), GMIA (Irrigation – Global Map of irrigated areas FAO, United Nations, and International Geosphere and Biosphere Programme (GBP) (human population density and Crop mosaic), projected that the invasion of this mosquito into African urban environments could place an additional 126 million people at malaria risk (Sinka *et al.* 2020). EO data is essential to design effective surveillance systems to monitor areas suitable for *An. stephensi.*

5.3 *Detection of surface-water bodies for effective mosquito larvae control*

For vectors with an aquatic life stage, systematic identification of dynamic hydrological systems can be valuable in identifying breeding sites and inform larval source management. While both satellite and aerial-based EO can be used to identify breeding sites, an increasing number of studies are using drones due to the high spatial resolution, ability to detect breeding sites within a specified time frame and ownership of these systems by disease control organisations.

In Unguja, Zanzibar Archipelago, a Spatial Intelligence System (SIS) was designed to identify all surface water bodies within malaria transmission hotspots over a wide area, defined using satellite radar and optical EO imagery (Hardy *et al.* 2017). In this study, off-the-shelf DJI Phantom 4 drones, fitted with a standard 4k RGB (Red-Green-Blue) camera, were used to collect detailed imagery of potential breeding sites at a high spatial resolution (0.1 m/pixel). Temporal resolution was determined by the hydrological conditions of the study area with new drone surveys being commissions where rainfall events led to a significant change in surface water extent. Surface water were very varied, including large inundated rice paddies, natural swamps with aquatic vegetation, and small (<2 m in diameter) ponding of water in tyre ruts and paths where soil infiltration rates are low. This complex array of water bodies was mapped using manual digitising assisted using a freely available region growing tool (Hardy *et al.* 2022a). Subsequent information on water body location and extent was uploaded to a smartphone app (Zzapp Malaria: https://www.zzappmalaria.com/) which was used by field operatives to locate and systematically treat potential *Anopheles sp.* breeding sites.

In Cote d'Ivoire, a technical workflow was established to integrate satellite data and drone surveys with mosquito larval sampling to identify large, semi-permanent water bodies that provide potential breeding sites for malaria vector *Anopheles funestus* (*Byrne et al. 2021b*). Using Sentinel-2 high-resolution multispectral satellite imagery, the study area was stratified into four environmental strata according to spectral profiles and derived vegetation indices from satellite data and sampled proportionally to identify semi-permanent water bodies across variable rural landscapes. Red-Green-Blue (RGB) mapping of areas surrounding surface water bodies was conducted using an off-the-shelf DJI Phantom 4 drone. To achieve the required spatial resolution for fine-scale mapping, drones were flown at 150 m altitude, generating a high resolution of 0.04 m/pixel. With the aim to develop a systematic approach and inform deep-learning approaches to EO data classification, this illustrates drone surveys conducted in a spatially representative sampling frame developed in conjunction with freely available satellite datasets.

In Maynas Province, Peru, the use of drone-based imagery has also been demonstrated in identification of *Nyssorhynchus darlingi* aquatic breeding sites in malaria hotspots (Carrasco-Escobar *et al.* 2019). Here, local vector ecology, the hydrological context and research aims determine a different set of requirements. To identify the most productive water bodies in a riverine environment, the study prioritised high-resolution images over a small study area (~1 km) and multispectral imagery. Conventional RGB imagery was captured using a DJI Phantom 4 Pro quadcopter with a DJI 4K RGB flown at an altitude of 100 m to give a spatial resolution of 0.1 m/pixel. In addition, multispectral imagery was collected using a 3DR Solo quadcopter, fitted with a Parrot Sequoia sensor composed of single-band cameras (Green, Red, Red Edge and Near Infrared – NIR). The 3DR Solo was flown at an altitude of 50 m, which gives a ground sampling distance of 0.02 m/pixel. This demonstrates the flexibility and richness of data available with tailored use of UAV technology and specific sensors. The study design itself provided proof-of-concept for using high-resolution imagery from UAV to differentiate the spectral profiles of productive water bodies where *Ny. darlingi* is likely to breed in Amazonian Peru, an innovation which could be applied to integrating larval source management in malaria elimination strategies.

5.4 *Early warning systems and automated mosquito surveillance using Earth observation*

EO data is also widely used to develop predictive models enabling deployment of targeted control measures. In the last decade, the emergence and re-emergence of VBD reinforced the need for an effective early warning, surveillance and control of vectors and preparedness (Weaver 2013). Due to arthropod vectors being especially sensitive to changes in climate, forecasting systems driven by EO data have been useful for predicting disease risk and to guide epidemiological surveillance and decision-making process (Thomson *et al.* 2006, Thomson *et al.* 2008). The publication of guidelines of Malaria Early Warning Systems for Africa by the WHO, offered a valuable framework for integrated approach response strategies and epidemic preparedness (DaSilva *et al.* 2004, Thomson and Connor 2001, World Health Organisation 2001). Social, environmental and epidemiological factors are involved in malaria epidemics prediction and together with weather monitoring and seasonal climate forecasts, can be incorporated in malaria early warning systems (Thomson *et al.* 2006, World Health Organisation 2001). Dengue ecology and its strong relationship with climate variation is another example of how risk prediction studies and modelling approaches could help in the forecast of outbreaks (Colón-González *et al.* 2018, Colon-Gonzalez *et al.* 2021, Lauer *et al.* 2018, Lowe *et al.* 2016, Petrova *et al.* 2019) (see Finch *et al.* Chapter 12 for detailed environmental EO predictors and EWS in VBD).

Other innovative approaches for VBD surveillance using EO, automated sensors and algorithms/machine learning are still underway. For instance, VECTRACK (https://vectrack.avia-gis.com/) is an Earth Observation service for preventive control of insect disease vectors. This project seeks to generate an automated surveillance system combining an Earth Observation (EO) Sentinel service and satellite data with a network of ground optoelectronic sensors and traps to enable fully remote and automated counting and classification of the target mosquitoes (McEntaggart *et al.* 2020). This combined data will then feed into spatial models, and along with data on meteorological and environmental conditions, this can be used to generate large-scale risk maps. The use of this approach might help to significantly reduce costs and time of monitoring and surveillance and allows for more rapid intervention; however, this has yet to be fully evaluated.

5.5 *Use of Earth observation data to map animal reservoirs and human populations at risk*

The use of EO data in ecological or conservation studies is already well established; for example, in aerial surveys of large wild mammals over sparse areas (Koh and Wich 2012). However, in the study of vector-borne diseases with sylvatic life cycles in wildlife reservoirs, ecology intersects with public health and EO data of human and animal hosts can also provide critical information on transmission cycles and potential distribution of disease.

Yellow Fever (YF) is a zoonotic disease endemic in neotropical forests, transmitted by *Haemagogus* spp. mosquito vectors and with reservoirs of Yellow Fever Virus (YFV) circulating in non-human primate hosts. In Brazil, satellite-derived EO data has been used to estimate the distribution of the primate host species *Alouatta caraya* and *A. guariba clamitans*, which is then built into ecological niche models using maximum entropy modelling (Maxent) to identify geographic areas at risk of sylvatic outbreaks and human populations at risk (de Almeida *et al.* 2019). Explanatory variables include topography derived from the SRTM (Jarvis *et al.* 2022) and climatic variables derived from WorldClim (e.g. rainfall, temperature, solar radiation, water vapor pressure, wind speed), which uses meteorological station data validated by MODIS-derived satellite data (Fick and Hijmans 2017) at 1 km resolution. Here, use of satellite EO data to predict the distribution of reservoir species provides a valuable tool in building spatial risk models to inform public health interventions.

EO data has also be used to provide detailed estimations of human populations for VBD surveillance and management (Tatem *et al.* 2012). Sub-national metrics for population density are vital to mitigate VBD, with population denominator data required to define infection rates, allocate resources and measure the impact of interventions. However, accurate population data can be lacking in resource-poor settings. In addition, non-uniform distributions of people within administrative boundaries can lead to miscalculations. Recent computational approaches have been used to map population density as a continuous surface, using available survey/census data and drawing on high-resolution satellite-derived remote sensing variables (e.g. topography, elevation, mean reflectance in specific bands, vegetation indices) to create a gridded population distribution (Qiu *et al.* 2022). Advances in high-quality and high-resolution (<10 m) satellite imagery has further improved global estimates, allowing human-built structures to be identified, counted and incorporated into models to generate spatially disaggregated estimates of human population distribution at resolutions of 90 m (Lloyd *et al.* 2017, Wardrop *et al.* 2018). In geographic areas that are at risk of VBD transmission but lack the infrastructure for updated or fine-scale demographic information, WorldPop population distribution surfaces can be vital in ensuring accurate risk mapping and targeted interventions.

At more localised spatial scales, UAVs can be used to map animal reservoirs of VBDs. Rift Valley Fever (RVF) is a viral zoonotic disease of wild ungulates in sub-Saharan Africa, that can be transmitted to humans through infective fluids or through bites from mosquito vectors. In Kenya, the commercially available senseFly eBee drone was used to identify the density and distribution of livestock and wildlife hosts of RVF (https://www.zooniverse.org/projects/rfv-drones/rift-valley-fever-drones). The UAV was fitted with the senseFly S.O.D.A sensor, a drone-specific photogrammetry camera that can capture sharp images and 3D digital surface models. From this, orthomosaic images were produced with a resolution of 0.03 m/pixel. This study required high resolution imagery across large study areas, with a view to identifying goats, camels and cattle and managing the disease reservoir. Imagery of this kind can be used to train machine learning algorithms to track and identify key mammal species in sparse landscapes that are integral to disease transmission cycles.

In Kinabatangan, Malaysia, a study aimed to identify and count the roosting sites of non-human primates (Jumail *et al.* 2021). Non-human primates are a reservoir for *Plasmodium knowlesi*, the aetiological agent of zoonotic malaria across Southeast Asia and most notably in East Malaysia. Unlike the broad swathes of savannah imaged in the previous example, this study looked at fine-scale 1 km transects of riverine forest. To obtain the required data, teams used a custom built hexacopter drone fitted with a FLiR Thermal Camera. Thermal images could then be used for visual identification of monkeys and counting of roosts across the transects. This is an example of the adaptability and user customisation possible with UAV technology, with equipment and sensors selected and modified to meet the requirements of both the ecological context and research aims.

6 Considerations for use of Earth observation data for VBD surveillance

Although these examples highlight how EO data can contribute to VBD surveillance, EO data remains underutilised in many VBD-endemic countries. While many sources of EO data are now freely available, one of the primary barriers to uptake remains technical expertise on remote sensing within disease control departments. This can be further challenged by the wide array of data sources and analysis platforms currently available. Decisions on EO data sources and analysis methods should be guided by local knowledge of vector ecology and the control strategies to be deployed. Factors to be considered include the following.

6.1 *Area of interest*

The geographical location and extent of the target area of interest will have determine the applicability of different data types. For example, fine-scale mapping may use targeted drone surveys while more extensive risk-mapping at larger spatial scales requires satellite-based EO data. Additionally, specific countries or regions may have targeted satellite or aerial EO data collection, such as through satellites run through national mapping services. The location also determines the feasibility of using different data sources; optical satellite data coverage may be limited in tropical forested areas with high cloud cover and drones may not be feasible in cities or areas with military activities.

6.2 *Mapping objectives*

The choice of EO data and analysis methods are also highly dependent on the objective of the mapping exercise and the corresponding features to be detected. For many risk mapping exercises, this may consist of a list of potential environmental covariates associated with a particular vector or VBD distribution. In other cases, the objective may be to detect specific vector breeding sites to deploy larval source control measures or to locate houses to plan a survey. In all cases, the specific features to be detected, and the characteristics of these features, should be identified. This may also consider specific types of EO data frequently used to detect these features, e.g. LIDAR data to measure canopy structure or optical data including NIR to calculate NDVI as a measure of greenness.

6.3 *Spatial and temporal resolution*

The spatial and temporal resolutions of these features should inform the selection of EO data with corresponding resolutions. For example, *An. funestus* typically breeds in large, semi-permanent water bodies which can be detected by coarser satellite-based EO data collected at irregular intervals. Other studies aiming to map the distribution of short-lived temporary water bodies, such as the breeding sites for *An. arabiensis*, or movements of disease hosts would be required to identify EO data with higher temporal resolutions to capture these dynamic features. Similar factors should be considered when mapping changing environments such as actively deforested areas. This should identify the temporal and spatial resolutions needed to capture these changes. Conversely, much coarser data may be required for large-scale mapping to capture broad environmental trends. Studies should consider the minimum resolutions of EO data required and trade-offs between computational requirements and higher resolution data.

6.4 *Cost and logistics*

Despite many sources of EO data being freely available, all mapping exercises require resources, such as personnel time, expertise, computing infrastructure or equipment purchase. These costs may increase when specialised equipment or data is required. For example, this may include the purchase of drones and sensors or tasking commercial satellites to cover specific areas. For studies requiring field activities, such as drone mapping or collection of ground-truthing data, these will require resources to support field staff, local transport and other consumables. Additionally, these studies typically require advanced permissions to collect samples, personnel data or to conduct drone mapping. This will often require permissions from Civil Aviation Authorities or other mapping agencies as well as local community acceptance and consent (Hardy *et al.* 2022b).

6.5 *Availability of training data*

One of the main determinants of analysis methods to be used is the availability of training data used to fit supervised models (such as machine learning and Artificial Intelligence approaches). The types and characteristics of training data needed are highly dependent on the target features to be identified. For example, algorithms designed to detect breeding sites of specific vector species are largely dependent on data from ground-based entomological surveys. Studies aiming to identify wider habitat types (e.g. forests or large water bodies) may be able to generate training data remotely by labeling high resolution imagery using GIS or specialised software tools. For specific applications, additional labelled training datasets may be available through online repositories (e.g. labelled agricultural data through Radiant Earth, https://www.radiant.earth/). The amount of training data required is dependent on the complexity of the feature to be identified as well as the type of algorithm used and may be a limiting factor in choosing specific algorithm types. However, there are example studies where training data has been generated automatically for machine learning models applied to satellite EO data providing an end-to-end automated mapping system, although such approaches have not yet been applied to drone-EO data (Hardy *et al.* 2019).

6.6 *Technical expertise and computing infrastructure*

Decisions on the types of EO data and analysis methods should also consider the availability of technical expertise needed to process EO data and develop algorithms. This should also assess how the data will be used, the time frames required and the primary end user. For example, if local health departments need to use information from drone surveys immediately after flights are conducted, the most feasible approaches may be manually digitising images in field settings offline. In other cases where mapping is repeatedly conducted over wide areas, it may be more feasible and cost-effective to develop deep-learning algorithms to automatically identify target features. Specific governments agencies or research programmes may additionally have access to dedicated servers or infrastructure to support repeated data analysis. In contrast, other smaller research projects or disease control agencies may need to rely on local infrastructure or cloud-based computing. The level of technical expertise available should be considered when planning any mapping activities and may impact the feasibility of different approaches.

7 Conclusions

Most VBD are governed by geographical components and decisions made in terms of controlling these diseases are often made a large (regional or national) scales. As such, EO has, and will continue to play a vital role in tackling VBDs. The rapid expansion of EO data and analysis methods offers new opportunities for VBD surveillance, from tracking habitats of invasive vector species to developing early warning systems or planning vector control activities. Rapidly changing environmental conditions increase the need for these methods and data sources to characterise changing VBD epidemiology. Within this chapter, we have given an overview of EO data sources and analysis methods as well as example applications. We have additionally outlined key considerations for the integration of EO data into VBD surveillance and priorities for determining the feasibility of different data sources and analysis strategies. While these technologies have the potential to transform VBD surveillance, EO data applications need to be designed to be appropriate for specific contexts and ecological settings.

Acknowledgements

This project was supported by a Sir Henry Dale fellowship jointly funded by the Wellcome Trust and the Royal Society (Grant no. 221963/Z/20/Z). Additional funding was provided by the project 'International collaborative network for the integration, standardisation and assessment of the use of drones in malaria vector control strategies' funded by the Global Challenges Research Fund (GCRF) Networking Grant (GCRFNGR4\1140). AJH received support from the Bill and Melinda Gates Foundation Innovation Fund INV-010583 through a grant managed by the Innovative Vector Control Consortium (IVCC). ML would like to acknowledge support from the National Institute of Health (USA) grant R03AI156580. The authors thank Antony Barja for processing the satellite data sources and availability and Edson J. Ascencio, Enrique A. Hernandez-Bustamante, Ximena J. Parraga, and Carmen Sofia Uribe Calama for their contribution to the scoping review in this chapter.

References

Ahmed A, Khogali R, Elnour M-AB, Nakao R and Salim B (2021) Emergence of the invasive malaria vector *Anopheles stephensi* in Khartoum State, Central Sudan. Parasites & vectors 14: 511. 10.1186/s13071-021-05026-4.

Baeza A, Santos-Vega M, Dobson AP and Pascual M (2017) The rise and fall of malaria under land-use change in frontier regions. Nat Ecol Evol 1: 108. 10.1038/s41559-017-0108.

Bergquist R, Luvall JC and Malone JB (2021) The changing risk of vector-borne diseases: Global satellite remote sensing and geospatial surveillance at the forefront. Geospat Health 16. 10.4081/gh.2021.1047.

Bhatt S, Gething PW, Brady OJ, Messina JP, Farlow AW, Moyes CL, Drake JM, Brownstein JS, Hoen AG, Sankoh O, Myers MF, George DB, Jaenisch T, Wint GR, Simmons CP, Scott TW, Farrar JJ and Hay SI (2013) The global distribution and burden of dengue. Nature 496: 504–507. 10.1038/nature12060.

Bravo DT, Lima GA, Alves WAL, Colombo VP, Djogbenou LS, Pamboukian SVD, Quaresma CC and Alves de Araujo S (2021) Automatic detection of potential mosquito breeding sites from aerial images acquired by unmanned aerial vehicles. Comput Environ Urban Syst 90.

Burke M, Driscoll A, Lobell DB and Ermon S (2021) Using satellite imagery to understand and promote sustainable development. Science 371. 10.1126/science.abe8628.

Byrne I, Aure W, Manin BO, Vythilingam I, Ferguson HM, Drakeley CJ, Chua TH and Fornace KM (2021a) Environmental and spatial risk factors for the larval habitats of *Plasmodium knowlesi* vectors in Sabah, Malaysian Borneo. Sci Rep 11: 11810. 10.1038/s41598-021-90893-1.

Byrne I, Chan K, Manrique E, Lines J, Wolie RZ, Trujillano F, Garay GJ, Del Prado Cortez MN, Alatrista-Salas H, Sternberg E, Cook J, N'Guessan R, Koffi A, Ahoua Alou LP, Apollinaire N, Messenger LA, Kristan M, Carrasco-Escobar G and Fornace K (2021b) Technical Workflow Development for Integrating Drone Surveys and Entomological Sampling to Characterise Aquatic Larval Habitats of *Anopheles funestus* in Agricultural Landscapes in Côte d'Ivoire. J Environ Public Health 2021: 3220244. 10.1155/2021/3220244.

Caminade C, McIntyre KM and Jones AE (2019) Impact of recent and future climate change on vector-borne diseases. Ann N Y Acad Sci 1436: 157–173. 10.1111/nyas.13950.

Caminade C, Medlock JM, Ducheyne E, McIntyre KM, Leach S, Baylis M and Morse AP (2012) Suitability of European climate for the Asian tiger mosquito *Aedes albopictus*: recent trends and future scenarios. J R Soc Interface 9: 2708–2717. 10.1098/rsif.2012.0138.

Carrasco-Escobar G, Manrique E, Ruiz-Cabrejos J, Saavedra M, Alava F, Bickersmith S, Prussing C, Vinetz JM, Conn JE, Moreno M and Gamboa D (2019) High-accuracy detection of malaria vector larval habitats using drone-based multispectral imagery. PLoS neglected tropical diseases 13: e0007105. 10.1371/journal.pntd.0007105.

Carter TE, Yared S, Gebresilassie A, Bonnell V, Damodaran L, Lopez K, Ibrahim M, Mohammed S and Janies D (2018) First detection of *Anopheles stephensi* Liston, 1901 (Diptera: culicidae) in Ethiopia using molecular and morphological approaches. Acta Trop 188: 180–186. https://doi.org/10.1016/j.actatropica.2018.09.001.

Cheng G, Xie X, Han J, Guo L and Xia G (2020) Remote sensing image scene classification meets deep learning: challenges, methods, benchmarks and opportunities. IEEE Journal of Selected Topics in Applied Earth Observations and Remote Sensing 13: 3735–3756.

Cline BL (1970) New eyes for epidemiologists: aerial photography and other remote sensing techniques. Am J Epidemiol 92: 85–89. 10.1093/oxfordjournals.aje.a121188.

Colón-González FJ, Harris I, Osborn TJ, Bernardo CSS, Peres CA, Hunter PR, Warren R, Vuurene Dv and Lake IR (2018) Limiting global-mean temperature increase to 1.5–2 °C could reduce the incidence and spatial spread of dengue fever in Latin America. Proceedings of the National Academy of Sciences 115: 6243–6248. doi:10.1073/pnas.1718945115.

Colon-Gonzalez FJ, Soares Bastos L, Hofmann B, Hopkin A, Harpham Q, Crocker T, Amato R, Ferrario I, Moschini F, James S, Malde S, Ainscoe E, Sinh Nam V, Quang Tan D, Duc Khoa N, Harrison M, Tsarouchi G, Lumbroso D, Brady OJ and Lowe R (2021) Probabilistic seasonal dengue forecasting in Vietnam: A modelling study using superensembles. PLoS medicine 18: e1003542. 10.1371/journal.pmed.1003542.

DaSilva J, Garanganga B, Teveredzi V, Marx SM, Mason SJ and Connor SJ (2004) Improving epidemic malaria planning, preparedness and response in Southern Africa. Report on the 1st Southern African Regional Epidemic Outlook Forum, Harare, Zimbabwe, 26–29 September, 2004. Malaria journal 3: 37. 10.1186/1475-2875-3-37.

de Almeida MAB, Dos Santos E, Cardoso JDC, da Silva LG, Rabelo RM and Bicca-Marques JC (2019) Predicting Yellow Fever Through Species Distribution Modeling of Virus, Vector, and Monkeys. EcoHealth 16: 95–108. 10.1007/s10393-018-1388-4.

de Castro MC, Monte-Mor RL, Sawyer DO and Singer BH (2006) Malaria risk on the Amazon frontier. Proceedings of the National Academy of Sciences of the United States of America 103: 2452–2457. 10.1073/pnas.0510576103.

Deblauwe V, Droissart V, Bose R, Sonké B, Blach-Overgaard A, Svenning J-C, Wieringa JJ, Ramesh BR, Stévart T and Couvreur TLP (2016) Remotely sensed temperature and precipitation data improve species distribution modelling in the tropics. Global Ecology and Biogeography 25: 443–454. https://doi.org/10.1111/geb.12426.

Dicko AH, Lancelot R, Seck MT, Guerrini L, Sall B, Lo M, Vreysen MJB, Lefrançois T, Fonta WM, Peck SL and Bouyer J (2014) Using species distribution models to optimize vector control in the framework of the tsetse eradication campaign in Senegal. Proceedings of the National Academy of Sciences 111: 10149–10154. doi:10.1073/pnas.1407773111.

Faulde MK, Rueda LM and Khaireh BA (2014) First record of the Asian malaria vector *Anopheles stephensi* and its possible role in the resurgence of malaria in Djibouti, Horn of Africa. Acta Trop 139: 39–43. https://doi.org/10.1016/j.actatropica.2014.06.016.

Fick SE and Hijmans RJ (2017) Worldclim 2: New 1-km spatial resolution climate surfaces for global land areas. International Journal of Climatology.

Finer M, Novoa S, Weisse MJ, Petersen R, Mascaro J, Souto T, Stearns F and Martinez RG (2018) Combating deforestation: From satellite to intervention. Science 360: 1303–1305. 10.1126/science.aat1203.

Fornace KM, Diaz AV, Lines J and Drakeley CJ (2021) Achieving global malaria eradication in changing landscapes. Malaria journal 20: 69. 10.1186/s12936-021-3599-0.

Fornace KM, Drakeley CJ, William T, Espino F and Cox J (2014) Mapping infectious disease landscapes: unmanned aerial vehicles and epidemiology. Trends in parasitology 30: 514–519. 10.1016/j.pt.2014.09.001.

Fornace KM, Surendra H, Abidin TR, Reyes R, Macalinao MLM, Stresman G, Luchavez J, Ahmad RA, Supargiyono S, Espino F, Drakeley CJ and Cook J (2018) Use of mobile technology-based participatory mapping approaches to geolocate health facility attendees for disease surveillance in low resource settings. International journal of health geographics 17: 21. 10.1186/s12942-018-0141-0.

Franke J, Gebreslasie M, Bauwens I, Deleu J and Siegert F (2015) Earth observation in support of malaria control and epidemiology: MALAREO monitoring approaches. Geospat Health 10: 335. 10.4081/gh.2015.335.

Gorris ME, Bartlow AW, Temple SD, Romero-Alvarez D, Shutt DP, Fair JM, Kaufeld KA, Del Valle SY and Manore CA (2021) Updated distribution maps of predominant *Culex* mosquitoes across the Americas. Parasites & vectors 14: 547. 10.1186/s13071-021-05051-3.

Gray PC, Fleishman AB, Klein DJ, McKown MW, Bezy VS, Lohmann KJ and Johnston DW (2019) A convolutional neural network for detecting sea turtles in drone imagery. Methods in Ecology and Evolution 00: 1–11.

Hansen MC, Potapov PV, Moore R, Hancher M, Turubanova SA, Tyukavina A, Thau D, Stehman SV, Goetz SJ, Loveland TR, Kommareddy A, Egorov A, Chini L, Justice CO and

Townshend JR (2013) High-resolution global maps of 21st-century forest cover change. Science 342: 850–853. 10.1126/science.1244693.

Hardy A, Ettritch G, Cross DE, Bunting P, Liywalii F, Sakala J, Silumesii A, Singini D, Smith M, Willis T and Thomas CJ (2019) Automatic Detection of Open and Vegetated Water Bodies Using Sentinel 1 to Map African Malaria Vector Mosquito Breeding Habitats. Remote Sensing 11: 593.

Hardy A, Makame M, Cross D, Majambere S and Msellem M (2017) Using low-cost drones to map malaria vector habitats. Parasites & vectors 10: 29. 10.1186/s13071-017-1973-3.

Hardy A, Oakes G, Hassan J and Yussuf Y (2022a) Improved use of drone imagery for malaria vector control through technology-assisted digitising (TAD). Remote Sensing 14.

Hardy A, Proctor M, MacCallum C, Shawe J, Abdalla S, Ali R, Abdalla S, Oakes G, Rosu L and Worrall E (2022b) Conditional trust: Community perceptions of drone use in malaria control in Zanzibar. Technology in Society 68: 101895. https://doi.org/10.1016/j.techsoc.2022.101895.

Hay SI (2000) An overview of remote sensing and geodesy for epidemiology and public health application. Advances in parasitology 47: 1–35.

Hay SI, Snow RW and Rogers DJ (1998) Predicting malaria seasons in Kenya using multitemporal meteorological satellite sensor data. Transactions of the Royal Society of Tropical Medicine and Hygiene 92: 12–20.

Iwamura T, Guzman-Holst A and Murray KA (2020) Accelerating invasion potential of disease vector *Aedes aegypti* under climate change. Nature communications 11: 2130. 10.1038/s41467-020-16010-4.

Jarvis A, Reuter A and Nelson EG (2022) Hole-filled SRTM for the globe version 4.0. In: Database C-CSm, ed.

Jones KE, Patel NG, Levy MA, Storeygard A, Balk D, Gittleman JL and Daszak P (2008) Global trends in emerging infectious diseases. Nature 451: 990–993. 10.1038/nature06536.

Jumail A, Liew TS, Salgado-Lynn M, Fornace KM and Stark DJ (2021) A comparative evaluation of thermal camera and visual counting methods for primate census in a riparian forest at the Lower Kinabatangan Wildlife Sanctuary (LKWS), Malaysian Borneo. Primates 62: 143–151. 10.1007/s10329-020-00837-y.

Kattenborn T, Eichel J and Fassnacht FE (2019) Convolutional Neural Networks enable efficient, accurate and fine-grained segmentation of plant species and communities from high resolution UAV imagery. Sci Rep 9.

Keiser J, De Castro MC, Maltese MF, Bos R, Tanner M, Singer BH and Utzinger J (2005) Effect of irrigation and large dams on the burden of malaria on a global and regional scale. The American journal of tropical medicine and hygiene 72: 392–406.

Koh L and Wich S (2012) Dawn of drone ecology: low-cost autonomous aerial vehicles for conservation. Tropical Conservation Science 5: 121–132.

Kraemer MUG, Reiner RC, Jr., Brady OJ, Messina JP, Gilbert M, Pigott DM, Yi D, Johnson K, Earl L, Marczak LB, Shirude S, Davis Weaver N, Bisanzio D, Perkins TA, Lai S, Lu X, Jones P, Coelho GE, Carvalho RG, Van Bortel W, Marsboom C, Hendrickx G, Schaffner F, Moore CG, Nax HH, Bengtsson L, Wetter E, Tatem AJ, Brownstein JS, Smith DL, Lambrechts L,

Cauchemez S, Linard C, Faria NR, Pybus OG, Scott TW, Liu Q, Yu H, Wint GRW, Hay SI and Golding N (2019) Past and future spread of the arbovirus vectors *Aedes aegypti* and *Aedes albopictus*. Nat Microbiol 4: 854–863. 10.1038/s41564-019-0376-y.

Lauer SA, Sakrejda K, Ray EL, Keegan LT, Bi Q, Suangtho P, Hinjoy S, Iamsirithaworn S, Suthachana S, Laosiritaworn Y, Cummings DAT, Lessler J and Reich NG (2018) Prospective forecasts of annual dengue hemorrhagic fever incidence in Thailand, 2010–2014. Proceedings of the National Academy of Sciences 115: E2175–E2182. doi:10.1073/pnas.1714457115.

Lippi CA, Stewart-Ibarra AM, Loor M, Zambrano JED, Lopez NAE, Blackburn JK and Ryan SJ (2019) Geographic shifts in *Aedes aegypti* habitat suitability in Ecuador using larval surveillance data and ecological niche modeling: Implications of climate change for public health vector control. PLoS neglected tropical diseases 13: e0007322. 10.1371/journal.pntd.0007322.

Liu D and Fan X (2010) Assessing object-based classification: advantages and limitations. Remote Sensing Letters 1: 187–194.

Lloyd CT, Sorichetta A and Tatem AJ (2017) High resolution global gridded data for use in population studies. Sci Data 4: 170001. 10.1038/sdata.2017.1.

Lowe R, Bailey TC, Stephenson DB, Jupp TE, Graham RJ, Barcellos C and Carvalho MS (2013) The development of an early warning system for climate-sensitive disease risk with a focus on dengue epidemics in Southeast Brazil. Stat Med 32: 864–883. 10.1002/sim.5549.

Lowe R, Coelho CA, Barcellos C, Carvalho MS, Catao Rde C, Coelho GE, Ramalho WM, Bailey TC, Stephenson DB and Rodo X (2016) Evaluating probabilistic dengue risk forecasts from a prototype early warning system for Brazil. Elife 5. 10.7554/eLife.11285.

Mather PM and Koch M (2010) Computer processing of remotely-sensed images (4th edition). Chichester, Wiley.

McEntaggart K, Fillet J, Marinoiu B, Quaresma H and de Paolis S (2020) The use of emerging technologies for regulation, Department for Business, Energy and Industrial Strategy.

Messina JP, Brady OJ, Golding N, Kraemer MUG, Wint GRW, Ray SE, Pigott DM, Shearer FM, Johnson K, Earl L, Marczak LB, Shirude S, Davis Weaver N, Gilbert M, Velayudhan R, Jones P, Jaenisch T, Scott TW, Reiner RC, Jr. and Hay SI (2019) The current and future global distribution and population at risk of dengue. Nat Microbiol 4: 1508–1515. 10.1038/s41564-019-0476-8.

Metcalf CJE, Walter KS, Wesolowski A, Buckee CO, Shevliakova E, Tatem AJ, Boos WR, Weinberger DM and Pitzer VE (2017) Identifying climate drivers of infectious disease dynamics: recent advances and challenges ahead. Proc Biol Sci 284. 10.1098/rspb.2017.0901.

Minakawa N, Munga S, Atieli F, Mushinzimana E, Zhou G, Githeko AK and Yan G (2005) Spatial distribution of anopheline larval habitats in Western Kenyan highlands: effects of land cover types and topography. The American journal of tropical medicine and hygiene 73: 157–165.

NASA (1973) The use of remote sensing in mosquito control, National Aeronautics and Space Administration, Lyndon B. Johnson Space Center, Houston, USA.

Noor AM, Alegana VA, Gething PW and Snow RW (2009) A spatial national health facility database for public health sector planning in Kenya in 2008. International journal of health geographics 8: 13. 10.1186/1476-072X-8-13.

Pareyn M, Rutten A, Merdekios B, Wedegärtner REM, Girma N, Regelbrugge L, Shibru S and Leirs H (2020) High-resolution habitat suitability model for Phlebotomus pedifer, the vector of cutaneous leishmaniasis in southwestern Ethiopia. Parasites & vectors 13: 467. 10.1186/s13071-020-04336-3.

Patz JA, Daszak P, Tabor GM, Aguirre AA, Pearl M, Epstein J, Wolfe ND, Kilpatrick AM, Foufopoulos J, Molyneux D, Bradley DJ, Working Group on Land Use C and Disease E (2004) Unhealthy landscapes: policy recommendations on land use change and infectious disease emergence. Environ Health Perspect 112: 1092–1098.

Pekel JF, Cottam A, Gorelick N and Belward AS (2016) High-resolution mapping of global surface water and its long-term changes. Nature 540: 418–422. 10.1038/nature20584.

Peterson AT (2014) Mapping Disease Transmission Risk. Baltimore, USA, Johns Hopkins University Press.

Petrova D, Lowe R, Stewart-Ibarra A, Ballester J, Koopman SJ and Rodó X (2019) Sensitivity of large dengue epidemics in Ecuador to long-lead predictions of El Niño. Climate Services 15: 100096. https://doi.org/10.1016/j.cliser.2019.02.003.

Phillips SJ, Anderson RP and Schapire RE (2006) Maximum entropy modeling of species geographic distributions. Ecol Modell 190: 231–259. https://doi.org/10.1016/j.ecolmodel.2005.03.026.

Qiu Y, Zhao X, Fan D, Li S and Zhao Y (2022) Disaggregating population data for assessing progress of SDGs: methods and applications. International Journal of Digital Earth 15: 2–29. 10.1080/17538947.2021.2013553.

Ryan SJ, Carlson CJ, Mordecai EA and Johnson LR (2019) Global expansion and redistribution of *Aedes*-borne virus transmission risk with climate change. PLoS neglected tropical diseases 13: e0007213. 10.1371/journal.pntd.0007213.

Seyfarth M, Khaireh BA, Abdi AA, Bouh SM and Faulde MK (2019) Five years following first detection of *Anopheles stephensi* (Diptera: Culicidae) in Djibouti, Horn of Africa: populations established – malaria emerging. Parasitol Res 118: 725–732. 10.1007/s00436-019-06213-0.

Simpson R, Page KR and De Roure D (2014) Zooniverse: observing the world's largest citizen science platform. Proceedings of the 23rd International Conference on the World Wide Web: 1049–1054.

Sinka ME, Golding N, Massey NC, Wiebe A, Huang Z, Hay SI and Moyes CL (2016) Modelling the relative abundance of the primary African vectors of malaria before and after the implementation of indoor, insecticide-based vector control. Malaria journal 15: 142. 10.1186/s12936-016-1187-8.

Sinka ME, Pironon S, Massey NC, Longbottom J, Hemingway J, Moyes CL and Willis KJ (2020) A new malaria vector in Africa: Predicting the expansion range of *Anopheles stephensi* and identifying the urban populations at risk. Proceedings of the National Academy of Sciences 117: 24900–24908. doi:10.1073/pnas.2003976117.

Stresman GH, Stevenson JC, Owaga C, Marube E, Anyango C, Drakeley C, Bousema T and Cox J (2014) Validation of three geolocation strategies for health-facility attendees for research and public health surveillance in a rural setting in western Kenya. Epidemiol Infect 142: 1978–1989. 10.1017/S0950268814000946.

Tatem AJ, Adamo S, Bharti N, Burgert CR, Castro M, Dorelien A, Fink G, Linard C, John M, Montana L, Montgomery MR, Nelson A, Noor AM, Pindolia D, Yetman G and Balk D (2012) Mapping populations at risk: improving spatial demographic data for infectious disease modeling and metric derivation. Population Health Metrics 10: 8. 10.1186/1478-7954-10-8.

Tatem AJ, Goetz SJ and Hay SI (2008) Fifty Years of Earth Observation Satellites: views from above have lead to countless advances on the ground in both scientific knowledge and daily life. Am Sci 96: 390–398. 10.1511/2008.74.390.

Thomson MC and Connor SJ (2001) The development of Malaria Early Warning Systems for Africa. Trends in parasitology 17: 438–445. 10.1016/s1471-4922(01)02077-3.

Thomson MC, Doblas-Reyes FJ, Mason SJ, Hagedorn R, Connor SJ, Phindela T, Morse AP and Palmer TN (2006) Malaria early warnings based on seasonal climate forecasts from multi-model ensembles. Nature 439: 576–579. 10.1038/nature04503.

Thomson MC, Garcia-Herrera R and Beniston M (2008) Seasonal forecasts, climate change and human health, Advances in Global Change Research. Dordrecht, Springer.

Union of Concerned Scientists (2021) UCS Satellite Database.

Vittor AY, Pan W, Gilman RH, Tielsch J, Glass G, Shields T, Sanchez-Lozano W, Pinedo VV, Salas-Cobos E, Flores S and Patz JA (2009) Linking deforestation to malaria in the Amazon: characterization of the breeding habitat of the principal malaria vector, *Anopheles darlingi*. The American journal of tropical medicine and hygiene 81: 5–12.

Wagner VE, Hill-Rowley R, Narlock SA and Newson HD (1979) Remote sensing: a rapid and accurate method of data acquisition for a newly formed mosquito control district. Mosquito News 39: 283–287.

Wardrop NA, Jochem WC, Bird TJ, Chamberlain HR, Clarke D, Kerr D, Bengtsson L, Juran S, Seaman V and Tatem AJ (2018) Spatially disaggregated population estimates in the absence of national population and housing census data. Proceedings of the National Academy of Sciences of the United States of America 115: 3529–3537. 10.1073/pnas.1715305115.

Weaver SC (2013) Urbanization and geographic expansion of zoonotic arboviral diseases: mechanisms and potential strategies for prevention. Trends Microbiol 21: 360–363. 10.1016/j.tim.2013.03.003.

Weiss DJ, Lucas TCD, Nguyen M, Nandi AK, Bisanzio D, Battle KE, Cameron E, Twohig KA, Pfeffer DA, Rozier JA, Gibson HS, Rao PC, Casey D, Bertozzi-Villa A, Collins EL, Dalrymple U, Gray N, Harris JR, Howes RE, Kang SY, Keddie SH, May D, Rumisha S, Thorn MP, Barber R, Fullman N, Huynh CK, Kulikoff X, Kutz MJ, Lopez AD, Mokdad AH, Naghavi M, Nguyen G, Shackelford KA, Vos T, Wang H, Smith DL, Lim SS, Murray CJL, Bhatt S, Hay SI and Gething PW (2019) Mapping the global prevalence, incidence, and mortality of *Plasmodium falciparum*, 2000–17: a spatial and temporal modelling study. Lancet 394: 322–331. 10.1016/S0140-6736(19)31097-9.

Weiss DJ, Mappin B, Dalrymple U, Bhatt S, Cameron E, Hay SI and Gething PW (2015) Re-examining environmental correlates of *Plasmodium falciparum* malaria endemicity: a data-intensive variable selection approach. Malaria journal 14: 68. 10.1186/s12936-015-0574-x.

Wimberly MC, de Beurs KM, Loboda TV and Pan WK (2021) Satellite Observations and Malaria: New Opportunities for Research and Applications. Trends in parasitology 37: 525–537. 10.1016/j.pt.2021.03.003.

World Health Organisation (2001) Malaria Early Warning Systems: Concepts, Indicators and Partners: A Framework for Field Research in Africa, World Health Organisation, Roll Back Malaria, Technical Support Network for Prevention and Control of Malaria, Geneva.

World Health Organisation (2019) Meeting report of the WHO technical consultation on the spread of *Anopheles stephensi*, World Health Organisation, Geneva.

Yared S, Gebressielasie A, Damodaran L, Bonnell V, Lopez K, Janies D and Carter TE (2020) Insecticide resistance in *Anopheles stephensi* in Somali Region, eastern Ethiopia. Malar J 19: 180. 10.1186/s12936-020-03252-2.

CHAPTER 12

Early warning systems for vector-borne diseases: engagement, methods and implementation

Emilie Finch[1,2*], *Martín Lotto Batista*[3,4], *Tilly Alcayna*[1,2,5], *Sophie A. Lee*[1,2], *Isabel K. Fletcher*[6] *and Rachel Lowe*[1,2,4,7*]

[1]Centre for Mathematical Modelling of Infectious Diseases, London School of Hygiene & Tropical Medicine, Keppel Street, WC1E 7HT, London, United Kingdom; [2]Centre on Climate Change and Planetary Health, London School of Hygiene & Tropical Medicine, Keppel Street, WC1E 7HT, London, United Kingdom; [3]Epidemiology Department, Helmholtz Centre for Infection Research (HZI), Inhoffenstraße 7, 38124 Braunschweig, Germany; [4]Barcelona Supercomputing Center (BSC), Plaça d'Eusebi Güell 1–3, 08034 Barcelona, Spain; [5]Red Cross Red Crescent Climate Centre, Anna van Saksenlaan 50, 2593 HT The Hague, the Netherlands; [6]Data for Science & Health, Wellcome Trust, 215 Euston Road, WC1E 6BP, London, UK; [7]Catalan Institution for Research and Advanced Studies (ICREA), Passeig Lluís Companys 23, 08010 Barcelona, Spain; *emilie.finch1@lshtm.ac.uk; rachel.lowe@bsc.es

Abstract

Vector-borne diseases, such as dengue and malaria, cause substantial morbidity and mortality around the globe, particularly in low- and middle-income countries located in the tropics and sub-tropics. With growing computational capacity and improved remote sensing technology, climate services can be coupled with forecasting models to provide early warning of disease outbreaks. In this chapter, we propose a series of steps necessary for the co-creation of a fully functional climate-informed early warning system. We aim to initiate a discussion about the strategies and challenges associated with building partnerships, data acquisition, model development, and tool implementation and evaluation. Finally, we provide cross-cutting recommendations focused on facilitating the shift from academic forecasting research to the implementation of climate-informed early warning systems at global, national and local scales.

Keywords

climate services – epidemic modelling – forecasting – co-creation – evaluation – outbreak risk – model validation

1 Introduction

Vector-borne diseases (VBDs) account for more than 17% of all infectious diseases and, according to the World Health Organization (WHO), cause more than 700,000 deaths each year, as well as substantial global economic burden (Sarma *et al.* 2019; Shepard *et al.* 2016). Climate change, international travel and trade, and rapid urbanisation, are shifting patterns in the transmission and burden of VBDs (Ryan *et al.* 2019). Dengue cases have increased substantially in recent decades with an 8-fold increase in the number of cases reported to the WHO between 2000 to 2019, alongside an over 4-fold increase in the number of deaths reported between 2000 and 2015. Following initial outbreaks in the Pacific, the emergence of chikungunya virus in the Americas in 2013 and Zika virus in 2015 resulted in major outbreaks in many countries leading to substantial morbidity and mortality, and, in some cases, overwhelming health systems (Puntasecca *et al.* 2021). Despite significant elimination efforts, malaria continues to be responsible for the majority of the global burden of VBDs, with nearly half of the world's population thought to be at risk of malaria in 2020 (World Malaria Report, 2021).

Climate-informed early warning systems (EWS) integrate climate data to predict the risk of an infectious disease outbreak. These systems offer the potential for advanced warning of disease outbreaks, with longer lead times for public health action than decision-support systems based solely on outbreak detection through epidemiological surveillance. The timescale of forecasts produced by a climate-driven EWS typically range from short-term predictions (e.g. days or weeks ahead) to sub-seasonal or seasonal predictions from several weeks to several months ahead. As such, a climate-informed EWS can improve the timeliness and impact of public health response to outbreaks, and will become increasingly crucial as the climate crisis leads to more frequent climatic extremes. While traditional infectious disease monitoring systems focus on detecting and predicting infectious disease risk, it is important that an EWS is also linked to appropriate response mechanisms such that timely action can be taken to prevent an outbreak from occurring or mitigate potential disease (World Health Organization 2021). Depending on stakeholder needs and capacity, a climate-informed EWS could provide support for public-health decision making on when or where to begin vector-control activities, enhance surveillance, or increase hospital capacity. Climate-informed EWS are an example of a climate service, defined by the World Meteorological Organization (WMO) as a decision aide derived from climate information that assists individuals and organisations in society to make improved ex-ante decision-making (World Meteorological Organization 2015). Despite the established use of EWS in other fields, such as for the prediction of natural hazards for disaster risk reduction or prediction of food security risk in the humanitarian sector, the integration of

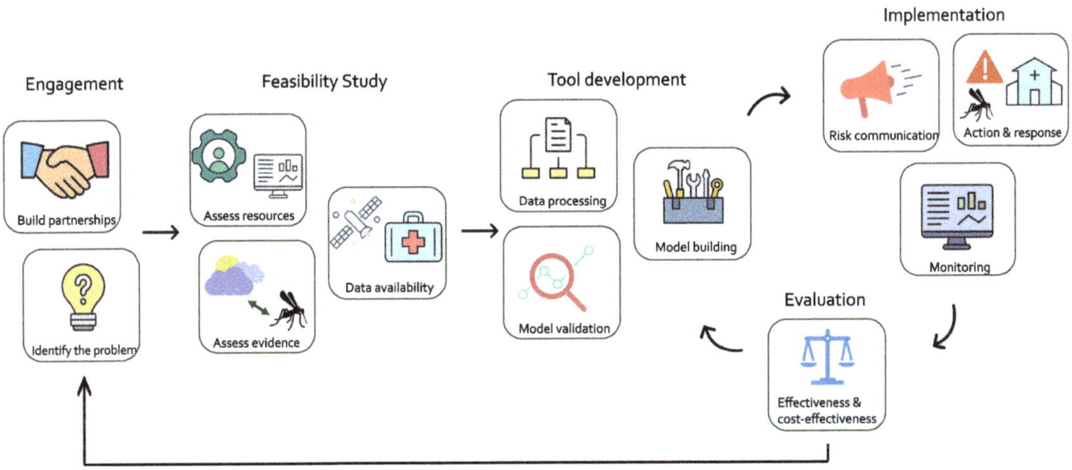

FIGURE 1 End-to-end overview of the stages involved in the co-creation of an early warning system for vector-borne disease

climate-informed EWS within the health sector remains limited to date. A recent review of software tools for predicting outbreaks of climate-sensitive infectious diseases found few operationalised tools, and suggested that research in this field is rarely translated into usable decision-support tools for early-warning (Ryan *et al.* 2023).

In this chapter, we provide an end-to-end overview of the stages involved in the development of an EWS for vector-borne diseases, drawing on insights from the epidemic forecasting community and those from researchers and institutions working on the application of climate services for health. We will focus on the following stages in the development of an EWS: (1) engagement, (2) conducting a feasibility study, (3) tool development, (4) implementation and monitoring, and (5) evaluation (Figure 1). While we hope this series of steps provides a useful overview of the process of co-design and development of an EWS for vector-borne diseases, it is not intended to be prescriptive. In fact, the process of EWS development and implementation is likely to evolve as research and implementation leads to new learning, improved communication, and public health action.

1.1 *Engagement*

Developing an EWS which can be integrated into public health planning and lead to an improved public health response to outbreaks is a complex transdisciplinary process, and building partnerships between key stakeholders is essential. Co-creation should be central to the development of an EWS and engagement between different partners, including decision-makers and tool developers, should happen at all stages of EWS development. Once these partnerships have been established, the co-creation process can begin with partners jointly identifying the public health needs and priorities and setting out the broad aims for an EWS tool.

1.1.1 Build partnerships

The co-creation of an EWS requires well-coordinated interaction from transdisciplinary stakeholders spanning governmental institutions, academia, the private sector, and civil society organisations to ensure the end-to-end functionality of the system (UNDP 2018) (Figure 1).

Building strong partnerships at the outset of EWS development is important to establish trust (both in the EWS and between partners), improve confidence in the EWS, create a sense of ownership of the final product, promote institutionalisation of the EWS, and, importantly, ensure warnings are used to prevent an outbreak (where possible) or to attempt to reduce the rate of transmission and mitigate the impact of an outbreak (Githeko *et al.* 2018; Hussain-Alkhateeb *et al.* 2021; UNDP 2018). For example, a recent multi-year project by climate and health practitioners to build a dengue EWS for Barbados employed a co-creation approach and highlighted the importance of co-learning to build strong partnerships between the different actors required to translate scientific knowledge into public health action (Stewart-Ibarra *et al.* 2022). The team described how their co-creation process spanned all stages of EWS development, from identification of the problem to model building and implementation. They found that this engagement process built trust and shared ownership in the EWS, which are crucial to the system's ultimate implementation and usefulness in informing public health action. Ultimately, only trusted EWS, which provide clear and useful warnings to decision-makers can lead to meaningful action.

1.1.1.1 *Who needs to be convened?*

Researchers, including environmental epidemiologists, spatial data experts, meteorologists, climate scientists, modellers, entomologists and infectious disease specialists, among others, provide the core analysis needed to develop an early-warning tool able to forecast future health risks, and to co-develop the technical guidance and standardised methodologies to interpret warnings. Early engagement of policymakers at the appropriate level from different ministries and agencies, such as, but not limited to, the Ministry of Health, national meteorological services and emergency services, ensure a greater chance of the EWS being used for a public health response, whereby the warning can be translated into widespread action. Government involvement is critical for the institutionalisation of any EWS. Ultimately only governments have the authority to create the institutional arrangements and legal frameworks, determine the mandates, roles, and responsibilities of interacting partners, disseminate early warning alerts to the public or take national-level public health action (IFRC 2012; UNDP 2018). In particular, the current lack of formal partnerships between health and climate sectors in many countries has been highlighted as a key barrier to the implementation of climate-informed early-warning systems. To date, few health and climate sectors have the mandate to focus on climate services for health and there is an urgent need to build stronger partnerships between these sectors in many countries, to facilitate research and implementation of EWS (Stewart-Ibarra *et al.* 2022).

Other important partners include the private sector, civil society organisations, non-governmental organisations, and the public themselves. The private sector may provide expertise in technology, infrastructure, data, or telecommunication and media to support the dissemination of warnings (UNDP 2018). Civil society organisations or the Red Cross Red Crescent Movement and their network of community-based volunteers are often highly trusted by communities and play a vital role in many countries before and during emergencies, including health emergencies. Finally, it's important that the public trust the EWS and understand what action they should take on the warnings that are received, in a similar way to how the public understand and act upon probabilistic weather forecasts. It will often also be crucial to involve the public in the development of an EWS, for instance in helping to define the locally appropriate solutions, participating in risk assessments, identifying particular at-risk groups, informing response initiatives and emergency plans, and providing feedback and evaluation on how to improve the system (IFRC 2012; UNDP 2018).

1.1.2 Identify the problem

EWS usually target epidemic or outbreak-prone infectious diseases, as these can exhibit rapid surges in case numbers that threaten significant morbidity, mortality and pressure on the health systems (World Health Organization 2005). Common vector-borne diseases targeted by EWS include; dengue, chikungunya, Japanese encephalitis, Rift Valley fever, West Nile virus, Ross River virus, malaria, Murray Valley fever, Lyme disease, and Yellow fever.

Public health decision-makers may be interested in a range of policy questions that could be informed by a climate-informed EWS. These could include questions on when and where to target interventions (primarily vector control efforts), when to begin enhanced surveillance of a vector-borne disease, or what the most effective or cost-effective intervention may be in various scenarios. The forecasting targets of the EWS (that is, the epidemiological output of interest from a forecasting model) should align with the policy questions of interest to ensure that the EWS is able to provide relevant and usable warnings to decision-makers. Forecasting targets should also be well-defined at the outset of the co-creation process and well-documented in the reporting of EWS forecasts to allow for clear and rigorous statistical evaluation of the predictive accuracy of forecasts, and to facilitate comparison with alternative EWS models (Pollett *et al.* 2021). For instance, during the Dengue Forecasting Challenge in 2015, teams generated forecasts for three epidemiological targets representing key features of dengue outbreaks: the overall number of cases in a season (season incidence); the intensity of the epidemic peak (peak incidence) and the timing of peak incidence (Johansson *et al.* 2019). However, other relevant targets may be of interest to stakeholders, such as the probability of exceeding a user-defined outbreak threshold. Different forecasting targets may inform different response actions. For example, predictions about the timing of peak incidence in a season could inform decisions on when to begin vector control efforts, while predictions about the magnitude of peak and season intensity could inform decisions on whether to employ emergency vector control efforts or increase medical supplies and treatment capacity.

The geographical extent of the EWS should also be defined. EWS can provide warnings of disease risk at the national, regional or local level, depending on the spatial and temporal resolution required for decision-making (Macherera and Chimbari 2016). Moreover, within a country, certain areas may be more prone to outbreaks than others. For example, an EWS for malaria may be more useful in certain highland areas where conditions are rarely suitable for malaria transmission, than neighbouring lowland areas where transmission can occur all year round (World Health Organization 2005). That being said, as climate change shifts transmission zones and erodes natural barriers to transmission, it will become increasingly crucial for an EWS to be able to monitor and give warning of potential outbreaks in unexpected regions (Lee *et al.* 2021a). The geographical extent of an EWS should be regularly updated as climate change may create more favourable conditions over a wider geographical range.

1.2 *Feasibility study*

After identifying the target disease, the relevant public health decision-making questions and geographical scope of an EWS, the next stage involves an assessment of the feasibility of an EWS system for the setting and vector-borne disease being considered. Here, a joint identification and assessment is needed of the resources of key partners and institutions involved, the evidence on climate-health linkages relevant to the problem identified, and the data availability of relevant climate and epidemiological data.

1.2.1 Assess resources

Through engagement and collaboration, the co-creation of an EWS should build on existing capacity to maximise the feasibility of integrating the EWS into national programmes. However, a review of EWS found that most did not assess the feasibility of implementing the developed EWS into national programs ahead of development (Hussain-Alkhateeb *et al.* 2021). Ideally, EWS should be based on data the country has regular access to (such as local or regional meteorological stations or routine epidemiology data). This, to a large extent, is determined by the infrastructure and budget of a country. The type of EWS that can be implemented and maintained depends on the investments in technology (the surveillance system, data pipelines, dissemination means), the investments in human resources (such as the skill level of analysts), and the investments in preparedness plans (including training, drills, and mobilisation of responders) (UNDP 2018). Most EWS identified in a recent a systematic review demanded advanced analytical skills (Hussain-Alkhateeb *et al.* 2021) which may affect the sustainability of such systems in lower resourced settings and suggests there was insufficient co-design and engagement in the outset of the projects reviewed.

However, while EWS developed in research settings should consider the resources available to implement the tool at the country or local level, in many settings it is also imperative to advocate for increased financial and technical resources as well as capacity building, particularly within the health and climate sectors. This would enable the harmonization and mutual understanding of climate and epidemiological data sets between climate and health practitioners, allowing for better integration of climate data into health decision-making (Lowe *et al.* 2020b; Stewart-Ibarra *et al.* 2022). In particular, financial and technical investment is often needed to ensure the accessibility of historical climate and health data, which may be incomplete, use inconsistent formats, or be paper-based, and may require increased training or personnel devoted to data management (Lowe *et al.* 2020b). During a recent exploration of national stakeholder needs and perceptions in Barbados and Dominica, national climate and health stakeholders reported a lack of technical expertise in geographic information systems (GIS), statistics, modelling and computer programming (Stewart-Ibarra *et al.* 2019). As well as improving routine data analytics performed at a national or local level, this kind of technical training would aid in the development, operationalisation and interpretation of a climate-driven EWS.

1.2.2 Assess the evidence

There is a growing body of evidence describing and quantifying climate-health linkages; however, not all climatic indicators will be relevant in all settings and for all VBDs, and it is often logistically challenging to collect data on all possible climatic drivers of transmission and include them in potential models. As such, it is important to consider the evidence from the literature and previous EWS when making decisions on relevant data to collect and include in the model selection process.

Climate is an important driver in the transmission of many infectious diseases, influencing both human behaviour as well as the survival and life cycle of the pathogen (Myers *et al.* 2000; World Health Organization 2005). Climate is a particularly important driver of VBDs due to the additional impact of climate variability on natural history traits of the disease vector (including vector fecundity, development and survival) and transmission of VBDs is typically seasonal (Mordecai *et al.* 2017;

Ryan *et al.* 2019). Ultimately, the suitability of a VBD for a climate-informed early warning system will depend on its sensitivity to climate variation.

1.2.2.1 *Seasonal climate patterns*

Temperature is a key climatic predictor of vector-borne disease transmission, with important effects on the lifecycle of the pathogen and the vector, among other factors. For example, the effect of temperature on arboviral transmission occurs through effects on viral replication as well as on *Aedes* mosquito survival, breeding, host-seeking and blood-feeding patterns (Bellone and Failloux 2020; Reinhold *et al.* 2018). Consequently, for most VBDs, transmission cannot occur below or above specific temperature extremes. For instance, 16 °C is thought to be the lower limit for the development of the malarial parasite *Plasmodium falciparum* (Patz and Olson 2006), while temperatures in the range of 18–34 °C are favourable for dengue virus transmission, with optimal transmission between 26–29 °C (Macdonald 1957; Mordecai *et al.* 2017). Rainfall is another important climatic driver of vector-borne disease transmission; however, the effects of rainfall on transmission are nuanced and dependent on the vector and setting being considered. Increased rainfall results in wet and humid conditions ideal for vector breeding and the creation of larval habitats, as in the case of *Anopheles* mosquitoes, which require monthly precipitation above 80 mm (Grover-Kopec *et al.* 2006). However, in some cases, excessive rainfall can also reduce transmission by washing larval habitats away entirely. This has been documented for dengue, as urban *Aedes* mosquito vectors typically lay eggs in small domestic water containers (Benedum *et al.* 2018; Koenraadt and Harrington 2008).

1.2.2.2 *Extreme climatic events*

Compared with seasonal fluctuations in temperature and rainfall, the effect of extreme climatic events (ECEs) on vector-borne disease transmission remains relatively understudied (Alcayna *et al.* 2022; McMichael 2015). However, ECEs such as flooding, drought or tropical storms can increase the risk of vector-borne disease outbreaks in some settings through the creation of larval habitats. For instance, droughts can, perhaps unintuitively, increase the risk of vector-borne disease transmission if they result in an increase in uncovered water storage containers in a particular setting. Both drought and excessive rainfall were found to increase the risk of a dengue outbreak, with differing delays, in Barbados and Brazil (Lowe *et al.* 2018, 2021).

The risk of a vector-borne disease outbreak can be further amplified by downstream impacts of ECEs such as population displacement or disruption to public health services, and disease outcomes could be worsened by the effects of concurrent food shortages or famine (Kovats *et al.* 2003). Understanding the linkages between ECEs and outbreaks of climate-sensitive infectious diseases is increasingly crucial as the climate emergency continues to increase both the frequency and magnitude of ECEs (Romanello *et al.* 2021). These insights can be incorporated into climate-informed EWS aiming to prevent or mitigate the harms from infectious disease outbreaks.

1.2.2.3 *El Niño Southern Oscillation*

El Niño Southern Oscillation (ENSO) is an irregular interannual climatic phenomena involving changes in sea-surface temperatures in the Pacific Ocean, which influences weather patterns around the world. ENSO oscillations can result in an El Niño event, with an anomalous temperature increase, or a contrasting anomalous temperature decrease, known as a La Niña event. El Niño and La Niña events are associated with an increased intensity of ECEs across the globe. El Niño events are associated with an average temperature increase globally of 0.5°C and an increased risk of drought in areas including Southern Africa, Southeast Asia, Indonesia and Australia, among others, and increased risk of extreme rainfall along the western coast of South America. Contrastingly, La Niña events have been associated with increased risk of flooding in the western Pacific and an increased frequency of tropical storms in areas such as the Caribbean and the Gulf of Mexico (Anyamba *et al.* 2019; Kovats *et al.* 2003). ENSO events can thus lead to increased vector-borne disease transmission through changes in temperature, rainfall or ECEs experienced in a particular setting.

Understanding the associations between interannual climate fluctuations and vector-borne disease transmission is valuable as it could allow for advanced warning of particularly high or low transmission seasons into a forecasting model, through the inclusion of an ENSO indicator (Kovats *et al.* 2003). Similarly, alternative indices such as the Indian Ocean Dipole (IOD), which measures oscillations in sea surface temperature in the Indian Ocean, are also associated with shifts in climatic patterns and subsequently with vector-borne disease risk, and may be more relevant than ENSO indicators in certain geographical settings (Chuang *et al.* 2017).

1.2.2.4 *Non-climatic drivers*

When considering relevant climate-disease linkages to incorporate into a climate-informed forecasting model it is also critical to evaluate other key drivers that may have a substantial impact on disease dynamics. The level of population immunity to a pathogen over time, which is continually shifting as new susceptibles enter the population and, in some cases, protective immunity wanes, is often a key determinant of the magnitude and timing of outbreaks. This is particularly evident when considering emerging diseases that are introduced into entirely susceptible populations. For instance, during the Zika and chikungunya outbreaks in Latin America, research has shown that lack of immunity to the pathogens was a dominant factor driving transmission in the Dominican Republic, with emergence occurring earlier in the year than optimal seasonal climatic conditions (Petrone *et al.* 2021). For pathogens with multiple serotypes, such as dengue virus, shifts in the dominant serotype in a setting can result in a change in the magnitude and timing of outbreaks (Rajarethinam *et al.* 2018).

Similarly, environmental or socioeconomic factors play an important role in the interaction of pathogens with vectors and humans. Certain characteristics of the environment can influence the likelihood of an outbreak occurring, including land cover characteristics, the level of urbanisation, the degree of environmental degradation, and the connectivity between regions, among others (Lee *et al.* 2021a; Semenza 2015; Ryan *et al.* 2023). The spread of the dengue vector from urban centres to neighbouring rural areas and urbanised forests in Brazil has been strongly associated with changes in the spatial connectivity, as well as forest degradation (Lee *et al.* 2021a; Lowe *et al.* 2020a). Where relevant, these variables can also be incorporated into modelling frameworks to improve the predictive power of models (Lowe *et al.* 2021). Additionally, incorporating climatic and non-climatic drivers within a single modelling framework can help to understand how, say, serological or environmental factors mediate climate-disease relationships and gain a better understanding of how multiple drivers work in combination to shape VBD risk.

1.2.3 Data availability

After considering the evidence on relevant climate-disease linkages and other non-climatic drivers for the particular problem targeted by a proposed EWS, model developers will need to consider the data streams and products available for a given setting. In practice, thinking about the available data streams will often occur in parallel to discussions about the ideal forecasting model structure for the problem at hand, and available data streams will shape the prediction tools. For instance, longer time-series are often required for statistical modelling approaches and will be particularly necessary for climatic drivers which experience significant inter-annual variability and in settings that may experience several unusually heavy rainy seasons in a row (Lee *et al.* 2021b).

In ideal circumstances, stakeholders should have open and equitable access to data which is updated regularly (Hussain-Alkhateeb *et al.* 2021; Ryan *et al.* 2023). In this section, we will describe the available data sources commonly used for developing forecasting models for EWS.

1.2.3.1 *Climate data*

As the evidence grows on the impact of climate, and of increasingly frequent climatic extremes, on human health, the availability of climate products for use in the health sector has increased (Fletcher *et al.* 2021). These services are informed by Earth observations, which comprise space or ground based climatic information describing atmospheric, oceanic or terrestrial conditions. Earth observations can be collected via local meteorological stations and using remote-sensing technologies such as satellite imagery (Fletcher *et al.* 2021).

Although many countries have networks of local meteorological stations, global coverage from local meteorological station data is patchy, can vary in quality, is often not easily accessible, and is often not directly applicable in large scale models (Ceccato *et al.* 2018). Satellite-derived climate products are valuable complements for local ground observations, as they provide continuous spatiotemporal historical observations (Fletcher *et al.* 2021). These datasets include a range of variables and vary in their resolution and spatiotemporal coverage (Table 1). When selecting the appropriate data product for analysis, there is often a trade-off to be made between the temporal and spatial resolution of data (sometimes referred to as the data granularity), the length of time-series available, and associated costs of data products that are not open-access. As an example, while the ERA5-Land products range from 1950 until the present at a 9 km resolution (Muñoz-Sabater *et al.* 2021), Landsat products offer 10-year time series at 30 metre resolution ('Landsat Missions, U.S. Geological Survey.,' 2022).

The choice of the gridded climate products should be informed by their ability to represent the local weather conditions and by considering the geographical scale of the problem at hand. For instance, fine scale data (i.e. 10 km^2) can allow for detailed studies of how local microclimates may affect disease risk, while coarser data may be more appropriate to characterise climate-disease linkages across regions containing varied microclimates. Fletcher and colleagues recommended comparing global products with local observations where possible, and applying bias correction techniques to correct for data nuances (Fletcher *et al.* 2021). Collaboration with local meteorologists can help model developers understand discrepancies between satellite and ground-truth data and which bias correction or downscaling techniques might be more appropriate. This is an important step in EWS development as the use of a data product which is not well suited to the study area, or which contains systematic biases, may affect the characterisation of the climate-disease relationship being modelled, and subsequently impact the quality of model forecasts for early warning.

The most commonly used variables for modelling climate-sensitive VBDs are temperature (usually recorded as the mean, maximum, minimum temperature or temperature range in a given time unit) and rainfall (typically recorded as cumulative rainfall in a given time unit), because of their well-established impact on vector survival and breeding (Ryan *et al.* 2023). However, additional variables such as absolute or relative humidity, wind speed and direction, and diurnal temperature range, and alternative climate indicators, such as the Standardized Precipitation Index (SPI), have also proven useful in assessing risk of vector-borne disease (Colón-González *et al.* 2021; Lowe *et al.* 2018; Pley *et al.* 2021; Romanello *et al.* 2021).

Additionally, indicators summarising anomalous conditions in the Pacific Ocean, such as the Oceanic Niño Index (ONI) (a 3-month running average of sea surface temperatures in the Nino 3.4 region) have also been used in VBD modelling studies (Lowe *et al.* 2017).

1.2.3.2 *Lags and lead-time*

The goal of a climate-informed EWS is to give warnings of increased outbreak risk with enough lead-time to deploy interventions that can mitigate the impact of an outbreak (Runge-Ranzinger *et al.* 2016). This can be achieved either by incorporating lagged weather variables in the model (such that temperature or rainfall in the previous month, say, is used to predict the number of cases this month), or through access to climate forecast products which can then be used as inputs for infectious disease forecasting models (Morin *et al.* 2018). Climate forecast products are available at local and global levels, and it is possible to test model performance using different forecast horizons (Colón-González *et al.* 2021). Uncertainty in climate forecasts can also be incorporated into the modelling framework, and this may be particularly important when considering infectious disease forecasts with several months lead time. One example of this can be found in a study conducted by Lowe and colleagues which used climate forecasts to predict the 2016 dengue season in Machala, Ecuador. Here, the authors used an ensemble of 24 seasonal climate forecasts (each obtained by perturbing initial conditions) as an input into the modelling framework, thereby incorporating the uncertainty in forecasted precipitation and minimum temperature into predictions of dengue cases from 1 to 11 months ahead (Lowe *et al.* 2017).

1.2.3.3 *Epidemiological and demographic data*

At their core, most forecasting models for EWS rely on surveillance data from routine surveillance systems capturing weekly or monthly reported cases (as well as deaths or severe outcomes) from a particular disease, often stratified by age or geographical units. Surveillance systems can also provide information about the conditions that enable transmission that may be useful for developing control strategies. In the case of vector borne diseases, vector species and pathogens can also be monitored (Braks *et al.* 2019). Cases reported through surveillance systems may be suspected cases, confirmed cases via epidemiological link, or laboratory confirmed cases.

Epidemiological data from surveillance systems has several key limitations, including delays in reporting, changes in reporting mechanisms over time and missing values or errors in data entry (Hussain-Alkhateeb *et al.* 2021). Additionally, for pathogens that result in a large proportion of asymptomatic or mild disease, such as dengue virus, surveillance systems may only detect a small proportion of overall infections. These limitations mean that interpreting patterns in surveillance data can be challenging.

TABLE 1 Global climate datasets openly available online (updated from Fletcher *et al.* 2021)

Source	Description	Temporal resolution	Spatial resolution	Time coverage	File format	Type
CHELSA v.2.1.3 (Karger *et al.* 2017; Karger *et al.* 2021)	Semi-mechanistic downscaling approach of global reanalysis data (ERA-Interim) to a high resolution	Monthly	1 km/0.008°	1979–2019	GeoTiff	Historic
CRU TS v.4.05 (Harris *et al.* 2020)	Estimates are produced using angular-distance weighting interpolation of climate anomalies from extensive global weather station observations	Monthly	55 km/0.5°	1901–2020	ASCII, NetCDF	Historic
ERA5-Land (Muñoz-Sabater *et al.* 2021)	A reanalysis dataset based on climate models of land surfaces	Hourly/ Monthly	9 km/0.08°	1950–2/3 months before present	GRIB, NetCDF	Historic
TerraClimate (Abatzoglou *et al.* 2018)	Uses climatically aided interpolation and combines climatological normals from WorldClim with time-varying anomalies from CRU TS v.4.0 and Japanese 55-year Reanalysis (JRA55)	Monthly	4 km/0.04°	1958–2020	NetCDF	Historic and climate projections
WorldClim v.2.1 (Fick and Hijmands 2017)	Historical estimates of climate variables obtained by utilising the spatial coverage of CRU TS v.4.03 downscaled using WorldClim v.2	Monthly	21 km/0.2°	1970–2020	GeoTiff	Historic and climate projections

When available, demographic information is useful to understand the underlying structure of the population at risk. Population sizes change over time, and it is necessary to account for these changes when creating forecasting tools. Census data is the primary source of demographic information, this is typically collected by governmental institutions and made available to the public. However, as these are not performed every year, population projections are necessary to complete the time series. Alternatively, there are gridded products, such as WorldPop, that provide population estimates in raster format ('WorldPop,' 2022). Contact patterns, population mobility, age structure and socio-economic conditions, among other variables, can also be incorporated into forecasting models to better capture pathogen spread in a population and the resultant burden of disease.

Epidemiological information from scientific literature can also be incorporated into forecasting models. For instance, estimates on the force of infection, Ro, case fatality ratio, or hospitalisation fatality ratio in a particular setting can provide information to parameterise mechanistic models (Lee *et al.* 2021b; Lessler *et al.* 2016).

1.2.3.4 *Environmental data*

Spatial information is also available on environmental or socioeconomic factors, such as land cover, urbanisation or environmental degradation. In these datasets, spatial units or grid cells are categorised into different classes based on satellite imagery of the Earth's surface. Land cover datasets describe the physical material on the surface of a country or region, for instance showing whether areas are covered by cropland, grasslands, forest or lakes. These may be static or dynamic, depending on whether they consider changes in land cover over time. Land use datasets also contain information on how people use different physical land types, for instance, classifying areas as industrial, agricultural, or recreational. Land use can modulate climate-disease relationships in important ways as discussed in a study by Fletcher and colleagues, which found that mining activity was associated with hotspots in malaria transmission in southern Venezuela, and that the influence of temperature on malaria differed depending on the intensity of mining activity (Fletcher *et al.* 2022).

A commonly used index is the Normalised Difference Vegetation Index (NDVI), which indicates the 'amount of greenness' in a certain area, which can be useful, for instance, in detecting forest areas compared with built-up urban areas. The Copernicus Global Land Service is an example of a data source that offers land cover products that monitor vegetation, water and energy cycle and the terrestrial cryosphere (Buchhorn *et al.* 2020). Additionally, there are products that track changes in urban development throughout time, which are useful for historic reconstruction of disease drivers and future projections (Liu *et al.* 2020). Local partners may also have access to local monitoring services of land cover/use data most relevant to the setting and establishing partnerships with local institutions or universities could provide high quality products, ready for model building.

1.2.3.5 *Common barriers to accessing data*

Climate-informed EWS require collaborative data generation between global and local stakeholders (Ryan *et al.* 2023), and therefore will rely on legislation or regulations in place surrounding data ownership and sharing (Pley *et al.* 2021; Ryan *et al.* 2023). A recent review of tools for modelling climate-sensitive infectious diseases found that the sharing of datasets was a key barrier to tool development and implementation, but noted that climate datasets were generally more easily accessible than epidemiological or health data, which were often found to be difficult to access due to privacy concerns (Ryan *et al.* 2023). Formalised collaborations between climate and health sectors, for instance through Memoranda of Understanding (MoUs) between different governmental departments or agencies, could help to overcome these barriers and pave the way for the development and implementation of EWS involving multiple governmental bodies (Stewart-Ibarra *et al.* 2022).

1.3 *Developing the tool*

Once the feasibility of an EWS has been investigated, considering the resources, evidence and data available to address the problem, the next step in the co-creation process is to develop the forecasting tool. This involves data processing, including the cleaning and harmonising of required data streams, as well as model building, and model validation, where the predictive ability of the forecasting model is assessed.

1.3.1 Data processing

The goal of data processing is to harmonise the spatiotemporal structure of all variables, so that they can be used as inputs for a forecasting tool. Usually, surveillance systems report the number of cases that occurred in an administrative unit per epidemiological week or month (for instance at the district or health centre level). Environmental and climate data products are typically provided in a grid format, which does not align with administrative-level summaries of epidemiological data. As such, it is necessary to process and summarise climate data used so it can be harmonised with the structure of the epidemiological data available. There are multiple ways of summarising spatial information into administrative units, including calculating an arithmetic mean or a population weighted mean. For example, Fletcher and colleagues took the mean value of gridded data per *cantón* when modelling malaria in Ecuador (Fletcher *et al.* 2020). The underlying assumption of working with averages is that there is a homogeneous distribution of the variable across the administrative unit, which becomes more of a limitation when working over larger or more diverse areas.

Temporal summaries require careful thought, as not all averages are equally informative. For example, it might be more appropriate to work with accumulated precipitation instead of average precipitation for a given disease outcome. Some studies have benefited from using climate indicators such as the Standardised Precipitation Index (SPI), which is used to characterise drought conditions over a range of timescales (Lowe *et al.* 2018).

1.3.1.1 *Bias correction and downscaling*

Global scale gridded climate products contain inherent biases which can result in systematic error when these products are downscaled to smaller administrative units, masking fine-scale ground conditions (Fletcher *et al.* 2021). In some cases, data from global scale climate products are consistently different from local observations, for instance, containing too many rainy days or temperatures that are consistently too high. There are a wide range of bias correction methods which are useful for overcoming these constraints. Bias correction methods generally use observed values to compute an adjustment factor. For example, the Delta change method, commonly used for climate change impact modelling, incorporates long term systematic deviances into historic observations. Additionally, the resolution of some products is coarser than that required by users, requiring downscaling to a finer resolution. Statistical downscaling is common practice and often occurs alongside bias correction. The monthly WorldClim products, for example, are a downscaled version of the CRU time series, simultaneously using the WorldClim v.2 product as reference for bias correction (Fick and Hijmans 2017).

1.3.2 Building the model

At the core of an EWS is a forecasting tool that is able to use information on the interaction between climate and disease to create predictions based on current or future climatic conditions (Morin *et al.* 2018). The goal of a forecasting tool is to provide warnings with sufficient lead time to deploy control strategies, to prevent or minimise occurrence of outbreaks. However, increased lead time of warnings often comes at the expense of increased uncertainty in model predictions. This trade-off will need to be evaluated during the co-creation of the tool, and time horizons can vary from short-term predictions, over days or weeks, to predictions for an entire season, to years or decades (Colón-González *et al.* 2021). Fundamentally, effective tools must include climate and epidemiological information, produce an output that can give warning of future disease risk, be well described and validated in a transparent manner, be clearly communicated to decision-makers to allow for public health action, and, ideally, be named and open source (Pollett *et al.* 2021; Ryan *et al.* 2023).

Forecasting tools include mechanistic, statistical, and machine learning approaches (Table 2 and 3). The choice of modelling approach will depend on the aim of the study, the type of data available and what is needed from the model output (Lee *et al.* 2021). Additionally, modern model building techniques often incorporate or blend together different aspects of statistical, mechanistic or machine learning approaches. In this section, we will give an overview to commonly used statistical and mechanistic modelling approaches. Machine learning approaches are detailed elsewhere (Bzdok *et al.* 2017).

Historically, the use of complex spatiotemporal Bayesian statistical models, and the fitting of mechanistic models to data has been limited because of the long computation times required for statistical inference of model parameters. However, techniques such as Markov Chain Monte Carlo (MCMC) and alternative computational methods have allowed for the more efficient estimation of a posterior distribution of model parameters. One example commonly used in Bayesian spatiotemporal statistical modelling is the use of integrated nested Laplace approximation (INLA) for posterior estimation, which can be easily implemented using the R-INLA package in the R programming language (Rue *et al.* 2009).

In recent years, researchers in the infectious disease modelling community have emphasised the importance of accurately incorporating uncertainty surrounding forecasts, in a similar way to the routine reporting of uncertainty associated with climate forecasts. As such, model forecasts are moving from deterministic point predictions (where predictions of incidence or outbreak risk have no associated uncertainty) to probabilistic forecasts, which include an associated probability distribution of the modelled outcome (Colón-González *et al.* 2021; Held *et al.* 2017).

TABLE 2 Common modelling approaches used to forecast outbreak risk for VBDs

Model class	Model description	Examples of model outputs	Advantages	Limitations	References
Statistical	Regression models, including:	Predictions of disease incidence	Widely used modelling approach, models are relatively easy to build and operate through standard statistical packages and software.	Often reliant on long time series for predictive power.	Colón-González *et al.* 2021; Lowe *et al.* 2021; Lowe *et al.* 2018; Chen *et al.* 2018; Shi *et al.* 2016
	Generalised Linear Model (GLM)	Probability of exceeding an outbreak threshold	Flexible approach that can be extended to account for important variation in the data due to unobserved processes.		

TABLE 2 Common modelling approaches used to forecast outbreak risk for VBDS (*cont.*)

Model class	Model description	Examples of model outputs	Advantages	Limitations	References
	Generalised Additive Model (GAM), also known as fixed-effects models, and their extensions GLMM and GAMM, also referred to as mixed-effects models or hierarchical models	Risk maps	Useful where causal relationships underlying disease transmission are not fully understood.		
Statistical	Autoregressive integrated moving average (ARIMA) model / seasonal autoregressive integrated moving average (SARIMA) model/ time series models	Predictions of disease incidence	Simple model framework with useful predictive ability. Can incorporate unmeasured confounders through autoregressive term.	Difficult to interpret the relationships between the outcome variable and other variables in the model and so will give limited insight into the causal pathways underlying transmission. May struggle to predict changes in trend if only based on past surveillance data. May also have poorer predictive ability at longer lead times if only dependent on surveillance data.	Eastin *et al.* 2014

TABLE 2 Common modelling approaches used to forecast outbreak risk for VBDs (*cont.*)

Model class	Model description	Examples of model outputs	Advantages	Limitations	References
Environmental threshold models		Reproduction number estimates Environmental suitability indices estimates (e.g. Index P) Mosquito population estimates Risk maps	Generate simple indices that can be easily understood by policy-makers and may be sufficient for decisions about when to implement vector-control.	Environmental suitability is necessary but not sufficient for transmission to occur and so these models only predict a proxy for the risk of transmission.	AeDES (Muñoz *et al.* 2020) MVSE (Obolski *et al.* 2019)
Mechanistic	Agent-based model or Individual-based model	Predictions of disease incidence Mosquito population estimates Impact of interventions	Able to incorporate individual-level stochasticity. Able to incorporate movement of people or vectors if this is known to be an important driver of disease.	Often too computationally complex to be fit to data; challenging to calibrate and to appropriately quantify uncertainty in predictions.	OpenMalaria (Smith *et al.* 2006) ANOSPEX (Oluwagbemi *et al.* 2013)
Mechanistic	Compartmental model Also referred to as: dynamical model; transmission dynamic model; SIR/SEIR model	Predictions of disease incidence			

TABLE 2 Common modelling approaches used to forecast outbreak risk for VBDs (*cont.*)

Model class	Model description	Examples of model outputs	Advantages	Limitations	References
		Predictions of epidemic years or exceeding an outbreak threshold	Can include multiple data streams within a single modelling framework	Quality of the results is dependent on the assumptions used to structure and parameterise the model.	Yamana *et al.* 2016
		Reproduction number estimates Estimated impact of interventions	Can model the impact of different interventions.	Can be computationally intensive to fit complex compartmental models to data.	
	Metapopulation model	As above	As above		
Semi-mechanistic		Predictions of disease incidence Reproduction number estimates	Can capture changes in transmission due to unobserved processes – useful in cases where a fully mechanistic model cannot be parameterised (e.g. in an outbreak of an emerging disease or when considering a pathogen whose transmission dynamics are not well characterised.	May be less successful in predicting points in epidemics where the transmission rate is changing. May be less informative for modelling the impact of interventions than a fully parameterised mechanistic model.	Epidemia (Scott *et al.* 2020)

TABLE 2 Common modelling approaches used to forecast outbreak risk for VBDs (*cont.*)

Model class	Model description	Examples of model outputs	Advantages	Limitations	References
Machine Learning	Including classification and regression algorithms, such as support vector machines (SVM), random forests	Predictions of disease incidence	Do not rely on assumptions about the transmission process or about the probability distribution underlying observed data.	Difficult to gain insight into the causal mechanisms underlying transmission and cannot be used to understand the potential impact of interventions.	Stolerman *et al.* 2019
		Predictions of epidemic years or exceeding an outbreak threshold		Typically reliant on more extensive datasets than statistical or mechanistic approaches.	

1.3.2.1 *Statistical models*

Statistical models are mathematical models able to make inferences from a sample regarding the entire population, under a set of assumptions about the probability distribution giving rise to the observed data (Cox 2006). These models are able to explore relationships between one or more variables when sufficient data are available and are useful for making predictions or inferences about an outcome of interest. Statistical regression models are flexible and relatively easy to build and operate, which is reflected in the frequency of their use in forecasting tools (Lee *et al.* 2021b; Morin *et al.* 2018; Ryan *et al.* 2023).

In their simplest form, regression models are able to quantify the associations between covariates and the risk of disease. In practice, it's often not possible to measure and access all the variables associated with a disease and it is necessary to use additional elements to account for excess variation in the outcome variable, such as random effects. Hierarchical or mixed-effect models can include terms to account for seasonality in the data or interannual variation, for instance due to changes in control interventions over time. Advanced spatially-explicit models can also take into account the underlying spatial structure of the data, using a range of assumptions about the dynamics between locations (Lee *et al.* 2021b).

Often there are many potential model formulations, particularly when considering multiple climatic variables at different lead times (for instance monthly rainfall with a 1:6-month lag), and model selection criteria can be used to determine the most appropriate candidate model. For example, information criteria such as Widely Applicable Bayesian Information Criterion (WAIC), Deviance Information Criterion (DIC) or Bayesian Information Criterion (BIC), aim to identify the most parsimonious model, balancing model simplicity with the need to minimise distance from the fitted and observed values (Schwarz 1978; Spiegelhalter *et al.* 2002; Watanabe 2013).

1.3.2.1.1 Statistical models for VBDs

The use of spatial and spatiotemporal models in infectious disease modelling has increased in the last decade as a result of higher computational capacity and the increased availability of gridded environmental and demographic datasets. Hierarchical generalised linear mixed models and Bayesian algorithms are often used when modelling risk of climate-sensitive VBDs because of their flexibility (Hussain-Alkhateeb *et al.* 2021). For example, temporal random effects can be used to recreate seasonality in the data and account for interannual variations (Figure 2, Lowe *et al.* 2018), whereas spatial random effects allow models to 'borrow strength' from neighbouring regions.

As an example of this kind of approach, Lowe and colleagues used a Bayesian temporal modelling framework to forecast outbreaks in Barbados. Their model used temporal monthly and yearly random effects to account for seasonality and interannual variation in the data (Figure 2) (Lowe *et al.* 2018). This work followed an earlier space-time modelling approach developed by Lowe and colleagues to

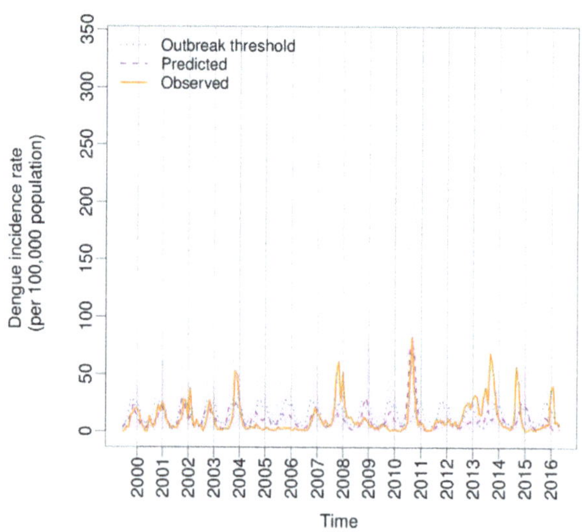

FIGURE 2
Predicted dengue incidence in Barbados between 2000 and 2016 with 95% credible intervals, compared to the observed incidence in the same period. Predictions were produced with a hierarchical mixed model using a Bayesian framework (Lowe *et al.* 2018)

forecast dengue risk in Brazil, which was later validated to consider its application in a prototype EWS (Lowe *et al.* 2016, 2014). Colón-Gonzalez and colleagues further extended this method by incorporating a superensemble approach to forecast dengue outbreaks in Vietnam, which was operationalised into an EWS called D-MOSS, see Case Study #3 below, (Colón-González *et al.* 2021).

1.3.2.1.2 Limitations of statistical models

The power of statistical models depends on the extent and quality of the data used to inform them. Large amounts of data are necessary for obtaining precise estimates, which makes them suitable for endemic diseases, although less useful for (re-) emerging diseases for which high-quality data is often lacking (Lee *et al.* 2021b; Stewart-Ibarra *et al.* 2022). Additionally, data quality is often a major constraint when developing statistical prediction models (Hussain-Alkhateeb *et al.* 2021). Furthermore, statistical models are only able to reliably make predictions within the scope of the used data, which narrows their ability to make out of sample predictions.

1.3.2.2 *Mechanistic models*

1.3.2.2.1 Mechanistic modelling approaches

Mechanistic modelling approaches, also referred to as dynamic modelling approaches, explicitly model disease states, and track changes in these disease states through time at either an individual or population level (Heesterbeek *et al.* 2015). One of the most common types of mechanistic model is the compartmental, or SIR model, which, in its simplest form, divides the population into compartments of 'Susceptible', 'Infected' and 'Recovered' individuals and tracks how individuals in the population move between compartments over time during an epidemic. At the other end of the spectrum are individual-based models, which track the disease state of individuals in a population, each of whom has particular associated demographic information and potentially an associated contact network. For VBDs, individual-based models can track humans in a particular setting, or model disease vectors. In addition to this, mechanistic models can be deterministic, where rerunning the model with the same initial parameters will always result in the same model outcome, or stochastic, where the role of chance in the processes driving transmission is considered and model outcomes over subsequent runs will vary (Heesterbeek *et al.* 2015). Overall, the appropriate level of model complexity, and the extent to which models incorporate stochasticity, will depend on the research question being considered.

Mechanistic models aim to capture the underlying processes driving infectious disease transmission and can incorporate information on population immunity, contact patterns, population mobility and control measures. As a result of this, mechanistic models offer the potential to improve forecasting of vector-borne disease incidence, particularly when considering diseases or settings where there are multiple important drivers of transmission (Lessler *et al.* 2016). The ability to consider multiple drivers of disease transmission within a single modelling framework also allows us to avoid incorrectly attributing variation in disease risk to a single variable, for instance a climatic variable, and instead gain understanding in how transmission is shaped by multiple important drivers working in combination.

Similarly, by explicitly modelling the underlying biological mechanisms driving transmission, mechanistic approaches can be used to provide policy makers with information on what may happen if certain public health actions are or aren't taken during the course of an outbreak. For instance, to inform how the imposition or timing of control measures or the introduction of a vaccination program might affect disease burden and transmission in a particular setting. Indeed, a recent report landscape mapping available tools for climate-sensitive infectious disease modelling found that the majority of identified tools used mechanistic or dynamical population modelling approaches, with varying structures, highlighting the wide applicability of mechanistic approaches in the modelling of climate-sensitive infectious diseases (Wellcome Trust 2022).

1.3.2.2.2 Mechanistic models for vector-borne diseases

Mechanistic models for vector-borne diseases can explicitly model human disease states, mosquito disease states, or both, with varying levels of complexity. For instance, several mechanistic models of dengue transmission use a simplified model structure based on direct host-to-host transmission (Andraud *et al.* 2012). Models describing human and vector disease states are often based on the Ross-Macdonald theory, originally developed to describe mosquito-borne pathogen transmission and model vector control strategies (Reiner *et al.* 2013). Additionally, for instances where the research question is focused on the spatial structure of transmission, metapopulation models can be used. These model infectious disease transmission between different 'patches' or populations based on assumptions of human or vector movement between populations.

1.3.2.2.3 Limitations of mechanistic models

Mechanistic models rely on assumptions about the transmission process of the VBD in question, and as such are less suitable for instances where the causal pathways underlying transmission are poorly characterised. Furthermore, complex mechanistic models, with many individuals or compartments, can be computationally costly to fit to data, posing challenges for model verification and validation and appropriate uncertainty quantification. Mechanistic models are not typically as widely used to forecast VBDs and in the 2015 Dengue Forecasting Challenge, mechanistic models were found to perform less well than statistical models which didn't incorporate information on the biological mechanisms underlying transmission (Johansson *et al.* 2019). However, mechanistic models have shown great utility in other epidemic scenarios and continuing research into the causal pathways underlying transmission will lead to the development of improved mechanistic models, which can also incorporate multiple data streams to improve their predictive ability.

1.3.2.3 *Semi-mechanistic and ensemble modelling*

1.3.2.3.1 Semi-mechanistic

While we have presented statistical and mechanistic methods as two separate modelling approaches, in reality many models will incorporate statistical and mechanistic elements. For instance, mechanistic approaches are reliant on statistical inference of model parameters. Moreover, semi-mechanistic approaches, which further blend mechanistic and statistical model frameworks, have been applied when forecasting infectious disease dynamics. For instance, Funk and colleagues used a semi-mechanistic framework to produce forecasts during the 2013–2016 West African Ebola epidemic where a compartmental mechanistic framework was combined with a time-varying stochastic rate of transmission between individuals (Funk *et al.* 2019). In this instance, a semi-mechanistic approach was able to provide more timely and accurate forecasts, as researchers were unable to parameterise a fully mechanistic model in real time during an evolving outbreak (Funk *et al.* 2019).

1.3.2.3.2 Ensembles

It has been argued that the dynamics of disease transmission are too complex to be entirely captured by one model. As an alternative, data-assimilation methods have been proposed as a tool for combining multiple model forecasts to produce more accurate predictions (Colón-González *et al.* 2021). Such techniques have been tested for forecasting outbreaks of dengue in Vietnam, which showed a meaningful improvement compared to the individual models (Colón-González *et al.* 2021). The Dengue Forecasting challenge, where different teams of researchers submitted dengue forecasts for San Juan, Puerto Rico and Iquitos, Peru during multiple dengue seasons, found that groups that used ensemble approaches had improved forecasting ability and calibration than other groups. Additionally, an average of all the forecasts submitted was found to routinely outperform other models for all the forecasting targets considered at each time point (Johansson *et al.* 2019). This makes intuitive sense, as different modelling approaches are associated with different assumptions and limitations, so an ensemble could in theory leverage the different strengths of each. Ensemble models are also able to better quantify uncertainty by considering where component models have high levels of disagreement compared with where models give very similar predictions. Particularly, ensembles including both mechanistic and statistical approaches may leverage the advantages of each, and allow for improved predictive ability.

However, it should be noted that model averages (for instance by weighting predictions from each model equally or with weighting based on previous performance) may not be the best option when the forecast target is concerned with the likelihood of an extreme event occurring. For instance, an outbreak of sufficient size that a health system is completely overwhelmed. Here, understanding the extremes of individual model predictions included in the ensemble may be more useful to inform public health planning, in a similar way to how ensemble modelling of extreme weather events is conducted by meteorological teams.

1.3.3 Model validation

1.3.3.1 *Out-of-sample testing*

Once a forecasting model has been developed, the most important test of the model's forecasting ability is its performance in predicting out-of-sample data, usually from the end of the time-series being considered. Out-of-sample testing data can be prospective data that had not yet been collected at the time of model development or data that has already been collected but is deliberately withheld from the model building phase in order to test the model. This train-test approach to model building, where one set of data is used to train the model and another is used to test its performance, is a common approach used to evaluate machine learning algorithms. This approach helps to assess if a model is underfitting – where the model does not learn enough from past data to predict future disease incidence – or overfitting – where the model fits too closely to noise in past data and is unable to generalise to unseen data and predict future disease incidence.

1.3.3.2 *Cross-validation*

In cases where, due to data constraints, it is not possible to leave a substantial testing data set out of the model building process, cross-validation techniques can be implemented. Cross-validation allows for a full use of the data, as each data point is used for both testing and training (Bergmeir and Benítez 2012). For instance, in a leave-one-out cross-validation approach, blocks of the dataset are left out at a time (for instance, a year of data or spatial unit) and the model's ability to predict each block is assessed (Lowe *et al.* 2016). One limitation of this approach is that it can cause difficulties with time-ordered data, as data from later years or months may be used to predict outcomes in earlier time points. Other methods such as Time-Series Cross Validation (TSCV) can also be used, where training sets only contain observations occurring prior to data in the training sets (Hyndman and Athanasopoulos 2021).

1.3.3.3 *Metrics for model evaluation*

Traditional metrics used to evaluate the epidemic model forecasts have focused on measuring goodness-of-fit, or how close model point predictions are to the true outcomes that occur. For instance, metrics such as the Mean Absolute Error (MAE) or Root Mean Squared Error (RMSE) which quantify the error of the model fit to data (Chowell 2017). However, a successful probabilistic forecast should also be able to correctly quantify uncertainty or confidence in predictions. In recent years, efforts have been made by researchers in the infectious disease modelling community to incorporate techniques already commonly used in weather and economic forecasting, to evaluate the success of model forecasts based on the entire probability distribution of forecasts, rather than specific point estimates. This allows forecasts to be evaluated based on both their ability to select between different possible outcomes and also to accurately quantify the uncertainty associated with their predictions (Held *et al.* 2017).

With this in mind, model evaluation should aim to assess the predictive performance of a model according to the paradigm of 'maximising the sharpness of the predictive distribution, subject to calibration' (Gneiting *et al.* 2007). Here calibration refers to the ability of a model to correctly quantify its own uncertainty in making predictions, while sharpness refers to how concentrated those predictions are within a narrow range (Funk *et al.* 2019).

Strictly proper scoring rules jointly assess calibration and sharpness and can be used as a metric of overall forecast skill (Gneiting and Raftery 2007). Commonly used metrics include the logarithm score, the continuous ranked probability score (CRPS) and the Brier score.

1.3.3.4 *Choice of reference model*

During model validation, the predictive ability of the candidate forecasting model should be compared to the current best-practice model available. In practice, this is often a seasonal model (i.e. where the cases in a given week or month are compared with cases at the same time in previous seasons), or a simple model to detect trends in surveillance data (i.e. whether cases are increasing or decreasing compared to previous weeks). In particular, comparisons should be made with any current early-warning models or signals used by the Ministry of Health and other partners to trigger response activities. The implementation of an EWS is a time-consuming and potentially costly endeavour and it is therefore essential that the relative benefit of a climate-informed EWS is well-established during the co-creation process.

1.4 *Implementation and monitoring*

Implementation of an EWS at the regional, national or global level relies on institutional arrangements for data sharing between relevant partners, as well as upon standard operating procedures to consistently track forecasting model outputs in time and space to identify warning signals of increased outbreak risk (Hussain-Alkhateeb *et al.* 2021). Currently, many promising EWS models are developed purely as academic research and are not operationalised within local climate and health sectors. As part of the co-creation process, consideration should be given from the outset as to how the EWS will be handed over from model developers to local public health authorities, and data scientists/managers and software engineers responsible for longer term maintenance, development and interpretation of the forecasting model.

EWS warning signals are meaningless unless they catalyse action. Risk communication creates meaning from information, prompting an appropriate public health response. Historically, most failures in EWS occurred due to miscommunication rather than any other failure in the system (UNDP 2018).

During the co-creation process, researchers should work in collaboration with key partners and stakeholders to understand how best to communicate model outputs to partners, relevant institutions and the general public. The construction of a user-friendly interface or application, using clear and accessible language or graphics, has been highlighted as a strategy to improve engagement with, and the impact of, a climate-informed EWS (Wellcome Trust 2022). Ultimately, the communication strategy (flow and frequency of warnings) and the technology used to disseminate warnings (SMS, social media, television news, radio broadcasts, local loudspeaker) will determine the reach and speed of the system (UNDP 2018). Commonly, a three staged progressive warning, which may be colour coded (green, amber, red), is used to communicate increasing risk. Typically, this might be 'be aware/watch/be alert'; followed by 'be prepared'; followed by 'take action'. Ideally, alert messages will combine the level certainty in the predictions with the potential impact of the outbreak using a decision-matrix, to allow for clear and actionable communication to public health decision-makers (Stewart-Ibarra *et al.* 2022).

Depending on the stage of the warning, different actions may be required by a variety of actors, ranging from government advisors, health managers, to the general public. Advanced planning and anticipation are key to putting in place effective public health responses (Semenza 2015; UNDP 2018). In cases where a climate-informed EWS gives a warning of increased VBD risk, public health actions that could be taken include; increased entomological or epidemiological surveillance, vector control activities, public awareness campaigns or preparations to increase hospital or treatment capacity (Semenza 2015). Importantly, EWS warnings of increased outbreak risk should have associated plans which recommend changes from the activities that would normally have taken place for a 'typical' VBD season (Lowe *et al.* 2016).

2 Case study 1. Dengue early warning systems in Singapore.

One example of a successfully operationalised climate-driven EWS can be found in the dengue EWS developed by the Singaporean National Environment Agency and collaborating universities (Shi *et al.* 2016). The EWS is based on a statistical forecasting model where multiple sub-models predict dengue cases 1:12 weeks ahead, with input variables chosen using a LASSO regression approach. Forecasting sub-models incorporate case data, population data, meteorological data including temperature variables (weekly mean temperature, maximum hourly temperature, number of hours of high temperature each week) and humidity variables (absolute and relative humidity), and vector surveillance data monitoring the prevalence of *Aedes aegypti* in Singapore. The model was assessed using out-of-sample testing and outperformed simpler model approaches based on the mean average percentage error. Crucially, although forecast accuracy was found to decrease with longer lead-times, Shi and colleagues found they were able to predict dengue outbreaks in 2013 and 2014 more than 10 weeks in advance, allowing the government to prepare hospital and diagnostic capacity, intensify vector control efforts and conduct a public communication campaign to mitigate the impact of the outbreak (Seltenrich 2016; Shi *et al.* 2016).

3 Case study 2. InfoDengue in Brazil.

InfoDengue in Brazil is a successful nowcasting system developed jointly by the Brazilian National Health Ministry, city-level health authorities and various research institutions (Codeco *et al.* 2018). The system integrates epidemiological, climate and social media data with a pipeline to clean, filter and integrate relevant datasets. The underlying modelling framework uses Bayesian methods to account for reporting delays and to estimate current dengue incidence and the effective reproductive number for dengue. Warnings are communicated using a colour-coded risk classification; green indicates poor conditions for transmission, yellow indicates favourable transmission conditions, orange indicates sustained transmission and red indicates high incidence. The strength of the InfoDengue system lies in streamlining the process of collecting and harmonizing local and national-level data and integrating relevant data streams to provide city-level warnings and situational awareness which can be acted upon by local health agencies responsible for disease prevention and mitigation efforts. Efforts are underway to expand the nowcasting system into an early-warning system able to give advance notice of dengue outbreaks by incorporating tailored seasonal and subseasonal forecasts. This will build on previous work by Lowe and colleagues developing a prototype dengue EWS to produce dengue forecasts ahead of the football World Cup in 2014, expanding this to provide seasonal and subseasonal forecasts to participating Brazilian cities (Lowe *et al.* 2014, 2016).

4 Case study 3. D-MOSS in Vietnam.

D-MOSS is a dengue EWS funded by the UK Space Agency and co-created by a collaboration of teams in the UK, Vietnam, and other countries. The underlying Bayesian spatiotemporal forecasting model uses Earth observations, seasonal climate forecasts provided by the UK Met Office, and lagged dengue cases in a superensemble of probabilistic dengue models which aim to predict dengue cases up to 6 months ahead (Colón-González *et al.* 2021; HR Wallingford 2022). Colón-González and colleagues demonstrated that the predictive ability of the superensemble outperformed a baseline model both when considering predictions of dengue incidence (evaluated using the continuous rank probability score, CRPS) and the outbreak detection capability of the model (evaluated using the Brier score) for Vietnamese provinces 1:6 months in advance (Colón-González *et al.* 2021). Model predictions are communicated to stakeholders through a user-friendly interface with graphs of anticipated dengue cases by month and province as well as maps of the distribution of dengue in neighbouring provinces. D-MOSS has been operational in Vietnam from 2019, Malaysia and Sri Lanka since 2020 and is in the process of being implemented in Cambodia, Laos, Thailand, and The Philippines. Stakeholders in Vietnam currently using the D-MOSS EWS have reported how D-MOSS is 'supporting to bridge the gap between early warning and early action' (HR Wallingford 2022). For instance, the National Institute of Hygiene and Epidemiology (NIHE) were able to use model predictions to anticipate a dengue outbreak in Nghe An province and implement enhanced disease response measures including environmental cleaning and spraying, as well as organising training on entomological surveillance and spraying methods for local public health officials.

4.1 *Evaluate the early warning systems*

4.1.1 Iteration and model tuning

Climate-informed EWS should be continually updated with appropriate corrections to reflect changes in VBD risk over space and time, as well as changes in technology and in user-experience. Evaluation of an EWS and iteration based on the lessons learnt is crucial for the continual improvement of the EWS. Evaluations of EWS which have been implemented in real-world settings, should include: (1) evaluation of the overall effectiveness of the system; (2) evaluation of the system components; and (3) an economic assessment of the cost-effectiveness and affordability of the system (Ebi and Schmier 2005). User experience has rarely been evaluated in EWS but, as highlighted at the beginning of this chapter, convening partners, and understanding how they will use the system is important for the institutionalisation of forecasting tools and the overall effectiveness of the system in preventing or reducing outbreaks (Hussain-Alkhateeb *et al.* 2021).

4.1.1.1 *Overall effectiveness of the system*

The first challenge is deciding which benchmark to evaluate the EWS against. Typically, the counterfactual (i.e. what has not happened) does not exist as an effective early warning with early action should have precluded the outbreak from occurring, or been able to reduce the epidemic peak. To overcome this, the reference standard is usually previous outbreaks with high reporting quality (Zhang *et al.* 2014).

There are two types of error that should be evaluated in an EWS – false alarms (predicting an outbreak that does not materialise) and missed events (failing to predict an outbreak). The consequences for which are very different. Trust in the system can be undermined if warning systems repeatedly call for early action when it is not needed. However, trust can equally be lost if the system fails to trigger a warning while substantial morbidity and mortality could occur in situations that could have been prevented. EWS should include checks and routines to minimise the risk of false alarms and improve the overall specificity of the system, without sacrificing the ability to detect events, or specificity (UNDP 2018). Finally, evaluations should consider the user-friendliness of the EWS for all stakeholders involved, the appropriateness of the EWS in terms of implementation, its coordination and coverage, efficiency (timeliness), impact, and sustainability (Hussain-Alkhateeb *et al.* 2021).

4.1.1.2 *System components*

Improvements may only be needed to certain components of the EWS, based on an identification of where a failure or inefficiency arose. EWS can and will fail for different reasons at different points (IFRC 2012). For example, delays in data availability, human error, misclassification, decision-makers not understanding and acting on the information (Hussain-Alkhateeb *et al.* 2021; IFRC 2012; Zhang *et al.* 2014). As previously mentioned, miscommunication has tended to contribute to the main failure in an EWS. This can be mitigated through the early engagement and co-learning between key stakeholders during the co-creation of an EWS. However, it may also be advisable to ensure redundancy exists in certain parts of the system to reduce the risk of EWS failure. For example, IFRC guidance suggests ensuring redundancy in two key areas by monitoring multiple indicators or outputs from a forecasting tool, and utilising multiple communication channels used to send warning messages (IFRC 2012).

4.1.1.3 *Cost-benefit*

Limited research exists on cost-benefit assessments of EWS for VBDs. Cost-benefit assessments for EWS of natural hazards, show that for every $1 spent on flood EWS and disaster risk reduction initiatives, $5 is saved in future losses (Mechler and Bouwer 2018). The ratio of benefits to costs for hurricane warnings is around 3:1, and 2,500:1 for heat waves in densely populated urban areas (e.g. Philadelphia) (Teisberg and Weiher 2009; UNDP 2018). Less is known about the cost-benefit of EWS for infectious diseases. The economic costs of false alarms (i.e. triggering a response for an outbreak which does not materialise) can be high, but difficult to quantify as it is not possible to be certain that actions may have helped prevent the outbreak. Cost-benefit analyses which assess the economic costs of false alarms vs missed events should be carried out to define the optimum alert trigger threshold (Colón-González *et al.* 2021; Lowe *et al.* 2016). These should be performed by the public health services based on health economic modelling so that EWS evaluations can be comparable to other health interventions (Ebi and Schmier 2005). Suggested cost-benefit assessments include: the cost per event (e.g. death, hospitalization) avoided (Ebi and Schmier 2005); the costs per reported event; the operating costs per surveillance unit per year (Ding *et al.* 2015). Furthermore, when establishing an EWS it is important to consider the total costs included in set-up (system development and training) and operating costs (data collection, quality control and signal verification) based on the available budget of the country (Ding *et al.* 2015).

5 Conclusions

Climate-informed EWS offer great potential for public-health decision-makers to prevent or mitigate the harms of outbreaks of VBDs and adapt to the harmful health impacts of climate change. With advances in the computational capacity needed to run complex forecasting models, as well as in the scientific knowledge of climate-health linkages, the time has come for a shift from academic EWS research to the implementation of climate-informed EWS at global, national, and local scales. The effects of climate change on the magnitude and frequency of VBD outbreaks are already clear in certain settings, and, as climate change continues to shift patterns of transmission, climate-informed EWS with good predictive ability and well characterised uncertainty surrounding their predictions will become increasingly crucial as a climate change adaptation measure. In this chapter we have given an overview of the stages involved in the co-creation of an EWS for vector-borne diseases, bringing together insight from epidemic forecasting and climate services for health communities of practice.

6 Recommendations

Recommendation	Description
Co-creation	Co-creation of EWS at all stages of development, and in particular engaging both climate and health sectors, is essential to ensure trust and shared ownership of the final tool, and that warnings generated are used by decision-makers and translated into meaningful action.
Uncertainty	The appropriate quantification and communication of uncertainty in predictions is essential, this should be considered during model design and validation, and consideration should be given as to how uncertainty in model predictions will be communicated (verbally and visually) to partners and decision-makers. This will allow decisions on appropriate response actions to be informed by both the impact of a potential outbreak and the level of certainty in the predictions, and also for expectations of the predictive ability of an EWS to be managed.
Operationalization	Currently, much work on climate-informed forecasting of infectious diseases occurs in a purely academic setting. EWS development should focus on the operationalization of tools from the outset, considering how a clear and user-friendly interface can be created for end-users of an EWS tool.
	A move from the development of EWS models in an academic context towards the operationalization of EWS will require funding streams dedicated to the development, translation and implementation of EWS tools in settings where they are most needed.
Evaluation	There is a need for improved evaluation methodology to assess the overall effectiveness and cost-effectiveness of EWS for VBDs. This will allow a greater understanding of what works in EWS to prevent or mitigate outbreaks of VBDs, and the levels of investment needed.

Acknowledgements

EF was funded by the Medical Research Council (grant number MR/N013638/1). RL was supported by a Royal Society Dorothy Hodgin Fellowship. SAL was supported by a Royal Society Research Grant for Research Fellows PhD studentship. MLB and RL were supported by the European Union's Horizon Europe programme (Grant Agreement: 101057554 IDAlert and 101086640 E4Warning). We would like to thank the LSHTM Planetary Health and Infectious Diseases lab and the BSC Global Health

Resilience group for their input and support, as well as Erin Coughlan de Perez and Adam Kucharski for providing valuable feedback on the initial conceptualizations and drafts of this book chapter.

References

Alcayna T, Fletcher I, Gibb R, Tremblay L, Funk S, Rao B and Lowe R (2022) Climate-sensitive disease outbreaks in the aftermath of extreme climatic events: A scoping review. One Earth 5: 336–350.

Andraud M, Hens N, Marais C and Beutels P (2012) Dynamic epidemiological models for dengue transmission: A systematic review of structural approaches. PLOS ONE 7: e49085.

Anyamba A, Chretien J-P, Britch SC, Soebiyanto RP, Small JL, Jepsen R, Forshey BM, Sanchez JL, Smith RD, Harris R, Tucker CJ, Karesh WB and Linthicum KJ (2019) Global disease outbreaks associated with the 2015–2016 El Niño event. Scientific Reports 9: 1930.

Bellone R and Failloux A-B (2020) The role of temperature in shaping mosquito-borne viruses transmission. Frontiers in Microbiology 11: 2388.

Benedum CM, Seidahmed OME, Eltahir EAB and Markuzon N (2018) Statistical modeling of the effect of rainfall flushing on dengue transmission in Singapore. PLOS Neglected Tropical Diseases 12: e0006935.

Bergmeir C and Benítez JM (2012) On the use of cross-validation for time series predictor evaluation. Information Sciences 191: 192–213.

Braks M, Giglio G, Tomassone L, Sprong H and Leslie TE (2019) Making vector-borne disease surveillance work: New opportunities from the SDG perspectives. Frontiers in Veterinary Science 6: 232.

Buchhorn M, Smets B, Bertels L, Roo BD, Lesiv M, Tsendbazar N-E, Herold M and Fritz S (2020) Copernicus global land service: Land cover 100m: Collection 3: Epoch 2019: Globe.

Bzdok D, Krzywinski M and Altman N (2017) Machine learning: A primer. Nature Methods 14: 1119–1120.

Ceccato P, Ramirez B, Manyangadze T, Gwakisa P and Thomson MC (2018) Data and tools to integrate climate and environmental information into public health. Infectious Diseases of Poverty 7: 126.

Chen Y, Ong JHY, Rajarethinam J, Yap G, Ng LC and Cook AR (2018) Neighbourhood level real-time forecasting of dengue cases in tropical urban Singapore. BMC Medicine 16: 129.

Chowell G (2017) Fitting dynamic models to epidemic outbreaks with quantified uncertainty: a primer for parameter uncertainty, identifiability, and forecasts. Infectious Disease Modelling 2: 379–398.

Chuang T-W, Chaves LF and Chen P-J (2017) Effects of local and regional climatic fluctuations on dengue outbreaks in southern Taiwan. PLOS ONE 12: e0178698.

Codeco C, Coelho F, Cruz O, Oliveira S, Castro T and Bastos L (2018) Infodengue: a nowcasting system for the surveillance of arboviruses in Brazil. Revue d'Épidémiologie et de Santé Publique 66: S386.

Colón-González FJ, Bastos LS, Hofmann B, Hopkin A, Harpham Q, Crocker T, Amato R, Ferrario I, Moschini F, James S, Malde S, Ainscoe E, Nam VS, Tan DQ, Khoa ND, Harrison M, Tsarouchi G, Lumbroso D, Brady OJ and Lowe R (2021) Probabilistic seasonal dengue forecasting in Vietnam: A modelling study using superensembles. PLOS Medicine 18: e1003542.

Cox DR (2006) Principles of statistical inference, Cambridge University Press, 7 pp.

Ding Y, Sauerborn R, Xu B, Shaofa N, Yan W, Diwan VK and Dong H (2015) A cost-effectiveness analysis of three components of a syndromic surveillance system for the early warning of epidemics in rural china. BMC Public Health 15: 1127.

Eastin MD, Delmelle E, Casas I, Wexler J and Self C (2014) Intra- and interseasonal autoregressive prediction of dengue outbreaks using local weather and regional climate for a tropical environment in Colombia. The American Journal of Tropical Medicine and Hygiene 91: 598–610.

Ebi KL and Schmier JK (2005) A stitch in time: improving public health early warning systems for extreme weather events. Epidemiologic Reviews 27: 115–121.

Fick SE and Hijmans RJ (2017) Worldclim 2: new 1-km spatial resolution climate surfaces for global land areas. International Journal of Climatology 37: 4302–4315.

Fletcher IK, Stewart-Ibarra AM, García-Díez M, Shumake-Guillemot J and Lowe R (2021) Climate services for health: From global observations to local interventions. Med 2: 355–361.

Fletcher IK, Stewart-Ibarra AM, Sippy R, Carrasco-Escobar G, Silva M, Beltran-Ayala E, Ordoñez T, Adrian J, Sáenz FE, Drakeley C, Jones KE and Lowe R (2020) The relative role of climate variation and control interventions on malaria elimination efforts in El Oro, Ecuador: A modeling study. Frontiers in Environmental Science 8.

Funk S, Camacho A, Kucharski AJ, Lowe R, Eggo RM and Edmunds WJ (2019) Assessing the performance of real-time epidemic forecasts: a case study of Ebola in the Western Area region of Sierra Leone, 2014–15. PLOS Computational Biology 15: e1006785.

Githeko A, Ototo E, Muange P, Zhou G, Yan G and Sang J (2018) The launch and operation of the malaria epidemic early warning system in Kenya. Science Publishing Group Journal 1 (2).

Gneiting T, Balabdaoui F and Raftery AE (2007) Probabilistic forecasts, calibration and sharpness. Journal of the Royal Statistical Society: Series B (Statistical Methodology) 69: 243–268.

Gneiting T and Raftery AE (2007) Strictly proper scoring rules, prediction, and estimation. Journal of the American Statistical Association 102: 359–378.

Grover-Kopec EK, Blumenthal MB, Ceccato P, Dinku T, Omumbo JA and Connor SJ (2006) Web-based climate information resources for malaria control in Africa. Malaria Journal 5: 38.

Heesterbeek H, Anderson RM, Andreasen V, Bansal S, Angelis DD, Dye C, Eames KTD, Edmunds WJ, Frost SDW, Funk S, Hollingsworth TD, House T, Isham V, Klepac P, Lessler J, Lloyd-Smith JO, Metcalf CJE, Mollison D, Pellis L, Pulliam JRC, Roberts MG, Viboud C and Collaboration INII (2015) Modeling infectious disease dynamics in the complex landscape of global health. Science 347(6227): aaa4339. https://doi.org/10.1126/science.aaa4339.

Held L, Meyer S and Bracher J (2017) Probabilistic forecasting in infectious disease epidemiology: The 13th armitage lecture. Statistics in Medicine 36: 3443–3460.

Hussain-Alkhateeb L, Ramírez TR, Kroeger A, Gozzer E and Runge-Ranzinger S (2021) Early warning systems (ewss) for chikungunya, dengue, malaria, yellow fever, and Zika outbreaks: what is the evidence? A scoping review. PLOS Neglected Tropical Diseases 15: e0009686.

Hyndman RJ and Athanasopoulos G (2021) Forecasting: Principles and practice (3rd edition), OTexts, 380 pp.

IFRC (2012) Community early warning systems: Guiding principles, IFRC.

Johansson MA, Apfeldorf KM, Dobson S, Devita J, Buczak AL, Baugher B, Moniz LJ, Bagley T, Babin SM, Guven E, Yamana TK, Shaman J, Moschou T, Lothian N, Lane A, Osborne G, Jiang G, Brooks LC, Farrow DC, Hyun S, Tibshirani RJ, Rosenfeld R, Lessler J, Reich NG, Cummings DAT, Lauer SA, Moore SM, Clapham HE, Lowe R, Bailey TC, García-Díez M, Carvalho MS, Rodó X, Sardar T, Paul R, Ray EL, Sakrejda K, Brown AC, Meng X, Osoba O, Vardavas R, Manheim D, Moore M, Rao DM, Porco TC, Ackley S, Liu F, Worden L, Convertino M, Liu Y, Reddy A, Ortiz E, Rivero J, Brito H, Juarrero A, Johnson LR, Gramacy RB, Cohen JM, Mordecai EA, Murdock CC, Rohr JR, Ryan SJ, Stewart-Ibarra AM, Weikel DP, Jutla A, Khan R, Poultney M, Colwell RR, Rivera-García B, Barker CM, Bell JE, Biggerstaff M, Swerdlow D, Mier-y-Teran-Romero L, Forshey BM, Trtanj J, Asher J, Clay M, Margolis HS, Hebbeler AM, George D and Chretien J-P (2019) An open challenge to advance probabilistic forecasting for dengue epidemics. Proceedings of the National Academy of Sciences 116: 24268–24274.

Koenraadt CJM and Harrington LC (2008) Flushing effect of rain on container-inhabiting mosquitoes *Aedes aegypti* and *Culex pipiens* (Diptera: Culicidae). Journal of Medical Entomology 45: 28–35.

Kovats RS, Bouma MJ, Hajat S, Worrall E and Haines A (2003) El Niño and health. The Lancet 362: 1481–1489.

Lee SA, Economou T, Barcellos C, Catão R, Carvalho MS and Lowe R (2021a) Effect of climate change, connectivity, and socioeconomic factors on the expansion of the dengue virus transmission zone in 21st century Brazil: An ecological modelling study. The Lancet Planetary Health 5: S14.

Lee SA, Jarvis CI, Edmunds WJ, Economou T and Lowe R (2021b) Spatial connectivity in mosquito-borne disease models: A systematic review of methods and assumptions. Journal of The Royal Society Interface 18: 20210096.

Lessler J, Azman AS, Grabowski MK, Salje H and Rodriguez-Barraquer I (2016) Trends in the mechanistic and dynamic modeling of infectious diseases. Current Epidemiology Reports 3: 212–222.

Liu X, Huang Y, Xu X, Li X, Li X, Ciais P, Lin P, Gong K, Ziegler AD, Chen A, Gong P, Chen J, Hu G, Chen Y, Wang S, Wu Q, Huang K, Estes L and Zeng Z (2020) High-spatiotemporal-resolution mapping of global urban change from 1985 to 2015. Nature Sustainability 3: 564–570.

Lowe R, Barcellos C, Coelho CAS, Bailey TC, Coelho GE, Graham R, Jupp T, Ramalho WM, Carvalho MS, Stephenson DB and Rodó X (2014) Dengue outlook for the world cup in Brazil: an early warning model framework driven by real-time seasonal climate forecasts. The Lancet Infectious Diseases 14: 619–626.

Lowe R, Coelho CA, Barcellos C, Carvalho MS, Catão RDC, Coelho GE, Ramalho WM, Bailey TC, Stephenson DB and Rodó X (2016) Evaluating probabilistic dengue risk forecasts from a prototype early warning system for Brazil. as 5: e11285.

Lowe R, Gasparrini A, Meerbeeck CJV, Lippi CA, Mahon R, Trotman AR, Rollock L, Hinds AQJ, Ryan SJ and Stewart-Ibarra AM (2018) Nonlinear and delayed impacts of climate on dengue risk in Barbados: A modelling study. PLOS Medicine 15: e1002613.

Lowe R, Lee S, Lana RM, Codeço CT, Castro MC and Pascual M (2020a) Emerging arboviruses in the urbanized Amazon rainforest. BMJ 371: m4385.

Lowe R, Lee SA, O'Reilly KM, Brady OJ, Bastos L, Carrasco-Escobar G, Catão RdC, Colón-González FJ, Barcellos C, Carvalho MS, Blangiardo M, Rue H and Gasparrini A (2021) Combined effects of hydrometeorological hazards and urbanisation on dengue risk in Brazil: a spatiotemporal modelling study. The Lancet Planetary Health 5: e209–e219.

Lowe R, Ryan SJ, Mahon R, Van Meerbeeck CJ, Trotman AR, Boodram L-LG, Borbor-Cordova MJ and Stewart-Ibarra AM (2020b) Building resilience to mosquito-borne diseases in the Caribbean. PLOS Biology 18: e3000791.

Lowe R, Stewart-Ibarra AM, Petrova D, García-Díez M, Borbor-Cordova MJ, Mejía R, Regato M and Rodó X (2017) Climate services for health: predicting the evolution of the 2016 dengue season in Machala, Ecuador. The Lancet Planetary Health 1: e142–e151.

Macdonald G (1957) The epidemiology and control of malaria, Oxford University Press, 280 pp.

Macherera M and Chimbari MJ (2016) A review of studies on community based early warning systems. Jàmbá: Journal of Disaster Risk Studies 8: 206.

McMichael AJ (2015) Extreme weather events and infectious disease outbreaks. Virulence 6: 543–547.

Mechler R and Bouwer L (2018) Climate loss and damage? Perspectives on the science and policy debate. 20th EGU General Assembly, EGU2018, Proceedings from the conference held 4–13 April, 2018 in Vienna, Austria: 9794.

Mordecai EA, Cohen JM, Evans MV, Gudapati P, Johnson LR, Lippi CA, Miazgowicz K, Murdock CC, Rohr JR, Ryan SJ, Savage V, Shocket MS, Ibarra AS, Thomas MB and Weikel DP (2017) Detecting the impact of temperature on transmission of Zika, dengue, and chikungunya using mechanistic models. PLOS Neglected Tropical Diseases 11: e0005568.

Morin CW, Semenza JC, Trtanj JM, Glass GE, Boyer C and Ebi KL (2018) Unexplored opportunities: Use of climate- and weather-driven early warning systems to reduce the burden of infectious diseases. Current environmental health reports 5: 430–438.

Muñoz ÁG, Chourio X, Rivière-Cinnamond A, Diuk-Wasser MA, Kache PA, Mordecai EA, Harrington L and Thomson MC (2020) AeDES: A next-generation monitoring and forecasting system for environmental suitability of *Aedes*-borne disease transmission. Scientific Reports 10: 12640.

Muñoz-Sabater J, Dutra E, Agustí-Panareda A, Albergel C, Arduini G, Balsamo G, Boussetta S, Choulga M, Harrigan S, Hersbach H, Martens B, Miralles DG, Piles M, Rodríguez-Fernández NJ, Zsoter E, Buontempo C and Thépaut J-N (2021) Era5-land: A state-of-the-art global reanalysis dataset for land applications. Earth System Science Data 13: 4349–4383.

Myers MF, Rogers DJ, Cox J, Flahault A and Hay SI (2000) Forecasting disease risk for increased epidemic preparedness in public health. Advances in Parasitology 47: 309–330.

Obolski U, Perez PN, Villabona-Arenas CJ, Thézé J, Faria NR and Lourenço J (2019) MVSE: An R-package that estimates a climate-driven mosquito-borne viral suitability index. Methods in Ecology and Evolution 10: 1357–1370.

Oluwagbemi OO, Fornadel CM, Adebiyi EF, Norris DE and Rasgon JL (2013) ANOSPEX: A stochastic, spatially explicit model for studying anopheles metapopulation dynamics. PLOS ONE 8: e68040.

Patz JA and Olson SH (2006) Malaria risk and temperature: Influences from global climate change and local land use practices. Proceedings of the National Academy of Sciences 103: 5635–5636.

Petrone ME, Earnest R, Lourenço J, Kraemer MUG, Paulino-Ramirez R, Grubaugh ND and Tapia L (2021) Asynchronicity of endemic and emerging mosquito-borne disease outbreaks in the Dominican Republic. Nature Communications 12: 151.

Pley C, Evans M, Lowe R, Montgomery H and Yacoub S (2021) Digital and technological innovation in vector-borne disease surveillance to predict, detect, and control climate-driven outbreaks. The Lancet Planetary Health 5: e739–e745.

Pollett S, Johansson MA, Reich NG, Brett-Major D, Valle SYD, Venkatramanan S, Lowe R, Porco T, Berry IM, Deshpande A, Kraemer MUG, Blazes DL, Pan-ngum W, Vespigiani A, Mate SE, Silal SP, Kandula S, Sippy R, Quandelacy TM, Morgan JJ, Ball J, Morton LC, Althouse BM, Pavlin J, Panhuis Wv, Riley S, Biggerstaff M, Viboud C, Brady O and Rivers C (2021) Recommended reporting items for epidemic forecasting and prediction research: The EPIFORGE 2020 guidelines. PLOS Medicine 18: e1003793.

Puntasecca CJ, King CH and LaBeaud AD (2021) Measuring the global burden of chikungunya and Zika viruses: A systematic review. PLOS Neglected Tropical Diseases 15: e0009055.

Rajarethinam J, Ang L-W, Ong J, Ycasas J, Hapuarachchi HC, Yap G, Chong C-S, Lai Y-L, Cutter J, Ho D, Lee V and Ng L-C (2018) Dengue in Singapore from 2004 to 2016: Cyclical epidemic patterns dominated by serotypes 1 and 2. The American Journal of Tropical Medicine and Hygiene 99: 204–210.

Reiner RC, Perkins TA, Barker CM, Niu T, Chaves LF, Ellis AM, George DB, Le Menach A, Pulliam JRC, Bisanzio D, Buckee C, Chiyaka C, Cummings DAT, Garcia AJ, Gatton ML, Gething PW, Hartley DM, Johnston G, Klein EY, Michael E, Lindsay SW, Lloyd AL, Pigott DM, Reisen WK, Ruktanonchai N, Singh BK, Tatem AJ, Kitron U, Hay SI, Scott TW and Smith DL (2013) A systematic review of mathematical models of mosquito-borne pathogen transmission: 1970–2010. Journal of the Royal Society Interface 10: 20120921.

Reinhold JM, Lazzari CR and Lahondère C (2018) Effects of the environmental temperature on *Aedes aegypti* and *Aedes albopictus* mosquitoes: A review. Insects 9: 158.

Romanello M, McGushin A, Napoli CD, Drummond P, Hughes N, Jamart L, Kennard H, Lampard P, Rodriguez BS, Arnell N, Ayeb-Karlsson S, Belesova K, Cai W, Campbell-Lendrum D, Capstick S, Chambers J, Chu L, Ciampi L, Dalin C, Dasandi N, Dasgupta S, Davies M, Dominguez-Salas P, Dubrow R, Ebi KL, Eckelman M, Ekins P, Escobar LE, Georgeson L, Grace D, Graham H, Gunther SH, Hartinger S, He K, Heaviside C, Hess J, Hsu S-C, Jankin S, Jimenez MP, Kelman I, Kiesewetter G, Kinney PL, Kjellstrom T, Kniveton D, Lee JKW, Lemke B, Liu Y, Liu Z, Lott M, Lowe R, Martinez-Urtaza J, Maslin M, McAllister L, McMichael C, Mi Z, Milner J, Minor K, Mohajeri N, Moradi-Lakeh M, Morrissey K, Munzert S, Murray KA, Neville T, Nilsson M, Obradovich N, Sewe MO, Oreszczyn T, Otto M, Owfi F, Pearman O, Pencheon D, Rabbaniha M, Robinson E, Rocklöv J, Salas RN, Semenza JC, Sherman J, Shi L, Springmann M, Tabatabaei M, Taylor J, Trinanes J, Shumake-Guillemot J, Vu B, Wagner F, Wilkinson P, Winning M, Yglesias M, Zhang S, Gong P, Montgomery H, Costello A and Hamilton I (2021) The 2021 report of the lancet countdown on health and climate change: Code red for a healthy future. The Lancet 398: 1619–1662.

Rue H, Martino S and Chopin N (2009) Approximate Bayesian inference for latent Gaussian models by using integrated nested Laplace approximations. Journal of the Royal Statistical Society: Series B (Statistical Methodology) 71: 319–392.

Runge-Ranzinger S, Kroeger A, Olliaro P, McCall PJ, Sánchez Tejeda G, Lloyd LS, Hakim L, Bowman LR, Horstick O and Coelho G (2016) Dengue contingency planning: From research to policy and practice. PLOS Neglected Tropical Diseases 10: e0004916.

Ryan SJ, Carlson CJ, Mordecai EA and Johnson LR (2019) Global expansion and redistribution of *Aedes*-borne virus transmission risk with climate change. PLOS Neglected Tropical Diseases 13: e0007213.

Ryan SJ, Lippi CA, Caplan T, Diaz A, Dunbar W, Grover S, Johnson S, Knowles R, Lowe R, Mateen B, Thomson M, Stewart-Ibarra AM. (2022). The current landscape of software tools for the climate-sensitive infectious disease modelling community. *The Lancet Planetary Health* 7: e527–36 (https://doi.org/10.1016/S2542-5196(23)00056-6.

Sarma N, Patouillard E, Cibulskis RE and Arcand J-L (2019) The economic burden of malaria: Revisiting the evidence. The American Journal of Tropical Medicine and Hygiene 101: 1405–1415.

Schwarz G (1978) Estimating the dimension of a model. The Annals of Statistics 6: 461–464.

Scott JA, Gandy A, Mishra S, Unwin J, Flaxman S and Bhatt S (2020) Epidemia: Modeling of epidemics using hierarchical Bayesian models. R package version 1.0.0. 2020.

Seltenrich N (2016) Singapore success: New model helps forecast dengue outbreaks. Environmental Health Perspectives 124: A167.

Semenza JC (2015) Prototype early warning systems for vector-borne diseases in europe. International Journal of Environmental Research and Public Health 12: 6333–6351.

Shepard DS, Undurraga EA, Halasa YA and Stanaway JD (2016) The global economic burden of dengue: A systematic analysis. The Lancet Infectious Diseases 16: 935–941.

Shi Y, Liu X, Kok S-Y, Rajarethinam J, Liang S, Yap G, Chong C-S, Lee K-S, Tan SSY, Chin CKY, Lo A, Kong W, Ng LC and Cook AR (2016) Three-month real-time dengue forecast models:

An early warning system for outbreak alerts and policy decision support in Singapore. Environmental Health Perspectives 124: 1369–1375.

Smith T, Killeen GF, Maire N, Ross A, Molineaux L, Tediosi F, Hutton G, Utzinger J, Dietz K and Tanner M (2006) Mathematical modeling of the impact of malaria vaccines on the clinical epidemiology and natural history of *Plasmodium falciparum* malaria: overview. The American Journal of Tropical Medicine and Hygiene 75: 1–10.

Spiegelhalter DJ, Best NG, Carlin BP and Van Der Linde A (2002) Bayesian measures of model complexity and fit. Journal of the Royal Statistical Society: Series B (Statistical Methodology) 64: 583–639.

Stewart-Ibarra AM, Rollock L, Best S, Brown T, Diaz AR, Dunbar W, Lippi CA, Mahon R, Ryan SJ, Trotman A, Van Meerbeeck CJ and Lowe R (2022) Co-learning during the co-creation of a dengue early warning system for the health sector in Barbados. BMJ global health 7: e007842.

Stewart-Ibarra AM, Romero M, Hinds AQJ, Lowe R, Mahon R, Van Meerbeeck CJ, Rollock L, Gittens-St. Hilaire M, St. Ville S, Ryan SJ, Trotman AR and Borbor-Cordova MJ (2019) Co-developing climate services for public health: Stakeholder needs and perceptions for the prevention and control of *Aedes*-transmitted diseases in the Caribbean. PLOS Neglected Tropical Diseases 13: e0007772.

Stolerman LM, Maia PD and Kutz JN (2019) Forecasting dengue fever in Brazil: An assessment of climate conditions. PLOS ONE 14: e0220106.

Teisberg T, J and Weiher R, F (2009) Background paper on the benefits and costs of early warning systems for major natural hazards. Submitted to the world bank group, global facility for disaster reduction and recovery (gfdrr).

U.S. Geological Survey (2022) Landsat missions. Available at.

UNDP (2018) Five approaches to build functional early warning systems.

Wallingford H (2022) D-MOSS: Dengue forecasting model satellite-based system. Available at.

Watanabe S (2013) A widely applicable bayesian information criterion. Journal of Machine Learning Research 14: 867–897.

World Health Organization (2005) Using climate to predict infectious disease epidemics, Geneva.

World Health Organization (2021a) Quality criteria for the evaluation of climate-informed early warning systems for infectious diseases.

World Health Organization (2021b) World malaria report.

World Meteorological Organization (2015) What do we mean by climate services? Available at.

WorldPop (2022) Open spatial demographic data and research. Available at: https://www.worldpop.org/.

Yamana TK, Kandula S and Shaman J (2016) Superensemble forecasts of dengue outbreaks. Journal of The Royal Society Interface 13: 20160410.

Zhang H, Li Z, Lai S, Clements ACA, Wang L, Yin W, Zhou H, Yu H, Hu W and Yang W (2014) Evaluation of the performance of a dengue outbreak detection tool for China. PLOS ONE 9: e106144.

CHAPTER 13

Impacts of climate change on malaria vector control in Africa

Heather M. Ferguson[1,2*] *and Nicodem J. Govella*[1,2]

[1]School of Biodiversity, One Health and Veterinary Medicine, University of Glasgow, Graham Kerr Building Glasgow G12 8QQ, United Kingdom; [2]Environmental Health, and Ecological Sciences Department, Ifakara Health Institute, Kiko Avenue, P.O. Box 78373, Mikocheni, Dar es Salaam, United Republic of Tanzania, *heather.ferguson@glasgow.ac.uk

Abstract

There has been extensive consideration of how climate change may impact the distribution of vector-borne diseases; with a particular focus on malaria risk in Africa. Such analyses primarily consider how the 'malaria map' will shift in response to changes in the environmental determinants of transmission, but rarely consider the equally if not more important question of whether climate change will impact the effectiveness of vector control measures. Here we hypothesize that the efficacy and ability to implement core vector control interventions for malaria could be significantly impacted by climate change due to direct and indirect impacts on mosquito vectors and interventions. We review current knowledge on the environmental dependency of current core interventions for malaria vector control including Insecticide Treated Nets, Indoor Residual Spraying and larviciding. We explore how anticipated changes in temperature, rainfall and humidity could impact vector ecology, behaviour and resistance mechanisms; and the knock on effects of these changes for intervention efficacy. Finally we review potential indirect impacts of climate change on the ability to finance, implement and sustain vector control; with a focus on changes in human behaviour, land use, socioeconomic conditions and health systems. We conclude by highlighting the need to build 'climate-proof' strategies into future vector control planning.

Keywords

Anopheles – climate change – mosquito behaviour – malaria interventions – insecticide treated nets – indoor residual spraying – temperature

 | DOI:10.3920/9789004688650_015

1 Introduction

Climate change and infectious disease present some of the greatest challenges of our age. Their devastating impacts are increasingly clear (McMichael 2013), and have potential to impact every aspect of life including ecosystem function, human and veterinary health, food security, economic and political stability. While the independent impacts of climate change and infectious disease are sizeable; the greatest threats may arise from their interaction whereby the occurrence of one directly impedes ability to address the other.

We hypothesize this scenario is highly likely to arise in the context of mosquito vector-borne diseases (VBDs). VBDs such as malaria are a leading source of mortality and morbidity within Low and Middle Income Countries. Amongst the VBDs, malaria has the largest mortality burden; causing 627,000 deaths in 2021 alone (WHO 2021). This burden is disproportionately concentrated in sub-Saharan Africa where more than 96% of malaria-related deaths occur; mostly in young children under 5 years old (WHO 2021). While the upscaling of vector control interventions including Insecticide Treated Nets (ITNs) and Indoor Residual Spraying (IRS) have significantly contributed to the halving of malaria prevalence in Africa since the year 2000 (Bhatt *et al.* 2015), this disease still poses an unacceptable public health burden. Of particular concern, progress towards elimination has stagnated in recent years; with malaria prevalence and mortality staying level or even increasing in some African countries since 2015 (Noor and Alonso 2022). The causes for this slow down are complex, but likely principally driven by a combination of biological challenges such as insecticide resistance and outdoor biting in malaria vectors, and reduced investment, economic constraints, and disruption due to COVID (WHO 2018, Lindsay *et al.* 2021, Weiss *et al.* 2021, Sherrard-Smith *et al.* 2019).

Numerous studies have demonstrated that malaria transmission is highly sensitive to climate (e.g. (Kelly-Hope and Thomson 2005, Mabaso *et al.* 2007, Caminade *et al.* 2014, Reiner *et al.* 2015, Fall *et al.* 2022)). This dependency arises because the survival, reproduction and behaviour of the major African malaria vectors (*Anopheles arabiensis, An.coluzzii, An. gambiae* and *An. funestus*) are highly sensitive to environmental conditions such temperature, humidity and rainfall (Afrane *et al.* 2012, Charlwood 2019; Parham *et al.* 2012). Also, malaria parasite development within vectors is temperature dependent (Paaijmans and Thomas 2013). Notably, temperature influences almost all mosquito life-history (Christiansen-Jucht *et al.* 2015, Agyekum *et al.* 2021) and demographic processes (Parham *et al.* 2012). The sporogonic success (development of infectious stages) of malaria parasites within vectors is also temperature dependent; with the length of the extrinsic incubation period decreasing with temperature up to a maximum threshold beyond which sporogony fails (Beier 1998; Murdock *et al.* 2016). The environmental dependencies of these key mosquito vector and parasite processes make malaria transmission highly likely to change with climate.

While the potential impacts of climate change on malaria have received much attention (Martens *et al.* 1999, Tanser *et al.* 2003, Thomas 2004, Gething *et al.* 2010, Ermert *et al.* 2013, Yamana and Eltahir 2013, Caminade *et al.* 2014, Diouf *et al.* 2021), there is another crucial question that has been largely overlooked: how effective will malaria vector control and elimination strategies be under modified climates? Here we hypothesize that the efficacy and ability to implement core vector control interventions for malaria could be significantly reduced by climate change due to direct and indirect impacts on mosquito vectors and interventions. If confirmed, such climate-mediated impacts could slow or even reverse progress towards malaria elimination even as the geographical area suitable for transmission in Africa may fall. To explore the potential for such a scenario, we first briefly review knowledge on how climate is expected to change in Africa, and its potential impact on transmission.

1.1 *Future climate change predictions for Africa*

While the effects of climate change will be global, it is hypothesized that sub-Saharan Africa is particularly vulnerable to severe and catastrophic impacts due to extreme reliance on small-scale rain-fed agriculture, socio-economic constraints and other factors (Connolly-Boutin and Smit 2016). Many studies have attempted to characterize and forecast the types of climate change anticipated in different regions of Africa; with predictions often varying between regions. Such predictions are generally derived from fitting a range of different Global Circulation Models (GCMs) to a series of Representative Concentration Pathways (RCPs) as proposed by the Intergovernmental Panel on Climate Change to reflect plausible future greenhouse gas emission scenarios (IPCC 2020). Key outputs of such forecasts are expected temperatures and precipitation patterns.

It is expected that temperatures in southern Africa may rise faster than the global average; generating a much higher frequency of heatwaves and droughts (Chersich *et al.* 2018). For example, a model developed for the Eerste River in South Africa predicted that climate change in the 'near' (2022–57) and 'far' (2058–2093) future will increase evaporation and decrease rainfall by 2% and 8% respectively, leading to a reduction in water availability between 8–18% (Du Plessis and Kalima 2021). Similar modelling of the hydrology of the Kabombo sub-basin within the Zambezi Basin indicates that stream flow will become much more variable; and decrease by up to 3% even under intermediate scenarios (RCP 4.5) (Ndhlovu and Woyessa 2021). Thus the overall assessment for southern Africa is much warmer and drier conditions.

Predicted impacts of climate change are more variable across the East African region. Specifically, predictions of the magnitude and direction of climate impacts vary somewhat between different GCM and RCP scenarios. Many East African countries are already classified as 'water stressed', and are expected to become increasingly so as climate changes. For example, per capita water availability is expected to fall below scarcity levels in Ethiopia, Kenya, Malawi, Mozambique, Rwanda,

Uganda, Tanzania and Zambia by the end of the century (Adhikari *et al.* 2015). This is based on predictions of temperature rises between 0.9–3.4 °C by the 2060s, and 1.3–5.5 °C by 2090s (Adhikari *et al.* 2015). However, there is some discrepancy between predictions depending on the modelling approach, focal area and scale applied. One study of future rainfall over the Lake Victoria region of East Africa predicted no significant change in mean monthly rainfall by the 2040s, and only a slight increase by 2075 (Akurut *et al.* 2014). While changes to precipitation across East Africa may be locally variable, there is consensus that temperatures will rise.

Analysis of time series data from the in Sahel region of west Africa indicate there has already been a substantial long-term decline in rainfall and increasing temperature between 1970–2000 (Ben Mohamed 2011). The ability to predict future climate is uncertain given some existing models do not fit well to historical data (Ben Mohamed 2011). However mean temperatures are expected to rise by at least 1–1.5 °C in the medium term (Amoussou, Awoye *et al.* 2020, Diedhiou, Bichet *et al.* 2018), and potentially considerably more in some areas (Chou *et al.* 2020). Predictions about rainfall are more variable, but there is an expectation of substantial alterations in frequency, seasonal duration and intensity of precipitation. For example, daily extremes in rainfall are expected to rise in the Mono Basin in Togo (Amoussou *et al.* 2020). More heatwaves of longer duration are predicted throughout the region, but with an intensification of rainfall in some areas and considerable drying and increase in drought conditions in others (Diedhiou *et al.* 2018). General trends and differences are evident between the four agro-ecological zones in Sahel region (UNHCR 2022). Higher temperature increases are projected for arid and semi-arid zones in the North compared to subhumid and tropical zones. However the subhumid and semi-arid zones will experience the largest increase in the proportion of 'very hot days' (e.g. temperature >35 °C, UNHCR 2022). Finally while the number of heavy precipitation days will decline in the northwest, pronounced increases are expected in the eastern Sahel (e.g. Northern Chad, Niger, Nigeria and Cameroon). Although predictions for specific regions are variable, substantial changes to climate are expected across the continent as whole; characterized by rising temperature, substantial shifts in rainfall and a higher frequency of extreme weather events.

1.2 *Predicted impacts of climate change on malaria in Africa*

The potential impacts of climate change on malaria in Africa have been investigated for more than 20 years (Martens *et al.* 1999, Tanser *et al.* 2003). Early work focussed on the use of biological models to estimate the geographical area suitable for malaria transmission based primarily on temperature requirements of mosquitoes and parasites (Martens *et al.* 1999). Such models predicted that climate change would lead to substantial increases in malaria distribution and people at risk. For example, one model estimated that approximately 300 and 150 million more people would be a risk of *P. falciparum* and *P. vivax* respectively by 2080 due to climate change (Martens *et al.* 1999). However, these models were subsequently questioned due to their failure or incomplete incorporation of other key environmental drivers of transmission (e.g. rainfall). Later work using more complex spatiotemporal models predicted less dramatic changes to the African malaria map; with little change predicted in the latitudinal range, but altitudinal increases (Tanser *et al.* 2003). This and other work indicated a more complex pattern of epidemiological impacts; including predictions of significant reductions in transmission in some parts of sub-Saharan Africa (Thomas 2004, Thomas *et al.* 2004, Lafferty 2009, Gething *et al.* 2010, Ermert *et al.* 2013). The need to incorporate more detailed consideration of related changes in land use, urbanization and socioeconomic factors has also been highlighted (Gething *et al.* 2010, Yamana and Eltahir 2013, Caminade *et al.* 2014).

Recent models have attempted to incorporate greater complexity and detail on the specific nature of metereological changes. Early models based on simplified assumptions and generalization of rainfall effects have been replaced by more sophisticated approaches based on explicit consideration of hydrology (e.g. water flow, concentration and evaporation across landscapes), land use change, and with predictions made at a finer scale. Such models have reinforced the prediction that increasingly warmer and drier conditions will reduce the length of the malaria transmission season in West Africa, but will increase the risk of highland malaria in East Africa (Alonso *et al.* 2011, Ermert *et al.* 2013, Caminade *et al.* 2014, Leedale *et al.* 2016, Yamana *et al.* 2016, Diouf *et al.* 2021). As an an example, one study in the Western Ugandan Highlands found that that extreme flooding was associated with a 30% increase in the risk of a person having a positive malaria test (Boyce *et al.* 2016); highlighting the additional risk expected in areas where climate change is expected to increase these events.

In combination, this body of work indicates that the geographical area in which malaria transmission can occur in Africa is unlikely to significantly expand due to climate change; with substantial contractions possible in some areas. However, most models so far have primarily focussed on the direct biological impacts of climate change on parasites and vectors, and not the wider impacts on control activities and health systems. Consideration of these factors may give a very different perspective on how the public health impact of malaria will respond to climate change. As highlighted by (Mordecai *et al.* 2020), the primary public health impact of climate change on VBDs may arise not through expansions of the 'malaria map', but increased exposure within stable areas of transmission. One economic analysis suggested the cost of in patient treatment for malaria as a proportion of annual health expenditures per 1,000 people could rise by up to 20% within some African countries (Egbendewe-Mondzozo *et al.* 2011). Whether detrimental impacts of this magnitude or greater will arise will ultimately depend on if and how climate change will impact the efficacy and ability to implement surveillance, control and treatment.

2 Impacts of climate change on vector ecology and transmission ability

2.1 *Importance of temperature to vector fitness and transmission potential*

Climate change is expected to alter the distribution, abundance and species composition of African malaria vectors because their reproduction, survival, behaviour and pathogen transmission capacity are highly sensitive to environmental conditions. Notably, temperature influences almost all mosquito life-history (Christiansen-Jucht *et al.* 2015, Agyekum *et al.* 2021) and demographic processes (Parham *et al.* 2012). Temperature effects are often curvilinear – with a fitness trait or demographic rate increasing with temperature up to maximum followed by a rapid decline (Agyekum *et al.* 2021). For example, the speed of larval development in the laboratory accelerates with temperature; with development period of *An. gambiae sl.* being ~10 days shorter at 36 °C compared to 25 °C. However, development is significantly impaired at higher temperatures, with no larvae surviving at ≥38 °C (Bayoh and Lindsay 2003, Bayoh and Lindsay 2004, Agyekum *et al.* 2022). At the adult stage, survival, fecundity and the length of the gonotrophic are reduced at high temperatures (Agyekum *et al.* 2021). Climate change is expected to increase not only mean temperatures across Africa, but also variability in daily temperatures. Increased temperature variability is difficult for ectotherms to cope with (Paaijmans *et al.* 2013); and may further impair population viability under climate change.

Rising temperatures may also affect the susceptibility and competence of vectors to malaria infection. The sporogonic success of malaria parasites is temperature dependent; with the length of the extrinsic incubation period (EIP) decreasing with temperature up to a maximum threshold beyond which sporogony fails (Ohm *et al.* 2018). For example, models fit to laboratory data indicate that the EIP of *P. falciparum* in *An. stephensi* falls from 16.1 to 8.8 days as temperature rises from 21 to 34 °C (Stopard *et al.* 2021); with no sporogonic development above 35 °C (Shapiro *et al.* 2017). Experimental studies indicate that temperature rises as expected under climate change will decrease the vectorial capacity of *An. gambiae* by reducing parasite sporogonic success. Laboratory experiments on *An. gambiae* and *An. stephensi* indicated that their vectorial capacity could be reduced by 51–89% with increases in mean temperature from 27 to 30 °C (Murdock *et al.* 2016). Furthermore, experimental studies show that *Anopheles* immune responses that might impair parasite development are also temperature dependent (Murdock *et al.* 2013, 2014). Taken together with projected impacts on mosquito demography, this suggests that temperature increases as expected under climate change will have complex and diverse impacts on malaria vector ecology and transmission potential.

While temperature rises will certainly influence malaria transmission, the specific nature of these impacts will vary between settings depending on whether they move local conditions either into or above the optimal threshold for mosquitoes and/or parasite development. Additionally, the effect of temperature may be offset or mitigated by concurrent changes in rainfall. As reviewed above, climate change may lead to much heavier rainfall and flooding in some areas of Africa, and considerable drying and drought conditions in others. Such changes could, for example, boost mosquito populations even in areas where temperature ranges were approaching the upper threshold for their survival. Additionally, the moving of climatic conditions into the optimal temperature range for sporogony may have little impact on transmission if this is accompanied by substantial drying and reduction of habitats for mosquito oviposition. In summary, while temperature will certainly play a crucial role in determining how malaria transmission will be altered by climate change; it's impacts must be evaluated within the wider context of concurrent conditions.

2.2 *Impact of climate change on malaria vector species composition*

Whilst all African malaria vectors will be exposed to climate change, impacts will likely vary between species due to differences in their innate habitat preferences and physiological tolerances. In addition to the four primary native African vector species (*An. arabiensis, An. coluzzii, An gambiae* and *An. funestus*), the major Asian malaria vector *An. stephensi* has now been detected in the Horn of Africa (Sinka *et al.* 2020). All of these vector species differ in ecology, behaviour and environmental adaptations in ways that could modulate their response to climate change (Table 1). First, changes to rainfall and humidity are likely to favour some vector species over others. This could arise through interspecific variation in physiological tolerance such as resistance to desiccation and capacity to store water being favoured (e.g. Table 1). It has been hypothesized that variation in these physiological traits explains why *An. gambiae* are more likely to be found in wet, saturated environments, and *An. arabiensis* in drier environments (Lindsay *et al.* 1998). Additionally, shifts in species composition could arise due to changes in the availability and diversity of aquatic larval habitats under climate change. Typically *An. gambiae* prefers to use small, temporary aquatic habitats for oviposition, while *An. funestus* is associated with larger and more permanent habitats (Kahamba *et al.* 2022). The invasive *An. stephensi* prefer artificial container habitats in urban settings (Sinka *et al.* 2020). In areas where climate change leads to drying, *An. funestus*, and *An. stephensi* may have an advantage because their larval habitats are most likely to persist (the former because it uses larger and more stable habitats and the latter because people may increasingly store water around houses when rainfall is limited). In contrast, a proliferation of small, temporary puddles in areas where climate change increases rainfall may benefit *An. gambiae*.

Changes in vector species composition due to climate change will also be determined by the extent of temperature rise. *Anopheles arabiensis* is generally considered better adapted to survival at high temperatures and more resistant to desiccation than *An. gambiae* (Table 1). *Anopheles funestus* may have similar or higher capacity

TABLE 1 Differences in thermal tolerances of current (*An. arabiensis, An. coluzzi, An. gambiae* and *An. funestus*) and recently invasive (*An. stephensi*) malaria vector species in Africa

Species	*An. arabiensis*	*An. coluzzii*	*An. gambiae*	*An. funestus*	*An. stephensi*	Source
Larval survival at high temperature	***			**		Lyons, Coetzee *et al.* 2012, Agyekum, Botwe *et al.* 2021
	***		**			Kirby and Lindsay 2009
Capacity for larval development at high temperature			*		**	Villena, Ryan *et al.* 2022
Resistance to dessication		***	**			Lee, Meneses *et al.* 2009
	***		**			Gray and Bradley 2005
	**			***		Lyons, Coetzee *et al.* 2014
Adult survival at high temperature	***		**			Kirby and Lindsay 2004
Persistence in the dry season				***		Charlwood, Vij *et al.* 2000

The number of * refers to the relative ability of each vector species. '*' = lower ability, '**' = intermediate ability; '***' = higher ability. Each row of the table is a different study

to endure high temperatures than *An. arabiensis* (Table 1). Few studies have directly compared the environmental tolerances of native African vector species with that of the invasive *An. stephensi*; probably because until recently they did not co-occur in the wild. However, a recent model based on data from seperate experiments suggests *An. stephensi* has a higher temperature optimum than *An. gambiae* (Villena *et al.* 2022), and is considered better adapted to warmer temperatures than *An. gambiae* (Mordecai *et al.* 2020).

Of all African vector species, *An. funestus* may be the best adapted to dry conditions due to its longer persistence throughout the dry season, higher dessication resistance than *An. arabiensis* (Table 1) and additional adaptations such as aestivation which can facilitate survival through prolonged hot, dry periods (Charlwood *et al.* 2000, Huestis and Lehmann 2014). However *An. stephensi* is also likely to thrive in the warmer and drier conditions expected with climate change. In the Horn of Africa, this species has now been detected year round including in extremely hot months in Djibouti (Seyfarth *et al.* 2019). Additionally unlike native African vector species, *An. stephensi* is highly adapted to urban environments (Mordecai *et al.* 2020). Consequently the concurrent impacts of climate change and increasing urbanization (Section 5.2) may drive the expansion of this highly efficient vector across urban settings in Africa

In addition to variation in climate responses between vector species, there can also be substantial intraspecific variation in environmental tolerances between populations. Several studies have documented associations between dessication resistance and chromosomal inversions within African vector species (Gray *et al.* 2009, Fouet *et al.* 2012). This inter- and intraspecific variation in mosquito adaptations means that malaria vector communities under future climate change scenarios in Africa are likely to be radically different from those at present.

Several modelling studies have attempted to predict how the species composition and distribution of malaria vectors will respond to climate change in Africa (e.g. (Drake and Beier 2014, Tonnang *et al.* 2014, Akpan *et al.* 2019, Olabimi *et al.* 2021). Key themes have been assessment of whether there will be a major shift towards more 'dry' or 'higher temperature' adapted species. For example, climate change has been hypothesized to favour *An. arabiensis* within the *An. gambiae* s.l group because it is the best adapted to dry conditions (Drake and Beier 2014). As this species is more exophagic and zoophilic than other members of the group (*An. coluzzii* and *An gambiae*; Lyimo and Ferguson 2009), a shift in this direction could reduce the suitability of indoor interventions such as ITNs and IRS. However, a study using ecological niche modelling predicted that climate change will significantly reduce the distribution of *An. arabiensis* by 2050 (Drake and Beier 2014). Thus *An. arabiensis* may not expand its range with climate change but could become an increasingly prominent vector within remaining foci of transmission. In contrast, a more localized modelling study suggested climate change will increase the range and density of both *An. arabiensis* and *An. gambiae* s.s. in Nigeria; primarily by facilitating increased expansion of Sahel and Sudan savannas within northern States (Akpan *et al.* 2019). It may not be possible to generalize about the predicted nature of shifts in African vector composition with climate change, as this likely depends on national and sub-national ecology and geography.

2.3 *Implications of changes in malaria vector species composition for control*

The nature and extent of climate-driven changes in malaria vector species composition could have significant impacts on the efficacy of interventions. Of particular concern is the potential for changes that favour vector species, genotypes and/or at behaviours with reduced susceptibility to interventions. There is evidence that the impact of the core indoor interventions of ITNs and IRS varies between African vector species (Sinka *et al.* 2016). In particular, there has been extensive analysis of differences in the impacts of ITNs between highly endophagic and anthrophilic species like *An. gambiae* and *An. funestus* compared to the more zoophagic and exophilic *An. arabiensis* (Kiware *et al.* 2012, Kiware *et al.* 2012, Killeen 2014, Killeen *et al.* 2014). Modelling indicates that the magnitude of transmission reduction expected from ITNs varies substantially between these species on account of differences in their innate host preference, the presence of alternative hosts (cattle), and degree of outdoor biting (e.g. (Killeen 2014)). Such impacts are complex; while more zoophagic species like *An. arabiensis* have lower vectorial capacity than highly anthrophilic species, they are also harder to suppress with indoor interventions like ITN and IRS because their behaviour means they come into contact with them less frequently. These theoretical predictions have been empirically supported by combined analysis of data from intervention trials; confirming that *An. funestus* is most heavily impacted by indoor insecticide-based interventions, followed by *An. coluzzii/gambiae* and then *An. arabiensis* (Sinka *et al.* 2016). Even if the geographic range of *An. arabiensis* decreases with climate change ((Drake and Beier 2014), its potential dominance within remaining transmission settings could pose a challenge for current core interventions.

Finally, the impact of current interventions could also be eroded if *An. stephensi* continues to emerge and expand across African cities (Sinka *et al.* 2020). Like *An. arabiensis*, this vector is quite exophilic and exophagic (Sinka *et al.* 2020, Balkew *et al.* 2021), and often bites early in the evening (e.g. before 10 pm, (Reisen and Aslamkhan 1978)). These behaviours will like reduce the impact of indoor interventions including ITNs. If climate change enhances the establishment of *An. stephensi*, there will be a need to expand the focus of control activities from rural to urban settings. The need to invest and implement in additional supplementary control measures will ultimately depend on which vector species are favoured under future climate scenarios.

3 Environmental dependency of vector control interventions

Climate change could directly affect control by modifying the efficacy and quality of interventions. Such effects could arise through environmental dependencies that are additional to those created by local vector ecology and insecticide resistance, and instead due to variation in product performance in different climates. Here we consider the potential for such effects with current WHO-recommended core (ITN and IRS) and supplementary (larviciding) vector control interventions.

3.1 *Insecticide treated nets and indoor residual spraying*

Both ITNs and IRS work by targeting adult mosquitoes with insecticides inside houses. ITNs target adult females during host seeking, and IRS the females and males that rest indoors. Until recently, pyrethroids were the only class of insecticides approved for use on ITNs. Products based on pyrethroids, organochlorines, organophosphates, carbamates and neonicotinoids have been approved for IRS (WHO 2022). Whilst ITNs and IRS are recommended as core general interventions, there is considerable heterogeneity in their impact between African settings. For example, in recent trials the IRS compound Actellic (pirimiphos-methyl) was associated with an 88% reduction of *An. funestus* in Kenya (Abong'o *et al.* 2020) but only 48% reduction of the same species in Mozambique (Wagman *et al.* 2021). Such differences may be due to variation in insecticide resistance and local vector ecology, but could also be due to local environmental conditions that impact product performance, durability and residual efficacy. Currently, the World Health Organization pre-qualifies vector control products including insecticides and treated nets on the basis of submission of evidence demonstrating impact on target vectors within environmental conditions of intended deployment settings (WHO 2021). Whether similar efficacy and durability would be maintained under altered climatic conditions is unknown; and may vary between products and intervention classes. Studies from agricultural entomology indicate that the immediate and residual efficacy of some insecticide classes vary with temperature (Arthur 2013, Arthur *et al.* 2019) and humidity conditions (Ranabhat and Wang 2020, Gerken *et al.* 2021). As reviewed by (Sibanda *et al.* 2011), the stability of compounds used in IRS also varies with temperature, ultraviolet light and other environmental variables. Consequently it is reasonable to expect that environmental conditions contribute to local heterogeneity in vector control product efficacy; however the nature and epidemiological relevance of such effects are unknown. The WHO has highlighted investigation of the environmental contribution to vector control impact as a key priority for research, particularly in the context of mosquito behaviour and outdoor transmission (WHO 2022).

Variation in insecticide performance could be linked to temperature. As reviewed by Glunt *et al.* the toxicity of insecticides used in vector control often depends on ambient temperature (Glunt *et al.* 2013). This is hypothesized to be a function of temperature impacts on mosquito metabolism and nervous system function (Glunt *et al.* 2013). It has been further suggested that the standard temperatures used in WHO insecticide bioassays (25±2 °C for ITNs, and 27±2 °C for IRS) may overestimate the temperatures at which mosquitoes are exposed to these interventions in the field (Glunt *et al.* 2013). The impact of temperature on toxicity appears to vary between insecticides classes (Glunt *et al.* 2013, Glunt *et al.* 2014, Glunt *et al.* 2018), with some potentially increasing with warming conditions and others falling or remaining stable. A recent systematic review supports a trend of decreasing toxicity at higher temperatures (Agyekum *et al.* 2021); which could lead to a deterioration of efficacy with climate change. As highlighted by (Glunt *et al.* 2013), more explicit consideration of the temperature profile of insecticide products and their fit to the environment of deployment could help mitigate against this. As discussed (Section 5.1), these potential impacts of temperature on insecticides may interact below with the willingness of people to use interventions like ITNs. This interplay between direct and indirect impacts on product efficacy and use will determine the impact of these interventions in warming conditions.

3.2 *Larviciding*

Larviciding is the regular application of microbial or chemical insecticides to water bodies or containers to kill the aquatic immature stages of mosquitoes (larvae and pupae). Larviciding is widely accepted as a supplement to the core interventions or ITNs and IRS. Several malaria endemic countries in Africa are now implementing larviciding; motivated by the need to incorporate additional approaches that also target exophilic, early biting and pyrethroid resistant vector populations (Tusting *et al.* 2013). Several larvicide products are non-chemically based (e.g. the bacteria *Bacillus thurigenesis*), and thus not impaired by pyrethroid resistance. Evidence on the effectiveness of ground larviciding application for malaria control is well-established (Tusting *et al.* 2013, Derua *et al.* 2019). Notable examples include the use of the chemical Paris Green to eliminate *Anopheles gambiae* in Brazil and Egypt in 1940 and 1945s respectively (Soper and Wilson 1943, Shousha 1948), and a 90% reduction in malaria prevalence following larviciding in Sri-Lanka (Tusting *et al.* 2013). Despite this rich evidence base in support of this intervention, there has been limited consideration of how climate change may impact its impact and feasibility.

African malaria vectors spend between 7 to 27 days (Fillinger *et al.* 2003, Majambere *et al.* 2007, Ng'habi *et al.* 2010, Nartey *et al.* 2013, Ngowo *et al.* 2021) in aquatic habitats before transforming into terrestrial adults. During this period, larvae can be targeted by a range of methods including chemical insecticides, bacteria (e.g. *Bacillus thuringiensis israelensis* and *bacillus sphaericus*), surface oils and films, Spinosyns (metabolites extracted from the bacterium *Saccharopolyspora spinosa*) and insect growth regulators (e.g. novaluron and pyriproxyfen)(WHO 2013). These larvicides can be delivered through ground application (by hand or using conventional sprayers) or aerial application. Ground based larviciding is the most common delivery mechanism in sub Saharan Africa (Choi *et al.* 2019). The feasibility and impact of larviciding is highly environmentally dependent; and is recommended for use only in settings where larval habitats are 'few', 'fixed' and 'findable' (WHO 2022). There are several reasons why these criteria may be impacted by climate change. First, climate change will lead to heavy and prolonged precipitation and extensive flooding in some African settings. Ground delivery of larvicides may be hampered by extensive flooding which could limit access to aquatic habitats, dilute and wash away product (the latter may not be a concern if larvae are also washed out). Heavy precipitation and rainfall can also generate cryptic breeding habitats that are too numerous to treat. Additionally more frequent periods of heavy rainfall will necessitate repeated re-application of larvicides that is beyond the capacity of control programmes to deliver. The impact of larvicides in reducing malaria vector density is linearly correlated with coverage (Smith *et al.* 2013). Thus if larval populations are increasingly dispersed across a larger number of small and hard to reach habitats, the overall impact of larviciding will be compromised. This was observed in a programme in a flood zone in The Gambia, where larviciding had limited impact largely because ground teams were unable to reach and treat breeding habitats in a timely manner (Majambere *et al.* 2010). An explosion in the number of larval habitats due to prolonged precipitation will also make larviciding prohibitively expensive to implement at appropriate coverage.

In contrast to challenges posed by extreme rainfall, the prolonged drought conditions created in some parts of Africa due to climate changes may be advantageous for larviciding. Extreme drought would eliminate most small and ephemeral aquatic habitats; with mosquito populations being restricted only to a few remaining large and more stable habitats. These larger habitats fit more closely to the paradigm of 'few, fixed and findable', and will be easier to identify, access and treat. For example, a study by Charlwood *et al.* (2000) in the Kilombero Valley of Tanzania found that malaria vector larvae only persisted along the edge of river systems and larger permanent water bodies in the dry season. The concentration of larvae into these more limited and recognizable habitats as conditions become drier will make ground larviciding a more practical and cost effective intervention.

Another challenge for larviciding will be the increasing unpredictability of seasonal rains under climate change. The implementation of larviciding is easiest in the dry season when aquatic habitats are at their fewest. However, both the timing and duration of dry periods are less predictable as climate changes. For example, the monsoon season in parts of India may be lengthening with climate change (Karmakar and Pradhan 2020), thus decreasing the window over which larviciding is feasible.

Finally as with insecticides used for adult control, there is evidence that the efficacy of larvicides is influenced by the micro-climatic conditions under which they are deployed. *Aedes vexans* larvae collected from a field population in Germany were much more likely to be killed by Bti at warm (25 °C) than cooler temperatures (5–20 °C); (Becker *et al.* 1992). However, another study found that Bti had a lower impact on *Ae. stimulans* in cool temperatures; presumably because larval feeding rates and thus biocontrol uptake was reduced (Walker 1995). To our knowledge, the impact of high temperatures on the efficacy of larvicides used for African malaria control is not well known.

3.3 *Novel vector control approaches*

The efficacy of other novel vector control products currently in the development process could also be highly sensitive to local micro-climatic conditions, and thus vulnerable to change with climate. For example, the performance of spatial repellents is dependent on temperature, humidity and airflow conditions within the treated space (Ogoma *et al.* 2012). Studies in rural Tanzania (Ogoma *et al.* 2017) and Vietnam (Kawada *et al.* 2006) indicate spatial repellency is higher at warmer than cooler temperatures. This potential benefit of increased efficacy at higher temperatures could be offset off by faster evaporation and thus lower residual efficacy.

Attractive Target Sugar Baits (ATSBs) is another promising new vector control intervention whose efficacy is likely to be environmentally-dependent (Fraser *et al.* 2021). This intervention consists of device baited with an attractant lure and sugar source containing an insecticide. The effectiveness of this intervention likely depends on the attractiveness of ATSBs relative to other sugar sources fed on by mosquitoes in the environment (plants, flowers, etc.); with early work showing this intervention has high entomological impact in arid areas with limited vegetation (e.g. Mali (Traore *et al.* 2020); Israel (Beier *et al.* 2012)). Trials are currently underway to evaluate the epidemiological impact of ATSBs in differing eco-epidemiological settings (Eisele *et al.* 2022); and will show whether impact is reduced when deployed in more vegetation rich settings. If so, this intervention may have greater impact under warmer, drying conditions that may arise under climate change.

Several novel (endectocides) and existing (insecticide-treatment) interventions are targeted at exophagic vector species that feed on cattle (e.g. *An. arabiensis* and *An. stephensi*). An example is Ivermectin; an endectocide that can be used to treat helminths and other parasitic infections in humans and livestock, and also kills mosquitoes that feed on treated hosts (e.g. (Sylla *et al.* 2010). Mass drug administration of ivermectin to humans and/or cattle is being considered as a vector control tool. Preliminary trial results and modelling indicate this intervention will be most effective in areas of highly seasonal transmission (Slater *et al.* 2020). Climate-driven changes in malaria seasonality, and/or livestock husbandry and movement patterns could thus modify the likely coverage and feasibility of this strategy.

Climate change could also impact the effectiveness of existing and novel (e.g. eave tubes) housing-based vector control interventions. These interventions usually involve screening or closing of mosquito entry points such as the open eave space between the roof and wall. In the case of Eaves Tubes, the eave space is filled in and PVC 'tubes' coated with insecticidal netting are inserted as points of air flow between the inside and outside of the house. Odours from people sleeping inside the house disseminate out through the Eaves Tubes; causing mosquitoes to be lured towards them and killed when landing on their surface. A recent epidemiological trial in Cote d'Ivoire indicated this intervention reduced malaria infection risk in children by 38% (Sternberg *et al.* 2021). In some cases, these interventions may increase indoor temperatures by reducing indoor air flow. Under warming conditions, the discomfort due to even small reductions in indoor airflow may reduce the acceptability of these interventions. This could be mitigated through additional house design modifications to ensure the comfort of the indoor microclimate.

As shown using these representative examples, microclimatic and other environmental conditions within the settings where novel vector control interventions are deployed are likely to affect their performance. Greater understanding of how new and existing products for malaria vector control will perform under future climate scenarios is needed.

4 Mosquito resistance strategies

There is growing evidence that resistance strategies mounted by mosquitoes are environmentally dependent. Focussing on ITNs and IRS, mosquito vectors have developed a variety of physiological resistance (Black *et al.* 2021) and behavioural avoidance strategies including early and outdoor biting and resting (Sherrard-Smith *et al.* 2019). There is extensive evidence from agricultural entomology that the efficiency of physiological resistance to insecticides is temperature dependent; with the implications for future climate scenarios already well recognized (Pu *et al.* 2020). Notably, while some studies found physiological resistance in agricultural pests was impaired at high temperature, others reported an enhancement (Pu *et al.* 2020). This increased resistance at higher temperature was hypothesized to be due to pleiotropy or increased enzymatic activity in warmer conditions (Pu *et al.* 2020). In contrast, there has been relatively limited consideration of the impacts of temperature on insecticide resistance in malaria vectors. A recent systematic review suggested there may be a positive association between physiological resistance and temperature in *Anopheles* vectors (Agyekum, Botwe *et al.* 2021); suggesting mosquitoes will be less susceptible to insecticides in warmer climates. However, there is considerable heterogeneity in findings between studies. One laboratory study found that an insecticide resistant strain of *An. arabiensis* lived longer than a susceptible control line under high temperatures (Oliver and Brooke 2017); suggesting that climate could modify or even reverse the fitness cost of resistance mechanisms. However, another study showed that a resistant line of *An. funestus* exposed to Bendiocarb was more likely to die at high than intermediate temperatures, whilst deltamethrin was least likely to kill a resistant line of *An. arabiensis* at intermediate temperature than either hot or cold extremes (Glunt *et al.* 2018). The manner in which temperature impacts physiological resistance is thus complex, and may vary between mechanisms, species and insecticide classes.

In addition to physiological resistance, malaria vectors employ a range a behavioural avoidance strategies to evade indoor interventions. These can include a shift to biting earlier in the evening or in the morning when people are not protected by ITNs (Moiroux *et al.* 2014), increased zoophily and outdoor resting (Kreppel *et al.* 2020), and outdoor biting (Govella and Ferguson 2012; Reddy *et al.* 2011, Russell *et al.* 2011). Similar to physiological resistance, these behavioural adaptations may be shaped by local environmental and microclimatic conditions. Recent work has shown that outdoor biting and resting can vary seasonally and in response to temperature. For example, *An. arabiensis* in Tanzania became more exophilic when temperatures indoors became warmer relative to outdoors (Ngowo *et al.* 2017), during the hot season (Kulkarni *et al.* 2006, Kreppel *et al.* 2019), and *An. gambiae sl* in Burkina Faso are more likely to rest indoors during the wet than dry season (Sanou 2020). Should such seasonal variation reflects how African malaria vectors could adapt their behaviour to warming conditions, suggesting there may be an increased need for outdoor interventions under future climate change scenarios.

5 Indirect impacts of climate change on vector control

In addition to the potential direct impacts described above, there are multiple ways through which the ability to implement vector control will be indirectly impacted by the wider social, ecological, economic and political consequences of climate change. Such indirect effects will be widespread and complex, and may have a larger impact on intervention strategy and efficacy than any of the more direct impacts outlined above. Here we highlight a few factors that may have the greatest bearing on malaria vector control.

5.1 *Human behaviour and use of interventions*

Climate change could impact vector control efficacy by changing the human behavioural factors that influence intervention coverage and uptake. For example, the degree of protection obtained from ITNs is crucially dependent on usage. The decision to use an ITN is associated with micro-climatic conditions (Pulford *et al.* 2011, von Seidlein *et al.* 2012, Ahorlu *et al.* 2019). Specifically, users perceive ITNs to be less comfortable under warmer indoor temperatures and higher humidity (von Seidlein *et al.* 2012). ITN usage may fall during hotter periods of the year when people prefer to sleep outside where it is cooler (Guglielmo *et al.* 2021). Similar effects could lead to a reduction in ITN usage with the warmer conditions brought by climate change.

In addition to influencing the decision of whether to use an ITN or not, climate change may influence the amount of time people are likely to spend under a net. Exposure to malaria vectors in outdoor settings in Africa happens in evening hours (e.g. <10 pm, before people go indoors to sleep); when people are engaged in outdoor activities such as cooking, eating or socializing (Finda *et al.* 2019, Monroe *et al.* 2019). Prolonged exposure longer into the night can also happen when people are engaged in specific types of outdoor work or socio-cultural events (Monroe *et al.* 2019). The total time spent outdoors in the evening and late night period is also influenced by microclimatic conditions. One study showed that residents of rural communities in Burkina Faso went indoors to sleep at later hours during the hotter period of the year (Guglielmo *et al.* 2021). By delaying the time of night at which users first go under an ITN, warming conditions could reduce the total amount of protection received from it. Improved understanding of the environmental factors that influence human behaviours and decisions on ITN use (Monroe *et al.* 2021) are needed.

5.2 *Land use and urbanization*

One of the largest expected impacts of climate change is on land use (IPCC 2020). Climate change is predicted to lead to large changes in land quality and use across the globe; including erosion and degradation in some coastal areas, and expansion of drylands with increasing desertification. Drying conditions combined with shorter more intense rainfall and extreme flooding events will increase erosion and diminish soil quality (IPCC 2020). Changes to land type and soil quality will fundamentally impact patterns of land use and human activities; with several consequences for vector control strategies.

Most directly, these changes will impact agriculture and food security. It is estimated that ~90% of agriculture in sub-Saharan Africa is dependent on rain and managed by small holders (Abraham 2018). Staple crops such as maize and wheat have already been negatively affected by recent climate change (IPCC 2020); with yields at further risk in the future. Additionally, reductions in water availability and distribution will impact livestock husbandry. This is in turn could impact the efficacy and feasibility of livestock-based vector control methods such as zooprophylaxis and endectocides (Donnelly *et al.* 2015) Adaptations such as crop diversification and irrigation will be required to mitigate against the most negative consequences of these changes (Abraham 2018). However, these strategies could also influence the efficacy and feasibility of vector control. For example, irrigation schemes and dams are known to have complex associations with malaria risk in Africa (Ijumba and Lindsay 2001, Keiser *et al.* 2005, Kibret *et al.* 2017, Kibret, McCartney *et al.* 2021) Analysis of the literature indicates that dams may lead to increased transmission in highland or semi-arid areas of unstable transmission, but may be less important in areas of endemic transmission (Kibret *et al.* 2017). The creation of large irrigated areas may increase mosquito breeding sites, and make larval control more difficult (Karch *et al.* 1992).

Another mitigation response to diminishing crop yields arising from unpredictable weather conditions is heavier pesticide use. For example, small scale farmers in Rwanda reported increased use of pesticides as one of several common responses to mitigate the adverse impacts of increased drought and floods on their crops (Helwig *et al.* 2020). Pesticides used in agriculture are a major source of selection for insecticide resistance in malaria vectors (Nkya *et al.* 2013, Nkya *et al.* 2014, Chouaibou *et al.* 2016); thus their intensified use in response to climate change could erode the efficacy of ITNs and other insecticide-based approaches. Such an interplay will increase the already great need for stronger intersectoral collaboration between agriculture and public health under future climate scenarios.

Diminishing returns from small scale agriculture as a result of climate change have been linked to increasing migration to urban centres in several areas of Africa (Henderson *et al.* 2014, 2017, Serdeczny *et al.* 2017). Currently urbanization is happening faster in Africa than anywhere else in the world; with up to 2/3 of the total population expected to live in urban areas by 2050 (OECD *et al.* 2020). Climate change poses specific risks to urban populations, particularly those living in informal settlements that are at increased risk of flood damage, socioeconomically deprived, and poorly connected to electricity and water infrastructure (Abraham 2018). These housing conditions could generate increased exposure to malaria and other vector-borne diseases (Mordecai *et al.* 2020). For example, rapid urbanization in Soweto led to more people living in flood plain areas (Abraham 2018); with these being ideal habitats for mosquito vectors. Urban dwellers, and particularly those living in peri-urban and informal settlements may increasingly turn to market gardening to enhance food security (Eigenbrod and Gruda 2015). This could increase malaria exposure in those living close to market gardens (e.g.(Yadouleton *et al.* 2010)); possibly due to the generation of larval breeding sites through agricultural activities.

Poor housing conditions in informal urban settlements may not only increase malaria risk (Tusting *et al.* 2015), but may make it more difficult to implement standard vector control measures including installation of ITNs and IRS. Some interventions such as larviciding may be more feasible and cost effective to implement in urban settings (Worrall and Fillinger 2011), whilst others like ITNs and IRS have lower usage in urban than rural settings (Ministry of Health, (Zanzibar) *et al.* 2018). As described in Section 2, the recent invasion of *An. stephensi* in East Africa poses an additional risk for malaria control in urban African settings (Sinka *et al.* 2020). Unlike native African vector species, *An. stephensi* is highly adapted to urban environments (Mordecai *et al.* 2020). The unique ecology and behaviour of this vector, combined with it higher transmission efficiency, could require more tailored vector control interventions in urban settings. Sustaining vector control under future climate scenarios will require adapting current approaches to socio-economically disadvantaged populations in urban environments.

5.3 *Economic and political factors*

The ability to finance and implement large scale vector surveillance is fundamentally dependent on strong political will, governance infrastructure and economic security. As illustrated by the recent overwhelming resurgence of vector-borne diseases in Venezuela, even countries with a long and successful history of vector control can see rapid reversals during socio-economic and humanitarian crises (Grillet *et al.* 2019). Climate change is likely to increase vulnerability to such socio-economic shocks and lead to corresponding constraints on health systems and vector control programmes. These constraints may be further exacerbated by increased conflict (Freeman 2017, Adaawen *et al.* 2019), migration and increases in other infectious (Ahmed *et al.* 2018, Adekiya *et al.* 2020, Bryson *et al.* 2020, Charnley *et al.* 2022) and non-communicable diseases (Amegah *et al.* 2016).

The United Nations High Commission on Refugees estimates that 21.5 million people have been forcibly displaced each year since 2008 due to extreme weather events including floods, storms, wildlife and extreme temperature (Bilak *et al.* 2016). This number is expected to increase with climate change; with as many as 86 million internal climate migrants expected in sub Saharan Africa by 2050 (Clement *et al.* 2021). Refugees often face a considerably higher risk of malaria exposure and severe outcomes due to a myriad of factors including poor and insecure housing, infrastructure and limited access to prevention and treatment (e.g. (Hauser *et al.* 2023 Anderson *et al.* 2011, Charchuk *et al.* 2016)). There is some evidence that migration can lead to malaria spillover across border areas and local upsurges in areas where transmission was under control (e.g. (Rodriguez-Morales *et al.* 2019). Thus in the absence of access to healthcare including diagnosis and treatment, climate refugees may increasingly strain malaria control and compromise elimination activities. Development and implementation of more tailored diagnostics, treatments and vector control interventions for emergency contexts will be needed to sustain progress under climate change.

Sustaining and expanding malaria vector control under these more complex and economically constrained circumstances will be challenging. Already funding for malaria control is substantially below the level needed to meet global elimination targets, and has largely plateaued since 2012 (Lindsay *et al.* 2021). If health systems become even more stretched as climate changes, vector control programmes will increasingly be asked to deliver more effective interventions with less funding. Mass distribution of efficacious but relatively higher cost interventions that are recommended for use now (e.g. some Next Generation Nets) may become increasingly unaffordable. Clearly, maintaining malaria vector control will require the adaptation of current approaches and development of new ones that are both effective and affordable under future climate scenarios.

6 Conclusions and recommendations

Consideration of the potential impacts of climate change on vector-borne diseases has so far focussed almost exclusively on assessment of the environmental determinants of transmission. Such analyses provide an essential foundation to understand how the area at 'risk' of transmission may expand or contract; but on their own are insufficient to predict the nature of public health impacts. An equally important yet largely neglected question is how well our current and prospective control measures will function under altered climates; and how our ability to implement and sustain these approaches will be shaped by shifts in wider socio-environmental, economic and political factors that accompany this change. Within the context of malaria vector control in Africa; we have highlighted several routes through which the efficacy of interventions could be modified by the types of climate change predicted. A key theme is that climate change will have diverse and complex impacts across different regions of Africa, so that there may be no universal impact in all settings. Through synthesis of the varied biological and indirect impacts considered here, it is clear that climate change could have wide-ranging impacts on the implementation, feasibility and efficacy of vector control interventions in Africa. The overall impact of these changes on malaria control will depend on to what extent conditions for the 'worst' vs 'best' case scenarios are realized, as exemplified by the representative example in Box 1. At one end of the spectrum, climate change may enhance vector control through causing malaria vector populations to contract and reduce in abundance, and increasing the efficacy of some control methods. Alternatively, climate change could substantially erode vector control through favouring vector species and phenotypes that are harder to tackle with existing interventions, enhancing capacity for resistance, reducing the acceptability and use of interventions, and generating economic constraints that make it harder to deliver control programmes. The degree to which potential challenges can be offset by such advantages will fundamentally depend on the robustness of public health and other socioeconomic infrastructure. Clearly, there is a need to 'future-proof' vector control strategies through more anticipation and integration of potential climate impacts into future planning. This will require going beyond modifications and tailoring of existing and currently developing interventions, to more 'blue sky' and integrated approaches that are able to mitigate the impacts of climate change on malaria and other environmental hazards at the same time. Just as there has been extensive consideration of adaptation of agricultural systems to climate change, similar forethought is required for adaptation of vector control strategies. In particular, the addition of new control strategies that may be less sensitive to the environmental conditions of deployment (e.g. malaria vaccines) could greatly supplement and bolster control. While we focus on malaria in Africa, many of the issues raised here apply to the control of other mosquito-borne diseases that are controlled through use of similar interventions (e.g. *Aedes* vectors of arboviruses).

To better prepare and mitigate against the most negative impacts, we advocate for consideration of climate change impacts to be built into future vector control and public health planning.

Box 1: Speculative 'best' and 'worst' case examples of how climate change may impact malaria vector control interventions in Africa, based on information reviewed in this chapter

		'Best case'	'Worst case'
Direct Biological Impacts	Vector ecology	Contraction of vector distribution and abundance with drying	Increased mosquito vector abundance and longer seasonal activity in areas receiving increased rainfall
		Reduction in vector survival and length of seasonal activity period due to unfavourable temperature and rainfall	Shifts in vector species composition with drying towards species that are better adapted to dry conditions but harder to target with indoor interventions (e.g. *An. arabiensis* and *An. stephensi*)
		Shifts in vector species composition towards species that are better adapted to dry conditions but easier to target with some interventions (e.g. *An. funestus* by larviciding and indoor interventions)	Spread of invasive *An. stephensi* (urban adapted, efficient transmission at high temperatures)
	Interventions	Larval habitats may become fewer and more 'findable' under drying conditions; improving the feasibility of larviciding	Reduced toxicity and residual efficacy of some chemical and biological insecticides at higher temperatures
		Possible enhancement of some novel vector control tools (e.g. ATSBS) under drier conditions	Lower coverage and need for more frequent application of larvicides with increasing rainfall /extreme weather events
			Possible reduced feasibility or acceptability of some novel control strategies at higher temperature/lower rainfall
	Vector Resistance Strategies	Reduced ability for vectors to mount energetically costly resistance mechanisms under environmental stress	More effective physiological resistance to insecticides due to enhanced expression of detoxification genes at higher temperatures
			Emergence of mosquito adaptations to warming conditions that also enhance insecticide resistance (e.g. cuticle thickening as a strategy for desiccation resistance)
			Shift to outdoor biting by mosquito vectors where warmer conditions reduce the suitability of indoor microclimatic conditions

Box 1: Speculative 'best' and 'worst' case examples (*cont.*)

		'Best case'	'Worst case'
Indirect Impacts	Human Behaviour		Lower usage and effective coverage of ITNs due to changes in human behaviour and sleeping patterns at warmer temperatures
	Land use	Changes in livestock keeping practices that reduce mosquito vector populations Increasing urbanization enhances the feasibility and implementation of some vector control interventions	Changes in livestock keeping practices that reduce potential for livestock-based interventions Higher selection for insecticide resistance due to intensification of pesticide use as a strategy for minimizing agricultural losses due to adverse weather and drought conditions Increase of urban migrants who are exposed to malaria vectors due to insecure housing, limited infrastructure and exposure to environmental risks
	Political and economic	Climate-driven reductions in malaria reduce the costs needed to run vector control programmes	Rise in climate refugees who are at greater risk of malaria Constraints on health systems due to rises in other health issues Reduction in financing for control due to national and global economic constraints Increased conflict and political insecurity impeding health services and control programmes

Acknowledgements

NJG and HMF were supported by joint funding from the UK Medical Research Council (MRC, MR/T008873/1) and the UK Foreign, Commonwealth & Development Office (FCDO) under the MRC/FCDO Concordat agreement which is also part of the EDCTP2 programme supported by the European Union.

References

Abong'o B, Gimnig JE, Torr SJ, Longman B, Omoke D, Muchoki M, ter Kuile F, Ochomo E, Munga S, Samuels AM, Njagi K, Maas J, Perry RT, Fornadel C, Donnelly MJ and Oxborough RM (2020) Impact of indoor residual spraying with pirimiphos-methyl (Actellic 300CS) on entomological indicators of transmission and malaria case burden in Migori County, western Kenya. Sci Rep 10. https://doi.org/10.1038/s41598-020-61350-2.

Abraham EM (2018) Understanding climate change adaptation in Africa: key considerations. Management of Environmental Quality 29: 165–179. https://doi.org/10.1108/meq-01-2017-0001.

Adaawen S, Rademacher-Schulz C, Schraven B and Segadlo N (2019) Drought, migration, and conflict in sub-Saharan Africa: what are the links and policy options? In: Mapedza E, Tsegai D, Bruntrup M and McLeman R eds., Drought Challenges: Policy Options for Developing Countries, Current Directions in Water Scarcity Research, pp. 15–31. https://doi.org/10.1016/b978-0-12-814820-4.00002-x.

Adekiya TA, Aruleba RT, Oyinloye BE, Okosun KO and Kappo AP (2020) The Effect of climate change and the snail-schistosome cycle in transmission and bio-control of schistosomiasis in Sub-Saharan Africa. International Journal of Environmental Research and Public Health 17. https://doi.org/10.3390/ijerph17010181.

Adhikari U, Nejadhashemi AP and Herman MR (2015) A review of climate change impacts on water resources in East Africa. Transactions of the ASABE 58: 1493–1507.

Agyekum TP, Arko-Mensah J, Botwe PK, Hogarh JN, Issah I, Dwomoh D, Billah MK, Dadzie SK, Robins TG and Fobil JN (2022) Effects of elevated temperatures on the development of immature stages of *Anopheles gambiae* (s.l.) mosquitoes. Tropical Medicine & International Health 27(4): 338–346. https://doi.org/10.1111/tmi.13732.

Agyekum TP, Botwe PK, Arko-Mensah J, Issah I, Acquah AA, Hogarh JN, Dwomoh D, Robins TG and Fobil JN (2021) A systematic review of the effects of temperature on *Anopheles* mosquito development and survival: implications for malaria control in a future warmer climate. International Journal of Environmental Research and Public Health 18. https://doi.org/10.3390/ijerph18147255.

Ahmed SA, Florez MG and Karanis P (2018) The impact of water crises and climate changes on the transmission of protozoan parasites in Africa. Pathogens and Global Health 112: 281–293. https://doi.org/10.1080/20477724.2018.1523778.

Ahorlu CS, Adongo P, Koenker H, Zigirumugabe S, Sika-Bright S, Koka E, Tabong PTN, Piccinini D, Segbaya S, Olapeju B and Monroe A (2019) Understanding the gap between access and use: a qualitative study on barriers and facilitators to insecticide-treated net use in Ghana. Malaria Journal 18. https://doi.org/10.1186/s12936-019-3051-0.

Akpan GE, Adepoju KA and Oladosu OR (2019) Potential distribution of dominant malaria vector species in tropical region under climate change scenarios. PLoS One 14. https://doi.org/10.1371/journal.pone.0218523.

Akurut M, Willems P and Niwagaba CB (2014) Potential Impacts of Climate Change on Precipitation over Lake Victoria, East Africa, in the 21st Century. Water 6: 2634–2659. https://doi.org/10.3390/w6092634.

Alonso D, Bouma MJ and Pascual M (2011) Epidemic malaria and warmer temperatures in recent decades in an East African highland. Proceedings of the Royal Society B-Biological Sciences 278: 1661–1669. https://doi.org/10.1098/rspb.2010.2020.

Amegah AK, Rezza G and Jaakkola JJK (2016) Temperature-related morbidity and mortality in Sub-Saharan Africa: a systematic review of the empirical evidence. Environment International 91: 133–149. https://doi.org/10.1016/j.envint.2016.02.027.

Anderson J, Doocy S, Haskew C, Spiegel P and Moss WJ (2011) The burden of malaria in post-emergency refugee sites: a retrospective study. Conflict and Health 5: (19 September 2011).

Arthur FH (2013) Dosage rate, temperature, and food source provisioning affect susceptibility of *Tribolium castaneum* and *Tribolium confusum* to chlorfenapyr. Journal of Pest Science 86: 507–513. https://doi.org/10.1007/s10340-013-0495-9.

Arthur FH, Starkus LA and McKay T (2019) Degradation and residual efficacy of betacyfluthrin as a surface treatment for control of *Tribolium castaneum* Herbst: Effects of temperature and environment. Journal of Stored Products Research 84. https://doi.org/10.1016/j.jspr.2019.101514.

Bayoh MN and Lindsay SW (2003) Effect of temperature on the development of the aquatic stages of *Anopheles gambiae sensu stricto* (Diptera : Culicidae). Bulletin of Entomological Research 93: 375–381.

Bayoh MN and Lindsay SW (2004) Temperature-related duration of aquatic stages of the Afrotropical malaria vector mosquito *Anopheles gambiae* in the laboratory. Medical and Veterinary Entomology 18: 174–179. https://doi.org/10.1111/j.0269-283X.2004.00495.x.

Becker N, Zgomba M, Ludwig M, Petric D and Rettich F (1992) Factors influencing the activity of *Bacillus-thuringiensis* var *israelensis* treatments. Journal of the American Mosquito Control Association 8: 285–289.

Beier JC (1998) Malaria parasite development in mosquitoes. Annual Review of Entomology 43: 519–543.

Beier JC, Muller GC, Gu WD, Arheart KL and Schlein Y (2012) Attractive toxic sugar bait (ATSB) methods decimate populations of *Anopheles* malaria vectors in arid environments regardless of the local availability of favoured sugar-source blossoms. Malaria Journal 11. https://doi.org/10.1186/1475-2875-11-31.

Ben Mohamed A (2011) Climate change risks in Sahelian Africa. Regional Environmental Change 11: S109–S117. https://doi.org/10.1007/s10113-010-0172-y.

Bhatt S, Weiss DJ, Cameron E, Bisanzio D, Mappin B, Dalrymple U, Battle KE, Moyes CL, Henry A, Eckhoff PA, Wenger EA, Briet O, Penny MA, Smith TA, Bennett A, Yukich J, Eisele TP, Griffin JT, Fergus CA, Lynch M, Lindgren F, Cohen JM, Murray CL, Smith DL, Hay SI, Cibulskis RE and Gething PW (2015) The effect of malaria control on *Plasmodium falciparum* in Africa between 2000 and 2015. Nature 526: 207–211. https://doi.org/10.1038/nature15535.

Bilak A, Cardona-Fox G, Ginnett J, Rushing EJ, Scherer, I, Swain M, Walicki N and Yonetani M (2016) Grid 2016: Global Report on Internal Displacement, Internal Displacement Monitoring Centre.

Black WC, Snell TK, Saavedra-Rodriguez K, Kading RC and Campbell CL (2021) From global to local-new insights into features of pyrethroid detoxification in vector mosquitoes. Insects 12: 19. https://doi.org/10.3390/insects12040276.

Boyce R, Reyes R, Matte M, Ntaro M, Mulogo E, Metlay JP, Band L and Siedner MJ (2016) Severe flooding and malaria transmission in the Western Ugandan Highlands: implications for disease control in an era of global climate change. Journal of Infectious Diseases 214: 1403–1410. https://doi.org/10.1093/infdis/jiw363.

Bryson JM, Bishop-Williams KE, Berrang-Ford L, Nunez EC, Lwasa S, Namanya DB, Harper SL and Indigenous Hlth Adaptation C (2020) Neglected tropical diseases in the context of climate change in East Africa: a systematic scoping review. American Journal of Tropical Medicine and Hygiene 102: 1443–1454. https://doi.org/10.4269/ajtmh.19-0380.

Caminade C, Kovats S, Rocklov J, Tompkins AM, Morse AP, Colon-Gonzalez FJ, Stenlund H, Martens P and Lloyd SJ (2014) Impact of climate change on global malaria distribution. Proceedings of the National Academy of Sciences of the United States of America 111: 3286–3291. https://doi.org/10.1073/pnas.1302089111.

Charchuk R, Paul MKJ, Claude KM, Houston S and Hawkes MT (2016) Burden of malaria is higher among children in an internal displacement camp compared to a neighbouring village in the Democratic Republic of the Congo. Malaria Journal 15. https://doi.org/10.1186/s12936-016-1479-z.

Charlwood JD, Vij R and Billingsley PF (2000) Dry season refugia of malaria-transmitting mosquitoes in a dry savannah zone of east Africa. Am J Trop Med Hyg 62: 726–732.

Charnley GEC, Kelman I and Murray KA (2022) Drought-related cholera outbreaks in Africa and the implications for climate change: a narrative review. Pathogens and Global Health 116: 3–12. https://doi.org/10.1080/20477724.2021.1981716.

Chersich MF, Wright CY, Venter F, Rees H, Scorgie F and Erasmus B (2018) Impacts of climate change on health and wellbeing in South Africa. International Journal of Environmental Research and Public Health 15. https://doi.org/10.3390/ijerph15091884.

Choi L, Majambere S and Wilson AL (2019) Larviciding to prevent malaria transmission (Review). Cochrane Database Syst Rev. https://doi.org/10.1002/14651858.CD012736.pub2.

Chou SC, Lyra AdA, Gomes JL, Rodriguez DA, Martins MA, Resende NC, Tavares PDS, Dereczynski CP, Pilotto IL, Martins AM, Alves de Carvalho LF, Lima Onofre JL, Major I, Penhor M and Santana A (2020) Downscaling projections of climate change in Sao Tome and Principe Islands, Africa. Climate Dynamics 54: 4021–4042. https://doi.org/10.1007/s00382-020-05212-7.

Chouaibou MS, Fodjo BK, Fokou G, Allassane OF, Koudou BG, David JP, Antonio-Nkondjio C, Ranson H and Bonfoh B (2016) Influence of the agrochemicals used for rice and vegetable cultivation on insecticide resistance in malaria vectors in southern Cote d'Ivoire. Malaria Journal 15: (24 August 2016)–(2024 August 2016).

Christiansen-Jucht CD, Parham PE, Saddler A, Koella JC and Basanez MG (2015) Larval and adult environmental temperatures influence the adult reproductive traits of *Anopheles gambiae* s.s. Parasites & Vectors 8. https://doi.org/10.1186/s13071-015-1053-5.

Clement V, Rigaud K, A dS, Jones B, S A, J S, N S and Shabahat E (2021) Groundswell Part 2: Acting on Internal Climate Migration. World Bank, Washington, DC. https://openknowledge.worldbank.org/handle/10986/36248.

Connolly-Boutin L and Smit B (2016) Climate change, food security, and livelihoods in sub-Saharan Africa. Regional Environmental Change 16: 385–399. https://doi.org/10.1007/s10113-015-0761-x.

Derua YA, Kweka EJ, Kisinza W, Githeko AK and Mosha FW (2019) Bacterial larvicides used for malaria vector control in sub-Saharan Africa: review of their effectiveness and operational feasibility. Parasit Vectors 12: 426.

Diouf I, Adeola AM, Abiodun GJ, Lennard C, Shirinde JM, Yaka P, Ndione J-A and Gbobaniyi EO (2021) Impact of future climate change on malaria in West Africa. Theoretical and Applied Climatology. https://doi.org/10.1007/s00704-021-03807-6.

Donnelly B, Berrang-Ford L, Ross NA and Michel P (2015) A systematic, realist review of zooprophylaxis for malaria control. Malaria Journal 14. https://doi.org/10.1186/s12936-015-0822-0.

Drake JM and Beier JC (2014) Ecological niche and potential distribution of *Anopheles arabiensis* in Africa in 2050. Malaria Journal 13: (3 June 2014).

Du Plessis JA and Kalima SG (2021) Modelling the impact of climate change on the flow of the Eerste River in South Africa. Physics and Chemistry of the Earth 124. https://doi.org/10.1016/j.pce.2021.103025.

Egbendewe-Mondzozo A, Musumba M, McCarl BA and Wu X (2011) Climate change and vector-borne diseases: an economic impact analysis of malaria in Africa. International Journal of Environmental Research and Public Health 8: 913–930. https://doi.org/10.3390/ijerph8030913.

Eigenbrod C and Gruda N (2015) Urban vegetable for food security in cities. A review. Agronomy for Sustainable Development 35: 483–498. https://doi.org/10.1007/s13593-014-0273-y.

Eisele TP, Kleinschmidt I, Sarrassat S, TerKuile F, Miller J, Chanda J, Silumbe K, Samuels A, Janssen J, Ogwang C, Bradley J, Orange E, Yukich J, Ashton R, Kyomuhangi I, Harris AF, Doumbia S, Toure M, Moumine M, Majambere S, Mburu MM, Mwaanga G, Simubali L, Simulundu E, Bennett A, Slutsker L, Muller G, Ochomo E, Gimnig J, Johnson PCD, Wagman J, Litrell M and Attractive Targeted Sugar Bait P (2022) Attractive targeted sugar bait phase III trials in Kenya, Mali, and Zambia. Trials 23. https://doi.org/10.1186/s13063-022-06555-8.

Ermert V, Fink AH and Paeth H (2013) The potential effects of climate change on malaria transmission in Africa using bias-corrected regionalised climate projections and a simple malaria seasonality model. Climatic Change 120: 741–754. https://doi.org/10.1007/s10584-013-0851-z.

Fall P, Diouf I, Deme A and Sene D (2022) Assessment of Climate-Driven Variations in Malaria Transmission in Senegal Using the VECTRI Model. Atmosphere 13. https://doi.org/10.3390/atmos13030418.

Fillinger U, Knols BGJ and Becker N (2003) Efficacy and efficiency of new *Bacillus thuringiensis* var. *israelensis* and Bacillus sphaericus formulations against Afrotropical anophelines in Western Kenya. Trop Med Int Health 8: 37–47. https://doi.org/10.1046/j.1365-3156.2003.00979.x.

Finda MF, Moshi IR, Monroe A, Limwagu AJ, Nyoni AP, Swai JK, Ngowo HS, Minja EG, Toe LP, Kaindoa EW, Coetzee M, Manderson L and Okumu FO (2019) Linking human behaviours and malaria vector biting risk in south-eastern Tanzania. PLoS One 14. https://doi.org/10.1371/journal.pone.0217414.

Fouet C, Gray E, Besansky NJ and Costantini C (2012) Adaptation to Aridity in the Malaria Mosquito *Anopheles gambiae*: Chromosomal Inversion Polymorphism and Body Size Influence Resistance to Desiccation. PLoS One 7. https://doi.org/10.1371/journal.pone.0034841.

Fraser KJ, Mwandigha L, Traore SF, Traore MM, Doumbia S, Junnila A, Revay E, Beier JC, Marshall JM, Ghani AC and Muller G (2021) Estimating the potential impact of Attractive Targeted Sugar Baits (ATSBs) as a new vector control tool for *Plasmodium falciparum* malaria. Malaria Journal 20. https://doi.org/10.1186/s12936-021-03684-4.

Freeman L (2017) Environmental Change, Migration, and Conflict in Africa: A Critical Examination of the Interconnections. Journal of Environment & Development 26: 351–374. https://doi.org/10.1177/1070496517727325.

Gerken AR, Scully ED, Campbell JF and Morrison WR, III (2021) Effectiveness of long-lasting insecticide netting on *Tribolium castaneum* is modulated by multiple exposures, biotic, and abiotic factors. Pest Management Science 77: 1235–1244. https://doi.org/10.1002/ps.6134.

Gething PW, Smith DL, Patil AP, Tatem AJ, Snow RW and Hay SI (2010a) Climate change and the global malaria recession. Nature 465: 342–U394. https://doi.org/10.1038/nature09098.

Gething PW, Smith DL, Patil AP, Tatem AJ, Snow RW and Hay SI (2010b) Climate change and the global malaria recession. Nature 465: 342–345. https://doi.org/10.1038/nature09098.

Glunt KD, Blanford JI and Paaijmans KP (2013) Chemicals, Climate, and Control: Increasing the Effectiveness of Malaria Vector Control Tools by Considering Relevant Temperatures. Plos Pathogens 9: e1003602. https://doi.org/10.1371/journal.ppat.1003602

Glunt KD, Oliver SV, Hunt RH and Paaijmans KP (2018) The impact of temperature on insecticide toxicity against the malaria vectors *Anopheles arabiensis* and *Anopheles funestus*. Malaria Journal 17. https://doi.org/10.1186/s12936-018-2250-4.

Glunt KD, Paaijmans KP, Read AF and Thomas MB (2014) Environmental temperatures significantly change the impact of insecticides measured using WHOPES protocols. Malaria Journal 13. https://doi.org/10.1186/1475-2875-13-350.

Gray EM and Bradley TJ (2005) Physiology of desiccation resistance in *Anopheles gambiae* and *Anopheles arabiensis*. American Journal of Tropical Medicine and Hygiene 73: 553–559. https://doi.org/10.4269/ajtmh.2005.73.553.

Gray EM, Rocca KAC, Costantini C and Besansky NJ (2009) Inversion 2La is associated with enhanced desiccation resistance in *Anopheles gambiae*. Malaria Journal 8. https://doi.org/10.1186/1475-2875-8-215.

Grillet ME, Hernandez-Villena JV, Llewellyn MS, Paniz-Mondolfi AE, Tami A, Vincenti-Gonzalez MF, Marquez M, Mogollon-Mendoza AC, Hernandez-Pereira CE, Plaza-Morr JD, Blohm G, Grijalva MJ, Costales JA, Ferguson HM, Schwabl P, Hernandez-Castro LE, Lamberton PHL, Streicker DG, Haydon DT, Miles MA, Acosta-Serrano A, Acquattela H, Basanez MG, Benaim G, Colmenares LA, Conn JE, Espinoza R, Freilij H, Graterol-Gil MC, Hotez PJ, Kato H, Lednicky JA, Martinez CE, Mas-Coma S, Morris JG, Navarro JC,

Ramirez JL, Rodriguez M, Urbina JA, Villegas L, Segovia MJ, Carrasco HJ, Crainey JL, Luz SLB, Moreno JD, Gonzalez OON, Ramirez JD and Alarcon-de Noya B (2019) Venezuela's humanitarian crisis, resurgence of vector-borne diseases, and implications for spillover in the region. Lancet Infect Dis 19: E149–E161. https://doi.org/10.1016/s1473-3099(18)30757-6.

Guglielmo F, Ranson H, Sagnon N and Jones C (2021) The issue is not 'compliance': exploring exposure to malaria vector bites through social dynamics in Burkina Faso. Anthropol Med 28: 508–525. https://doi.org/10.1080/13648470.2021.1884185.

Hauser M, Kabuya JBB, Mantus M, Kamavu LK, Sichivula JL, Matende WM, Fritschi N, Shields T, Curriero F, Kvit A, Chongwe G, Moss WJ, Ritz N and Ippolito MM (2023) Malaria in Refugee Children Resettled to a Holoendemic Area of Sub-Saharan Africa. Clinical Infectious Diseases 76(3): e1104–e1113 https://doi.org/10.1093/cid/ciac417.

Helwig K, C H-OC, Mikulewicz M, Mugiraneza P and E C (2020) The Role of Microfinance in Climate Change Adaptation: Evidence from Rural Rwanda, Glasgow Caledonian University Glasgow.

Henderson JV, Storeygard A and Deichmann U (2014) 50 Years of urbanization in Africa: examining the role of climate change. Policy Research Working Paper – World Bank: 42 pp.

Henderson JV, Storeygard A and Deichmann U (2017) Has climate change driven urbanization in Africa? J Dev Econ 124: 60–82. https://doi.org/10.1016/j.jdeveco.2016.09.001.

Ijumba JN and Lindsay SW (2001) Impact of irrigation on malaria in Africa: paddies paradox. Medical and Veterinary Entomology 15: 1–11. https://doi.org/10.1046/j.1365-2915.2001.00279.x.

IPCC (2020) Climate Change and Land, Geneva.

Kahamba NF, Finda M, Ngowo HS, Msugupakulya BJ, Baldini F, Koekemoer LL, Ferguson HM and Okumu FO (2022) Using ecological observations to improve malaria control in areas where *Anopheles funestus* is the dominant vector. Malaria Journal 21. https://doi.org/10.1186/s12936-022-04198-3.

Karch S, Asidi N, Manzambi ZM and Salaun JJ (1992) Efficacy of *Bacillus-sphaericus* against the malaria vector *Anopheles-gambiae* and other mosquitos in swamps and rice fields in Zaire. Journal of the American Mosquito Control Association 8: 376–380.

Karmakar M and Pradhan MM (2020) Climate change and public health: a study of vector-borne diseases in Odisha, India. Nat Hazards 102: 659–671. https://doi.org/10.1007/s11069-019-03594-4.

Kawada H, Iwasaki T, Luu Le L, Tran Khanh T, Nguyen Thi Nhu M, Shono Y, Katayama Y and Takagi M (2006) Field evaluation of spatial repellency of metofluthrin-impregnated latticework plastic strips against *Aedes aegypti* (L.) and analysis of environmental factors affecting its efficacy in My Tho City, Tien Giang, Vietnam. American Journal of Tropical Medicine and Hygiene 75: 1153–1157. https://doi.org/10.4269/ajtmh.2006.75.1153.

Keiser J, De Castro MC, Maltese MF, Bos R, Tanner M, Singer BH and Utzinger J (2005) Effect of irrigation and large dams on the burden of malaria on a global and regional scale. American Journal of Tropical Medicine and Hygiene 72: 392–406. https://doi.org/10.4269/ajtmh.2005.72.392

Kelly-Hope L and Thomson MC (2005) Climate and infectious diseases. In: Climate, Climatic Change and Human Health Workshop, Sep 12–14, Wengen, Switzerland, Advances in Global Change Research.

Kibret S, McCartney M, Lautze J, Nhamo L and Yan GY (2021) The impact of large and small dams on malaria transmission in four basins in Africa. Sci Rep 11. https://doi.org/10.1038/s41598-021-92924-3.

Kibret S, Wilson GG, Ryder D, Tekie H and Petros B (2017) The Influence of Dams on Malaria Transmission in Sub-Saharan Africa. EcoHealth 14: 408–419. https://doi.org/10.1007/s10393-015-1029-0.

Killeen GF (2014) Characterizing, controlling and eliminating residual malaria transmission. Malar J 13. https://doi.org/10.1186/1475-2875-13-330.

Killeen GF, Kiware SS, Seyoum A, Gimnig JE, Corliss GF, Stevenson J, Drakeley CJ and Chitnis N (2014) Comparative assessment of diverse strategies for malaria vector population control based on measured rates at which mosquitoes utilize targeted resource subsets. Malar J 13: 338. https://doi.org/10.1186/1475-2875-13-338.

Kirby MJ and Lindsay SW (2004) Responses of adult mosquitoes of two sibling species, *Anopheles arabiensis* and *A. gambiae* s.s. (Diptera: Culicidae) to high temperatures. Bull Entomol Res 94: 441–448.

Kirby MJ and Lindsay SW (2009) Effect of temperature and inter-specific competition on the development and survival of *Anopheles gambiae sensu stricto* and *An. arabiensis larvae*. Acta Tropica 109: 118–123.

Kiware SS, Chitnis N, Devine GJ, Moore SJ, Majambere S and Killeen GF (2012a) Biologically meaningful coverage indicators for eliminating malaria transmission. Biol Lett 8: 874–877. https://doi.org/10.1098/rsbl.2012.0352.

Kiware SS, Chitnis N, Moore SJ, Devine GJ, Majambere S, Merrill S and Killeen GF (2012b) Simplified models of vector control impact upon malaria transmission by zoophagic mosquitoes. PLoS One 7: e37661. https://doi.org/10.1371/journal.pone.0037661.

Kreppel K, Caminade C, Govella N, Morse AP, Ferguson HM and Baylis M (2019) Impact of ENSO 2016–17 on regional climate and malaria vector dynamics in Tanzania. Environmental Research Letters 14. https://doi.org/10.1088/1748-9326/ab26c7.

Kulkarni MA, Kweka E, Nyale E, Lyatuu E, Mosha FW, Chandramohan D, Rau ME and Drakeley C (2006) Entomological evalution of malaria vectors at different altitudes in Hal District, Northeastern Tanzania. Journal of Medical Entomology 43: 580–588.

Lafferty KD (2009) The ecology of climate change and infectious diseases. Ecology 90: 888–900. https://doi.org/10.1890/08-0079.1.

Lee Y, Meneses CR, Fofana A and Lanzaro GC (2009) Desiccation resistance among subpopulations of *Anopheles gambiae* s.s. from Selinkenyi, Mali. Journal of Medical Entomology 46: 316–320. https://doi.org/10.1603/033.046.0216.

Leedale J, Tompkins AM, Caminade C, Jones AE, Nikulin G and Morse AP (2016) Projecting malaria hazard from climate change in eastern Africa using large ensembles to estimate uncertainty. Geospatial Health 11: 102–114. https://doi.org/10.4081/gh.2016.393.

Lindsay SW, Parson L and Thomas CJ (1998) Mapping the ranges and relative abundance of the two principal African malaria vectors, *Anopheles gambiae sensu stricto* and *An. arabiensis*, using climate data. Proc Biol Sci 265: 847–854.

Lindsay SW, Thomas MB and Kleinschmidt I (2021) Threats to the effectiveness of insecticide-treated bednets for malaria control: thinking beyond insecticide resistance. Lancet Global Health 9: E1325–E1331. https://doi.org/10.1016/s2214-109x(21)00216-3.

Lyimo IN and Ferguson HM (2009) Ecological and evolutionary determinants of host species choice in mosquito vectors. Trends in Parasitology 25: 189–196.

Lyons CL, Coetzee M, Terblanche JS and Chown SL (2012) Thermal limits of wild and laboratory strains of two African malaria vector species, *Anopheles arabiensis* and *Anopheles funestus*. Malaria Journal 11: (6 July 2012).

Lyons CL, Coetzee M, Terblanche JS and Chown SL (2014) Desiccation tolerance as a function of age, sex, humidity and temperature in adults of the African malaria vectors *Anopheles arabiensis* and *Anopheles funestus*. Journal of Experimental Biology 217: 3823–3833. https://doi.org/10.1242/jeb.104638.

Mabaso MLH, Craig M, Ross A and Smith T (2007) Environmental predictors of the seasonality of malaria transmission in Africa: The challenge. American Journal of Tropical Medicine and Hygiene 76: 33–38. https://doi.org/10.4269/ajtmh.2007.76.33.

Majambere S, Lindsay SW, Green C, Kandeh B and Fillinger U (2007) Microbial larvicides for malaria control in The Gambia. Malaria Journal 6:76. https://doi.org/10.1186/1475-2875-6-76.

Majambere S, Pinder M, Fillinger U, Ameh D, Conway DJ, Green C, Jeffries D, Jawara M, Milligan PJ, Hutchinson R and Lindsay SW (2010) Is Mosquito Larval Source Management Appropriate for Reducing Malaria in Areas of Extensive Flooding in The Gambia? A Cross-over Intervention Trial. Am J Trop Med Hyg 82: 176–184.

Martens P, Kovats RS, Nijhof S, de Vries P, Livermore MTJ, Bradley DJ, Cox J and McMichael AJ (1999) Climate change and future populations at risk of malaria. Global Environmental Change-Human and Policy Dimensions 9: S89–S107. https://doi.org/10.1016/s0959-3780(99)00020-5.

McMichael AJ (2013) Globalization, Climate Change, and Human Health REPLY. New England Journal of Medicine 369: 96–96.

Ministry of Health CD, Gender, Elderly and Children (Tanzania), (Zanzibar) MoH, (Tanzania) NBoS, Statistician OotCG and ICF (2018) Tanzania Malaria Indicator Survey 2017, Dar es Salaam.

Monroe A, Moore S, Koenker H, Lynch M and Ricotta E (2019) Measuring and characterizing night time human behaviour as it relates to residual malaria transmission in sub-Saharan Africa: a review of the published literature. Malaria Journal 18. https://doi.org/10.1186/s12936-019-2638-9.

Monroe A, Moore S, Olapeju B, Merritt AP and Okumu F (2021) Unlocking the human factor to increase effectiveness and sustainability of malaria vector control. Malaria Journal 20. https://doi.org/10.1186/s12936-021-03943-4.

Mordecai EA, Ryan SJ, Caldwell JM, Shah MM and LaBeaud AD (2020) Climate change could shift disease burden from malaria to arboviruses in Africa. Lancet Planetary Health 4: E416–E423.

Murdock CC, Sternberg ED and Thomas MB (2016) Malaria transmission potential could be reduced with current and future climate change. Sci Rep 6. https://doi.org/10.1038/srep27771.

Nartey R, Owusu-Dabo E, Kruppa T, Baffour-Awuah S, Annan A, Oppong S, Becker N and Obiri-Danso K (2013) Use of *Bacillus thuringiensis* var *israelensis* as a viable option in an Integrated Malaria Vector Control Programme in the Kumasi Metropolis, Ghana. Parasites & Vectors 6: 1–10.

Ndhlovu GZ and Woyessa YE (2021) Evaluation of Streamflow under Climate Change in the Zambezi River Basin of Southern Africa. Water 13. https://doi.org/10.3390/w13213114.

Ng'habi KR, Mwasheshi D, Knols BG and Ferguson HM (2010) Establishment of a self-propagating population of the African malaria vector *Anopheles arabiensis* under semi-field conditions. Malar J 9: 356. https://doi.org/10.1186/1475-2875-9-356.

Ngowo HS, Hape EE, Matthiopoulos J, Ferguson HM and Okumu FO (2021) Fitness characteristics of the malaria vector *Anopheles funestus* during an attempted laboratory colonization. Malaria Journal 20. https://doi.org/10.1186/s12936-021-03677-3.

Ngowo HS, Kaindoa EW, Matthiopoulos J, Ferguson HM and Okumu FO (2017) Variations in household microclimate affect outdoor-biting behaviour of malaria vectors. Wellcome open research 2: 102. https://doi.org/10.12688/wellcomeopenres.12928.1.

Nkya TE, Akhouayri I, Kisinza W and David J-P (2013) Impact of environment on mosquito response to pyrethroid insecticides: Facts, evidences and prospects. Insect Biochemistry and Molecular Biology 43: 407–416. https://doi.org/10.1016/j.ibmb.2012.10.006.

Nkya TE, Poupardin R, Laporte F, Akhouayri I, Mosha F, Magesa S, Kisinza W and David J-P (2014) Impact of agriculture on the selection of insecticide resistance in the malaria vector *Anopheles gambiae*: a multigenerational study in controlled conditions. Parasites & Vectors 7. https://doi.org/10.1186/s13071-014-0480-z.

Noor AM and Alonso PL (2022) The message on malaria is clear: progress has stalled. Lancet 399: 1777–1777. https://doi.org/10.1016/s0140-6736(22)00732-2.

OECD, Sahel and Club WA (2020) Africa's Urbanisation Dynamics 2020. https://doi.org/doi:https://doi.org/10.1787/b6bccb81-en.

Ogoma SB, Mmando AS, Swai JK, Horstmann S, Malone D and Killeen GF (2017) A low technology emanator treated with the volatile pyrethroid transfluthrin confers long term protection against outdoor biting vectors of lymphatic filariasis, arboviruses and malaria. PLoS Negl Trop Dis 11: e0005455.

Ogoma SB, Moore SJ and Maia MF (2012) A systematic review of mosquito coils and passive emanators: defining recommendations for spatial repellency testing methodologies. Parasites & Vectors 5. https://doi.org/10.1186/1756-3305-5-287.

Ohm JR, Baldini F, Barreaux P, Lefevre T, Lynch PA, Suh E, Whitehead SA and Thomas MB (2018) Rethinking the extrinsic incubation period of malaria parasites. Parasites & Vectors 11. https://doi.org/10.1186/s13071-018-2761-4.

Olabimi IO, Ileke KD, Adu BW and Arotolu TE (2021) Potential distribution of the primary malaria vector *Anopheles gambiae* Giles Diptera: Culicidae in Southwest Nigeria under current and future climatic conditions. Journal of Basic and Applied Zoology 82. https://doi.org/10.1186/s41936-021-00261-8.

Oliver SV and Brooke BD (2017) The effect of elevated temperatures on the life history and insecticide resistance phenotype of the major malaria vector *Anopheles arabiensis* (Diptera: Culicidae). Malaria Journal 16. https://doi.org/10.1186/s12936-017-1720-4.

Paaijmans KP, Heinig RL, Seliga RA, Blanford JI, Blanford S, Murdock CC and Thomas MB (2013) Temperature variation makes ectotherms more sensitive to climate change. Global Change Biology 19: 2373–2380. https://doi.org/10.1111/gcb.12240.

Parham PE, Pople D, Christiansen-Jucht C, Lindsay S, Hinsley W and Michael E (2012) Modeling the role of environmental variables on the population dynamics of the malaria vector *Anopheles gambiae sensu stricto*. Malaria Journal 11. https://doi.org/10.1186/1475-2875-11-271.

Pu J, Wang Z and Chung H (2020) Climate change and the genetics of insecticide resistance. Pest Management Science 76: 846–852. https://doi.org/10.1002/ps.5700.

Pulford J, Hetzel MW, Bryant M, Siba PM and Mueller I (2011) Reported reasons for not using a mosquito net when one is available: a review of the published literature. Malaria Journal 10. https://doi.org/10.1186/1475-2875-10-83.

Ranabhat S and Wang C (2020) Effect of moisture on efficacy of selected insecticide dusts against the common bed bug, *Cimex lectularius* (Hemiptera: Cimicidae). Journal of Economic Entomology 113: 1933–1939. https://doi.org/10.1093/jee/toaa122.

Reiner RC, Geary M, Atkinson PM, Smith DL and Gething PW (2015) Seasonality of *Plasmodium falciparum* transmission: a systematic review. Malaria Journal 14. https://doi.org/10.1186/s12936-015-849-2.

Rodriguez-Morales AJ, Suarez JA, Risquez A, Villamil-Gomez WE and Paniz-Mondolfi A (2019) Consequences of Venezuela's massive migration crisis on imported malaria in Colombia, 2016–2018. Travel Med Infect Dis 28: 98–99. https://doi.org/10.1016/j.tmaid.2019.02.004.

Sanou A (2020) The ecology and behaviour of insecticide resistant malaria vectors and implications for control in Burkina Faso, University of Glasgow.

Serdeczny O, Adams S, Baarsch F, Coumou D, Robinson A, Hare W, Schaeffer M, Perrette M and Reinhardt J (2017) Climate change impacts in Sub-Saharan Africa: from physical changes to their social repercussions. Regional Environmental Change 17: 1585–1600. https://doi.org/10.1007/s10113-015-0910-2.

Seyfarth M, Khaireh BA, Abdi AA, Bouh SM and Faulde MK (2019) Five years following first detection of *Anopheles stephensi* (Diptera: Culicidae) in Djibouti, Horn of Africa: populations established malaria emerging. Parasitology Research 118: 725–732. https://doi.org/10.1007/s00436-019-06213-0.

Shapiro LLM, Whitehead SA and Thomas MB (2017) Quantifying the effects of temperature on mosquito and parasite traits that determine the transmission potential of human malaria. Plos Biology 15. https://doi.org/10.1371/journal.pbio.2003489.

Sherrard-Smith E, Skarp JE, Beale AD, Fornadel C, Norris LC, Moore SJ, Mihreteab S, Charlwood JD, Bhatt S, Winskill P, Griffin JT and Churcher TS (2019) Mosquito feeding behavior and how it influences residual malaria transmission across Africa. Proceedings of the National Academy of Sciences of the United States of America 116: 15086–15095. https://doi.org/10.1073/pnas.1820646116.

Shousha AT (1948) Species-eradication. the eradication of *Anopheles gambiae* from Upper Egypt, 1942–1945. Bull World Health Organ 1: 309–353.

Sibanda MM, Focke WW, Labuschagne FJWJ, Moyo L, Nhlapo NS, Maity A, Muiambo H, Massinga P, Jr., Crowther NAS, Coetzee M and Brindley GWA (2011) Degradation of insecticides used for indoor spraying in malaria control and possible solutions. Malaria Journal 10. https://doi.org/10.1186/1475-2875-10-307.

Sinka ME, Golding N, Massey NC, Wiebe A, Huang Z, Hay SI and Moyes CL (2016) Modelling the relative abundance of the primary African vectors of malaria before and after the implementation of indoor, insecticide-based vector control. Malaria Journal 15. https://doi.org/10.1186/s12936-016-1187-8.

Sinka ME, Pironon S, Massey NC, Longbottom J, Hemingway J, Moyes CL and Willis KJ (2020) A new malaria vector in Africa: Predicting the expansion range of *Anopheles stephensi* and identifying the urban populations at risk. Proceedings of the National Academy of Sciences of the United States of America 117: 24900–24908. https://doi.org/10.1073/pnas.2003976117.

Slater HC, Foy BD, Kobylinski K, Chaccour C, Watson OJ, Hellewell J, Aljayyoussi G, Bousema T, Burrows J, D'Alessandro U, Alout H, Ter Kuile FO, Walker PGT, Ghani AC and Smit MR (2020) Ivermectin as a novel complementary malaria control tool to reduce incidence and prevalence: a modelling study. Lancet Infect Dis 20: 498–508. https://doi.org/10.1016/s1473-3099(19)30633-4.

Smith DL, Perkins TA, Tusting LS, Scott TW and Lindsay S (2013) Mosquito population regulation and larval source management in heterogeneous environments. PLoS One 8: e71247.

Soper FL and Wilson DB (1943) *Anopheles gambiae* in Brazil: 1930 to 1940. New York, The Rockefeller Foundation, 262 pp.

Sternberg ED, Cook J, Alou LPA, Assi SB, Koffi AA, Doudou DT, Aoura CJ, Wolie RZ, Oumbouke WA, Worrall E, Kleinschmidt I, N'Guessan R and Thomas MB (2021) Impact and cost-effectiveness of a lethal house lure against malaria transmission in central Cote d'Ivoire: a two-arm, cluster-randomised controlled trial. Lancet 397: 805–815. https://doi.org/10.1016/s0140-6736(21)00250-6.

Stopard IJ, Churcher TS and Lambert B (2021) Estimating the extrinsic incubation period of malaria using a mechanistic model of sporogony. Plos Computational Biology 17. https://doi.org/10.1371/journal.pcbi.1008658.

Sylla M, Kobylinski KC, Gray M, Chapman PL, Sarr MD, Rasgon JL and Foy BD (2010) Mass drug administration of ivermectin in south-eastern Senegal reduces the survivorship of wild-caught, blood fed malaria vectors. Malaria Journal 9. https://doi.org/10.1186/1475-2875-9-365.

Tanser FC, Sharp B and le Sueur D (2003) Potential effect of climate change on malaria transmission in Africa. Lancet 362: 1792–1798. https://doi.org/10.1016/s0140-6736(03)14898-2.

Thomas C (2004) Malaria – A changed climate in Africa? Nature 427: 690–691. https://doi.org/10.1038/427690b.

Thomas CJ, Davies G and Dunn CE (2004) Mixed picture for changes in stable malaria distribution with future climate in Africa. Trends in Parasitology 20: 216–220.

Tonnang HEZ, Tchouassi DP, Juarez HS, Igweta LK and Djouaka RF (2014) Zoom in at African country level: potential climate induced changes in areas of suitability for survival of malaria vectors. International Journal of Health Geographics 13: (20 May 2014).

Traore MM, Junnila A, Traore SF, Doumbia S, Revay EE, Kravchenko VD, Schlein Y, Arheart KL, Gergely P, Xue RD, Hausmann A, Beck R, Prozorov A, Diarra RA, Kone AS, Majambere S, Bradley J, Vontas J, Beier JC and Muller GC (2020) Large-scale field trial of attractive toxic sugar baits (ATSB) for the control of malaria vector mosquitoes in Mali, West Africa. Malaria Journal 19. https://doi.org/10.1186/s12936-020-3132-0.

Tusting LS, Ippolito MM, Willey BA, Kleinschmidt I, Dorsey G, Gosling RD and Lindsay SW (2015) The evidence for improving housing to reduce malaria: a systematic review and meta-analysis. Malaria Journal 14. https://doi.org/10.1186/S12936-015-0724-1.

Tusting LS, Thwing J, Sinclair D, Fillinger U, Gimnig JE, Bonner KE, Bottomley C and Lindsay S (2013) Mosquito larval source management for controlling malaria. Cochrane Database of Sytematic Reviews CD008923.

UNHCR (2022) Climate Risks Profile: Sahel, UN Refugee Agency.

Villena OC, Ryan SJ, Murdock CC and Johnson LB (2022) Temperature impacts the environmental suitability for malaria transmission by *Anopheles gambiae* and *Anopheles stephensi*. Ecology 103: e3685. https://doi.org/10.1002/ecy.3685.

von Seidlein L, Ikonomidis K, Bruun R, Jawara M, Pinder M, Knols BGJ and Knudsen JB (2012) Airflow attenuation and bed net utilization: observations from Africa and Asia. Malaria Journal 11. https://doi.org/10.1186/1475-2875-11-200.

Wagman JM, Varela K, Zulliger R, Saifodine A, Muthoni R, Magesa S, Chaccour C, Gogue C, Tynuv K, Seyoum A, Dengela D, Saute F, Richardson JH, Fornadel C, Linton YM, Slutsker L, Candrinho B and Robertson M (2021) Reduced exposure to malaria vectors following indoor residual spraying of pirimiphos-methyl in a high-burden district of rural Mozambique with high ownership of long-lasting insecticidal nets: entomological surveillance results from a cluster-randomized trial. Malaria Journal 20. https://doi.org/10.1186/s12936-021-03583-8.

Walker ED (1995) Effect of low-temperature on feeding rate of *Aedes stimulans* larvae and efficacy of *Bacillus-thuringiensis* var *israelensis* (H-14). Journal of the American Mosquito Control Association 11: 107–110.

Weiss DJ, Bertozzi-Villa A, Rumisha SF, Amratia P, Arambepola R, Battle KE, Cameron E, Chestnutt E, Gibson HS, Harris J, Keddie S, Millar JJ, Rozier J, Symons TL, Vargas-Ruiz C, Hay SI, Smith DL, Alonso PL, Noor AM, Bhatt S and Gething PW (2021) Indirect effects of the COVID-19 pandemic on malaria intervention coverage, morbidity, and mortality in Africa: a geospatial modelling analysis. Lancet Infect Dis 21: 59–69. https://doi.org/10.1016/s1473-099(20)30700-3.

WHO (2013) Larva source management: a supplementary measure for malaria vector control, WHO, Geneva.

WHO (2018) World Malaria Report, World Health Organization, Geneva.

WHO (2021a) Overview of the WHO Prequalification of Vector Control Products, Geneva.

WHO (2021b) World Malaria Report, 978-92-4-004049-6 Geneva.

WHO (2022) WHO Guidelines for Malaria, Geneva.

Worrall E and Fillinger U (2011) Large-scale use of mosquito larval source management for malaria control in Africa: a cost analysis. Malaria Journal 10. https://doi.org/10.1186/1475-2875-10-338.

Yadouleton A, N'Guessan R, Allagbe H, Asidi A, Boko M, Osse R, Padonou G, Kinde G and Akogbeto M (2010) The impact of the expansion of urban vegetable farming on malaria transmission in major cities of Benin. Parasites & Vectors 3. https://doi.org/10.1186/1756-3305-3-118.

Yamana TK, Bomblies A and Eltahir EAB (2016) Climate change unlikely to increase malaria burden in West Africa. Nature Climate Change 6: 1009-+. https://doi.org/10.1038/nclimate3085.

Yamana TK and Eltahir EAB (2013) Projected Impacts of Climate Change on Environmental Suitability for Malaria Transmission in West Africa. Environmental Health Perspectives 121: 1179–1186. https://doi.org/10.1289/ehp.1206174.

Conclusions

Kimberly M. Fornace, Leonardo Suveges Moreira Chaves, Maria Anice M. Sallum and Jan E. Conn

As seen throughout the chapters of this book, extensive changes to Earth's natural systems have profound effects on human health by altering vector-borne disease risks and impacts. Current levels of anthropogenic environmental change are unprecedented; these have disrupted existing ecosystems and climatic patterns, reduced global biodiversity, increased the frequency of extreme weather events and created new pressures on healthcare and food systems (IPCC 2022). It is becoming increasingly clear that environmental change is a health issue and there is a critical need for climate adaptation and mitigation measures to safeguard human health and well-being (Haines 2017).

Environmental changes, such as deforestation and changing land use, can create new breeding sites and lead to wider shifts in vector composition and disease risks (Chapter 1). The impacts of these changes are highly apparent in the Amazon regions of South America, a region with the highest rates of deforestation globally (Hansen *et al.* 2013). However, the impacts on specific disease risks and vector populations can be highly variable and environmental changes that increase risks of one disease may decrease risks of others (Chapter 1, 4). For example, as areas are cleared and developed, disease burdens may shift to more urban adapted vectors and diseases, for example increased global incidence of urban dengue (Chapter 4).

Critically, these impacts on vector-borne disease transmission do not occur in isolation. Coupled heterogeneities between vector-borne disease transmission and other wider environmental and societal changes may amplify impacts and create new challenges for control. Natural disasters, such as floods and extreme weather events, have the potential to cause severe disruptions through mass migration, destruction of housing and other infrastructure and weakened or overburdened health systems (Chapter 3). Other health emergencies, such as the COVID-19 pandemic, may similarly burden health systems and cause wider changes in mobility, health-seeking behaviours and exposure to vectors that affect disease risks (Chapter 8).

Similarly, economic crises, such as the one in Venezuela, may severely weaken health systems and vector control activities and create new economic pressures to undertake occupational activities in high-risk areas (Chapter 2). Informal settlements established to extract resources frequently operate largely outside of formal health systems. These settlements may also be associated with changing demographic distributions and increased susceptibility in migrant populations without existing immunity (Chapter 5). In all types of settlements, increased incidence of

 | DOI:10.3920/9789004688650_016

vector-borne diseases has major economic costs to both individuals and populations. These include both direct economic costs from morbidity and mortality as well as indirect costs on long term financial security and health (Chapter 6). These may lead to feedbacks where economic stresses drive disease risks and disease risks create new economic burdens.

These changing burdens and risks of vector-borne diseases have become the drivers of new approaches to study the linkages between environment and disease. Technologies, such as drones and satellites, enable monitoring of landscapes and meteorological factors (Chapters 7, 11, 12). Advances in machine learning approaches and rapid expansions in the quality and quantity of Earth Observation data collected create new opportunities for disease surveillance (Chapter 11). However, while the use of these technologies may reflect wider shifts towards environmental management of vector-borne diseases, these methods also require simplifying and flattening complex landscapes, reflecting existing biases (Chapter 7). There is a need for increased input from communities living within these environments to understand the dynamics shaping disease risks. Citizen science methods may offer new opportunities to both collect data but also to understand local perceptions of environment and engage with communities at risk (Chapters 8, 11).

Alongside developments in data sources, there have been major advances in statistical and mechanistic mathematical modelling methods to both understand drivers of disease risk and predict future risks (Chapters 10, 12). Environmental factors often impact disease risk in nonlinear ways at different spatial and temporal scales, necessitating more complex model structures and methods of communicating complexity and uncertainty. Challenges remain in obtaining sufficient data on disease and vector outcomes, identifying model structures, incorporating uncertainty in future environmental and climate predictions and translating models into policy (Chapter 10). Co-developing early warning systems with decision-makers and scientists is essential to develop usable predictive modelling systems to guide policy decisions (Chapter 12).

As well as integrating environmental data into surveillance systems, there is a need to assess how climate change will impact vector control measures. In some cases, environmental change may reduce disease risk; however, there is also the potential for environmental change to reduce efficacy or access to vector control (Chapter 13). Multi-sector engagement and cooperation is needed to identify potential solutions and co-benefits for environment and health. For example, agricultural practices can be modified to reduce mosquito breeding sites while supporting crop production (Chapter 9). There is a need for assessment of strategies to develop multi-functional landscapes to support human health and environmental goals.

The extent of global environmental change is now a major threat to human health that requires new, innovative solutions. The chapters of this book have demonstrated how these changes disrupt ecological and social systems in complex and often unpredictable ways. However, despite these challenges, we have new opportunities for solutions both to monitor these changing risks and identify sustainable control methods. The growing field of planetary health encompasses this wide range of disciplines and presents a research and policy agenda for how to address these global challenges to support human and ecosystem health.

References

Haines A (2017). Addressing challenges to human health in the Anthropocene epoch-an overview of the findings of the Rockefeller/Lancet Commission on Planetary Health. International Health 9: 269–271.

Hansen MC, Potapov PV, Moore R, Hancher M, Turubanova SA, Tyukavina A, Thau D, Stehman SV, Goetz SJ, Loveland TR, Kommareddy A, Egorov A, Chini L, Justice CO and Townshend JR (2013). High-resolution global maps of 21st-century forest cover change. Science 342: 850–853.

IPCC. 2022. Climate change 2022: impacts, adaptation and vulnerability. In Contribution of Working Group II to the Sixth Assessment Report of the Intergovernmental Panel on Climate Change. Cambridge University Press, Cambridge, UK and New York, NY, USA.

www.ingramcontent.com/pod-product-compliance
Lightning Source LLC
Chambersburg PA
CBHW080935240926
51849CB00004BA/466
9789004687684